To

Ara G. Tilkian, M.D.

In tribute to his excellence as a Cardiologist,
selfless concern for his patients,
innate sense of ethics, and wonderful sense of humor

Co-author, consultant, friend
"Thank you" never seems to be enough

UNDERSTANDING ELECTROCARDIOGRAPHY

MARY BOUDREAU CONOVER, RN, BSNed

Director of Education
Critical Care Conferences
Santa Cruz, California

SEVENTH EDITION

with 394 *illustrations*

Mosby

St. Louis   Baltimore   Boston   Carlsbad   Chicago   Naples   New York   Philadelphia   Portland
London   Madrid   Mexico City   Singapore   Sydney   Tokyo   Toronto   Wiesbaden

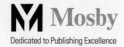

Mosby
Dedicated to Publishing Excellence

A Times Mirror Company

Publisher: Nancy Coon
Acquisitions Editor: Barry Bowlus
Developmental Editors: Brian Morovitz, Kathleen McDonald Sundt
Project Manager: Patricia Tannian
Production Editor: Melissa Mraz
Manuscript Editor: Mary McAuley
Book Design Manager: Gail Morey Hudson
Manufacturing Supervisor: Dave Graybill

SEVENTH EDITION

Printed in the United States of America
Composition by Clarinda Company
Printing/binding by Maple-Vail Book Mfg. Group

Mosby–Year Book, Inc.
11830 Westline Industrial Drive
St. Louis, Missouri 63146

Library of Congress Cataloging in Publication Data

Conover, Mary Boudreau
    Understanding electrocardiography / Mary Boudreau Conover.—7th ed.
      p.   cm.
    Includes bibliographic references and index.
    ISBN 0-8151-1927-5
    1. Electrocardiography. I. Title.
    [DNLM: 1. Electrocardiography. WG 140 C753u 1995]
  RC683.5E5C65 1995
  616.1′207547—dc20
  DNLM/DLC
  for Library of Congress
                                   95-32204
                                      CIP

95 96 97 98 99 / 9 8 7 6 5 4 3 2 1

Consulting Panel

HEIN J.J. WELLENS, M.D.

Professor and Chairman
Department of Cardiology
University of Limburg and Academic Hospital
Maastricht, The Netherlands

Director and Chairman
Scientific Council
Interuniversity Cardiology Institute The Netherlands (ICIN)
Utrecht, The Netherlands

ARA G. TILKIAN, M.D., F.A.C.C.

Assistant Clinical Professor of Medicine
University of California School of Medicine
Los Angeles, California

Director of Cardiology
Holy Cross Medical Center
Mission Hills, California

DOUGLAS P. ZIPES, M.D.

Distinguished Professor of Medicine
Professor of Pharmacology and Toxicology
Indiana University School of Medicine

Senior Research Associate
Krannert Institute of Cardiology
Indianapolis, Indiana

MASOOD AKHTAR, M.D.

Professor of Medicine
Associate Director
Cardiovascular Disease Section
University of Wisconsin Medical School
Milwaukee Clinical Campus

Director for Arrhythmia Services
Milwaukee Heart Institute of Sinai Samaritan Medical Center

Staff Electrophysiologist
Sinai Samaritan Medical Center
St. Luke's Medical Center,
Milwaukee, Wisconsin

ROGER A. WINKLE, M.D.

Director, Cardiac Surveillance Unit and
Electrophysiology Laboratory
Sequoia Hospital
Redwood City, California

Preface

Those of us who have the responsibility for evaluating and teaching electrocardiography and for making emergency and long-term decisions for our patients have a need for an ECG text that effectively links the study of electrocardiography with the new clinical realities.

The goal of this book is clearly an understanding of electrocardiography through an appreciation of the mechanisms of cardiac activation, normal and abnormal. When mechanisms are understood, ECG recognition is facilitated, clinical implications are understood, and better patient care is assured. Additionally, the seventh edition of this text has been made more practical and clinically useful with the addition of physical signs of arrhythmias and pediatric considerations. Atrial fibrillation and atrial flutter now have their own chapters for easier access. Every chapter has been extensively revised and some have been completely rewritten to reflect new information.

The text is divided into four sections:

I. **Introduction to the 12-lead electrocardiograms**

This section provides background and depth for an understanding of the 12-lead ECG. There is a chapter explaining unipolar and bipolar leads and another with a logical step-by-step demonstration of how the normal ECG is formed. An important chapter is electrical axis; an appreciation for how current flow relates to the axes of the leads is critical to the goals of this text.

II. **Arrhythmia recognition**

Here you find all of the exciting recent break-throughs put into clinical context. Each arrhythmia is discussed under the headings of ECG recognition, mechanism, clinical implications, pediatrics (when applicable), physical signs, and treatment, including emergency response and radiofrequency ablation.

III. **Abnormal 12-lead electrocardiograms**

In this section you encounter 12-lead ECGs as Wellens syndrome is explained, and the ECG recognition of WPW syndrome and its arrhythmias are discussed. The chapter on acute myocardial infarction emphasizes the importance of ECG identification of high-risk patients. The chapter on pulmonary embolism explains the emergency role of the ECG and echocardiogram in this often fatal condition, and offers a swift route from onset of symptoms to treatment. It is my hope that the chapter on diagnostic monitoring leads is a useful guide and convincingly illustrates that there should never be one standard monitoring lead. Rather they should be individually chosen to best monitor each patient's clinical problem.

IV. **Special diagnostic and therapeutic procedures**
The concept and clinical value of signal-averaged ECG is explained, and there is an excellent chapter on pacemaker therapies for bradycardias, expertly written by Dr. John Buysman.

No doubt about it, the electrocardiogram is a superior diagnostic and prognostic tool. Advances in the last 4 years in the field of cardiac electrophysiology, mapping, emergency treatment, and cures for tachyarrhythmias have been profound and have clarified the mechanisms and management of arrhythmias, particularly the tachycardias. The successful cures using radiofrequency catheter ablation for PSVT and idiopathic VT have been exciting and have changed the way these patients are evaluated, and it is only the beginning! The stunning findings of the CAST reports have dramatically changed the way patients with arrhythmias are managed. Mapping studies have given birth to the ECG criteria for VT, localization of its origin, and catheter ablation methods for both ventricular and supraventricular arrhythmias. Computerized ambulatory ECG recorders are now available as is signal-averaged ECG, which helps in risk stratification.

Because of these profound advances, the use of the ECG in clinical practice has never been so indispensable. The informed clinician can now respond with more confidence in emergency settings, offer patients a correct diagnosis, and know when to refer patients for further evaluation and a possible cure.

These are the exciting possibilities that are offered in the seventh edition of this book. I hope that you enjoy learning from it and learn to enjoy electrocardiography as I do. It is my purpose to help you to approach the diagnostic ECG with confidence and eagerness, especially in the emergency settings of tachycardia, profound bradycardia, and drug toxicity. Much good can be accomplished for our patients by an informed clinician and the well-informed teacher. My hope is that many of my readers will be both . . . clinician and teacher.

Mary Conover

Acknowledgments

A book written by a nurse that discusses the emergency and long-term treatment of arrhythmias, myocardial infarction, unstable angina, and acute pulmonary embolism should not be published without being reviewed by cardiovascular physicians who are experts in their field. I take very seriously the responsibility to seek the best for this purpose as a pledge to my readers to produce a book that can be trusted.

I would like to say thank you once again to my friend, co-author, and consultant, Hein J.J. Wellens, M.D., of the Netherlands, teacher, clinician, and scientist, who has been with me through five editions, and from whom I have learned so much through his many books and journal publications and from his personal guidance as my co-author.

Ara G. Tilkian, M.D., Van Nuys, California, to whom this book is dedicated, and to whom I owe many thanks, has once again responded without hesitation to my request for a review. I value his clinical expertise and his enthusiastic, firm, and expert additions and subtractions.

I am proud to announce three new additions to my consulting panel. I was very excited, a little scared, and felt extremely fortunate when these highly committed men who have earned international acclaim for excellence in their clinical work, scientific research, and publications agreed to evaluate parts of this book. Thank you

Douglas P. Zipes, M.D., Indianapolis, Indiana, for Chapter 13;
Masood Akhtar, M.D., Milwaukee, Wisconsin, for Chapter 14; and
Roger A. Winkle, M.D., Redwood City, California, for Chapter 8.

I would also like to thank Mr. Martin Collins of Colloquium International, Verulam House, United Kingdom, for his cheerful response to my many requests for Med-searches and for his dogged persistence in those searches.

Contents

PART I INTRODUCTION TO THE 12-LEAD
ELECTROCARDIOGRAM

1 The 12 Electrocardiogram Leads, 3

Frontal Plane Leads Compared With Horizontal Plane Leads, 3
Limb Leads, 4
Einthoven's Triangle, 4
Placement of Electrodes for Einthoven's Triangle, 5
    Lead I, 5
    Lead II, 5
    Lead III, 6
Unipolar Limb Leads, 6
Precordial Leads, 6
Right Chest Leads, 8
MCL Leads, 8
Placement of Electrodes for Multichannel Monitoring, 10
Summary, 11

2 Normal Electrical Activation of the Heart, 12

Depolarization, 13
Repolarization, 13
Sodium-Potassium Adenosine Triphosphatase Pump, 13
Automaticity, 13
Action Potential, 14
    Phase 0, 14
    Phase 1, 15
    Phase 2, 15
    Phase 3, 15
    Phase 4, 15
Normal Pacemaker and Conduction System of the Heart, 15
Atrioventricular Node and Atrioventricular Nodal Pathways, 15
Normal Electrocardiogram, 17
Step-By-Step Electrical Activation of the Heart (Lead I), 17
P Wave, 20
    Duration, 20
    Height, 20
    Polarity, 20
    Axis, 21
    Shape, 22
    Summary of the normal P wave, 22
Normal QRS Complex in the Limb Leads, 22

QRS Complexes in the Precordial Leads, 23
Transitional Zone, 24
Evaluating the QRS Complex, 24
   Duration, 24
   Measurement, 24
   Best leads for measuring, 25
   Amplitude, 26
   Polarity, 26
   Shape, 26
   Normal Q wave, 27
ST Segment, 27
   Level, 27
   Shape, 28
T Wave, 28
   Polarity of the normal T wave, 28
   Vulnerable period, 28
   Shape, 29
   Height, 29
U Wave, 29
Summary, 29

3 Measurement of Heart Rate and Intervals, 31

ECG Paper, 31
Calculation of Heart Rate, 31
PR Interval, 33
   PR segment, 33
   Influence of heart rate, 33
   Prolonged PR interval, 34
   Shortened PR interval, 34
QT Interval, 34
   Measuring the QT interval, 34
   Corrected QT interval, 34

4 Determination of the Electrical Axis, 36

Why Is It More Important to Learn Axis Determination? 36
   Cardiac emergencies, 36
   Understanding the 12-lead electrocardiogram, 37
Methods of Axis Determination, 37
Lesson Plan, 37
Instant-To-Instant Electrical Activation of the Heart, 37
Vectors and the Axis of the Heart, 37
Current Flow Related to the Lead Axis, 38
Normal Electrical Axis, 40
Axis at a Glance, 40
Easy Two-Step Method of Axis Determination, 41
Exercises for Axis Determination, 43
   Exercise 1: normal axis, 43
   Exercise 2: normal axis, 43
   Exercise 3: no man's land axis, 44
   Exercise 4: borderline axis of −30 degrees, 44
   Exercise 5: left axis deviation, 44
   Exercise 6: right axis deviation, 45
Use of Leads I and aV$_F$ in Axis Determination: The Quadrant Method, 45
Hexaxial Figure: A More Precise Method of Axis Determination, 47
Summary, 47

PART II   ARRHYTHMIA RECOGNITION

5   Mechanisms of Arrhythmias, 53

Arrhythmia or Dysrhythmia? 53
Reentry, 54
   Anatomic reentry, 55
   Functional reentry, 56
   Anisotropic reentry, 56
Reflection, 56
Altered Automaticity, 57
Triggered Activity, 58
Clinical Application, 59
Summary, 60

6   Arrhythmias Originating in the Sinus Node, 61

Normal Sinus Rhythm, 61
Sinus Tachycardia, 63
   ECG recognition, 63
   Mechanism, 65
   Clinical implications, 65
   Treatment, 65
Sinus Bradycardia, 65
   ECG recognition, 66
   Mechanism, 66
   Clinical implications, 66
   Treatment, 67
Sinus Arrhythmia and Heart Rate Variability, 67
   ECG recognition, 67
   Mechanism, 68
   Clinical implications, 68
   Symptoms, 68
   Treatment, 68
Two Types of Sinoatrial Block, 68
Sinoatrial Wenckebach (Type I Sinoatrial Block), 68
   ECG recognition, 70
   Mechanism, 70
   Clinical implications, 70
   Treatment, 71
Type II Sinoatrial Block, 71
   ECG recognition, 71
Sinus Arrest or Sinus Pause, 71
   ECG recognition, 71
   Treatment, 73
Permanent Atrial Standstill, 73
   ECG recognition, 73
   Mechanism, 73
Sinus Nodal Dysfunction (Sick Sinus Syndrome), 73
   ECG recognition, 74
   Mechanisms, 75
   Pathologic features, 75
   Treatment, 76
Sinus Nodal Reentry Tachycardia, 76
   ECG recognition, 76
   Mechanism, 77
   Clinical implications, 77

Differential diagnosis, 77
Treatment, 78
Wandering Pacemaker, 78
ECG recognition, 78
Summary, 79

7 Premature Atrial Complexes and Atrial Tachycardia, 81

Premature Atrial Complex, 81
"Walking out" the rhythm, 81
ECG recognition, 82
AV conduction following a PAC, 83
Overdrive suppression, 83
Mechanism, 84
Clinical implications and causes, 85
Treatment, 85
Types of Premature Atrial Complexes, 86
PACs that hide in T waves, 86
Bigeminal PACs, 86
Nonconducted PACs, 86
Bigeminal nonconducted PACs, 86
Differential diagnosis, 88
Atrial Tachycardia, 88
Pediatrics, 90
Automatic atrial tachycardia, 90
Reentrant atrial tachycardia, 91
ECG Recognition, 92
Clinical implications, 92
Physical findings, 93
Treatment, 93
Multifocal (Chaotic) Atrial Tachycardia, 93
ECG recognition, 93
Mechanism, 94
Clinical implications and causes, 94
Pediatrics, 94
Treatment, 94

8 Atrial Fibrillation, 96

ECG Recognition, 96
Risk, 98
Mechanism, 98
Clinical Features, 100
Paroxysmal, 100
Postoperative atrial fibrillation, 100
Vagally induced and catecholamine-sensitive atrial fibrillation, 100
Ventricular Response to Atrial Fibrillation: "Controlled" or "Uncontrolled"? 100
Concealed Conduction, 101
Causes, 101
Risk of Thromboembolism, 101
Pediatrics, 101
Symptoms, 101
Physical Assessment, 102
Treatment Goals and Categories, 102
Treatment of Acute Atrial Fibrillation, 102
Digoxin, 103
Beta blockers, 104

Calcium channel blockers, 104
DC cardioversion, 105
Treatment of Subacute Atrial Fibrillation, 105
Treatment of Chronic Atrial Fibrillation, 105
Rate control, 105
DC conversion, 106
Antithrombotic Therapy, 106
Radiofrequency Ablation, 106
Surgery, 106
Treatment of Postoperative Atrial Fibrillation, 106
Digitalis Toxicity in Atrial Fibrillation, 107
Atrial Fibrillation with an Accessory Pathway, 107
Summary, 107

9 Atrial Flutter, 111

Terminology, 111
ECG Recognition, 111
Differential Diagnosis, 114
Mechanism, 114
Type I atrial flutter, 114
Type II atrial flutter, 114
F-Wave Morphology, 115
Type I atrial flutter, 115
Type II atrial flutter, 115
Atrioventricular Conduction, 117
Mechanism of Wenckebach conduction in atrial flutter, 119
Clinical Setting and Incidence, 119
Pediatrics, 120
Physical Signs, 120
Emergency Treatment, 120
Long-Term Treatment, 120
Flutter-Fibrillation (Impure Flutter), 121
Summary, 121

10 Junctional Beats and Rhythms, 123

Terminology, 123
AV Junction, 124
Atrionodal (AN) region, 124
Nodal (N) region, 124
Nodal-His (NH) region, 124
Junctional rhythm, 125
Premature Junctional Complex, 125
ECG recognition, 126
Treatment, 126
Nonparoxysmal Junctional Tachycardia, 126
ECG recognition, 126
Mechanism, 128
Causes, 128
Pediatrics, 128
Physical signs, 128
Treatment, 128
Junctional Escape Beats and Rhythms, 129
ECG recognition, 129
Treatment, 129
Summary, 130

11   Paroxysmal Supraventricular Tachycardia, 132

Terminology, 132
Atrioventricular Nodal Reentry Tachycardia, 133
  Location of the fast and slow atrioventricular nodal pathways, 133
  Mechanism, 134
  ECG recognition, 135
  Clinical implications, 137
  Emergency treatment, 137
  Treatment with radiofrequency ablation, 137
  Uncommon form, 137
Circus Movement Tachycardia (Atrioventricular Reciprocating
  Tachycardia), 137
  Location of the accessory pathways, 137
  Mechanism, 137
  ECG recognition, 139
Circus movement tachycardia initiated by a premature ventricular
    complex, 140
  ECG signs negating the possibility of circus movement
    tachycardia, 141
  Clinical implications, 143
  Emergency treatment, 143
  Treatment (cure) with radiofrequency ablation, 143
Circus Movement Tachycardia With a Slowly Conducting Accessory
    Pathway, 143
Emergency Response to Paroxysmal Supraventricular Tachycardia, 144
  Hemodynamically stable patient, 144
Rationale of Emergency Response, 144
  Why multiple lead recordings? 144
  Interrupting the reentry circuit, 145
  Vagal maneuver, 145
  Adenosine (Adenocard), 146
  Verapamil, 147
  Procainamide (Pronestyl), 147
  Cardioversion, 147
  Recording the sinus rhythm, 147
  Taking a history, 147
Mechanism and Methods of Vagal Stimulation, 147
Carotid Sinus Massage, 148
  Effect of carotid sinus massage on supraventricular tachycardia, 150
  Caution, 150
  Procedure, 150
Symptoms of Paroxysmal Supraventricular Tachycardia, 150
Physical Signs of Paroxysmal Supraventricular Tachycardia, 151
  Pulse, blood pressure, and heart sounds, 151
  Polyuria, 151
  Syncope, 151
Pediatrics: Paroxysmal Supraventricular Tachycardia in the Fetus and
    Neonate, 152
Summary, 152

12   Premature Ventricular Complexes, 155

ECG Recognition, 155
Mechanism, 156
QRS Width, 157

QRS Shape, 157
Increases Amplitude, 158
T-Wave of Opposite Polarity, 158
The Full Compensatory Pause, 158
Overdrive Suppression, 160
Types of Premature Ventricular Complexes, 161
    The "ugly" premature ventricular complex, 161
    Unifocal premature ventricular complexes, 161
    Multifocal premature ventricular complexes, 161
    Bigeminy, trigeminy, quadrigeminy, and pairs, 163
    End-diastolic premature ventricular complexes, 164
    Interpolated premature ventricular complexes, 165
    Fascicular premature ventricular complexes, 166
    R-on-T phenomenon, 166
Rule of Bigeminy, 169
Pediatrics, 170
Physical Signs, 170
Clinical Implications, 170
    Nonsymptomatic patient with no structural heart disease, 170
    Apparently healthy middle-age men, 170
    Acute myocardial infarction, 170
Treatment, 171
Summary, 171

13   Monomorphic Ventricular Tachycardia, 173

Terminology, 173
Diagnosis, 174
Mechanism, 175
    Reentry, 176
    Abnormal automaticity, 176
    Triggered activity, 176
Incidence, 176
Prognosis and Clinical Implications, 176
    Nonsustained ventricular tachycardia, 176
    Sustained ventricular tachycardia, 176
Pediatrics, 177
Management of Sustained Broad-QRS Tachycardia With Hemodynamic
    Decompression, 177
Management of Sustained Broad-QRS Tachycardia Without Hemodynamic
    Decompensation, 177
    Procainamide versus lidocaine, 178
    Precordial thump, 178
When in Doubt, 178
Looks Like Ventricular Tachycardia, Heart Rhythm Irregular, Heart Rate
    Over 200 Beats/Min?, 178
If Supraventricular Tachycardia With Aberrancy Is Suspected, 178
Idiopathic Ventricular Tachycardia, 178
    History, 179
    Types of idiopathic ventricular tachycardia, 179
    ECG recognition of LBBB-shaped idiopathic ventricular tachycardia
        as compared with ischemic ventricular tachycardia or the
        ventricular tachycardia of right ventricular dysphasia, 180
    ECG recognition of RBBB-shaped idiopathic ventricular tachycardia
        as compared with ischemic ventricular tachycardia or the
        ventricular tachycardia of right ventricular dysplasia, 180
    Clinical implications, 181

Symptoms, 182
Emergency treatment of idiopathic ventricular tachycardia, 182
Long-term treatment of idiopathic ventricular tachycardia, 182
Bundle Branch Reentrant Ventricular Tachycardia, 183
ECG recognition, 183
Mechanism, 184
Pathophysiology, 186
Emergency treatment, 186
Long-term treatment (cure), 186
Prognosis, 186
Radiofrequency Ablation for Ventricular Tachycardia, 186
Idiopathic ventricular tachycardia, 186
Bundle branch reentry ventricular tachycardia, 187
Ventricular tachycardia late after myocardial infarction, 187
Treatment of Drug-Related Ventricular Tachycardia, 187
Torsades de pointes, 187
Sustained (incessant) monomorphic ventricular tachycardia induced
by antiarrhythmic drugs, 187
Signal-Averaged ECG in Patients With Sustained Ventricular
Tachycardia, 188
Ventricular Flutter and Ventricular Fibrillation, 188
ECG recognition, 188
Mechanisms, 189
Prognosis, 189
Symptoms, 189
Treatment: immediate electrical shock, 189

14   Aberration Versus Ectopy, 192

Aberrant Ventricular Conduction, 192
Phase 3 Block, 192
Retrograde Concealed Conduction, 193
Importance of Differentiating Among Broad QRS
Tachycardias, 194
Importance of Taking a History, 195
Atrioventricular Dissociation, 195
Physical signs, 195
ECG signs of atrioventricular dissociation, 196
Finding P Waves in the Broad QRS Tachycardia, 196
Exercise 1, 196
Exercise 2, 198
Retrograde Conduction to the Atria During Ventricular
Tachycardia, 199
ECG Diagnosis of Broad QRS Tachycardia, 200
QRS Width, 200
Axis, 200
Clinical correlations, 200
Summary of axis, 201
Capture Beats and Fusion Beats, 201
Concordant Pattern, 201
QRS Morphologic Appearance, 202
When lead V_1 is positive, 206
Pitfalls, 207
When lead V_1 is negative, 209
Value of a Baseline 12-Lead ECG, 212
When in Doubt, 213
Summary, 214

15 Torsades de Pointes and Polymorphic Ventricular Tachycardia, 216

Torsades de Pointes or Polymorphic Ventricular Tachycardia? The Difference Is Important, 216
    Torsades de pointes, 216
    Polymorphic ventricular tachycardia, 216
Torsade de Pointes, 217
    Torsade or torsades?, 217
    ECG diagnosis, 217
    Characteristic features of quinidine-related torsades de pointes, 221
    Mechanism, 221
    Causes of acquired torsade de pointes, 222
    Causes of congenital (idiopathic) torsades de pointes (long QT syndrome), 222
    Symptoms, 223
    Possible outcomes, 223
    Prevention, 223
    Emergency treatment of torsades de pointes in the setting of acquired long QT syndrome, 223
Emergency treatment of torsades de pointes in the setting of congenital long QT syndrome, 224
    Suggested dosage of regimens for magnesium chloride or $MgSO_4$, 224
    Contraindications for magnesium, 224
    Advantages of magnesium for torsades de pointes, 224
    Latent long QT syndrome, 225
    Corrected QT interval, 225
Polymorphic Ventricular Tachycardia (Without QT Prolongation), 225
    Chronic coronary artery disease, 225
    Acute myocardial ischemia, 228
Summary, 229

16 Accelerated Idioventricular Rhythm and Ventricular Escape, 232

Definition of accelerated idioventricular rhythm, 232
ECG identification of the area of reperfusion, 234
ECG recognition of accelerated idioventricular rhythm not related to reperfusion, 234
Clinical implications, 234
Mechanisms, 236
Treatment, 237
Ventricular Escape, 237

17 Digitalis-Induced Arrhythmias, 239

Acute Myocardial Uptake of Digoxin, 240
Mechanisms of Digitalis-Induced Tachyarrhythmias, 240
Systematic Approach, 242
Factors That Affect Digitalis Dosage Requirements, 242
Alerting Features of the Arrhythmias in Digitalis Intoxication, 242
Bigeminal Rhythms, 243
Sinus Bradycardia, 243
Sinoatrial Block, 243
Atrioventricular Block, 245
Atrial Tachycardia With block, 246
    ECG recognition, 246

Nonparoxysmal Junctional Tachycardia, 249
  ECG recognition, 249
  Terminology, 250
  Junctional tachycardia during atrial fibrillation, 250
Fascicular Ventricular Tachycardia, 253
  ECG recognition, 253
Bifascicular Ventricular Tachycardia, 254
  ECG recognition, 254
Double Tachycardias, 255
Noncardiac Signs of Digitalis Toxicity, 257
  Color vision, 257
  Gastrointestinal symptoms, 257
Treatment, 257
  Management of early manifestations, 257
  Aggressive management of patients with serious arrhythmias or
    hemodynamic compromise, 257
  Fab fragments of cardiac glycoside–specific antibodies, 258
Emergency Approach, 258
Summary, 258

18 Atrioventricular Block, 260

Pediatrics, 261
First-Degree Atrioventricular Block, 261
  ECG recognition, 261
  Mechanism, 261
  Clinical implications, 263
  Physical signs, 263
  Assessment of the jugular venous pulse, 263
  Pediatrics, 263
  Treatment, 263
Second-Degree Atrioventricular Block, 263
  Type I atrioventricular block (atrioventricular Wenckebach), 264
  Type II atrioventricular block, 267
  Two-to-one atrioventricular block, 269
Complete (Third-Degree) Atrioventricular Block, 271
  ECG recognition, 272
  Pathology, 272
  Clinical implications, 272
  Physical signs, 272
Noninvasive Evaluation of the Site of Block, 272
Treatment, 274
Summary, 274

19 Potassium Derangements, 276

Major Cellular Antiarrhythmic Functions of Potassium, 276
Hypokalemia, 276
  ECG recognition, 276
  Causes, 278
  Clinical implications, 278
  Signs and symptoms, 279
  Treatment, 279
  Prevention, 279
Hyperkalemia, 279
  ECG recognition, 279
  Treatment, 282
Summary, 283

20   Atrioventricular Dissociation, 284

Causes, 284
Physical Findings, 284
Treatment, 285
Sinus Bradycardia and Atrioventricular Dissociation, 285
  ECG recognition, 285
  Mechanism, 286
  Clinical implications, 286
Nonparoxysmal Junctional Tachycardia With Atrioventricular
    Dissociation, 287
  ECG recognition, 287
  Mechanism, 287
  Clinical implications, 287
Accelerated Idioventricular Rhythm With Atrioventricular
    Dissociation, 288
  ECG recognition, 288
  Mechanism, 288
  Clinical implications, 289
  Physical signs, 289
Atrioventricular Block and Atrioventricular Dissociation, 289
  ECG recognition, 289
  Mechanism, 290
  Clinical implications, 291
Summary, 291

21   Fusion Complexes, 292

Mechanisms, 292
ECG Recognition, 292
Ventricular Fusion, 293
Atrial Fusion, 295
Summary, 295

22   Parasystole, 296

ECG in Parasystole, 296
  No fixed coupling, 296
  Fusion beats, 296
  Interectopic intervals, 297
Modulated Parasystole, 297
Mechanism, 298
Clinical Implications, 300

PART III   ABNORMAL 12-LEAD ELECTROCARDIOGRAMS

23   Wolff-Parkinson-White and Other Preexcitation Syndromes, 303

Classification of the Preexcitation Syndromes, 303
Wolff-Parkinson-White Syndrome, 304
  Anatomic development, 304
  Historical background, 304
  Accessory pathway, 304
  Incidence, 305
  Genetics, 306
  ECG recognition (overt Wolff-Parkinson-White syndrome), 306

PR interval, 309
Delta wave, 309
Understanding the degree of preexcitation, 310
Maximal preexcitation, 313
Less than maximal preexcitation: the fusion beat, 314
The latent accessory pathway: no preexcitation, 314
T-wave changes, 317
Estimating the refractory period of the accessory pathway, 317
Concealed accessory pathway, 317
Arrhythmias in Wolff-Parkinson-White Syndrome, 318
Circus movement tachycardia, 318
Orthodromic circus movement tachycardia (using a rapidly
conducting accessory pathway), 318
Emergency response to paroxysmal supraventricular tachycardia, 319
Orthodromic circus movement tachycardia (using a slowly
conducting accessory pathway), 323
Antidromic circus movement tachycardia, 325
Circus movement tachycardia with two accessory pathways, 325
Atrial fibrillation, 328
Atrial fibrillation with two accessory pathways, 334
Locating the accessory pathway, 335
Radiofrequency Ablation, 335
Nodoventricular and Fasciculoventricular Fibers, 336
ECG during sinus rhythm, 336
Paroxysmal supraventricular tachycardia resulting from nodoventricular
fibers, 339
Short PR Syndrome (Intranodal Bypass Tract), 340
Summary, 340

24   Unstable Angina, Wellens Syndrome, and Left Main and
     Three-Vessel Coronary Artery Disease, 342

Unstable Angina, 342
Incidence, 342
Type of pain, 342
Identifying characteristics, 343
Anginal pain, 343
Patients' common descriptions of anginal pain, 343
Pain that is not anginal, 343
Pathogenesis, 344
Wellens Syndrome, 344
Historical background, 346
ECG recognition, 346
ECG during pain, 349
Time frame for the development of the typical ECG findings, 353
Diagnostic monitoring leads, 355
Emergency angiography, 358
Medical Treatment of Unstable Angina, 358
Why not thrombolysis?, 358
Left Main and Three-Vessel Coronary Artery Disease, 360
ECG recognition, 360
Summary, 360

25   Bundle Branch Block and Hemiblock, 362

Structure of the Trifascicular Specialized Conduction System, 362
Blood Supply to the Conduction System, 364
Bundle Branch Block in Acute Myocardial Infarction Treatment, 364

Chronic Bundle Branch Block, 365
Pediatrics, 365
Physical Findings, 365
Comparison of Right- and Left-Sided Bundle Branch Block in
    Lead V$_1$, 365
Normal Ventricular Activation Time (Intrinsicoid Deflection), 366
T-Wave Changes in Bundle Branch Block, 366
Right Bundle Branch Block, 367
    Mechanism, 367
    QRS complex in right bundle branch block with and without acute
        anteroseptal myocardial infarction, 368
    Intrinsicoid deflection in the right bundle branch block, 371
Complete Versus Incomplete Right Bundle Branch Block, 371
    Mechanism, 371
    ECG recognition, 371
    Incomplete bundle branch block in athletes, 371
Left Bundle Branch Block, 372
    Mechanism, 372
    QRS complex in left bundle branch block with and without acute
        anteroseptal myocardial infarction, 373
    ECG recognition of underlying cardiac disease in left bundle branch
        block, 376
Alternating Right- and Left-Sided Bundle Branch Block, 377
Anterior Hemiblock, 377
    Mechanism, 378
    ECG recognition, 378
    Clinical implications, 379
Posterior Hemiblock, 380
    Mechanism, 380
    ECG recognition, 380
    Clinical implications, 381
Hemiblock with Right Bundle Branch Block (Bifascicular Block), 381
    Mechanism, 381
    ECG recognition, 382
    Clinical implications, 382
Differential Diagnosis in Anterior Hemiblock, 382
    Inferior wall myocardial infarction, 382
    Anterior wall myocardial infarction, 383
Monitoring for Axis Shifts and for Right Bundle Branch Block, 383
Trifascicular Block, 385
Summary, 386

26   **Acute Myocardial Infarction**, 387

Pathophysiology of the Evolving Myocardial Infarction, 388
Prognosis, 389
Blood Supply to the Myocardium and Conduction System, 389
    Right coronary artery, 390
    Left coronary artery, 391
ECG Signs of Myocardial Infarction, 391
T Waves, 391
    Normal T wave, 392
    Ischemic T wave, 392
    T-wave inversions from causes other than myocardial infarction, 393
    Hyperacute T waves, 393
ST segment, 395
    Acute injury, 395
    ST-T changes not caused by myocardial infarction, 396

Q Waves, 398
  Normal q waves, 398
  Pathologic q waves, 398
  Q waves from causes other than myocardial infarction, 399
Locating the Infarct, 400
Anterior Wall Myocardial Infarction, 400
  Reflecting leads, 400
  ECG recognition, 402
  ECG identification of high-risk patients, 402
  Pathologic features, 406
  Conduction abnormalities, 407
Non-Q-Wave Acute Myocardial Infarction, 407
  Reflecting leads, 408
  ECG recognition, 408
  Pathologic features, 408
  Clinical significance, 408
Inferior Myocardial Infarction, 409
  Reflecting leads: II, III, aV$_F$, 409
  ECG recognition, 409
  High-risk patients, 410
  ECG identification of high-risk patients, 410
  Culprit coronary artery, 411
  Locating the occluded artery, 411
  Conduction abnormalities, 414
  "Benign reciprocal changes" or worse prognosis? 415
Right Ventricular Infarction, 415
  ECG diagnosis, 415
  Recording lead V$_{4R}$ in the coronary unit, 416
  Pathophysiology, 416
  Clinical implications: an overview, 416
Peri-Infarction Block in Inferior Myocardial Infarction, 417
  History, 417
  Clinical significance, 417
  ECG recognition, 418
Inferolateral Myocardial Infarction, 418
  ECG recognition, 418
  ECG identification of high-risk patients, 418
Acute Posterior Wall Myocardial Infarction, 418
  Reflecting leads, 418
  ECG recognition, 418
Atrial Infarction, 420
  ECG recognition, 420
  Clinical implications, 420
  Differential diagnosis, 420
Emergency Approach to Acute Myocardial Infarction, 420
Aggressive Therapy for High-Risk Patients, 421
ECG Evaluation of Successful Reperfusion, 421
  ST-segment changes, 422
  Reperfusion arrhythmias, 422
  Q waves and T-wave inversion, 422
Transporting Patients and Initiating Therapy, 422
Eliminating Unnecessary Delays, 423
Candidates for Thrombolysis, 424
Contraindications to Thrombolytic Therapy, 424
  Absolute contraindications, 424
  Relative major contraindications (individual evaluation of risk versus benefit), 425
  Relative minor contraindications, 425

Effects of Prophylactic Antiarrhythmic Drug Therapy in Acute
    Myocardial Infarction, 425
Differential Diagnoses, 426
    Acute pulmonary embolism, 426
    Wolff-Parkinson-White syndrome, 426
    Pericarditis, 426
    Aortic dissection, 427
    Pancreatitis and cholecystitis, 427
Summary, 427

27 Acute Pulmonary Embolism, 431

Common Risk Factors, 431
Pathophysiology, 432
Signs and Symptoms, 432
Physical Findings, 432
Value of the ECG, 432
Common ECG Findings in the Acute Phase, 433
Value of the Echocardiogram, 434
Other Available Tests, 436
    Nonuseful tests, 436
Differential Diagnosis, 436
Treatment, 436
Prevention, 437
    Pharmacologic prophylaxis, 437
    Nonpharmacologic prophylaxis, 437
Family history and young age, 437
Summary, 437

28 Hypertrophy, 439

Pathogenesis of Ventricular Hypertrophy, 439
Diagnostic Tools, 439
Left Ventricular Hypertrophy, 440
    ECG recognition, 440
    Left atrial involvement, 441
    Estes criteria and the use of Cornell voltage, 443
Right Ventricular Hypertrophy, 444
    ECG recognition, 444
Chronic Obstructive Lung Disease, 445
    ECG recognition, 445
Biventricular Hypertrophy, 446
    ECG recognition, 447
Normal P Wave, 447
Left Atrial Abnormality, 447
    ECG recognition, 447
Right Atrial Abnormalities: P Pulmonale, 449
    ECG recognition, 450
Right Atrial Hypertrophy, 451
    ECG recognition, 451

29 Expert Bedside Monitoring, 452

Digitalis Intoxication, 452
Paroxysmal Supraventricular Tachycardia, 452
Unstable Angina, 458
Broad QRS Tachycardia, 458
High-Risk Myocardial Infarction, 462

PART IV   SPECIAL DIAGNOSTIC AND THERAPEUTIC
          PROCEDURES

30 Signal-Averaged ECG and Fast Fourier Transform Analysis, 467

    Problems in Analyzing Small ECG Signals, 467
    Signal Averaging, 468
      Spatial averaging, 468
      Ensemble averaging (signal averaging), 468
    Time Domain Analysis of the Signal-Averaged ECG, 469
      Interpreting the time domain signal-averaged ECG, 469
    Frequency Domain Analysis of the Signal-Averaged ECG, 470
      Frequency domain, 471
      Methodology, 473
      Interpreting the frequency domain signal-averaged ECG, 475
    Other Analytic Methods, 475
    Summary, 476

31 Electrical Stimulation Therapies, 479

    Organization of Arrhythmias With Respect to Electrical Therapies, 479
    Goals of Electrical Therapies, 479
    Electrical Therapies of Bradycardia, 480
    Electrical Therapies for Tachycardias Resulting From Cellular
          Abnormalities, 481
      Prevention, 481
      Termination, 482
    Electrical Therapies for Tachycardia Resulting From Reentrant
          Loops, 482
      Prevention, 482
      Termination, 482
      Tiered therapy, 487
      Atrioventricular reciprocation tachycardia: a special case, 490
    Acknowledgment, 490

32 Pacemaker Therapies for Bradycardias, 491

    Pacing Concept, 492
      Stimulus artifacts on the ECG, 492
    Stimulation Concepts, 492
      Mechanisms of stimulation, 492
      Paced fusion and pseudofusion, 492
      Competitive pacing, 493
    Sensing Concepts, 494
      Mechanisms of sensing, 494
      Undersensing and oversensing, 494
    Pacemaker Timing, 494
      Intercycle timing, 494
      Timing mechanisms, 495
      Magnet mode, 497
    Advanced Pacing, 498
    Pacemakers That Provide a Responsive Heart Rate, 498
      Sensors, 499
      Rate prescriptions, 499
    Applications of Advanced Pacing Concepts, 499
      Matching the pacemaker to the patient, 501

Retrograde (Ventriculoatrial) Conduction, 505
   Effects of retrograde conduction, 505
   Managing retrograde conductions (ventriculoatrial conduction), 506
Tracking Limitations Caused by Atrioventricular Interval and
   Postventricular Atrial Refractory Period, 508
   Moderating the effects of 2:1 pacemaker block, 510
   Maintaining desirable heart rates during exercise, 511
Special Features, 513
   Pacemaker management of vasovagal and carotid sinus
     syndromes, 513
   Sleep rates, 513
Maximizing Atrioventricular Synchrony With Ventricular
   Pacemakers, 513
Obtaining Assistance, 514

PART

I

INTRODUCTION TO THE 12-LEAD ELECTROCARDIOGRAM

1

The 12 Electrocardiogram Leads

Frontal Plane Leads Compared with
   Horizontal Plane Leads   *3*
Limb Leads   *4*
Einthoven's Triangle   *4*
Placement of Electrodes for Einthoven's
   Triangle   *5*
Unipolar Limb Leads   *6*

Precordial Leads   *6*
Right Chest Leads   *8*
MCL Leads   *8*
Placement of Electrodes for Multichannel
   Monitoring   *10*
Summary   *11*

The heart is an electrical field in which currents flow in repetitive patterns with each cardiac cycle, consisting of electrical systole (depolarization and repolarization) and electrical diastole (the resting phase). The arms and legs are linear extensions of this electrical field. Therefore the electrical activity of the heart can be detected at the extremities by placing electrodes of opposite polarity on the skin at opposite poles of the heart's electrical field.

A lead is composed of two electrodes of opposite polarity (bipolar) or one electrode and a reference point (unipolar). It is attached to an amplifier within an oscilloscope or strip recorder (Fig. 1-1). This instrument, the *electrocardiograph,* accurately records the electrical activity of the heart, being influenced by the direction and magnitude of current flow. The recording of the cardiac electrical cycle is called the *electrocardiogram (ECG).*

There are 12 leads in the standard surface electrocardiogram, 3 bipolar and 9 unipolar. The only bipolar leads are on the limbs, and there are 3 unipolar limb leads as well; the remaining leads are on the chest (precordial). These leads record atrial activation (depolarization), ventricular activation (depolarization), and ventricular recovery (repolarization).

FRONTAL PLANE LEADS COMPARED WITH HORIZONTAL PLANE LEADS

The limb leads—I, II, III, aV_R, aV_L, and aV_F—are called *frontal plane leads* because they give information about current flow that is right, left, inferior, or superior. The precordial leads are called *horizontal plane leads* because they give information about current flow that is right, left, anterior, or posterior.

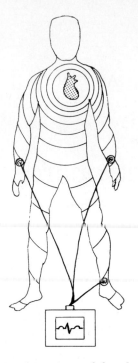

Fig. 1-1. The arms and legs are linear extensions of the electrical field of the heart. The current flow from each cardiac cycle is detected at the skin by electrodes, amplified, and displayed on an oscilloscope or written on a strip recorder.

LIMB LEADS

Half of the limb leads are bipolar (I, II, and III), and half are unipolar (aV_R, aV_L, and aV_F).

Bipolar leads have two electrodes (positive [+] and negative [-]) about equidistant from the heart, with each contributing equally to the tracing. An imaginary line drawn between the two electrodes is the *axis of the lead,* illustrated in Fig. 1-2; all currents generated by the heart relate to the axis of each lead.

Unipolar leads have a positive electrode and an indifferent connection, which is achieved by connecting the electrodes from the three bipolar limb leads, I, II, and III, through resistances, to a central terminal. The potential at the central terminal, which represents the center of the electrical field of the heart, is almost zero, so the contribution to the tracing is made solely by the positive electrode. The axes of unipolar limb leads are from the positive electrode on the limbs (*R,* right arm; *L,* left arm; *F,* left leg) to the zero potential at the center of the electrical field, the heart.

EINTHOVEN'S TRIANGLE

Willem Einthoven, as a young scientist and professor of physiology at Leiden University, first introduced the three bipolar limb leads (I, II, and III), whose axes form an equilateral triangle (Fig. 1-3). The sum of voltages in any closed path such as Einthoven's triangle equals zero. However, because Einthoven reversed the positive and negative electrodes of lead II in his triangle, in the equation you would

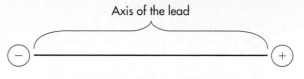

Fig. 1-2. The axis of a lead is an imaginary line drawn between the two electrodes of the bipolar lead or between the positive electrode and a reference point of the unipolar lead.

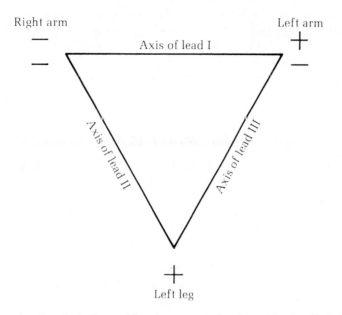

Fig. 1-3. Einthoven's triangle is formed by the axes of the three bipolar limb leads, I, II, and III. The diagram shows the placement of the positive and negative electrodes for each lead.

then subtract instead of add the voltage from lead II. That is, the voltages from lead I plus voltages from lead III, *minus* voltages from lead II equals zero (I + III − II = 0).

The zero potential created by the vector sum of these voltages is the virtual ground used as a reference point for the unipolar leads; that reference point is in the center of the triangle.

PLACEMENT OF ELECTRODES FOR EINTHOVEN'S TRIANGLE
Lead I

The negative electrode is on the right arm and the positive on the left arm. Thus the axis of lead I is from shoulder to shoulder.

Lead II

The negative electrode is on the right arm and the positive on the left leg. Thus the axis of lead II is from the right shoulder to the apex of the triangle.

NOTE: Although the placement of an electrode on the left leg makes the triangle seem out of balance, it is nevertheless an equilateral triangle because all electrodes are about equidistant from the electrical field of the heart.

Lead III

The negative electrode is on the left arm and the positive is on the left leg. Thus the axis of lead III is from the left shoulder to the apex of the triangle.

UNIPOLAR LIMB LEADS

The axes of the three unipolar limb leads, aV_R, aV_L, and aV_F are illustrated in Fig. 1-4. Note that a positive electrode in the R, L, and F positions is compared with the zero potential at the center of the heart's electrical field (i.e., the center of Einthoven's triangle). The letter *a* stands for augmented, a term added when it was discovered that eliminating a negative electrode resulted in the amplitude of the recording being augmented by 50%. The letter *V* indicates a unipolar lead. The letters *R*, *L*, and *F* indicate where the positive electrode is placed, that is, right arm, left arm, and left leg. In some records these leads are simply designated R, L, and F, instead of aV_R, aV_L, and aV_F.

PRECORDIAL LEADS

The axes of the precordial leads are illustrated in Fig. 1-5. This cross section of the thorax demonstrates how valuable these leads are in recording anterior and posterior; right and left forces.

The placement of the precordial electrodes is shown in Fig. 1-6. As with the limb leads, the letter *V* indicates a unipolar lead. The numbers 1 to 6 are codes for locations on the precordium. V_1 and V_2 are on either side of the sternum at the fourth intercostal space. V_4 is at the midclavicular line, fifth intercostal space. V_3 is halfway between V_2 and V_4. On the same level with V_4 are the two lateral chest leads, V_5 and V_6; they are placed in the anterior and midaxillary lines, respectively. Identify the placement for V_6 by first locating the fifth intercostal space at the sternal border and drawing a straight imaginary line across the chest to the midaxillary line.

Lead V1 looks into the right ventricle; leads V_2 to V_3 span the interventricular septum; lead V_4 is over the cardiac apex; and leads V_5 and V_6 reflect the left lateral wall of the heart.

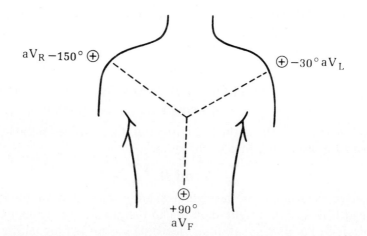

Fig. 1-4. The axes of the unipolar limb leads are from the positive electrode on each point of Einthoven's triangle to the center of the electrical field (the heart).

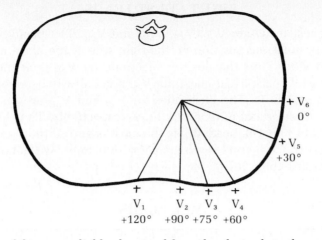

Fig. 1-5. The axes of the precordial leads extend from the electrode to the center of the heart's electrical field.

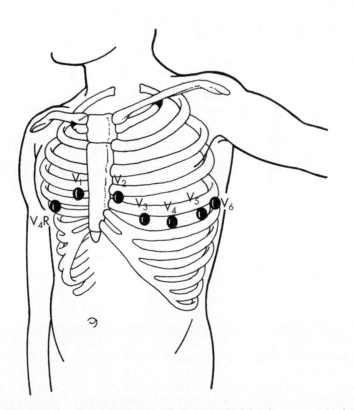

Fig. 1-6. Electrode sites for the chest leads. The precordial leads are on the left from V_1 on the right sternal border to V_6 at the left midaxillary line. One of the designated right chest leads is shown (V_{4R}), although V_1 is also a right chest lead. Please see text for exact placement of electrodes.

RIGHT CHEST LEADS

The right chest leads are V_{3R}, V_{4R}, V_{5R}, and V_{6R}. The positive electrodes for these leads are in the same position on the right side of the chest as their counterparts on the left side. Thus the positive electrode for V_{4R} is at the midclavicular line, fifth intercostal space, right chest; for V_{3R} it is halfway between V_{4R} and V_1 of the standard 12-lead ECG. The electrodes for V_{5R} and V_{6R} are on the same level with V_{4R}, in the anterior and midaxillary lines, respectively. The electrode position for V_{4R} is shown in Fig. 1-6. Lead V_{4R} is the most useful of the right chest leads in the emergency setting. It is used to evaluate risk in patients with acute inferior myocardial infarction (Chapter 26).

MCL LEADS

The older ECG equipment that does not offer the capability of simultaneous bipolar and unipolar monitoring leads creates a significant inconvenience and diagnostic challenge. Many times in such situations by the time the necessary leads are recorded the arrhythmia in question is no longer present, depriving the patient of a diagnosis.

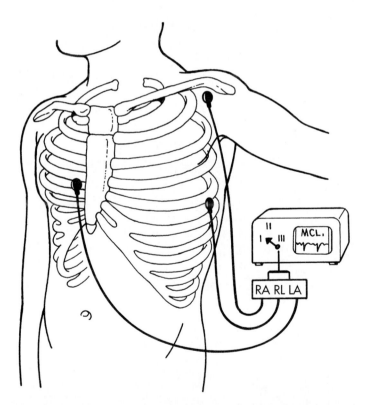

Fig. 1-7. Electrode placement for MCL_1 using the single-channel monitor with three lead-wire cables capable of recording only one bipolar lead. The bedside oscilloscope is usually marked with three choices, I, II, or III. To record MCL_1 turn the channel selector to lead I, causing the left arm *(LA)* lead wire to be positive and the right arm *(RA)* lead wire to be negative. Place the LA electrode at the V_1 position on the chest (fourth intercostal space, right sternal border) and the RA electrode below the clavicle toward the shoulder. The remaining lead wire (right leg [RL]) is a ground but can be attached in the V_6 position. When the oscilloscope dial is turned to lead II, it becomes positive and the LA wire becomes ground. This allows a quick switch from MCL_1 to MCL_6.

The MCL leads are bipolar precordial leads that simulate unipolar precordial leads. Before 1960 the ECG sometimes contained three bipolar chest leads with the positive electrode on the chest (C) and the negative electrode on an extremity (R, L, or F). With the introduction of the coronary care units in 1962, there was only one monitoring lead available. Dr. Henry Marriott modified the old bipolar CL lead, placing the positive electrode in the V_1 position and the negative electrode at the left shoulder, under the left clavicle (modified CL lead in the V_1 position, MCL_1). Dr. Marriott found that this placement simulated the complex seen in the unipolar V_1 position. Since then, this lead has been used for monitoring in certain clinical settings when V_1 is not available. Modern equipment with multiple monitoring leads eliminates the need for this useful lead.

To facilitate your use of the MCL leads it is important not to think in terms of colors (the color-coded lead cables), but to think in terms of + and −. For MCL_1 your goal is to have a negative electrode at the left shoulder and a positive electrode on the right sternal border in the V_1 position. These positions are illustrated in Fig. 1-7.

1. To record MCL_1 and MCL_6, place the electrodes in the positions illustrated in Fig. 1-7 (with one electrode in the V_1 position and another in the V_6 position; the third electrode is at the left shoulder).
2. Turn your lead selector to lead I, which means that the right arm cable is negative and the left arm cable is positive. (If you turned the lead selector to lead II, it would be the left leg cable that would be positive.) Thus the right arm cable goes to the left shoulder electrode and the left arm cable to the V_1

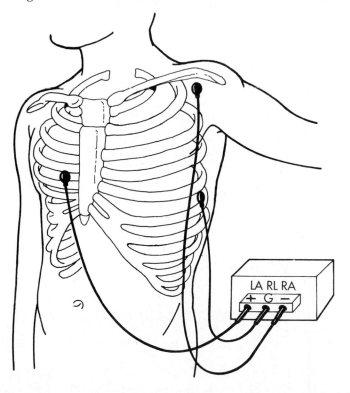

Fig. 1-8. Electrode placement for single-channel telemetry monitoring. Usually there is no selector dial for changing among leads I, II, and III. To record MCL_1 simply place the positive electrode in the V_1 position (fourth intercostal space, right sternal border) and the negative electrode below the clavicle toward the left shoulder.

position on the right sternal border; the third cable (RL) goes to the electrode in the V_6 position.

3. You are now recording the bipolar lead, MCL_1, a simulation of the unipolar lead, V_1.

4. If you turn your lead selector to lead II, you will be recording the bipolar lead, MCL_6, a simulation of the unipolar lead, V_6.

5. To record a simulated V_2 or V_3 lead, simply move the electrode at the right sternal border to those positions.

Many telemetry monitors have no selector dial for changing leads. In Fig. 1-8 the electrode positions for recording MCL_1 are illustrated. Should you wish to record a simulated V_2 or V_3, simply move the left arm electrode across the sternum to those positions.

PLACEMENT OF ELECTRODES FOR MULTICHANNEL MONITORING

Fig. 1-9 shows the correct placement for the electrodes of multichannel monitors with five lead-wire cables. Such an arrangement permits recording all the limb leads (I, II, III, aV_R, aV_L, aV_F) and one precordial lead. The precordial lead shown is V_1; however, it is possible to record other precordial leads by moving the chest (C) electrode to the desired position. Right chest leads may also be obtained by moving the C electrode to the V_{3R}, V_{4R}, V_{5R}, or V_{6R} positions.

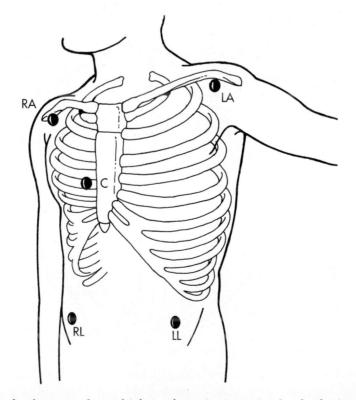

Fig. 1-9. Electrode placement for multichannel monitoring using five lead-wire cables capable of recording one or more limb leads and any one of the precordial leads. (V_1 is shown here.)

SUMMARY

The standard ECG consists of 12 leads, 6 frontal plane leads and 6 horizontal plane leads. There are only 3 bipolar leads; they are leads I, II, and III. The axes of these leads form an equilateral triangle around the heart's electrical field. The sum of the potentials from these 3 bipolar leads offers a zero potential in the center of the triangle. All unipolar leads use this zero potential as a reference point. Thus the axis of all unipolar leads is from the positive electrode to the center of the triangle. There are 3 unipolar limb leads, aV_R, aV_L, and aV_F, and 6 precordial leads from V_1, located on the right chest at the sternal border, to V_6 at the midaxillary line.

2

Normal Electrical Activation of the Heart

Depolarization   *13*

Repolarization   *13*

Sodium-Potassium Adenosine
   Triphosphatase Pump   *13*

Automaticity   *13*

Action Potential   *14*

Normal Pacemaker and Conduction
   System of the Heart   *15*

Atrioventricular Node and
   Atrioventricular Nodal Pathways   *15*

Normal Electrocardiogram   *17*

Step-By-Step Electrical Activation of the
   Heart (Lead I)   *17*

P Wave   *20*

Normal QRS Complex in the Limb
   Leads   *22*

QRS Complexes in the Precordial
   Leads   *23*

Transitional Zone   *24*

Evaluating the QRS Complex   *24*

ST Segment   *27*

T Wave   *28*

U Wave   *29*

Summary   *29*

The normal activation of the heart is initiated by the sinus node. In turn the atria depolarize, and during this time the atrioventricular (AV) node is also depolarized; the P wave represents atrial depolarization. The bundle of His, bundle branches, and Purkinje fibers are then activated; this is not seen on the ECG. Ventricular depolarization proceeds from endocardium to epicardium starting with the interventricular septum; the QRS complex represents ventricular depolarization. The ST segment is from the end of the QRS complex to the beginning of the T wave; it should be isoelectric and slightly slanted up. The T wave represents ventricular repolarization.

The electrical cardiac cycle consists of three phases: depolarization, repolarization, and resting. The resting myocardial cell is negatively charged to −90 mV. This negative charge is maintained until the cell is activated (depolarization) or activates itself (automaticity).

DEPOLARIZATION

Depolarization is the process by which a resting cell becomes more positive. A myocardial cell that is activated by an impulse from the sinus node instantly switches from its resting negative charge of -90 mV to a positive charge that momentarily reaches $+30$ mV.

REPOLARIZATION

Repolarization is the process by which a depolarized cell is restored to its resting state. The repolarization process begins immediately after rapid depolarization; a complicated interaction of current flow first maintains the membrane at a *plateau* of approximately 0 mV and then rapidly restores the membrane to its resting state of -90 mV. The plateau permits a *refractory period* during which the cell cannot be activated again.

SODIUM-POTASSIUM ADENOSINE TRIPHOSPHATASE PUMP

The sodium-potassium adenosine triphosphatase (ATPase) pump is an energy-driven mechanism located in the sarcolemma by which three sodium ions (Na^+) are pumped out for every two potassium ions (K^+) pumped in (Fig. 2-1). Adenosine triphosphate (ATP) and ATPase are involved in the energy production for this pump.

AUTOMATICITY

Automaticity is the ability of a cell to depolarize itself (slow depolarization), reach threshold potential, and produce a propagated action potential. The cells of the conduction system differ from those of the rest of the heart in that they are capable of spontaneous depolarization; that is, they possess the property of automaticity. Atrial and ventricular myocardial cells do not depolarize spontaneously. As long as they remain healthy, they await a stimulus from the sinus node or another pacing source to activate them.

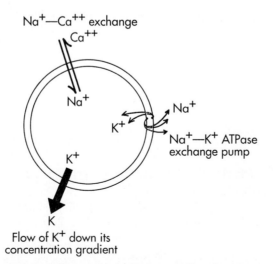

Fig. 2-1. A diagramatic representation of the sodium-potassium adenosine triphosphatase (ATPase) pump. The pump rids the inside of the cell of sodium ions and replenishes the potassium ions that are constantly being lost from the cell.

ACTION POTENTIAL

The action potential is a graph of the transmembrane potential of a single cell during the cardiac cycle. The different phases of the action potential (Fig. 2-2) represent rapid depolarization (phase 0), initial repolarization (phase 1), the plateau (phase 2), rapid repolarization (phase 3), and quiescence (phase 4). The property of automaticity (phase 4 depolarization) can be seen in the second action potential; the slow rise of phase 4 to a more positive value reflects slow diastolic depolarization (automaticity). This cell reaches threshold potential (−70 mV) without outside stimulus.

Phase 0

During phase 0, the depolarizing phase of the action potential is mediated in most cardiac fibers by the rapid influx of sodium ions via voltage dependent sodium channels. (Notable exceptions are the sinus and AV nodes.) In most cardiac fibers the fast sodium channels open at approximately −65 mV, the main cause of the phase 0 spike. A second inward current is initiated during phase 0 at about −60 to −50

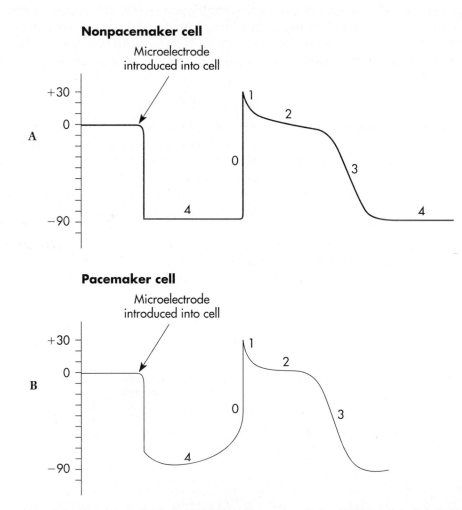

Fig. 2-2. A, An action potential from a ventricular myocardial cell. Phase 4 is flat, indicating lack of automaticity. **B,** An action potential from a pacemaker cell. In this case phase 4 slopes upward toward threshold potential, indicating the power of automaticity.

mV when the T-type calcium channels briefly open. At approximately −30 to −10 mV the L-type (slow) calcium channels open in clustered bursts and continue during phase 2.

Phase 1

Phase 1 is the rapid, brief, incomplete beginning of repolarization immediately following phase 0. It occurs because of a transient outward potassium current through fast-activating and transient potassium channels. This brief efflux sets the stage for the ion channels that will be active during phase 2.

Phase 2

Phase 2 is the plateau or phase of slow repolarization, most notable in the Purkinje fibers. During this time there is a balance of inward and outward ion fluxes across the membrane to maintain an equilibrium, the dominant ones being a calcium influx and a rising potassium permeability that ultimately repolarizes the cell. Thus far, at least seven functionally distinct potassium currents have been described. The reader is referred to the references for a detailed description of the channels active during the cardiac action potential.[1]

Phase 3

Phase 3 is the phase of late, rapid repolarization. During this phase the slow calcium channels close, accelerating the process of repolarization.

Phase 4

Phase 4 is electrical diastole when all the heart rests, except the pacemaker cells; at the end of phase 3, pacemaker cells begin the process that is intended to bring them to threshold potential. In the normal heart only the sinus node reaches that threshold.

NORMAL PACEMAKER AND CONDUCTION SYSTEM OF THE HEART

The pacing and conduction system is illustrated in Fig. 2-3. It is composed of the sinus node (pacemaker), the compact atrioventricular (AV) node with its anterior (fast) and posterior (slow) AV nodal fibers (not shown), and the His-Purkinje system (His bundle, bundle branches, and Purkinje fibers).

The sinus node, located high in the right atrium near the superior vena cava, normally activates the atria at a rate consistent with the needs of the body. Thus atrial activation is from superior to inferior and from right to left. The impulse reaches the compact AV node via the fast AV nodal pathway before atrial activation is completed. It is then conducted down the bundle of His and into the ventricles via the bundle branches and the Purkinje fibers (the His-Purkinje system). Because the His-Purkinje system is a subendocardial structure, the impulse is delivered to the endocardium of both ventricles and activates them from endocardium to epicardium.

ATRIOVENTRICULAR NODE AND ATRIOVENTRICULAR NODAL PATHWAYS

Anatomic and electrophysiologic studies suggest that the *slow AV nodal fibers* extend from the coronary sinus os region anteriorly along the tricuspid annulus to

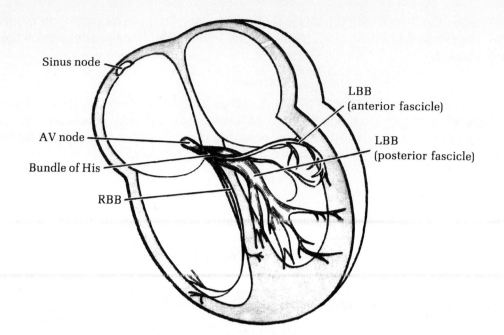

Fig. 2-3. The sinus node and conduction system. *AV,* Atrioventricular; *LBB,* left bundle branch; *RBB,* right bundle branch.

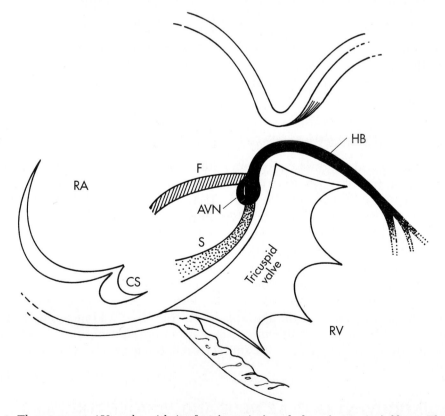

Fig. 2-4. The compact AV node with its fast (anterior) and slow (posterior) fibers. The slow pathway fibers extend from a broad area near the os of the coronary sinus and converge as a common pathway as they reach the compact AV node. The fast pathway fibers arise near the tendon of Todaro and enter the compact AV node superiorly. *RA,* Right atrium; *CS,* coronary sinus; *AVN,* atrioventricular node; *F,* fast pathway; *S,* slow pathway; *HB,* His bundle. *(Adapted from Keim S, Werner P, Jazayeri M et al: Circulation 86:919, 1992.)*

join the compact AV node. The *fast AV nodal fibers* are located superiorly along the compact AV node and exit into the atrial septum near the tendon of Todaro.[2,3] The fast and slow AV nodal pathways are diagramed in Fig. 2-4.

NORMAL ELECTROCARDIOGRAM

In Fig. 2-5 the normal ECG records atrial depolarization, represented by a small, rounded deflection called a *P wave;* ventricular depolarization, represented by a swift, angular deflection called a *QRS complex;* and ventricular repolarization, called the *ST segment* and *T wave.* A *U wave* is a very small deflection that follows the T wave and has the same polarity as the T. The PR interval represents atrial activation and the conduction time of the cardiac impulse as it passes down the AV node, His bundle, bundle branches, and Purkinje fibers.

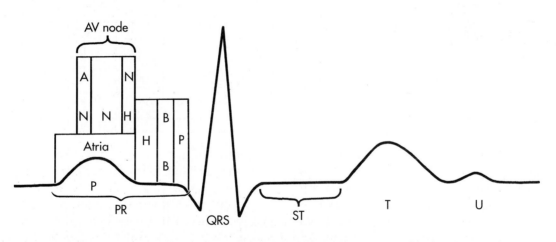

Fig. 2-5. The normal ECG: P wave, atrial depolarization; QRS, ventricular depolarization; ST segment and T wave, ventricular repolarization. The U wave is a small positive deflection. The PR interval reflects not only atrial depolarization, but also the conduction time through the AV node, His bundle *(H),* bundle branches *(BB),* and Purkinje fibers *(P). AN,* Atrionodal; *N,* compact AV node; *NH,* nodal His.

STEP-BY-STEP ELECTRICAL ACTIVATION OF THE HEART (LEAD I)

The following sequence of illustrations and text demonstrates the step-by-step electrical activation of the heart and how each step is reflected on lead I of the ECG. The axis of lead I is depicted to show how the current flow relates to that lead axis. When current flows toward the positive electrode, the ECG stylus moves up; when current flows toward the negative electrode, the stylus moves down.

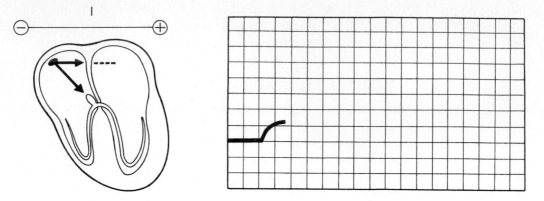

The first half of the *P wave* is inscribed in lead I when the sinus impulse activates the right atrium and reaches the AV node.

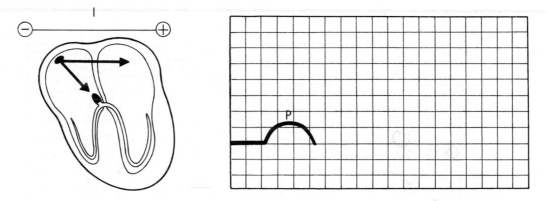

The left atrium and AV node have been activated by the time the P wave is completed. Note that the P wave represents both right and left atrial activation in sequence. Normally the P wave is smooth in contour, but if one or the other atrium is stretched or hypertrophied, the P wave can be distorted. It is also easy to see that the P wave would be negative instead of positive in lead I if it were activated from the left atrium instead of the right. At approximately the peak of the P wave the AV node is being activated. This is a "silent" event, not seen on the ECG because the currents involved are so small.

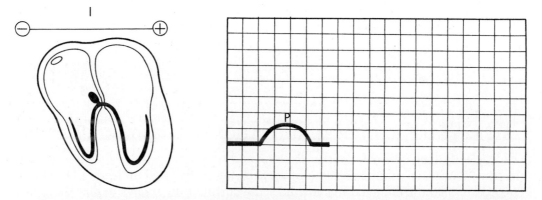

During the *PR segment* (end of the P wave to the beginning of the ventricular complex), the His-Purkinje system is being activated. This is another silent event, not seen on the surface ECG.

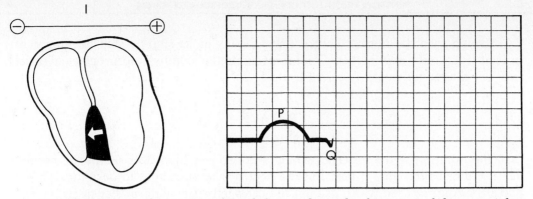

The interventricular septum from left to right is the first part of the ventricles to activate. Note that this current moves toward the negative electrode of lead I and produces a small, narrow, negative deflection called a *Q wave.* AV conduction is measured from the beginning of the P wave to the onset of the ventricular complex. This measurement is called the *PR interval,* although in this case it is actually a "PQ" interval. (This term is not used).

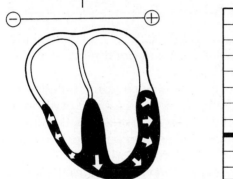

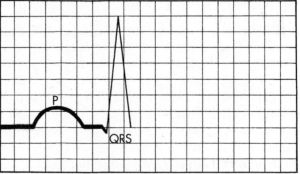

When the two ventricles are activated from endocardium to epicardium, a tall positive spike is recorded in lead I. Note that although current is flowing toward both the positive and the negative electrode, the stronger current is toward the positive electrode because of the relative thickness of the left ventricular walls. The ventricular complex is generically referred to as a *QRS complex.* If the complex in this lead were to be described more accurately, it would be called a qR complex, that is, a small initial negative deflection (q) followed by a large positive one (R).

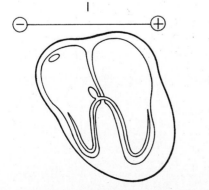

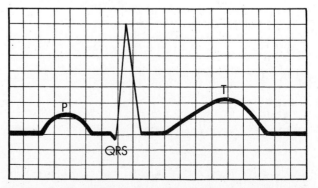

Electrical currents generated during repolarization of the ventricles are reflected in the *ST segment* and the *T wave.* The ST segment is the flat (isoelectric) portion following the QRS complex; it is followed by a slightly asymmetric curve (T wave).

Having seen the normal ventricular complex in its step-by-step development in lead I, it would now be beneficial to evaluate the step-by-step progress of atrial and ventricular activation in all 12 leads.

P WAVE
Duration

The duration of the P wave, which is not greater than 0.11 sec in the normal heart, indicates the time it takes for the depolarization current to pass through the two atria. An increased width usually indicates left atrial abnormality or right atrial hypertrophy.

Height

The normal P wave is not more than 3 mm in height. This is because the atria are thin-walled structures. If the P wave is taller than this, atrial enlargement is suspected and may indicate AV valvular problems, hypertension, cor pulmonale, or congenital heart disease.

Polarity

The polarity of the P wave in leads I, II, aV_F, and V_4 to V_6 (Fig. 2-6) is normally positive. This is because the P vector travels in a leftward, inferior direction toward the positive electrode of these leads.

In leads III, aV_L, and V_1 to V_3 (Fig. 2-7) the P wave may be upright, diphasic, flat, or inverted, depending on the position of the heart in the chest and on the orientation of the atrial vector to the positive terminals. The P wave is usually diphasic in leads V_1 and V_2 because the activation of the right atrium (anterior P vector) and the activation of the left atrium (posterior P vector) are recorded sequentially. In cases of left atrial enlargement, the second half of the P wave is significantly negative in lead V_1.

In lead aV_R the normal P wave is negative because the P vector travels away from the positive electrode of that lead (Fig. 2-8). The P wave is often positive but

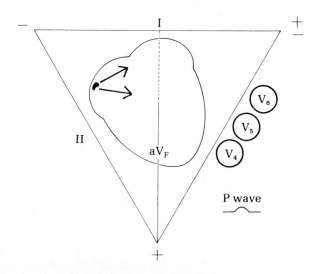

Fig. 2-6. The P vectors related to the axes of leads I, II, aV_F, and V_4 to V_6. The P wave is positive in these leads.

may normally be negative or diphasic in leads aV$_L$ and V$_1$ to V$_3$. A deeply negative, broad terminal trough in the P wave of V$_1$ indicates left atrial abnormality.

Axis

The normal P axis is about +60 degrees in the frontal plane.

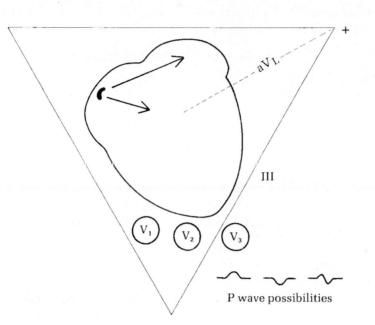

Fig. 2-7. The P vectors related to the axes of leads III and V$_1$ to V$_3$. The P wave may normally be positive, negative, or biphasic.

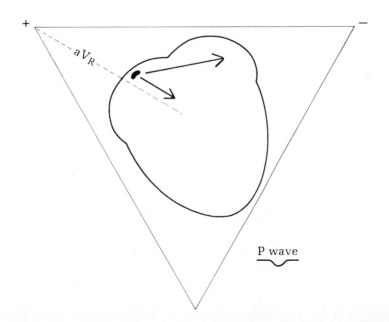

Fig. 2-8. The P vectors related to the axes of lead aV$_R$. The normal P wave is always negative in this lead.

Shape

The normal P wave is not notched or peaked. A notched P wave that is upright in leads I, II, and V_4 to V_6 indicates left atrial abnormality. A tall, peaked P wave in the inferior leads and sometimes in lead V_1 is called *P-pulmonale* and is probably caused by the increased sympathetic stimulation and the low position of the diaphragm associated with diffuse lung disease. The increased sympathetic stimulation causes increased P amplitude, and low position of the diaphragm causes the P axis to be rightward.

Summary of the Normal P Wave

1. Not broader than 0.11 sec
2. Not taller than 3 mm
3. Upright in leads I, II, aV_F, and V_4 to V_6
4. Inverted in aV_R
5. May be positive, negative, or diphasic in leads III, aV_L, and V_1 to V_3, but the negative component in V_1 should not be excessively broad or deep
6. Not notched or peaked

NORMAL QRS COMPLEX IN THE LIMB LEADS

Figs. 2-9 and 2-10 illustrate the step-by-step evolution of the QRS complex in the limb leads (bipolar and unipolar). Numbers are used instead of letters to illustrate how each instantaneous event is reflected in a particular lead. The numbers correspond to the numbered currents in the heart. The long arrow represents the

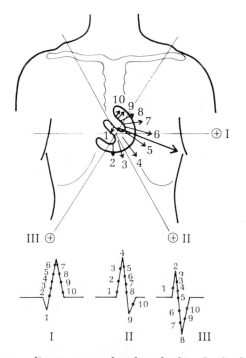

Fig. 2-9. Instant-to-instant cardiac vectors related to the bipolar limb leads. The numbers on the ventricular complexes correspond to the cardiac vectors. Septal activation is well defined in lead I (vector 1).

electrical axis of the heart (Chapter 4). These figures again illustrate that when the current is flowing toward a positive electrode, a positive deflection is recorded. The deflection is most positive when the current is parallel with the lead axis. When current flow is perpendicular to the lead axis, it is isoelectric (neither positive nor negative).

QRS COMPLEXES IN THE PRECORDIAL LEADS

The precordial chest leads give valuable information about anterior and posterior forces and, because of their proximity to the surface of the heart, are helpful in localizing pathologic changes in the myocardium. The six standard positive precordial electrodes form one fourth of a circle around the heart, beginning on the right side of the sternum, continuing over the right ventricle, and ending on the left lateral chest wall over the left ventricle (Fig. 2-11). From V_1 to V_6 the positive electrode gets closer and closer to current flow in the thick-walled left ventricle, and the R wave (positive component) becomes taller and taller. This normal R wave progression reflects intact anterior forces; if anterior forces are lost, so are the R waves. The R wave in V_6 may actually be smaller than that of V_5 because the V_6 electrode is farther from the heart.

In V_1 the initial little r wave reflects both septal and right ventricular forces. However, when right ventricular activation is still just beginning, the dominant leftward force of the left ventricle produces a deep S wave. Thus a narrow rS complex is normal for V_1, although the little r wave may be normally absent. In V_6 normal septal activation can easily be detected. It is reflected by the small, narrow q wave (as seen in lead I).

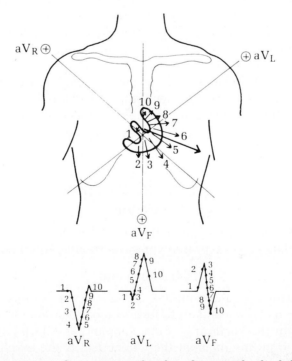

Fig. 2-10. Instant-to-instant cardiac vectors related to the unipolar limb leads. The numbers on the ventricular complexes correspond to the cardiac vectors.

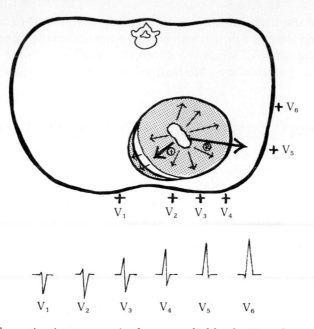

Fig. 2-11. Ventricular activation as seen in the precordial leads. Note the normal R-wave progression.

TRANSITIONAL ZONE

As the R wave becomes taller across the precordial leads, the S wave becomes smaller. Usually, between V₃ and V₄ the R and the S are equal. This equiphasic complex defines the *transitional zone.* If the transitional zone is to the left (toward V₆), there is clockwise rotation of the heart. If the shift is to the right (toward V₁), there is counterclockwise rotation of the heart.

A shift in the transitional zone to the left is one of the ECG signs of acute pulmonary embolism, right ventricular hypertrophy, and atrial septal defect. A shift to the right is seen in left ventricular hypertrophy. Fig. 2-12 illustrates the normal transitional zone compared with shifts to the right (counterclockwise rotation) and to the left (clockwise rotation).

EVALUATING THE QRS COMPLEX
Duration

In the adult the duration of the QRS complex is 0.05 to 0.10 sec; in the newborn it is 0.04 to 0.05 sec. It represents intraventricular conduction time.

Measurement

When measuring the QRS complex, be sure to take in any initial or terminal components (little q or s wave) and to look in more than one lead. Sometimes it is difficult to pinpoint the beginning of the complex. The duration of the QRS complex is measured from the moment the tracing leaves the baseline to the point at which it returns. In bundle branch block the duration is 0.12 sec or more; in ventricular hypertrophy it is 0.10 to 0.11 sec.

Transitional Zones

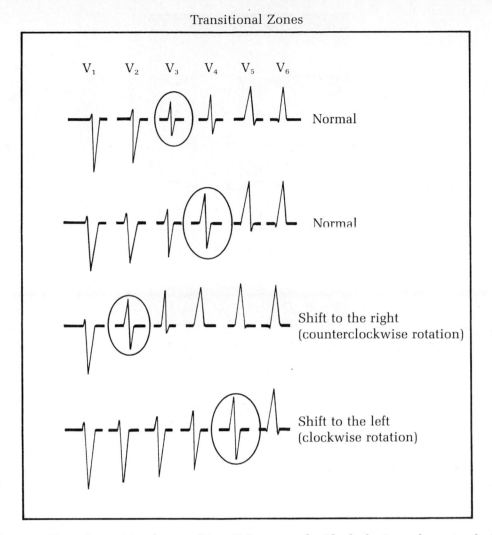

Fig. 2-12. Normal transitional zones (V_3 to V_4) compared with clockwise and counterclockwise rotation of the heart.

Best leads for measuring

The QRS complex may be narrower in one or two leads than it is in others. This is because either the initial vector or the terminal vector is perpendicular to that particular lead axis and the record remains on, or returns to, the isoelectric line. Wanderman et al[1] found a 5- to 20-ms delay in the onset of the QRS complex in one or two leads in almost half of more than 300 patients tested. Lead II was the lead that most frequently showed a delayed QRS onset and therefore would seem to be a poor choice for measuring the QRS duration. A right precordial lead (V_1 or V_2) was found to be most reliable for the actual QRS recording, and when this was combined with a simultaneous recording of a limb lead, the most accurate measurement was ensured. Fig. 2-13 illustrates the delay in onset of the QRS that is sometimes encountered. In this case the delay is in lead III. Note that the beginning of the QRS complex in lead II is slow, making it difficult to determine the precise point where it begins, unless the complex is recorded simultaneously with V_1.

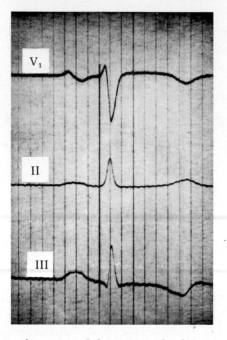

Fig. 2-13. Delay of 20 ms in the onset of the QRS in lead III as compared with V_1. *(From Wanderman KL et al: Circulation 63:933, 1981.)*

Amplitude

QRS voltage varies with age, being greater in the younger individual and in those with thin chest walls; depends on the mean frontal plane QRS axis, being greater in the lead whose axis is parallel with the mean current flow; and is less in obese individuals and in those with lung disease.

In the precordial leads the voltage of the QRS complex in a standardized ECG recording should not be less than the following:

6 mm in V_1 and V_6
8 mm in V_2 and V_5
10 mm in V_3 and V_4

The upper limit of normal in a precordial lead is accepted by most authors as 25 to 30 mm.

In the bipolar limb leads the amplitude of the QRS complex is considered to be too low if the total value (add the positive and negative components) of the QRS complex is less than 6 mm in leads I, II, and III. Some conditions causing low voltage are diffuse coronary disease, pericardial effusion, emphysema, myxedema, primary amyloidosis, and cardiac failure.

Polarity

Leads I, II, and V_3 to V_6: positive to equiphasic.
Leads aV_L and aV_F: positive, negative, or equiphasic
Lead aV_R: negative

Shape

The term *QRS* may be used to refer in general to the ventricular complex, whatever its shape. It is a generic term not intended to describe the morphology of the

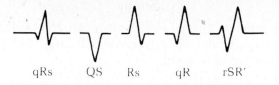

qRs   QS   Rs   qR   rSR′

Fig. 2-14. QRS deflections described using uppercase and lowercase letters. R or r waves are always positive. A negative component is either a Q or an S. A Q is before an R wave, an S follows an R.

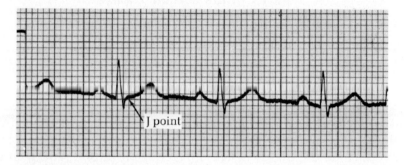

Fig. 2-15. The J point *(arrow)* defines the end of the QRS complex and the beginning of the ST segment.

complex. If it is necessary to describe precise deflections, uppercase and lowercase letters are used to indicate relative sizes of the components. All positive deflections are R or r waves. If there are two R (or r) waves in the same complex, the second is named R or r prime (R′ or r′). A negative component is either an uppercase or a lowercase Q or S; the Q is before the first R, and the S follows it. Fig. 2-14 illustrates a few possibilities.

Normal Q wave

A normal q wave is expressed with the small letter and is found in leads I, aV_L, and V_6. It is less than 0.04 sec in duration and has less than 25% of the amplitude of the R wave.

ST SEGMENT

The ST segment is part of the repolarization phase of the heart and is normally isoelectric, slanting slightly upward from the end of the QRS, into the T wave. The point where the QRS ends and the ST segment begins is called the *J point* (Fig. 2-15). Some causes of ST segment deviation (elevated or depressed) are tachycardia, digitalis effect, preexcitation, ventricular hypertrophy, conduction disturbances, and cardiac injury.

Level

Normally, the ST segment can be slightly elevated above the baseline (1 mm in leads I, II, and III and as much as 2 mm in some precordial leads), but it should never be depressed more than 0.5 mm in any lead. To determine ST elevation, draw a straight line from J point to J point in sequential cycles.

Shape

The normal ST segment curves very slightly into the beginning of the T wave. In fact, an absolutely horizontal ST segment, which forms a sharp angle with the T wave, is highly suggestive of ischemia.

T WAVE

The T wave is the result of current generated during rapid repolarization of the heart.

Polarity of the normal T wave

Leads I, II, and V₂ to V₆: Positive
Lead aV_R: Inverted
Leads aV_L and aV_F: Positive, but may be inverted if the QRS complex is less than 6 mm tall
Leads III and V₁: Varied

Isolated T wave inversion in asymptomatic adults is usually a normal variant.[4] In patients with unstable angina, progressive, deep, symmetric T wave inversion in V_2 and V_3 reflects critical proximal left anterior descending coronary artery occlusion[5-7] (Chapter 24) and is a sign of reperfusion in this setting and also following thrombolysis.[7a]

Although T wave change is the most sensitive indicator of infarction, it is the least specific.

Abnormal T wave shapes are seen in patients with long QT syndrome. The presence of "humps" near the apex or on the descending limb of upright T waves may suggest the presence of the long QT syndrome trait in symptomatic blood relatives with borderline QTc interval.[8]

Vulnerable period

The vulnerable period is at the peak of the T wave, offset slightly toward the end of the T wave. During this short time not all the fibers of the heart are refractory; some are able to accept a stimulus and produce a propagated impulse. The result may be electrical chaos when the current meets with fibers that are still refractory or conducting too slowly. The approximate location of the vulnerable period is shown in Fig. 2-16.

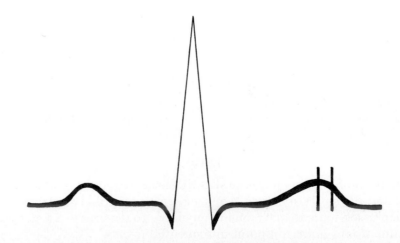

Fig. 2-16. Approximate location of the vulnerable period.

Shape

The normal T wave is rounded and asymmetric. It usually ascends more slowly than it descends. A notched T wave is normal in children but may also be found in adults with pericarditis. Whenever the depolarization process of the ventricles is abnormal, repolarization processes change as well. Examples of such conditions are bundle branch block, digitalis therapy, quinidine therapy, ischemia (slow conduction), ventricular ectopic beats, and ventricular hypertrophy. T-wave abnormalities are also sensitive indicators of a variety of conditions including hyperkalemia, hyperventilation, metabolic diseases, acid-base imbalance, and the presence of various drugs.

Height

The T wave should not exceed 5 mm in height in leads I, II, and III, or 1 mm in the precordial leads. Tall, pointed T waves reflect hyperkalemia or myocardial ischemia and are sometimes seen before the T-wave inversion of myocardial infarction. T-wave alternans may be seen in hypokalemia, hypocalcemia, hypomagnesemia, tachycardia, congestive heart disease, and pericardial disease.[9]

U WAVE

The U wave follows the T wave and is the same polarity as the T. It normally goes unnoticed because of its low voltage. Its mechanism is unknown. Some researchers believe that the U wave represents repolarization of Purkinje fibers; others believe it to be a reflection of a diastolic event. It becomes taller in hypokalemia and inverted in heart disease. Hypertension is the most common cause of a negative U wave.[10] Transient U-wave inversion can be caused by acute myocardial ischemia or a rise of blood pressure. Typically when associated with ischemia there is terminal U-wave inversion (inversion after positive U-wave deflection). When associated with hypertension only the initial part of the U wave is negative.[11]

SUMMARY

The normal activation of the heart is initiated by the sinus node. In turn the atria depolarize and during this time the AV node is also depolarized; the P wave represents atrial depolarization. The bundle of His, bundle branches, and Purkinje fibers are then activated; this is not seen on the ECG. Ventricular depolarization proceeds from endocardium to epicardium starting with the interventricular septum; the QRS complex represents ventricular depolarization. The ST segment is from the end of the QRS complex to the beginning of the T wave; it should be isoelectric and slightly slanted up. The T wave represents ventricular repolarization.

REFERENCES

1. Zipes DP, Jalife J, eds: *Cardiac electrophysiology: from Cell to bedside,* Philadelphia, 1995, WB Saunders.
2. Keim S, Werner P, Jazayeri M, et al: Localization of the fast and slow pathways in atrioventricular nodal reentrant tachycardia by intraoperative ice mapping, *Circulation* 86:919, 1992.
3. Moulton K, Miller B, Scott J, Woods WT Jr: Radiofrequency catheter ablation for AV nodal re-

entry: a technique for rapid transection of the slow AV nodal pathway, *PACE Pacing Clin Electrophysical* 16:760, 1993.
4. Okada M, Yotsukura M, Shimada T, Ishikawa K: Clinical implications of isolated T wave inversion in adults: electrocardiographic differentiation of the underlying causes of this phenomenon, *J Am Coll Cardiol* 24:739, 1994.
5. de Zwaan C, Bar RWHM, Wellens HJJ: Characteristic electrocardiographic pattern indicating

a critical stenosis high in left anterior descending coronary artery in patients admitted because of impending myocardial infarction, *Am Heart J* 103:730, 1982.

6. Wellens HJJ: The electrocardiogram 80 years after Einthoven, *J Am Coll Cardiol* 7:484, 1986.

7. de Zwaan C, Bär FW, Janssen JH, et al: Angiographic and clinical characteristics of patients with unstable angina showing an ECG pattern indicating critical narrowing of the proximal LAD coronary artery, *Am Heart J* 117:657, 1989.

7a. Doevendans PA, Gorgels AP, van der Zee R et al: Electrocardiographic diagnosis of reperfusion during thrombolytic therapy in acute myocardial infarction, *Am J Cardiol* 75:1206, 1995.

8. Lehmann MH, Suzuki F, Fromm BS, et al: T wave "humps" as a potential electrocardiographic marker of the long QT syndrome, *J Am Coll Cardiol* 24:746, 1994.

9. Vora AM, Dalvi B, Joshi M, et al: Ventricular tachycardia with retrograde 2:1 atrial activation masquerading as T wave alternans, *Am Heart J* 125:1197, 1993.

10. Fisch C: Evolution of clinical electrocardiogram, *J Am Coll Cardiol* 14:1127, 1989.

11. Miwa K, Miyagi Y, Fujita M, et al: Transient terminal U wave inversion as a more specific marker for myocardial ischemia, *Am Heart J* 125:981, 1993.

C H A P T E R

3

Measurement of Heart Rate and Intervals

ECG Paper   *31*   PR Interval   *33*
Calculation of Heart Rate   *31*   QT Interval   *34*

ECG PAPER

Time is measured on the horizontal plane. Each small square on the ECG paper is 1 mm in length and represents 0.04 sec in time. Each larger square, which is defined by the heavier lines, is 5 mm in length and represents 0.2 sec in time when the paper speed is 25 mm/sec.

Amplitude (voltage) is measured on the vertical plane. All diagnostic 12-lead ECGs are standardized so that 1 mV is equal to 10 mm (two large squares).

The single vertical lines above the ECG grid are 3 inches apart and represent 3-sec intervals (Fig. 3-1) when the paper speed is 25 mm/sec.

CALCULATION OF HEART RATE

Any of several methods can be used to calculate heart rate.

1. Count the number of cycles in a 6-sec strip and multiply by 10. This method, which is fast and simple, can be used when the rhythm is either regular or irregular (Fig. 3-2).
2. Count the number of large squares between two R waves and divide into 300. This method is accurate only if the rhythm is regular (Fig. 3-3).
3. Measure the time interval in seconds between two R waves and divide into 60. For example, if the distance between the R waves of two consecutive beats is 0.60 sec, the heart rate is 100 beats/min. This method is accurate only if the rhythm is regular.
4. For more rapid rhythms or to calculate a rapid atrial rate, count the number of small squares (0.04 sec) between R waves or P waves and divide into 1500. This method is accurate only if the rhythm is regular.

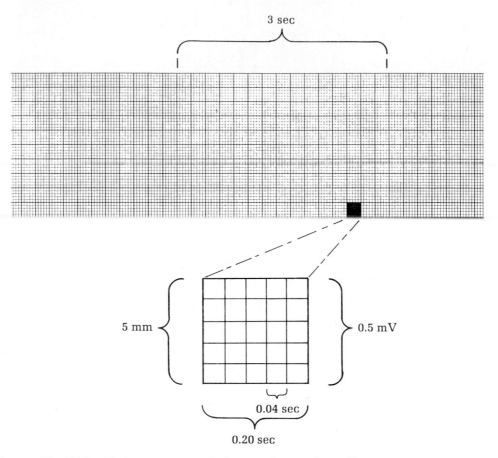

Fig. 3-1. The ECG grid. At a paper speed of 25 mm/sec, each small square represents 0.04 sec and each large square, 0.20 sec. In the standardized ECG, 5 mm equals 0.5 mV.

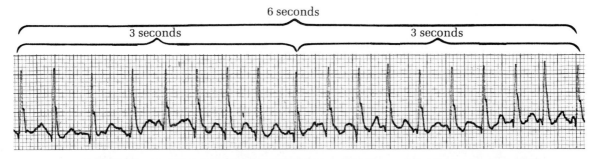

Fig. 3-2. When the rhythm is irregular, heart rate can be determined by counting the R waves in a 6-sec strip and multiplying by 10. (Paper speed is 25 mm/sec.)

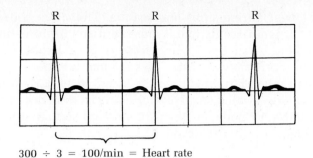

$$300 \div 3 = 100/\text{min} = \text{Heart rate}$$

Fig. 3-3. When the rhythm is regular, heart rate can be determined at a glance. Divide the number of small squares into 300.

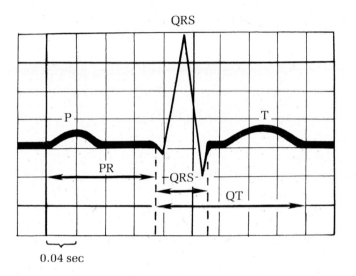

0.04 sec

Fig. 3-4. ECG complexes and intervals.

PR INTERVAL

The PR interval (Fig. 3-4) is normally between 0.12 and 0.20 sec. It represents the length of time it takes for the impulse to travel from the atria to the ventricles. The PR interval is measured from the very beginning of the P wave to the first ventricular deflection. The onset of the P wave is the beginning of atrial activation, just as the onset of the QRS complex is the beginning of ventricular activation. During the PR interval, the atrioventricular (AV) node and His-Purkinje system are also being activated.

PR segment

The PR segment is part of the PR interval. It is that segment from the end of the P wave to the beginning of the QRS complex (Fig. 3-4). The PR segment is normally isoelectric but may be displaced in atrial infarction and in acute pericarditis.

Influence of heart rate

Because the sinus node and the AV node are both under the control of the vagus nerve, the PR interval varies with heart rate, becoming shorter during sinus tachycardia and longer during sinus bradycardia. The sinus node responds to the needs of the body. It increases its rate if more cardiac output is necessary. The AV node responds in kind by shortening its refractory period so that the quicker sinus rate will be able to reach the ventricles. This tandem functioning of the two nodes is noticeably absent when atrial tachycardia is caused by a rhythm outside the sinus node (an ectopic rhythm). Instead of shortening its refractory period in response to the tachycardia, the AV node lengthens this period so that at least the ventricles are somewhat protected from the unwelcome tachycardia.

Prolonged PR interval

The PR interval may be prolonged because of AV block or hypothyroidism. However, a PR interval longer than the prescribed limits may be normal for a particular individual.

Shortened PR interval

The PR interval may be shortened because of preexcitation syndromes, AV junctional rhythms, glycogen storage disease, or hypertension. However, a PR interval that is shorter than the prescribed limit may be normal for a particular individual.

QT INTERVAL

The QT interval is the distance from the beginning of the ventricular complex to the end of the T wave (Fig. 3-4). It represents the sum of depolarization and repolarization periods in the heart (refractory period of the ventricles). Following myocardial infarction the longest QT interval is usually seen in leads V_2 to V_4.[1,2]

The QT interval is significantly influenced by heart rate and autonomic tone;[3] it also varies in males and females and with age. As the heart rate speeds up, the QT shortens; as the heart rate slows down, the QT lengthens. This response represents a fundamental physiologic phenomenon by which the heart is protected from stimulation before an adequate diastolic filling period can be achieved. QT prolongation reflects dispersion of repolarization within the myocardium, predisposing to a malignant polymorphous ventricular tachycardia known as torsades de pointes.

The QT interval may lengthen because of drugs, notably quinidine, procainamide, or disopyramide. It also lengthens, and the U wave is increased, with bradycardia, hypokalemia, and hypomagnesemia. The QT interval may be prolonged by 10% to 15% in trained athletes.[4]

Measuring the QT interval

The QT interval is measured in a lead where the end of the T wave is best seen (Fig. 3-4); this is often lead II. Measurement of the QT interval may be difficult when the T waves are flat, broad, or notched. A notched T wave could represent fusion of the T wave and the U wave. In such a case the duration of the QT interval cannot be exactly measured. The same problem exists when a P wave is superimposed on a T wave.

Corrected QT interval

Because the QT interval lengthens with tachycardia and shortens with bradycardia, it is corrected for heart rate, using Bazett's formula, which is based on the observation that the QT interval varies with the square root of the cycle length. (Divide the square root of the RR interval into the QT interval, measured in seconds.)

The corrected QT interval (OTc) is said to be 0.44 sec, but may be longer and differ slightly for men (0.46) and women (0.47) ±15% of the mean. However, a normal range for the QTc remains unsettled, a wide range being observed in normal subjects as in individuals with long QT syndrome.[2] It has been shown that correcting the QT for heart rate may mask ventricular repolarization abnormalities.[5] One study[6] has found that evaluating the QT-RR relationship by means of 24-hour ambulatory Holter ECG recording may be helpful in assessing ventricular repolarization abnormalities.

REFERENCES

1. Cowan JC, Yusoff K, Moore M, et al: Importance of lead selection in QT interval measurement, *Am J Cardiol* 61:83, 1988.
2. Schweitzer P: The values and limitations of the QT interval in clinical practice, *Am Heart J* 124:1121, 1992.
3. Surawicz B, Knoebel SB: Long QT: good, bad or indifferent? *J Am Coll Cardiol* 4:398, 1984.
4. Zehender M, Meinertz T, Keul J, and Just H: ECG variants and cardiac arrhythmias in athletes: clinical relevance and prognostic importance, *Am Heart J* 119:1378, 1990.
5. Ward DE: Is it appropriate to correct the QT interval for heart rate? In GS Butrous, PJ Schwartz, eds: *Clinical aspects of ventricular repolarization,* London, 1989, Farrand.
6. Fei L, Statters DJ, Anderson MH, et al: Is there an abnormal QT interval in sudden cardiac death survivors with a "normal" QTc? *Am Heart J* 128:73, 1994.

4

Determination of the Electrical Axis

Why is It Important to Learn Axis
  Determination? *36*
Methods of Axis Determination *37*
Lesson Plan *37*
Instant-To-Instant Electrical Activation
  of the Heart *37*
Vectors and the Axis of the Heart *37*
Current Flow Related to the Lead
  Axis *38*
Normal Electrical Axis *40*

Axis at a Glance *40*
Easy Two-Step Method of Axis
  Determination *41*
Exercises for Axis Determination *43*
Use of Leads I and aV$_F$ in Axis
  Determination: the Quadrant
  Method *45*
Hexaxial Figure: a More Precise Method
  of Axis Determination *47*
Summary *47*

WHY IS IT IMPORTANT TO LEARN AXIS DETERMINATION?

The ability to determine the electrical axis of the heart is important for two main reasons. It is a necessary skill in the intelligent response to several cardiac emergencies, and it gives depth to your understanding of the 12-lead ECG and monitoring leads.

Cardiac emergencies

In the cardiac emergency of wide QRS tachycardia, rapid axis determination is helpful in many cases and diagnostic in some. This skill is a mandate for the speedy identification of patients with hemiblock. In the cardiac emergency of broad QRS tachycardia, axis determination can sometimes be diagnostic. Axis determination is also useful in the recognition of life-threatening hyperkalemia. In narrow QRS tachycardia, an understanding of the QRS axis easily leads to an understanding of the P wave axis. This knowledge is diagnostic in some cases of paroxysmal supraventricular tachycardia (PSVT) not only for the mechanism of the tachycardia, but also for the location of an accessory pathway.

Understanding the 12-lead electrocardiogram

An understanding of the 12-lead ECG and the nonstandard monitoring leads is not possible without a clear appreciation of the instant-to-instant electrical vectors of the heart and how they relate to each lead axis. This knowledge provides an important foundation in electrocardiography. Once the axes of the six limb leads and the frontal plane axis of the heart are understood, the student easily understands why the P wave or QRS complex is negative in one lead and positive in another. An understanding of the relationship of mean current flow to the axes of the six limb leads has already provided depth in understanding (Chapter 2).

METHODS OF AXIS DETERMINATION

For the reasons mentioned earlier this text discusses several methods for axis determination, that is, axis at a glance (for emergencies) and two other methods (the easy two-step method and the quadrant method). This will assist in providing the depth of understanding necessary for an appreciation of the normal ECG and how the mechanisms of arrhythmias and other abnormalities such as preexcitation, bundle branch block, hemiblock, acute myocardial infarction, and chamber enlargement are reflected on the ECG.

For completeness the hexaxial figure is also included in this chapter, although I do not use it myself in teaching. It is an accurate, useful means of axis determination. However, I have found that although the student may understand the concept of the hexaxial figure in class, this understanding is generally not carried through to the pressured clinical setting. There is no doubt that visualizing the hexaxial wheel and plotting currents on it takes more time and requires a long-time familiarity. In the setting of cardiac emergencies, axis at a glance seems best.

LESSON PLAN

The 12 leads and their axes have already been discussed in Chapter 1. This chapter presupposes that knowledge and sequentially builds on these concepts:
1. The instant-to-instant electrical activation of the heart
2. The axis of the heart
3. How current flow relates to the lead axis
4. How instant-to-instant currents form the ventricular complex in specific leads
5. The easy two-step method and practice with this method
6. The quadrant method and its advantages and single disadvantage

INSTANT-TO-INSTANT ELECTRICAL ACTIVATION OF THE HEART

The impulse is delivered at the endocardial surface of the two ventricles almost simultaneously by the rapidly conducting His-Purkinje system. The impulse then travels from endocardium to epicardium; the numbers from 1 to 10 in Fig. 4-1 represent the sequence of impulse arrival at the epicardium. The whole process in the normal heart takes about 0.08 sec or less.

VECTORS AND THE AXIS OF THE HEART

Vectors are quantities that have both a magnitude and direction. We use vectors many times in everyday life. For example, if Aunt Sue lives 10 miles southeast

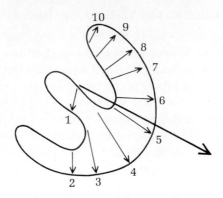

Fig. 4-1. Instant-to-instant currents *(1 to 10)* resulting from the orderly depolarization of the ventricular muscle mass. The prominent arrow between 5 and 6 represents the electrical axis of the heart.

of the post office; that is a vector. The magnitude is 10 miles and its direction is southeast. The direction can also be expressed in degrees; in this case it would be 135 degrees. Vectors can also be added together to give a resultant vector. In adding vectors we simply travel along the first and then along the second and see where we end up. The process is not unlike the sailboat that sails northeast for 10 miles and then tacks to sail to the southeast for 10 miles. Our intrepid mariners will end up due east of the starting point because the northerly component of their travel exactly cancels the southerly component, leaving only the easterly component. Although the total distance traveled is 20 miles, the sailors end up only about 14 miles east of the starting point. This can be easily verified by using a ruler to make a scale drawing. As with ordinary addition, when many numbers can be added together to get a result, many vectors can be vector-added to get a resultant vector.

Current flow can be represented by a vector, with the amount of current being the magnitude and the direction of flow being its direction. The small arrows in Fig. 4-1 represent the current flow vectors for the ventricles during activation. If we add all of these vectors, the resultant vector, represented by the long, darker arrow, is called the *axis of the heart.* It may also be called the *QRS axis.* Just as the total effort of our sailors' Sunday afternoon sail was a 14-mile trip to the east, the total electrical effort of the heart is a current flow along its axis, represented by the long arrow in Fig. 4-1. Because we are primarily interested in the direction of current flow, I will refer to "currents" rather than vectors and to "axis" rather than "QRS vector."

CURRENT FLOW RELATED TO THE LEAD AXIS

The currents generated by the heart cause certain deflections on the ECG, according to how they relate to the lead axis.

1. When the electrical axis is parallel to the lead axis, the resulting ECG complex is either the most positive or the most negative deflection of all, depending on whether it flows toward the positive or the negative electrode. This principle is illustrated in Fig. 4-2, where lead I is depicted; the negative electrode is on the right arm (RA), and the positive electrode is on the left arm (LA).

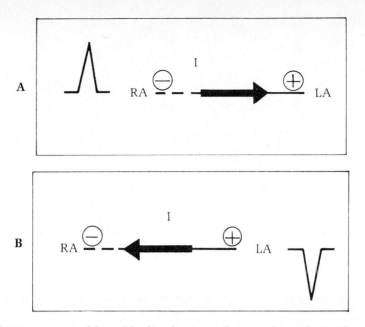

Fig. 4-2. Lead I is represented here (the line between the two electrodes). When current flow *(arrow)* is parallel to the axis of a lead (in this case, lead I) it results in, **A,** the tallest positive deflection or, **B,** the deepest negative deflection. *LA,* Left arm; *RA,* right arm.

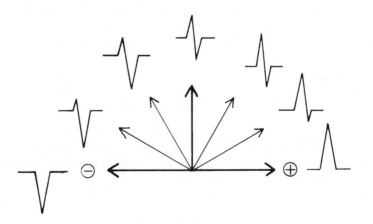

Fig. 4-3. Several electrical axes and their resultant ECG complex are represented. The arrows represent the electrical axes from seven different hearts. The lead axis is a straight line between the two electrodes. Take special note that a current perpendicular to the lead axis produces an equiphasic deflection and that a current parallel to the axis of the lead results in the tallest complex possible if the current flows toward the positive electrode and results in the deepest complex possible if the current flows toward the negative electrode.

1. When the main current flow of the heart is perpendicular to the axis of the lead, it is neither positive nor negative, and an isoelectric (equiphasic) deflection is written.

Fig. 4-3 shows lead I and illustrates complexes from seven different hearts, each with a different electrical axis. Remember in looking at Fig. 4-3 that the axis of the lead is a straight line between the two electrodes. Moving from left to right across

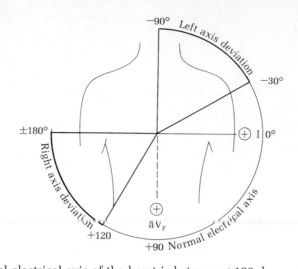

Fig. 4-4. The normal electrical axis of the heart is between +120 degrees and −30 degrees.

Fig. 4-3, notice that when the current is flowing toward the negative electrode and is parallel with the axis of the lead, the resulting ECG complex is more negative than any of the others. Beause the mean current is directed away from this parallel orientation, the sum of the ECG complex becomes less and less negative until the current is perpendicular to the axis of the lead and the ECG complex becomes iso-electric. As the current is directed into the positive half of the lead axis, the ECG complex becomes more and more positive until it is fully so when the current is parallel with the axis of the lead—this time flowing toward the positive electrode.

NORMAL ELECTRICAL AXIS

The normal electrical axis of the heart is illustrated in Fig. 4-4. It is between −30 degrees and +120 degrees. The axis is left, of course, when it is beyond 0 degrees. However, it is not an abnormal left axis deviation until it is beyond −30 degrees.

AXIS AT A GLANCE

Whether the easy two-step method, the quadrant method, or the hexaxial figure for axis determination is used, in the emergency setting knowing how to recognize an abnormal axis at a glance is most helpful. This is especially true when there is a broad QRS tachycardia or acute myocardial infarction.

Fig. 4-5 illustrates this useful shortcut to axis determination. Leads I and II are used:

Normal axis: I and II are upright (first three examples).
Left axis deviation: I is up; II is down.
Right axis deviation: I is down; II is up.
Northwest quadrant ("no man's land" or "indeterminate"): I and II are down.

Of course, when I is up and II is equiphasic, the axis is at −30 degrees. This is a borderline left axis deviation because if the complex in lead II were a little more negative, it would be left axis deviation.

Rapid axis determination

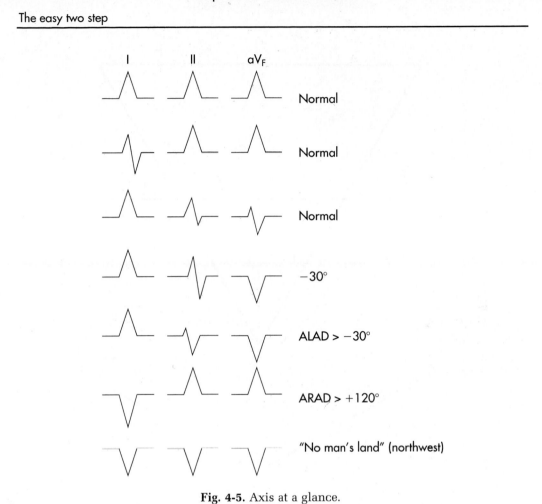

Fig. 4-5. Axis at a glance.

EASY TWO-STEP METHOD OF AXIS DETERMINATION

When the Y shape of the three unipolar limb leads, aV_R, aV_L, and aV_F, is combined in a drawing with the Δ shape formed by the three bipolar limb leads I, II, and III, as seen in Fig. 4-6, each bipolar lead axis is perpendicular to a unipolar lead axis, providing an excellent frame of reference in which to determine the electrical axis of the heart.

For example, if the heart's electrical axis is perpendicular to the lead axis of aV_R, it is also parallel to the lead axis of III. Thus when the equiphasic deflection is seen in one of these leads, a positive or negative deflection is seen in the other. Let us say that the equiphasic deflection is in lead aV_R (current flow is perpendicular to that lead axis). If the complex in lead III is positive, the axis is to the right; if the complex in lead III is negative, the axis is to the left. Thus you have the easy two-step method of axis determination:

1. Look for an equiphasic deflection; it tells you that current flow is perpendicular to that lead axis.

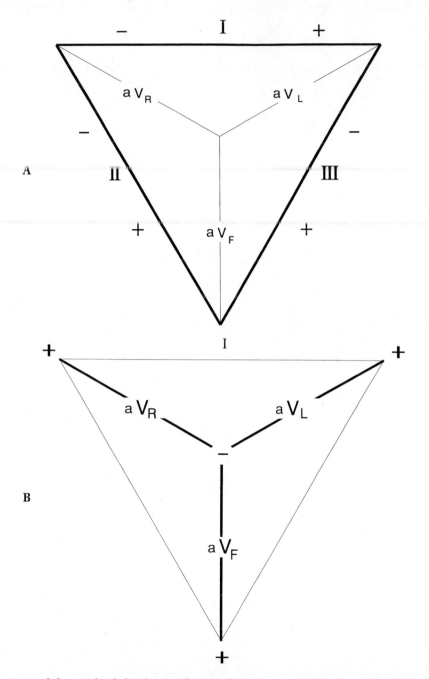

Fig. 4-6. Axes of the six limb leads. **A,** The (Δ) shape is created by the axes of the three bipolar limb leads, I, II, and III. **B,** The Y shape is formed by the axes of the three unipolar limb leads, aV$_R$, aV$_L$, and aV$_F$. The center of the triangle is the zero reference point and the assigned negative for the unipolar leads.

2. Now that the plane of current flow is known, look at the lead whose axis is parallel with the current flow to see whether current is flowing toward or away from its positive electrode.

EXERCISES FOR AXIS DETERMINATION

1. Place a piece of paper over all of the triangles on the right of the following exercises.
2. Draw your own triangle; then look for the equiphasic deflection. If it is in a unipolar lead, draw that lead axis too.
3. Draw a line indicating current flow, making the current flow line perpendicular to the axis of the lead where you found the equiphasic deflection.
4. Now evaluate the second lead of the easy two-step method. This will be the lead whose axis is parallel with the current flow. For example, if current flow is perpendicular to lead I, it will be parallel with lead aV_F.

Exercise 1: normal axis

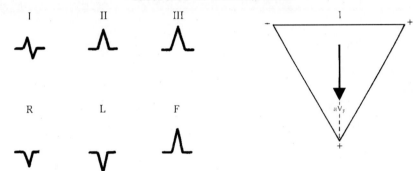

Step 1: Look for the equiphasic deflection. It is in lead I; therefore current flow is perpendicular to that lead axis.
Step 2: Note that the lead axis of aV_F is also perpendicular to the lead axis of I.
Conclusion: Since the ECG complex in lead III is positive, the mean current is flowing inferiorly toward the positive electrode of that lead. This is a normal axis.

Exercise 2: normal axis

Step 1: Look for the equiphasic deflection. It is in lead aV_L, therefore current flow

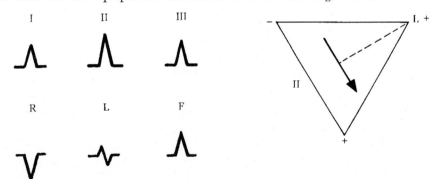

is perpendicular to that lead axis.
Step 2: Note that the lead axis of aV_L is also perpendicular to the lead axis of II.
Conclusion: Since the ECG complex in lead II is positive, the mean current is flowing inferiorly toward the positive electrode of that lead. This is a normal axis.

Exercise 3: no man's land axis

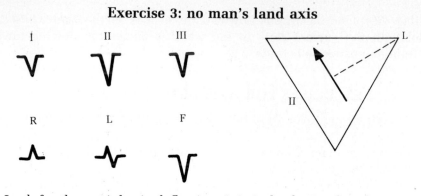

Step 1: Look for the equiphasic deflection. It is in lead aV_L; therefore current flow is perpendicular to that lead axis.

Step 2: Note that the lead axis of aV_L is also perpendicular to the lead axis of II.

Conclusion: Since the complex in lead II is negative, the mean current is flowing superiorly to the right and toward the negative electrode of lead II. This is commonly referred to as "no man's land," the northwest quadrant, or an indeterminate axis.

Exercise 4: borderline axis of −30 degrees

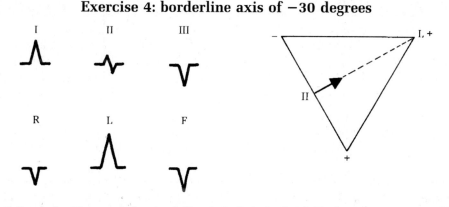

Step 1: Look for the equiphasic deflection. It is in lead II; therefore current flow is perpendicular to that lead axis.

Step 2: Note that the lead axis of II is also perpendicular to the lead axis of aV_L.

Conclusion: Since the ECG complex in lead aV_L is positive, the mean current is flowing horizontally toward the positive electrode of that lead. This is a borderline axis (−30 degrees). If lead II were any more negative, the axis would be beyond −30 degrees, an abnormal left axis.

Exercise 5: left axis deviation

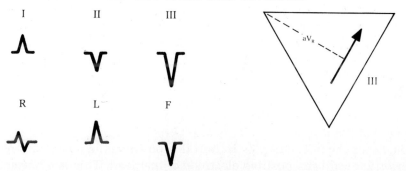

Step 1: Look for the equiphasic deflection. It is in lead aV$_R$; therefore current flow is perpendicular to that lead axis.

Step 2: Note that the lead axis of aV$_R$ is also perpendicular to the lead axis of III.

Conclusion: Since the ECG complex in lead III is negative, the mean current is flowing superiorly to the left and toward the negative electrode of lead III. This is an abnormal left axis (greater than −30 degrees).

Exercise 6: right axis deviation

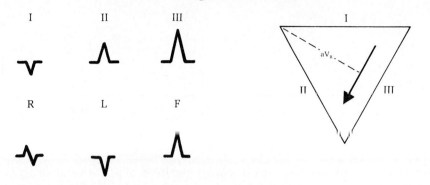

Step 1: Look for the equiphasic deflection. It is in lead aV$_R$; therefore current flow is perpendicular to that lead axis.

Step 2: Note that the lead axis of aV$_R$ is also perpendicular to the lead axis of III.

Conclusion: Since the complex in lead III is positive, the mean current is flowing inferiorly to the right and toward the positive electrode of lead III. This is an abnormal right axis deviation (greater than +120 degrees).

USE OF LEADS I AND aV$_F$ IN AXIS DETERMINATION: THE QUADRANT METHOD

Note that in Fig. 4-7 the axes of leads I and aV$_F$ divide the thorax into quadrants—normal, left, right, and northwest. The four examples that follow are meant

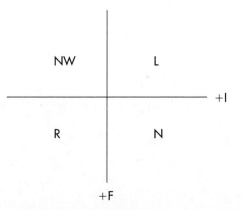

Fig. 4-7. The four quadrants defined by leads I and aV$_F$. *N*, Normal; *L*, left; *R*, right; *F*, aV$_F$; *NW*, northwest.

to point out the advantages of this method and its single disadvantage, that is, the inability to determine whether a left axis is normal (less than −30 degrees) or abnormal (at or greater than −30 degrees).

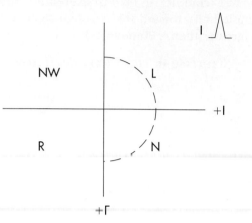

Note that the complex in lead I is mainly positive. Thus the axis must be to the left between +90 degrees and −90 degrees.

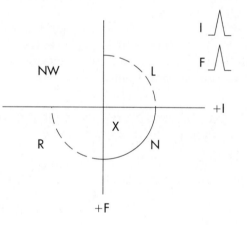

If the complex in lead aV$_F$ is also positive, the axis is inferior and located in the normal quadrant (between 0 degrees and +90 degrees), since this is the quadrant that I and aV$_F$ share when both are positive).

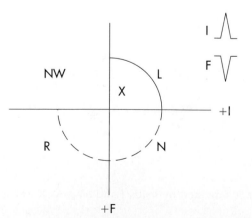

However, in the event of lead aV$_F$ being negative (and lead I positive), the axis would be superior and somewhere in the left quadrant (between 0 degrees and −90 degrees). From this information alone it is not known whether the axis is left but normal (0 degrees to −30 degrees) or abnormal (−30 degrees to −90 degrees). To obtain this information, lead II is needed (axis at a glance method). If the complex in II is mostly positive, the axis is normal; if equiphasic, the axis is −30 degrees; if negative, the axis is abnormal.

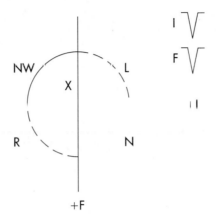

When the complex is negative in leads I and aV$_F$, the axis is in no man's land (northwest quadrant). In the setting of broad QRS tachycardia, such an axis is diagnostic of ventricular tachycardia.

HEXAXIAL FIGURE: A MORE PRECISE METHOD OF AXIS DETERMINATION

Once you have become comfortable and adept at determining the electrical axis using axis at a glance, the easy two-step method, and the quadrant method, you may wish to refine your skill by learning to work with the hexaxial figure, which provides an excellent reference system for estimating the axis in degrees.

The hexaxial figure is drawn by shifting the axes of the six limb leads so that they all pass through the zero potential of the heart's electrical field (Fig. 4-8). There are 30-degree increments between lead axes. Figs. 4-9 and 4-10 describe the use of the hexaxial figure.

SUMMARY

The normal electrical axis of the heart is between −30 degrees and +120 degrees. This axis may be quickly estimated by the polarity of the complexes in leads I and II; especially useful is the knowledge that the axis is normal if the complexes in leads I and II are upright. Leads I and aV$_F$ may also be used to determine which quadrant (normal, left, right, or northwest) the axis is in. Other methods requiring more figuring are the easy two-step method and plotting current flow on the hexaxial figure.

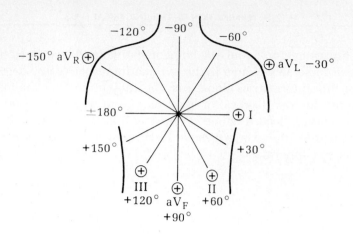

Fig. 4-8. Hexaxial figure. All of the limb lead axes are drawn through a central point. They are 30 degrees apart.

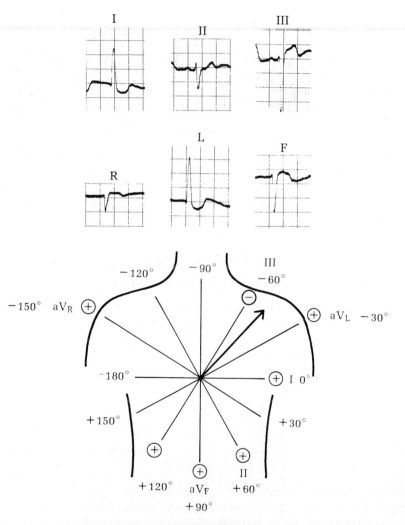

Fig. 4-9. The use of the hexaxial figure in determining electrical axis. Leads I and aV$_F$ reveal that the axis is in the left quadrant. Now look at the other two leads in this quadrant, III and aV$_L$. Lead III is more negative than lead aV$_L$ is positive; therefore the main current flow is closer to the axis of III than to that of aV$_L$, or at about -50 degrees, an abnormal left axis deviation.

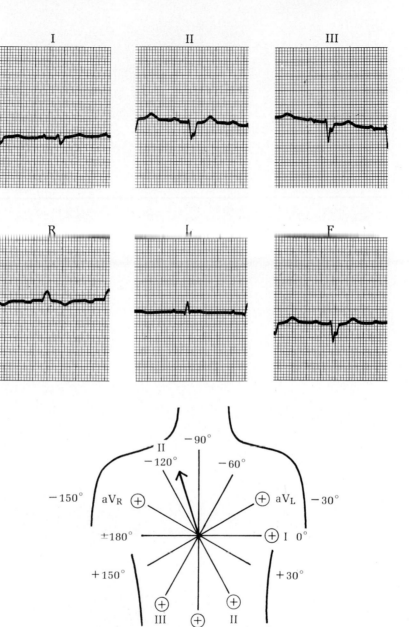

Fig. 4-10. Use of the hexaxial figure. In this illustration the axis is placed in "no man's land" (−90 degrees to ±180 degrees) because both I and aV_F are negative. When the axis is in this quadrant, it is either extreme right or extreme left axis deviation. Now look at the other two leads within this quadrant (II and aV_R). The complex in lead II is clearly more negative than aV_R is positive, placing the axis closer to II. However, if the main current were parallel to the axis of II, aV_L would be equiphasic. Because this is not the case, aV_L being positive, the axis is slightly to the right of −120 degrees, or −115 degrees.

ARRHYTHMIA RECOGNITION

C H A P T E R
5
Mechanisms of Arrhythmias

Arrhythmia or Disrhythmia?   *53*

Reentry   *54*

Reflection   *56*

Altered Automaticity   *57*

Triggered Activity   *58*

Clinical Application   *59*

Summary   *60*

An *arrhythmia* or *dysrhythmia* is an abnormal cardiac rhythm. It usually occurs when the sinus rhythm is interfered with by ectopic beats or rhythms or when atrioventricular (AV) conduction is compromised. Sinus rhythms that are too fast or too slow or that fail also qualify as arrhythmias. Two categories of arrhythmias have been described[1]: abnormalities of conduction (block; reentry; or reflection, a type of reentry) and abnormalities of impulse initiation (abnormal automaticity, enhanced normal automaticity, or triggered activity).

ARRHYTHMIA OR DYSRHYTHMIA?

Both terms are acceptable, despite the militant declaration that the traditional term "arrhythmia" be abandoned for the new "dysrhythmia",[2] insisting that the *a* prefix (alpha privative) means an "absence of." Marriott[21] has eloquently pointed out that the original meaning of the alpha privative often implied an "imperfection in" or "lack of" rather than the flat, negative absence of. In addition, the original *rhythmos* had much broader application than our anglicized word *rhythm*. Apart from original meanings, Marriott points out that the most important factor for retaining the term arrhythmia is "the sovereign role of usage," suggesting that both terms be accepted, "arrhythmia because it has tradition and no perceptible flaws, and dysrhythmia because it offers variety and satisfies spurious scholarship."

The determining factor may be Marriott's[21] usage theory. The term dysrhythmia has not "caught on" or even been considered as an option in the writings,[3-12] lectures, and scientific conversations of internationally known experts and world leaders in the field of cardiovascular medicine.

REENTRY

Reentry is the reactivation of fibers for a second time or repeatedly by the same wave front. Normally the cardiac impulse moves rapidly through the heart and is extinguished in its first pass because the entire heart becomes refractory and the impulse expires, having "no place to go."[13] The terms used to describe arrhythmias supported by reentry are circus movement, reciprocal or echo beats, reciprocating tachycardia, and, of course, reentry or reentrant tachycardia.

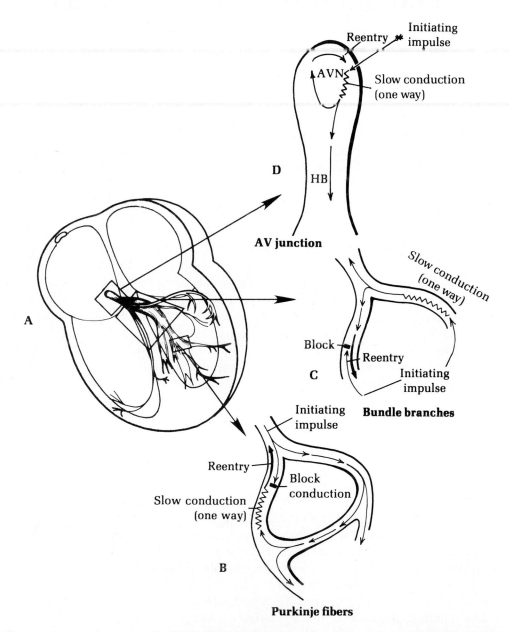

Fig. 5-1. Anatomic reentry, Purkinje fibers, atrioventricular (AV) node, and bundle branches. AV reentry with anterograde use of the AV node and retrograde use of an accessory pathway is not shown.

Given the right conditions, it is possible for any part of the myocardium or conductive network to support reentry circuits. Typically, reentry tachyardias are paroxysmal and may be terminated with a critically timed, paced beat or, in the case of paroxysmal supraventricular tachycardia (PSVT), with a vagal maneuver, adenosine, calcium channel blockers, or procainamide. In the following chapters you will become acquainted with reentry as a cause of atrial flutter and with PSVT because of sinoatrial (SA) nodal reentry, AV nodal reentry, and AV reentry using the AV node and an accessory pathway.

Three types of reentry have been described: anatomic, functional, and anisotropic.

Anatomic reentry

Anatomic reentry consists of an excitation wave that passes around an anatomic obstacle or obstacles; such reentry circuits are shown in Fig. 5-1, (AV nodal reentry, reentry using Purkinje fibers, bundle branches, the tricuspid annulus, and the AV node and an accessory pathway [not shown]) and in Fig. 5-2 (models of Mines and Lewis).

The Mines model. The earliest and simplest model of reentry, introduced by Mines[14] in 1913, shows an impulse that circles a large anatomic obstacle. The white part within the circle represents fibers that are nonrefractory. This "excitable gap" continues to move around the circle behind the refractory tissue (stippled area). The wave of excitation is thus propagated to produce a regular tachycardia.

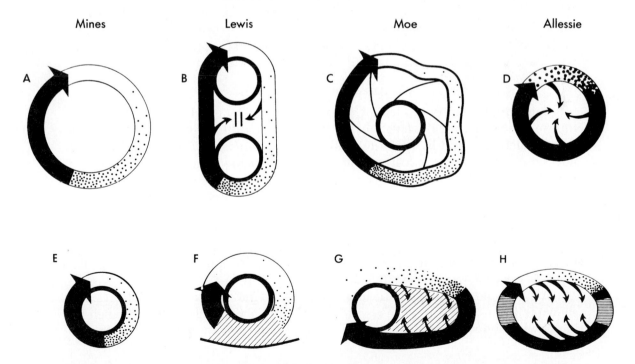

Fig. 5-2. Schematic representation of various types of reentry. The black arrows represent the crest of a circulating depolarization wave and the absolute refractory phase. The stippled areas indicate the refractory tail of the circuit. See text for description of **A** to **H**. *(From Allessie MA, Rensma W, Brugada J et al: In Touboul P, Waldo AL, eds: Atrial arrhythmias: current concepts and management, St Louis, 1990, Mosby.)*

The Lewis model. In 1920 Lewis[15] introduced a reentry loop whose pathway took in two anatomic obstacles (for example, venae cavae). Such a large circuit could result in the impulse crossing at the isthmus to establish a smaller circuit and a faster tachycardia.[16]

In the lower row of Fig. 5-2, *E, F,* and *G* are also models of anatomic reentry. In Fig. 5-2, *E,* the impulse wave length is shortened. Such an impulse may circle an anatomic obstacle and produce a stable reentry circuit. In Fig. 5-2, *F,* there is an area of depressed conduction between the two anatomic boundaries, which allows for an excitable gap in the normal myocardium. In Fig. 5-2, *G,* note an area of prolonged refractoriness next to an anatomic obstacle; the depolarization wave encircles both in a pathway that may be long enough to create an excitable gap in the normal myocardium. Such a circuit may pivot at slightly different points, allowing for different cycle lengths; such a reentrant tachycardia could last for an extended time.[17]

Functional reentry

Functional reentry does not require an anatomic structure to circle around; it depends on the local differences in conduction velocity and is characterized by the "leading circle" (Moe and Allessie models in Fig. 5-2).

Model of Moe et al. In 1980 Moe et al.[18] described a reentry circuit that was conducted at different velocities through the atria (for example, on Bachmann's bundle and the internodal muscle bands).

Model of Allessie et al. In 1977 Allessie et al.[19] described the "leading circle" type of reentry, in which the length of the pathway was not defined by an anatomic obstacle, but rather by the functional electrophysiologic properties of the myocardium. In this model the reentrant impulse conducts in partially refractory myocardium with the crest of activation constantly on the refractory tail of the circuit.

Anisotropic reentry

Anisotropic reentry is a circuit that is determined by the difference in conduction velocities through the length of the fiber as opposed to across its width. *Isotropic* conduction would be uniform in all directions; *anisotropic* conduction would not. Slow conduction in at least part of the reentrant pathway, although not required for reentry to occur, facilitates the mechanism, allowing time for recovery of tissue in the path of the circulating wave front. One-way conduction (unidirectional block) is an essential component of the reentry circuit; otherwise, the impulse would be canceled out by opposing traffic. The anisotropic properties of cardiac muscle, that is, that conduction is faster lengthwise in the fiber than it is crossways, contribute to slow conduction and unidirectional block. An anisotropic reentry circuit is diagramatically illustrated in Fig. 5-2, *H.*

A figure-of-8 reentry circuit in a patient late after a myocardial infarction is shown in Fig. 5-3.[4] Reentry can also occur with use of a damaged bundle branch for the slowly conducting arm and the undamaged bundle branch for the return circuit.[5]

REFLECTION

Reflection is another form of reentry that occurs in parallel pathways of Purkinje fibers or myocardial tissue that have depressed segments. Fig. 5-4 illustrates a reflected impulse. When the cardiac impulse reaches the severely depressed segment, it is blocked there but transmitted slowly in a less severely depressed neighboring fiber.

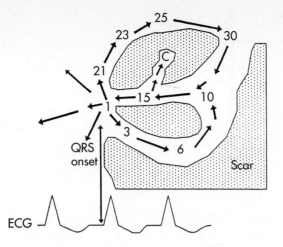

Fig. 5-3. Schematics of a figure-of-8 circuit through myocardial scar tissue late after a myocardial infarction. Sites 1 to 10 are the inner loop, sites 21 to 30 are the outer loop, and sites 10 to 20 are the common pathway. *(From Stevenson WG, Khan H, Sager P et al: Circulation 88:1647, 1993.)*

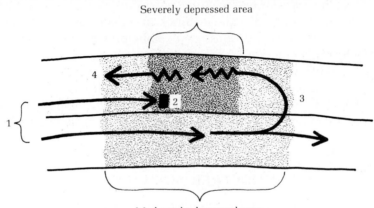

Fig. 5-4. Reflection, a type of reentry that occurs in depressed nonbranching Purkinje fibers. Impulse conduction *(1)* is blocked in a severely depressed segment *(2)* and is conducted slowly in a less severely depressed segment. It then returns to its origin *(3 and 4)* by traveling in a retrograde direction in the previously blocked segment.

Upon reaching the end of the segment, the impulse activates the surrounding tissue and returns in the retrograde direction through the severely depressed segment.[6,7]

ALTERED AUTOMATICITY

Altered automaticity is divided into two types (Fig. 5-5): enhanced normal automaticity and abnormal automaticity.

Enhanced normal automaticity may occur in His-Purkinje fibers that are functioning normally. However, catecholamines can cause a steepening of phase 4 in His-Purkinje fibers, resulting in an increase of firing rate to about 100 beats/min (rarely more rapid). Such fibers are readily suppressed by overdrive pacing.[8]

Abnormal automaticity is the spontaneous firing of cardiac cells because of such things as ischemia or electrolyte imbalance; both cause a reduction in membrane potential. When the membrane potential is sharply reduced to a critical level (−60 mV), spontaneous depolarization may occur. Abnormal automaticity can oc-

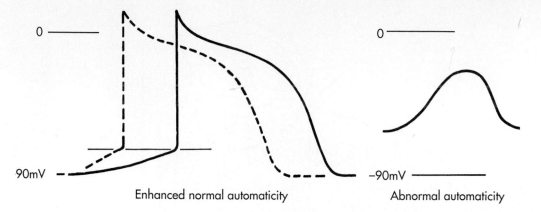

Fig. 5-5. The two types of altered automaticity. Enhanced normal automaticity is caused by catecholamines and occurs in pacemaker cells such as His-Purkinje cells. Abnormal automaticity is due to ischemia or injury and may occur anywhere in the heart.

cur anywhere in the myocardium or His-Purkinje system, even in fibers that did not have the capability of automaticity in health. The tachycardia that results is not readily suppressed by overdrive pacing.[9,10] A reduction in membrane potential may be the result of an increase in extracellular potassium, a decrease in intracellular potassium, an increase in sodium permeability, or a decrease in potassium permeability. Some of the clinical conditions responsible are ischemia, infarction, hypokalemia, hypocalcemia, and cardiomyopathy.

Although the sinus node normally suppresses latent pacemaker activity, it may not have that power over fibers with abnormal automaticity. As a result, although a long sinus cycle may not elicit normal escape beats, areas of abnormal automaticity may easily surface when the rate of the sinus node drops below that of the ectopic focus.[8]

TRIGGERED ACTIVITY

Triggered activity is the activity that arises as a result of afterdepolarizations.

Afterdepolarizations are oscillations of membrane potential that attend or follow the action potential and depend on preceding transmembrane activity for their manifestation.[9] When these oscillations depolarize the cell to threshold potential, they induce spontaneous action potentials (triggered activity) that are responsible for extrasystoles and tachycardias.[10-12] Afterdepolarizations are divided into two subclasses: early and delayed.

Early afterdepolarizations are oscillations of the membrane potential that interrupt or retard repolarization. This type of oscillation may occur during phase 2 or phase 3, or both, of the cardiac action potential. Triggered activity (tachycardia) induced by early afterdepolarizations is associated with the class IA drugs (quinidine, procainamide, and disopyramide) and with slow heart rates and hypokalemia. Other conditions that may cause early afterdepolarizations include myocardial stretch, hypothermia, hypoxia, acidosis, low blood calcium levels, catecholamines, sotalol, certain antihistamines, erythromycin, and bretylium tosylate.[13] Fig. 5-6 illustrates an early afterdepolarization that occurs during phase 3; upon reaching threshold potential, it produces a propagated action potential (dotted line), that is, a triggered beat. Pauses in the cardiac cycle can exacerbate this type of triggered activity. Conditions that predispose to early afterdepolarizations also predispose to reentry. Because of this, establishment of the mechanism of tachycardias is often difficult.[14] Further discussion of triggered activity that is a result of early afterdepolarizations can be found in Chapter 14.

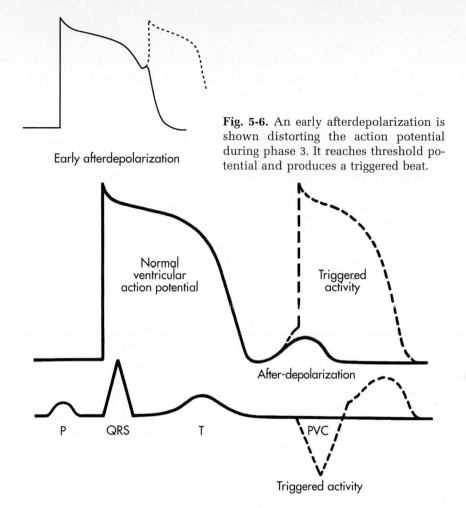

Fig. 5-6. An early afterdepolarization is shown distorting the action potential during phase 3. It reaches threshold potential and produces a triggered beat.

Fig. 5-7. A delayed afterdepolarization is shown following the action potential. It reaches threshold potential *(dotted line)* and produces a triggered beat. *PVC,* Premature ventricular complex.

Delayed afterdepolarizations are oscillations of the membrane potential that occur after completion of the action potential (i.e., following full repolarization). If the oscillation reaches threshold potential (dotted line in Fig. 5-7), it produces a propagated action potential (a triggered beat). Triggered activity induced by delayed afterdepolarizations is associated with drugs that cause increased intracellular levels of calcium.[15] This mechanism is discussed more completely in Chapter 17.

CLINICAL APPLICATION

ECG differentiation among the mechanisms of reentry, altered automaticity, and triggered activity is at best difficult and often impossible. Occasionally, however, ECG clues point to a particular mechanism, such as one of the following.

Automaticity is suspected when the following occur: gradual acceleration or gradual emergence of an arrhythmia, long coupling or variable coupling intervals, and an arrhythmia that is introduced by a fusion beat. Automatic rhythms include parasystole, escape rhythms, nonparoxysmal junctional tachycardia, and accelerated idioventricular rhythms.[20]

Reentry is suspected when the following occur: fixed coupling, abrupt termination of an arrhythmia by an extra beat, and, in the setting of prolonged conduction, the appearance of an ectopic rhythm.

Triggered activity is more difficult to recognize but is suspected to be the mechanism of long-QT ventricular tachycardia (torsades de pointes) and the tachycardias of digitalis toxicity.

SUMMARY

Two categories of arrhythmias have been described: abnormalities of conduction caused by conduction block, reentry, or reflection and abnormalities of impulse initiation caused by altered automaticity (enhanced "normal" automaticity or "abnormal" automaticity) or triggered activity (caused by early or delayed afterdepolarizations). Enhanced normal automaticity is caused by a steepening of phase 4 in His-Purkinje fibers, and abnormal automaticity occurs in myocardial fibers with abnormally reduced membrane potentials. Triggered activity is the result of afterdepolarizations; there are two types, early and delayed. Early afterdepolarizations are the result of prolonged QT intervals; delayed afterdepolarizations are the result of excess intracellular calcium.

REFERENCES

1. Hoffman BF, Cranefield PF: The physiological basis of cardiac arrhythmias, *Am J Med* 37:670, 1964.
2. Trommer PR: Cardiolocution and dysrhythmia *Am J Cardiol* 50:1198, 1982 (letter).
3. Zipes DP: Management of cardiac arrhythmias: pharmacological, electrical, and surgical techniques. In Braunwald E, ed: *Heart disease,* ed 4, Philadelphia, 1992, WB Saunders.
4. Zipes DP: Specific arrhythmias: diagnosis and treatment. In Braunwald E, ed: *Heart disease,* ed 4, Philadelphia, 1992, WB Saunders.
5. El-Sherif N: Reentrant mechanisms in ventricular arrhythmias. In Zipes DP, Jalife J, eds: *Cardiac electrophysiology from cell to bedside,* ed 2, Philadelphia, 1995, WB Saunders.
6. Franz MR: Stretch-activated arrhythmias. In Zipes DP, Jalife J, eds: *Cardiac electrophysiology from cell to bedside,* ed 2, Philadelphia, 1995, WB Saunders.
7. Zipes DP, Jalife J, eds: *Cardiac electrophysiology from cell to bedside,* ed 2, Philadelphia, 1995, WB Saunders.
8. Roelke M, Ruskin JN: Dilated cardiomyopathy: ventricular arrhythmias and sudden death. In Zipes DP, Jalife J, eds: *Cardiac electrophysiology from cell to bedside,* ed 2, Philadelphia, 1995, WB Saunders.
9. Perry JC, Garson A Jr: Arrhythmias following surgery for congenital heart disease. In Zipes DP, Jalife J, eds: *Cardiac electrophysiology from cell to bedside,* ed 2, Philadelphia, 1995, WB Saunders.
10. Stevenson WG, Middlekauff HR, Saxon LA: Ventricular arrhythmias in heart failure. In Zipes DP, Jalife J, eds: *Cardiac electrophysiology from cell to bedside,* ed 2, Philadelphia, 1995, WB Saunders.
11. Gillette PC, Zeigler VL, Case CL: Pediatric arrhythmias: are they different? In Zipes DP, Jalife J, eds: *Cardiac electrophysiology from cell to bedside,* ed 2, Philadelphia, 1995, WB Saunders.
12. Naccarelli GV, Willerson JT, Blomquist CG: Recognition and physiologic treatment of cardiac arrhythmias and conduction disturbances. In Willerson JT, Cohn JN, eds: *Cardiovascular medicine,* New York, 1995, Churchill Livingstone.
13. Zipes DP: Genesis of cardiac arrhythmias: electrophysiological considerations. In Braunwald E, ed: *Heart disease,* ed 4, Philadelphia, 1992, WB Saunders.
14. Mines GR: On dynamic equilibrium in the heart, *J Physiol (Lond)* 46:349, 1913.
15. Lewis T: Observations upon flutter and fibrillation. IV. Impure flutter: theory of circus movement, *Heart* 7:293, 1920.
16. Allessie MA, Rensma W, Brugada J et al: Modes of atrial reentry. In Touboul P, Waldo AL, eds: *Atrial arrhythmias: current concepts and management,* St Louis, 1990, Mosby.
17. Allessie MA, Rensma W, Brugada J et al: Modes of atrial reentry. In Touboul P, Waldo AL, eds: *Atrial arrhythmias: current concepts and management,* St Louis, 1990, Mosby.
18. Moe GK, Pastelin G, Mendez R: Circus movement excitation of the atria. In Little RC, ed: *Physiology of atrial pacemakers and conductive tissue,* New York, 1980, Futura.
19. Allessie MA, Bonke FIM, Schopman FJG: Circus movement in rabbit atrial muscle as a mechanism of tachycardia. III. The "leading circle" concept: a new model of circus movement in cardiac tissue without the involvement of an anatomic obstacle, *Circ Res* 41:9, 1977.
20. Fisch C: Evolution of the clinical electrocardiogram, *J Am Coll Cardiol* 14:1127, 1989.
21. Marriott HJL: Arrhythmia versus dysrhythmia, *Am J Cardiol* 53:628, 1984.

6

Arrhythmias Originating in the Sinus Node

Normal Sinus Rhythm   *61*

Sinus Tachycardia   *63*

Sinus Bradycardia   *65*

Sinus Arrhythmia and Heart Rate
   Variability   *67*

Two Types of Sinoatrial Block   *68*

Sinoatrial Wenckebach (Type I Sinoatrial
   Block)   *68*

Type II Sinoatrial Block   *71*

Sinus Arrest or Sinus Pause   *71*

Permanent Atrial Standstill   *73*

Sinus Nodal Dysfunction (Sick Sinus
   Syndrome)   *73*

Sinus Nodal Reentry Tachycardia   *76*

Wandering Pacemaker   *78*

Summary   *79*

Arrhythmias (or dysrhythmias) that originate in the sinus node are designated as such because the rate is too fast (sinus tachycardia) or too slow (sinus bradycardia), the sinus rhythm is irregular (sinus arrhythmia), or a sinus node impulse either does not form within the sinus node (sinus arrest) or fails to exit from the sinus node (sinoatrial [SA] block). Such arrhythmias are not necessarily abnormal. For example, sinus tachycardia is a physiologic response to the needs of the body (e.g., prompted by exercise, emotions, or fever), sinus bradycardia is common in athletes and during sleep, and sinus arrhythmia is associated with the vagal effect of respirations. When these arrhythmias are symptomatic or inappropriate, they are abnormal. Sinus nodal disease may manifest itself as SA block, sinus arrest, or sick sinus syndrome.

NORMAL SINUS RHYTHM

A normal sinus rhythm is recognized as a heart rate of 60 to 100 beats/min, a rate that has been generally agreed on for many years. However, in clinical practice most clinicians are alert to possible problems when the heart rate is faster than 90 beats/min and are not concerned unless the heart rate drops to less than 50 beats/min. In 500 consecutive normal adults the mean resting afternoon heart rates for

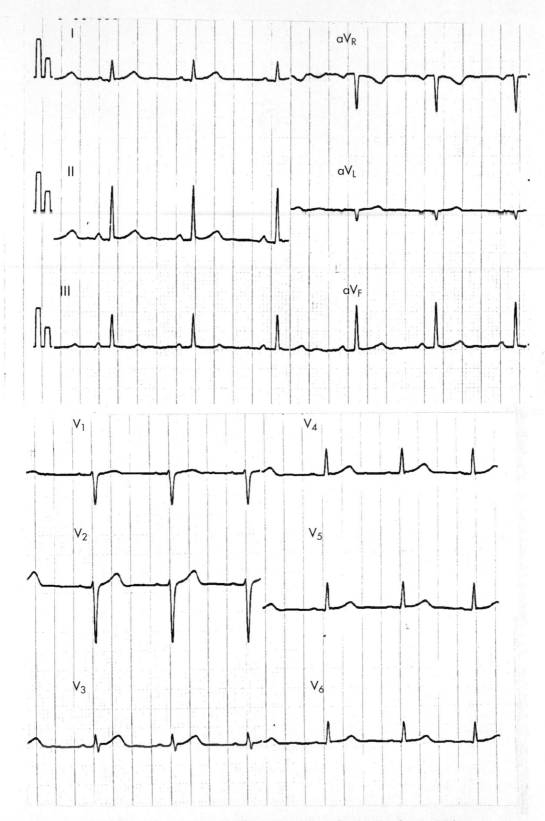

Fig. 6-1. Normal sinus rhythm. *(Courtesy Julie M. Boudreau, BS.)*

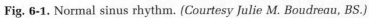

men and women were approximately 70 beats/min, with no significant difference because of age.[1] One group from the Cleveland Clinic[31] studied 536 consecutive healthy subjects and recommended that the normal sinus rate should be defined at 44 to 84 beats/min for males and 50 to 90 beats/min for females.

The autonomic nervous system controls the discharge rate of the sinus node; vagal stimulation decreases the rate and sympathetic stimulation increases the rate. Steady vagal stimulation dominates steady sympathetic stimulation.

Pediatrics: The younger the age, the faster the rate of the normal sinus rhythm. A rate of 200 beats/min may be the upper limit of normal for a 1-month-old infant but would be abnormal in an older child. Normal heart rate in the newborn varies from 110 to 200 beats/min; the variability decreases with age. In the first week of life the average rate is less than 140 beats/min; in the first year it is less than 120 beats/min.

Other features of a normal sinus rhythm include the appropriate polarity of the P waves for each recording lead. Mandatory shapes are upright in leads I, II, aV_F and V_4 to V_6, negative in lead aV_R. In leads III, aV_L, and V_1 to V_3 the P wave can be positive, negative, or biphasic. Fig. 6-1 is a normal sinus rhythm (rate 62 beats/min) from a 28-year-old woman. Note the normal frontal plane QRS axis (+80 degrees), normal PR interval (0.15 sec); normal QRS duration (0.09 sec), and normal QT and corrected QT (QTc) intervals (0.40 and 0.41 sec, respectively). In the precordial leads one looks for R-wave progression (reflecting normal anterior forces), septal activation (tiny q in leads I, V_5, and V_6), and a transitional zone somewhere between V_3 and V_4.

SINUS TACHYCARDIA

Sinus tachycardia is the rapid beating of the sinus node at rates of more than 100 beats/min, as seen in Fig. 6-2.

Pediatrics: Sinus tachycardia is a rate greater than 200 beats/min in an infant and between 140 and 200 beats/min in a child.

ECG recognition

Heart rate: Ranges from 100 to 180 beats/min; higher with exertion. Sinus tachycardia is generally described as more than 100 beats/min in the adult, although most clinicians would be suspicious of a resting heart rate of 90 beats/min. The rate of the sinus node rarely exceeds 180 beats/min, although rates of more than 200 are seen in healthy adults and children. During strenu-

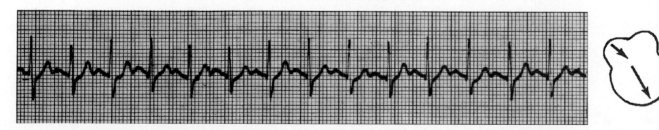

Fig. 6-2. Sinus tachycardia of 140 beats/min. The pacemaker is the sinus node, and conduction is normal. The undulating heights of the QRS complexes are caused by respirations.

ous physical exercise the maximal heart rate achieved decreases with age from nearly 200 beats/min to less than 140 beats/min.[2]

Rhythm: May be slightly irregular; gradually accelerates to a rapid, regular rhythm and then gradually decelerates when the physiologic needs no longer exist.

P waves: P waves are usually identical in shape to the P waves of slower, normal sinus rhythm. However, with the tachycardia it is possible for the pacing site within the sinus node itself to shift, causing the shape of the P wave to differ from that of a slower sinus rhythm.[3,4] Fig. 6-3 illustrates how the shape of the P wave can change with the heart rate during sinus rhythm.

PR interval: As the sinus rate accelerates, the PR interval shortens slightly. This is because the atrioventricular (AV) node is under the same control as the sinus node, and acceleration of the rate of sinus firing is accompanied by shortening of AV conduction.

QRS complex: The QRS complex during sinus tachycardia is identical in shape to the QRS at normal rates. Aberrant ventricular conduction (Chapter 14) does not usually occur during sinus tachycardia in the normal heart.

QT interval: The QT interval shortens with tachycardia and lengthens with bradycardia.

Response to carotid sinus massage: The sinus rate gradually and temporarily slows in response to vagal maneuvers. Sinus slowing is accompanied by a slowing or block of AV conduction (PR lengthens, or a P wave is not conducted). This inhibitory effect on heart rate of a given level of vagal activity is more pronounced the greater the prevailing level of sympathetic activity, a mechanism termed *accentuated antagonism.*[5]

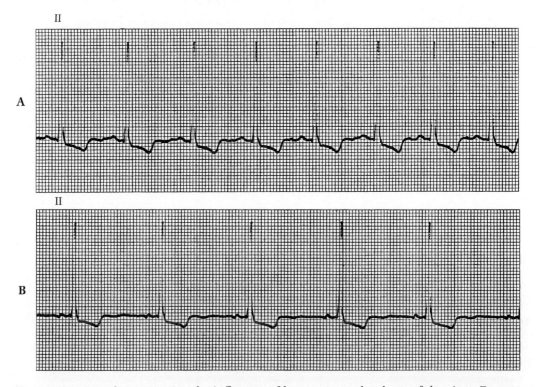

Fig. 6-3. Tracings demonstrating the influence of heart rate on the shape of the sinus P wave. The **A** and **B** are from the same patient.

Mechanism

The mechanism of sinus tachycardia is physiologically enhanced automaticity (steepening of phase 4 of the action potential) that is due to sympathetic stimulation or vagal block.[6] Instantaneous sinus tachycardia can be induced by an event such as the unexpected sound of gunfire at close range. This dramatic response is mediated by the sudden cessation of parasympathetic restraint on the sinus node, with sympathetic stimulation developing slightly later.[5]

Clinical implications

Sinus tachycardia is the body's normal response to exertion and to congestive heart failure, cardiogenic shock, acute pulmonary embolism, acute myocardial infarction, or infarct extension. In the setting of mitral stenosis or severe ischemia, sinus tachycardia may precipitate other arrhythmias. Inappropriate sinus tachycardia may be related to a primary sinus node abnormality.[7]

Sinus tachycardia occurs with exercise, emotion, pain, fever, inflammation, or any condition that increases sympathetic stimulation. Some of the drugs causing sinus tachycardia are atropine, catecholamines, thyroid, alcohol, nicotine, and caffeine.

Treatment

Sinus tachycardia itself is not treated. If the tachycardia is inappropriate or if the patient is symptomatic, the cause is identified and treated (e.g., hypovolemia or fever). In certain cases relief may be found in eliminating obvious causes such as tobacco, alcohol, or caffeine. An unsuspected cause may be the sympathomimetic agents in nose drops.

SINUS BRADYCARDIA

Sinus bradycardia is the slow beating of the sinus node at rates of less than 60 beats/min. Most clinicians would not be alarmed at a heart rate of 59 beats/min as long as the patient has hemodynamic stability. The sinus rate in Fig. 6-4 is about 38 beats/min. Sinus bradycardia is often associated with sinus arrhythmia.

Pediatrics: Sinus bradycardia is rare in normal, healthy children. It may be seen in hypothyroidism, hypothermia, hypopituitarism, obstructive jaundice, and typhoid fever. Transient sinus bradycardia may be seen in normal premature infants. Reflex sinus bradycardia occurs because of increased intracranial pressure or increased systemic blood pressure and, occasionally, during cardiac catheterization.

II

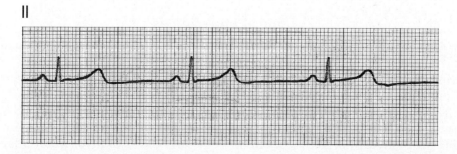

Fig. 6-4. Sinus bradycardia of 39 beats/min. The pacemaker is the sinus node, and conduction is normal.

Neonates can tolerate ventricular rates of 55 beats/min or greater if the heart is normal and 65 beats/min when associated with congenital heart disease. In addition, in the neonatal period there is little heart rate variability. (Sleeping and awake rates are similar.)[8]

ECG recognition

Heart rate: The heart rate is less than 60 beats/min in the adult, although a resting heart rate in the range of 50 beats/min in an athletic person is not abnormal.

Rhythm: Regular unless associated with sinus arrhythmia.

P waves: P waves are usually identical in shape to the P waves of normal sinus rhythm, or there may be a slight change in morphologic features because of a shift in pacing site within the sinus node.[3]

PR interval: Greater than 0.12 sec.

QRS complex: The QRS complex during sinus bradycardia is identical in shape to the QRS at normal rates.

QT interval: The QT interval lengthens with bradycardia.

Response to carotid sinus massage: The sinus rate gradually and temporarily slows.

Response to vagal block: Vagal block, such as with atropine, causes the normal sinus node to increase its rate, usually by more than 50% above baseline but not in excess of 120 beats/min. In fact, one of the signs of intrinsic sinus nodal dysfunction is that the heart rate does not exceed 90 beats/min following vagal block with 2 to 4 mg/kg of intravenous (IV) atropine.[9]

Mechanism

Sinus bradycardia may be caused by excessive vagal tone, decreased sympathetic tone, or anatomic changes. In most people vagal activity exerts a strong influence on the circadian variation in sinus rate that occurs during the normal sleep-wake cycle. Vagal activity also establishes a set point for mean sinus rate during inactivity. During sleep, enhanced vagal activity can result in sinus rates of less than 40 beats/min, and this is normal.[10] In fact, one of the ways sinus nodal disease is recognized is by the reduction of such circadian variation.[11]

Syncope is commonly considered an indication of severity in sinus bradycardia. Recent data suggest that in the majority of cases a patient with sinus bradycardia is symptomatic for syncope only if affected with an anomalous neural reflex in addition to the sinus node dysfunction, suggesting pharmacologic treatment of neurally mediated syncope over pacemaker implantation. Syncope is defined as a transient loss of consciousness with inability to maintain postural tone.[12]

Clinical implications

Sinus bradycardia is a relatively benign condition and occurs normally in trained athletes and during sleep. In acute myocardial infarction, especially of the inferior wall, sinus bradycardia is common (25% to 40%)[13] and may be beneficial by producing a longer diastole and increased ventricular filling time. Sinus bradycardia without hypotension is associated with an equal or lower mortality rate than if the heart rate had been faster,[14] although ventricular ectopy may be more frequent during the bradycardia that occurs in the very early phase of myocardial infarction. When the sinus bradycardia is profound and associated with hypotension in the setting of acute myocardial infarction, the prognosis is poor, especially if the deteriorating hemodynamic situation is not corrected rapidly.[15] Sinus bradycardia may occur during reperfusion with thrombolytic agents. If it occurs after resuscitation from cardiac arrest, it is associated with a poor prognosis.[16]

Treatment

Sinus bradycardia is not treated unless the patient is symptomatic; then atropine 0.04 mg/kg body weight is given. A temporary pacemaker may be indicated if the heart rate does not accelerate. A permanent pacemaker may be needed for patients with congestive heart failure or patients in whom the arrhythmia is chronic and associated with low cardiac output. This is because heart rate cannot be reliably and safely increased with drugs on a long-term basis.[16]

SINUS ARRHYTHMIA AND HEART RATE VARIABILITY

Sinus arrhythmia is the variation in heart rate (RR interval). It is often observed in clinical practice to be synchronized with breathing, slowing with expiration and accelerating with inspiration. In Fig. 6-5 the effect of respirations on a normal sinus rhythm is shown. Analysis of heart rate variability for prognostic purposes in patients with ischemic heart disease is accomplished by 24-hour Holter recordings and measurements in the time and frequency domain.

Pediatrics: Sinus arrhythmia is rare in the young infant but common in children and adolescents.

ECG recognition

Heart rate: In the classic form of sinus arrhythmia the heart rate slows with expiration and accelerates with inspiration. The slow phase may be less than 60 beats/min in the adult.

Rhythm: Irregular because of acceleration and deceleration of the heart rate.

P waves: Normal sinus P waves.

PP interval: Sinus arrhythmia is present when the difference between the shortest PP interval and the longest PP interval is greater than 0.12 sec. Respiratory sinus arrhythmia is quite pronounced in children (Fig. 6-5). In this tracing the difference between the longest and shortest PP interval is 0.26 sec. The rate, taken over a full minute, is normal at approximately 75 beats/min.

PR interval: The PR interval may change slightly as the heart rate changes.

QRS complex: The QRS complex is not affected by the sinus arrhythmia.

QT interval: The QT interval changes with heart rate, becoming longer during the slow phase of this rhythm.

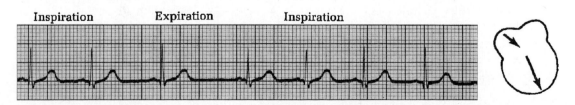

Fig. 6-5. Sinus arrhythmia in a 4-year-old.

Mechanism

Direct recordings from the sinus node have shown that sinus arrhythmia is associated not only with changes in sinus cycle length but also with changes in SA conduction time.[9] Sinus arrhythmia is most pronounced in the young and becomes less and less marked as a child becomes older.

In the healthy heart the sinus rhythm is not absolutely regular. Factors that cause heart rate variability include exercise, mental stress, respiration, blood pressure regulation, thermoregulation, actions of the renin-angiotensin system, some medications, and circadian rhythms. The effect of respirations on sinus rhythm is known to be an autonomic mechanism—a balance between sympathetic and parasympathetic tone—since it can be abolished by parasympathetic blockade, exercise, or heart transplant. Normally during sleep parasympathetic activity predominates, although in patients with anterior myocardial infarcts this may be suppressed by the relatively high sympathetic activity.[17]

Clinical implications

Decreased heart rate variability indices are reported to indicate abnormalities of autonomic input to the heart with increased susceptibility to ventricular arrhythmias. They are associated with an adverse outcome in patients with coronary artery disease and are an independent risk factor for mortality after myocardial infarction in patients with advanced congestive heart failure.[17-21]

A reduction in beat-to-beat heart rate variability during sinus rhythm is associated with aging,[22] postprandial hypotension,[23] diabetes, alcoholic cardiomyopathy, and sudden death syndromes. Women have relatively greater high-frequency heart rate fluctuations and greater overall complexity of sinus rhythm–heart rate variability than men.[24]

Symptoms

Symptoms are uncommon. However, excessively long pauses may result in dizziness or in some cases syncope, if not accompanied by an escape rhythm.[16]

Treatment

Sinus arrhythmia is not treated unless the bradycardia phase of the arrhythmia is marked, causing symptoms.

TWO TYPES OF SINOATRIAL BLOCK

Sinoatrial block is the failure of a sinus impulse to exit from the sinus node to activate the atria. There are two types of SA block, type I (SA Wenckebach) and type II. Both types are recognized because of dropped P waves. They are differentiated because type I SA block has the signs of Wenckebach and type II SA block has fixed PP intervals with the pause being an exact multiple. The two types of SA block are discussed separately.

Pediatrics: Second-degree SA block may be seen in infants (especially newborns) and children without heart disease. In adolescents it is usually caused by increased vagal tone.

SINOATRIAL WENCKEBACH (TYPE I SINOATRIAL BLOCK)

Sinoatrial Wenckebach is the progressive lengthening of SA conduction until P wave conduction fails for one beat and the sequence begins again. This results in

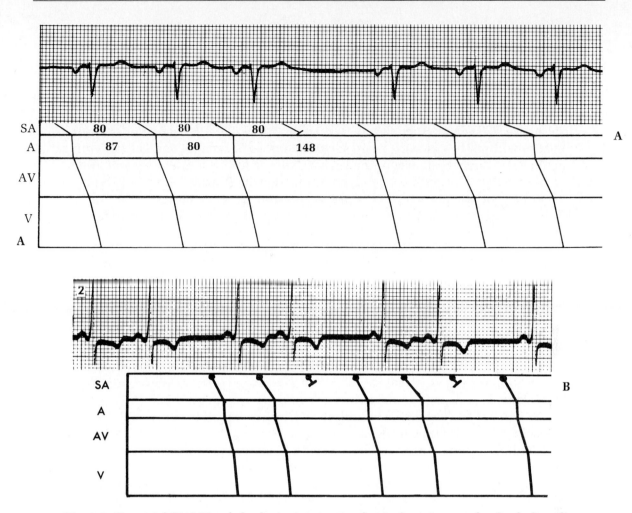

Fig. 6-6. Sinoatrial (SA) Wenckebach. **A,** A 4:3 ratio, that is, four sinus cycles (including the missing one) for three P waves. In **B,** A 3:2 ratio (i.e., three sinus cycles for two P waves).

group beating, shortening PP intervals, and pauses that are less than twice the shortest cycle (Dr. Marriott's "footsteps of Wenckebach"). In the case of SA Wenckebach visualize conduction between the sinus node and the atrial fibers surrounding it. The sinus discharge is not seen on the surface ECG; it is the atrial activation that produces the P wave. Thus it is possible for the sinus node to discharge and not produce a P wave. Sinoatrial Wenckebach is diagnosed because of its "footsteps." Fig. 6-6 shows two instances of SA Wenckebach, one with a 4:3 conduction ratio and the other with a 3:2 conduction ratio; this means that in Fig. 6-6, *A,* there are four discharges from the sinus node with three of them being conducted and in Fig. 6-6, *B,* there are three sinus node impulses with two being conducted. The best way to illustrate this mechanism is with a laddergram. There are four tiers in this particular laddergram. The top tier accommodates sinus node impulses and SA conduction; note that SA conduction time lengthens until one sinus impulse is not conducted.

ECG recognition

Heart rate: There may be bradycardia because of the pauses.

Rhythm: Group beating (usually groups of 2 or 3).

P waves: Normal sinus P waves.

PP interval: Shortens until there is a pause, and then the sequence begins again (shortening PP intervals and a pause).

The pause: Less than twice the shortest cycle. Although a P wave is missing, the pause will not be twice the shortest cycle because SA conduction is lengthening with every sinus beat, placing the P waves later in the cycle than they would normally appear. However, SA conduction time for the P wave following the pause is at its shortest, causing this P wave to be earlier than the others.

PR interval: Normal and fixed unless there is an associated AV conduction problem.

QRS complex: Normal unless associated with an intraventricular conduction problem.

Summary: The diagnosis of SA Wenckebach is made because of normal P waves, group beating, shortening PP intervals (except when there are only two P waves in the group), and pauses that are less than twice the shortest cycle.

Mechanism

The Wenckebach conduction phenomenon (lengthening conduction time until there is a nonconducted beat) can be found anywhere there are slow-response action potentials, normally in the two nodes and abnormally in ischemic tissue anywhere in the heart. Thus the mechanism of SA Wenckebach is easily explained because of the type of tissue involved. Sinus nodal cells are quite similar to AV nodal cells; both have slow-response action potentials, slow conduction, and similar conduction problems. Although the sinus node is capable of beating very rapidly, the conduction of an impulse through this tissue is at least as slow as conduction through the AV node. Sinoatrial exit block may result from drugs (e.g., quinidine, procainamide, or digitalis), acute myocarditis, myocardial infarction, fibrosis of the atrium, or excessive vagal stimulation.[16]

In SA Wenckebach there is not the tell-tale lengthening of the PR interval seen in AV Weckenbach (Chapter 18). The firing of the sinus node and the conduction time from that focus to the atrial tissue are concealed (not seen on the ECG). Therefore the problem is diagnosed by the tracks that it leaves on the ECG (its "footsteps").

Clinical implications

Sinoatrial block is usually a transient condition. Asymptomatic pauses of more than 2 sec have been noted in ambulatory patients, trained athletes, and healthy

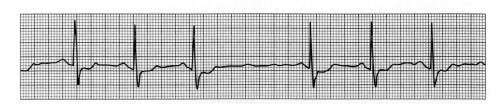

Fig. 6-7. Type II SA block. The PP interval spanning the pause is twice that of the sinus cycle.

young persons and do not necessarily carry a poor prognosis. Sinoatrial Wenckebach, when associated with other arrhythmias, may be part of the sick sinus syndrome.

Treatment

SA Wenckebach is not treated unless the pauses are symptomatic; then it is
managed as a sinus bradycardia.

TYPE II SINOATRIAL BLOCK

Type II SA block is the regular firing of the sinus node with periodic failure of
conduction. Unlike SA Wenckebach, this failure of conduction is not preceded by
increments in SA conduction time.

ECG recognition

Heart rate: Pauses in the sinus rhythm may cause bradycardia.
Rhythm: Regular before and after the pauses.
P waves: Normal sinus P waves.
PP interval: Fixed before and after the pauses.
The pause: Can be multiplied by an integer (a whole number). Unlike SA Wencke-
    bach, a P wave is dropped without increments in SA conduction.
PR interval: Normal and fixed unless there is an associated AV conduction prob-
    lem.
QRS complex: Normal unless associated with an intraventricular conduction prob-
    lem.
Summary: The diagnosis of type II SA block is made because of dropped P waves
    against a background of fixed PP intervals and pauses that are multiples of the
    uninterrupted sinus rhythm, as seen in Fig. 6-7.

SINUS ARREST OR SINUS PAUSE

Sinus arrest or sinus pause is a failure of impulse formation in the sinus node,
an event that is impossible to determine with certainty on the surface ECG. One
can, however, be suspicious of this condition if the PP intervals of the basic cycle
cannot be "walked out" across the pause, ending on a P wave. Fig. 6-8 shows two
examples of sinus arrest. In Fig. 6-8, A, during a long sinus pause there is an absence of an appropriate escape junctional beat. When another P wave appears, AV
conduction is a problem. The long pause without relief from the junction is a manifestation of sick sinus syndrome. In Fig. 6-8, B, the second pause is interupted by a
junctional escape beat and all P waves are conducted. Fig. 6-9 shows SA block or
sinus arrest compounded by other problems (sick sinus syndrome). The main dramatic concern for this patient was the long pauses unrelieved by a junctional escape beat. The pauses were due not only to the SA block, but to AV Wenckebach
and nonconducted premature atrial complexes (PACs), profound overdrive suppression, and failure of a junctional escape mechanism. Note in Fig. 6-9, A, the small
increments in PR intervals until there is a dropped beat (AV Wenckebach); in Fig.
6-9, B, a nonconducted premature atrial beat is seen just before the last pause.

ECG recognition

Heart rate: May be marked bradycardia because of long pauses.

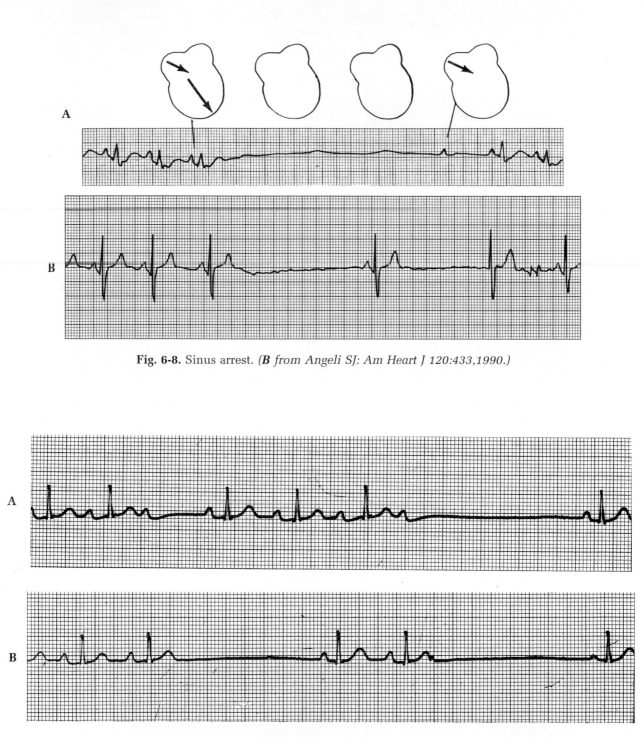

Fig. 6-8. Sinus arrest. *(**B** from Angeli SJ: Am Heart J 120:433,1990.)*

Fig. 6-9. Sick sinus syndrome consisting of SA block or sinus arrest, atrioventricular (AV) Wenckebach, nonconducted premature atrial complex (PAC), and profound overdrive suppression. The sinus arrest is seen in the long pauses. **A,** There are shortening PP intervals in the center, indicating incremental SA conduction time. The nonconducted PAC initiates the last pause in **B.**

Rhythm: Regular with pauses that have no numeric relationship to the basic cycle length.

P waves: There may be normal sinus P waves along with atrial escape beats.

PP interval: May be fixed before and after the pauses.

The pause: Not a multiple of a whole number. That is, the basic PP interval cannot be "walked out" across the pause and end on a P wave.

PR interval: Normal and fixed unless there is an associated AV conduction problem.

QRS complex: Normal unless associated with an intraventricular conduction problem.

Summary: The diagnosis of sinus arrest is made because of a pause or pauses in a sinus rhythm that are not a multiple of a whole number.

Treatment

SA block is not treated unless the pauses are symptomatic and complicated by other arrhythmias (sick sinus syndrome); then a pacemaker may be indicated.

PERMANENT ATRIAL STANDSTILL

Permanent atrial standstill is the inability of the atria to respond to stimuli. It is an infrequently recognized arrhythmia and has been diagnosed in three clinical settings: long-standing progressive cardiac disease, neuromuscular disease, and patients with vertigo or syncope. Not only are P waves absent in all leads of the surface ECG (Fig. 6-10) and in the atrial electrogram, but also the A waves are absent in the jugular venous pulse and right atrial pressure tracings.

ECG recognition

P waves: Absent in all leads, including right precordial leads and extreme left precordial leads.

QRS complex: Junctional or ventricular escape beats.

Summary: The diagnosis of permanent atrial standstill is made because the ECG and atrial electrogram have absent P waves, and pressure tracings from the jugular venous pulse and right atrium have absent A waves.

Mechanism

The atria are immobile on fluoroscopy and cannot be stimulated electrically, so it is possible that the sinus node may actually be firing but the atria are incapable of responding.

SINUS NODAL DYSFUNCTION (SICK SINUS SYNDROME)

Sinus nodal dysfunction (SND) or the so-called sick sinus syndrome (SSS) encompasses a broad range of abnormalities, including disorders of impulse generation and conduction, failure of latent pacemakers, and a susceptibility to paroxysmal or chronic atrial tachycardias.[25] There is a tendency in the literature to replace the phrase "sick sinus syndrome" with SND, sinoatrial disease, or sinoatrial dysfunction.

Pediatrics: Sick sinus syndrome is seen in children during the postoperative period, usually following extensive intraatrial surgery (especially surgery for transposition of the great vessels). The rhythms seen are profound sinus bra-

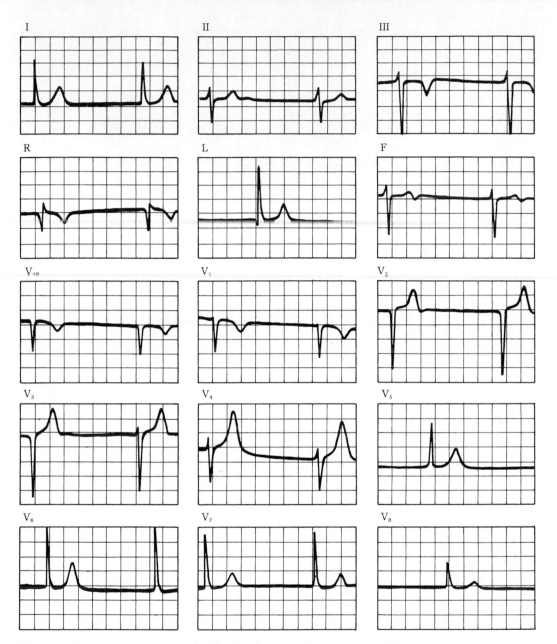

Fig. 6-10. Permanent atrial standstill. The absence of P waves in all leads is evident, including a right precordial lead (V$_{3R}$) and extreme left precordial leads V$_7$ and V$_8$. *(Courtesy Dr. James Wolliscroft, Ann Arbor, Mich.)*

dycardia, periods of sinus arrest, atrial or junctional rhythms, atrial flutter, and rarely atrial fibrillation. The focus may switch from one to another, especially during the immediate postoperative period.

ECG recognition

ECG manifestations of SSS include the following:
1. Profound sinus bradycardia
2. Sinus pauses or sinus arrest

V₁

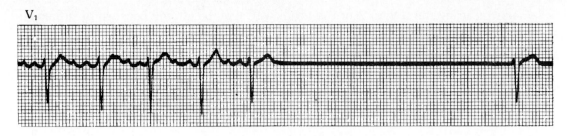

Fig. 6-11. Sick sinus syndrome caused by bradycardia-tachycardia. *(From Marriott HJL, Conover M: Advanced concepts in arrhythmias, St Louis, 1983, Mosby.)*

3. SA block
4. Chronic atrial tachyarrhythmias, especially atrial fibrillation associated with a slow ventricular response (unrelated to drugs)
5. Bradycardia that alternates with tachycardia, usually paroxysmal atrial fibrillation or flutter (bradycardia-tachycardia syndrome; Fig. 6-11)
6. Inappropriate sinus node response to exercise or stress

Sick sinus syndrome is often characterized by persistent sinus bradycardia and episodic sinus pauses that are due to sinus arrest or SA block and is frequently accompanied by episodic atrial fibrillation, atrial flutter, and atrial tachycardia.[26] In susceptible patients, transient marked sinus bradycardia or sinus pauses can result in syncope.

The bradycardia-tachycardia syndrome often precedes the development of chronic atrial fibrillation and is a common manifestation of SSS. The tachycardia phase is often paroxysmal atrial fibrillation or flutter but may be atrial ectopic or junctional. Often in the transition between the tachycardia and the bradycardia there are long pauses caused by overdrive suppression of the sinus node or the escape atrial pacemaker.

Mechanisms

A wide spectrum of abnormalities of both sinus node automaticity and SA conduction cause the long sinus pauses of SSS. Complete SA block with an atrial escape rhythm can occur. It has also been shown that although the sinus impulse may not be able to conduct to the atria, conduction in the opposite direction (atriosinus) can occur and suppress the sinus node. The long pauses following atrial tachyarrhythmias are the result of SA block and overdrive suppression of the sinus node.

Pathologic features

Sick sinus syndrome is an acquired condition. Drugs most often implicated as an extracardiac factor include cardiac glycosides, sympatholytic antihypertensive agents, beta blockers, calcium channel blockers, and membrane-active antiarrhythmic agents. Marked hypervagotonia, sometimes combined with certain drugs, may be implicated in some cases of SSS. There is still uncertainty regarding the disease processes that may cause intrinsic sinus nodal dysfunction. In adult patients coronary atherosclerosis is the most prominent one linked to SSS.

SSS is frequently intermittent and unpredictable and may occur in the absence of other cardiac disease. The sinus node itself may be partially or totally destroyed. There may be discontinuity between the SA node and atrial tissue; the nervous system surrounding the SA node or the atrial wall may be altered because of inflammatory or degenerative processes.[16]

Treatment

Treatment[25] is determined by the patient's symptoms and ECG findings. Important therapeutic considerations include the following:

1. Thromboembolism (anticoagulation and preservation of organized atrial activation)
2. Symptoms of exertional intolerance (chronotropic support when indicated)
3. Survival (enhanced by physiologic pacing therapy along with appropriate pharmacologic interventions)

When symptoms of dizziness and syncope are related to bradyarrhythmia in patients with SSS permanent cardiac pacemaker therapy is usually indicated.[16] There are also data supporting the beneficial use of oral theophylline in patients with SSS.[27,28]

SINUS NODAL REENTRY TACHYCARDIA

Sinus nodal reentry tachycardia is an uncommon cause (5% to 10%)[16,29] of paroxysmal supraventricular tachycardia (PSVT) sustained by a reentry circuit through the sinus node. It is recognized because of its paroxysmal nature, the shape of the P waves (sinus), and its termination with use of vagal maneuvers or adenosine.[30] It can consistently be initiated and terminated with programed electrical stimulation. Fig. 6-12 represents SA nodal reentry tachycardia.

ECG recognition

Heart rate: Ranging from 80 to 140 beats/min (average, 130 to 140 beats/min).
Rhythm: PSVT.
P waves: The P waves of the paroxysmal tachycardia are in front of the QRS complex and identical or similar in shape to the normal sinus beats.
PR interval: Normal and fixed; during the paroxysm of tachycardia the PR shortens slightly along with the cycle length.
QRS complex: Normal unless associated with an intraventricular conduction problem.

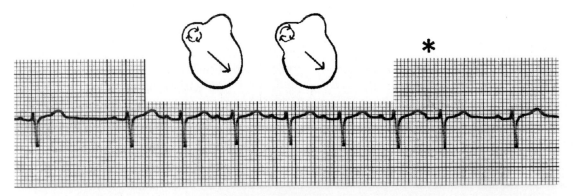

Fig. 6-12. Paroxysmal supraventricular tachycardia (PSVT) resulting from SA nodal reentry. The tachycardia is terminated by a single PAC (in the T wave with the asterisk).

AV conduction: AV block may be present, especially AV Wenckebach; the PSVT is not affected.

Summary: The diagnosis of SA nodal reentry tachycardia is made because of paroxysmal narrow QRS tachycardia in which the P waves immediately precede the QRS, are upright in lead II, and are the same shape as the normal sinus beats.

Mechanism

The precise mechanism of SA nodal reentry tachycardia is unclear. It may be a reentrant circuit completely confined to the sinus node, or the circuit may also involve surrounding atrial tissue. Such a reentry circuit may be initiated by a premature atrial complex or by a sinus beat. The possibility of a mechanism using the SA node as the slow pathway and surrounding atrial tissue to complete the circuit is illustrated in Fig. 6-13.

Clinical implications

Often this arrhythmia does not cause serious symptoms and individuals do not seek medical attention. In other cases this arrhythmia may be misdiagnosed as a sinus tachycardia resulting from anxiety.

Differential diagnosis

Sinoatrial nodal reentry tachycardia may easily be mistaken for sinus tachycardia because it is hemodynamically tolerated and has a heart rate similar to that of sinus tachycardia, and because the P waves are the same shape as normal sinus P waves. Thus SA nodal reentry tachycardia is often missed. It differs from sinus tachycardia in that it may be abruptly terminated with a vagal maneuver, whereas sinus tachycardia slows gradually. Sinoatrial nodal reentry may also be mistaken for a marked sinus arrhythmia; however, SA nodal reentry tachycardia does not fluctuate with respirations.

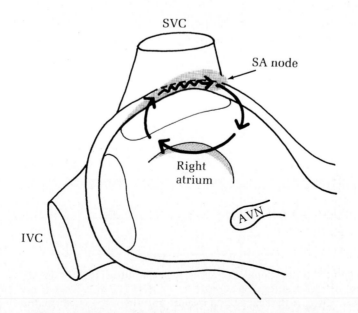

Fig. 6-13. Mechanism of SA nodal reentry tachycardia.

Treatment

Propranolol, verapamil, and digitalis may be effective.[16]

WANDERING PACEMAKER

A wandering pacemaker is a sinus arrhythmia with an escape atrial or junctional rhythm, often resulting in atrial fusion beats. Fig. 6-14 is a typical example of a wandering pacemaker. Sinus slowing occurs, permitting an atrial ectopic focus to escape at a rate of 50 beats/min. Notice that during the transition from sinus rhythm to junctional escape rhythm and back again, both the sinus node and the junction activate the atria at the same time, producing atrial fusion beats. Fusion beats result when currents from two independent sources collide within a heart chamber. The type of passive pacemaker shift seen in Fig. 6-14 occurs frequently in normal individuals and is of no consequence. What is sometimes incorrectly labeled "wandering" or "shifting" pacemaker is shown in Fig. 6-15. This tracing, however, is not an escape mechanism but an accelerated atrial ectopic rhythm at a rate of 77 beats/min. Because the ectopic P waves are negative in lead II, one may assume that the ectopic focus is in the low right atria. Three atrial fusion beats occur as the control of the heart shifts from the ectopic focus to the sinus node.

ECG recognition

Heart rate: Bradycardia.
Rhythm: Irregular.

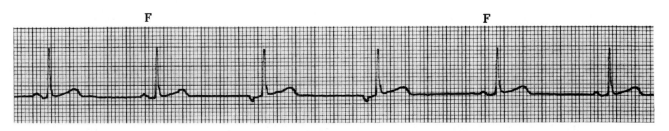

Fig. 6-14. Sinus slowing with a junctional escape rhythm (often called a *wandering pacemaker*). There is an atrial fusion beat *(F)* as the two foci (sinus and junctional) vie for control of the heart.

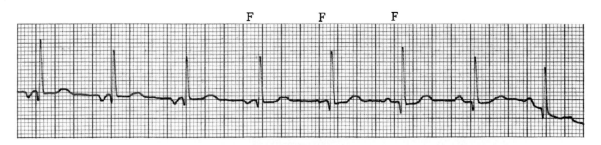

Fig. 6-15. An accelerated junctional rhythm of 77 beats/min. The junctional focus can be seen at the beginning of this tracing. The fourth P wave is a fusion beat *(F)* as the sinus node begins to regain control with a rate of 78 beats/min. There are atrial fusion beats *(F)* during the change of control.

P waves: Multiform with fusion beats.

PR or P′R intervals: Normal unless associated with an AV conduction problem.

QRS complex: Normal unless there is an intraventricular conduction problem.

Summary: The wandering pacemaker is recognized in the setting of sinus bradycardia when the escape pacemakers come from more than one focus or when the sinus rate and the atrial escape rate are similar, resulting in atrial fusion beats.

SUMMARY

The arrhythmias originating in the sinus node that are physiologic are sinus tachycardia (a response to exercise, emotions, fever, and the like), sinus bradycardia (common in athletes and during sleep), and sinus arrhythmia (associated with the vagal effect of respirations). When these arrhythmias are symptomatic or inappropriate, they are abnormal. Sinus nodal disease may manifest itself as SA block, sinus arrest, or sick sinus syndrome.

REFERENCES

1. Spodick DH: Normal sinus heart rate: sinus tachycardia and sinus bradycardia redefined, *Am Heart J* 124:1119, 1992.
2. Weisfeldt ML, Lakatta EG, Gerstenblith G: Aging and the heart. In Braunwald E, ed: *Heart disease,* ed 4, Philadelphia, 1992, WB Saunders.
3. Gomes JA, Winters SL: The origins of the sinus node pacemaker complex in man: demonstration of dominant and subsidiary foci, *J Am Coll Cardiol* 9:45, 1987.
4. Boineau JP, Schuessler RB, Roeske WR et al: The quantitative relation between sites of atrial impulse origin and cycle length, *Am J Physiol* 245:H781, 1983.
5. Braunwald E, Sonnenblick EH, Ross J: Mechanisms of cardiac contraction and relaxation. In Braunwald E, ed: *Heart disease,* ed 4, Philadelphia, 1992, WB Saunders.
6. Akhtar M: Supraventricular tachycardias: electrophysiologic mechanisms, diagnosis, and pharmacologic therapy. In Josephson ME, Wellens HJJ, eds: *Tachycardias: mechanisms, diagnosis, treatment,* Philadelphia, 1984, Lea & Febiger.
7. Morillo CA, Klein GJ, Thakur RK et al: Mechanism of "inappropriate" sinus tachycardia; role of sympathovagal balance, *Circulation* 90:873, 1994.
8. Gillette PC, Zeigler VL, Case CL: Pediatric arrhythmias: are they different? In Zipes DP, Jalife J, eds: *Cardiac electrophysiology from cell to bedside,* ed 2, Philadelphia, 1995, WB Saunders.
9. Reiffel JA: Clinical electrophysiology of the sinus node in man. In *Electrophysiology of the sinoatrial and atrioventricular nodes,* New York, 1988, Alan R Liss.
10. Brodsky M, Wu D, Denes P et al: Arrhythmias documented by 24-hour continuous electrocardiographic monitoring in 50 male medical students without apparent heart disease, *Am J Cardiol* 39:390, 1977.
11. Alboni P, Uberti ED, Codeca L et al: Circadian variations of sinus rate in subjects with sinus node dysfunction, *Chronobiologia* 9:173, 1982.
12. Alboni P, Menozzi C, Brignole M et al: An abnormal neural reflex plays a role in causing syncope in sinus bradycardia, *J Am Coll Cardiol* 22:1130, 1993.
13. Pasternak RC, Braunwald E, Sobel BE: Acute myocardial infarction. In Braunwald E, ed: *Heart disease,* ed 4, Philadelphia, 1992, WB Saunders.
14. Corr P, Gillis R: Autonomic neural influences on the dysrhythmias resulting from myocardial infarction, *Circ Res* 43:1, 1978.
15. Juma Z et al: Prognostic significance of the electrocardiogram in patients with coronary heart disease. In Wellens HJJ, Kulbertus HE, eds: *What's new in electrocardiography?* The Hague, 1981, Martinus Nijhoff.
16. Zipes DP: Specific arrhythmias: diagnosis and treatment. In Braunwald E, ed: *Heart disease,* ed 4, Philadelphia 1992, WB Saunders.
17. Stein PK, Bosner MS, Kleiger RE, Conger BM: Heart rate variability: a measure of cardiac autonomic tone, *Am Heart J* 127:1376, 1994.
18. Dreifus LS, Agarwal JB, Botvinick EH, et al: Heart rate variability for risk stratification of life-threatening arrhythmias, *J Am Coll Cardiol* 22:948, 1993.
19. Bigger JT Jr, Fleiss JL, Steinman RC et al: Correlations among time and frequency domain measures of heart period variability two weeks after myocardial infarction, *Am J Cardiol* 69:891, 1992.
20. Pipilis A, Flather M, Ormerod O, Sleight P: Heart rate variability in acute myocardial infarction and its association with infarct site

and clinical course, *Am J Cardiol* 67:1137, 1991.

21. Huikuri HV, Niemelä MJ, Ojala S et al: Circadian rhythms of frequency domain measures of heart rate variability in healthy subjects and patients with coronary artery disease: effects of arousal and upright posture, *Circulation* 90: 121, 1994.

22. Schwartz JB, Gibb WJ, Tran T: Aging effects on heart rate variation, *J Gerontol Med Sci* 46: M99, 1991.

23. Ryan SM, Goldberger AL, Ruthazer R et al: Spectral analysis of heart rate dynamics in elderly persons with postprandial hypotension, *Am J Cardiol* 69:201, 1992.

24. Ryan SM, Goldberger AL, Pincus SM et al: Gender- and age-related differences in heart rate dynamics: are women more complex than men? *J Am Coll Cardiol* 24:1700, 1994.

25. Benditt DG, Sakaguchi S, Goldstein MA et al: Sinus node dysfunction: pathophysiology, clinical features, evaluation, and treatment. In Zipes DP, Jalife J, eds: *Cardiac electrophysiol-ogy from cell to bedside,* ed 2, Philadelphia, 1995, WB Saunders.

26. Wu D, Yeh SJ, Lin FC et al: Sinus automaticity and sinoatrial conduction in severe symptomatic sick sinus syndrome, *J Am Coll Cardiol* 19:355, 1992.

27. Saito D, Matsubara K, Yamanari H et al: Effects of oral theophylline on sick sinus syndrome, *J Am Coll Cardiol* 21:1199, 1993.

28. Alboni P, Ratto B, Cappato R et al: Clinical effects of oral theophylline in sick sinus syndrome, Am Heart J 122:1361, 1991.

29. Sanders WE Jr, Sorrentino RA, Greenfield RA et al: Catheter ablation of sinoatrial node reentrant tachycardia, *J Am Coll Cardiol* 23:926, 1994.

30. Grifith MJ, Garratt CJ, Ward DE et al: The effects of adenosine on sinus node reentrant tachycardia, *Clin Cardiol* 12:409, 1993.

31. Yang XS, Beck GJ, Wilkoff BL: Redefining normal sinus heart rate, *J Amer Col Cardiol* 749-1:193A, 1995.

C H A P T E R

7

Premature Atrial Complexes and Atrial Tachycardia

Premature Atrial Complex   *81*
Types of Premature Atrial Complexes   *86*
Atrial Tachycardia   *88*

Multifocal (Chaotic) Atrial
Tachycardia   *93*

PREMATURE ATRIAL COMPLEX

A premature atrial complex (PAC) is an atrial impulse that emerges earlier than the next expected sinus beat and originates from a focus other than the sinus node. It is recognized because it is premature, it usually (not always) has a different shape from that of the sinus P wave, and its P′R interval is more than 0.12 sec (except, of course, in Wolff-Parkinson-White (WPW) syndrome). An ectopic P wave is called a P′ (P prime) wave. Fig. 7-1 illustrates the focus and resulting P wave of the normal sinus beat compared with the P′ wave of the PAC.

"Walking out" the rhythm

Irregularities, premature beats, and the presence or absence of atrioventricular (AV) dissociation are evaluated by using a caliper or a piece of paper and a sharp pencil to mark off ("walk out") the rhythm in question (sinus, junctional, or ventricular). Although the two premature atrial complexes in Fig. 7-1 are immediately apparent, this tracing can be used for practice. Mark off the first three P waves, and you will find that the PP intervals are identical and that the PAC is easily found. If you continue to walk out the sinus rhythm across the PAC, you will find that the sinus P wave after the PAC falls earlier than expected. This is because of the early discharge and resetting of the sinus node by the PAC. This shortened pause is referred to as a "noncompensatory" pause (i.e., less than a full compensatory pause). A *full compensatory pause* is seen when a premature ventricular beat does not disturb the regular sinus rhythm, but the P wave that occurs during or immediately following the premature beat is not conducted, creating a pause. The P waves are all on time when the PP intervals are walked out across the premature beat. Although a noncompensatory pause indicates atrial involvement, a full compensatory pause

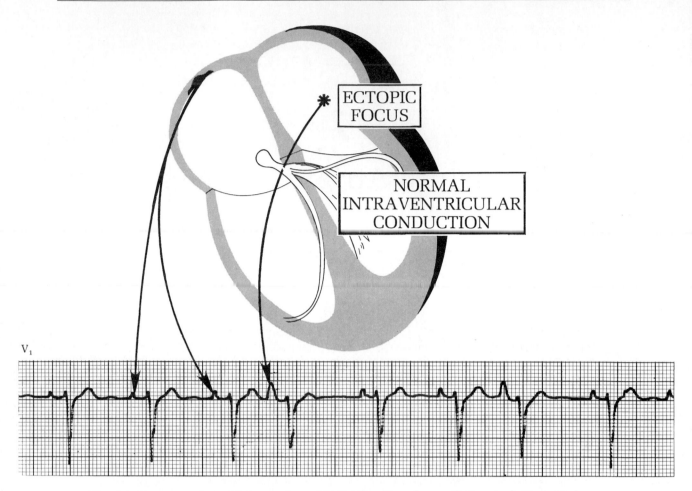

Fig. 7-1. Two premature atrial complexes (PACs) (fourth and seventh P waves). Sinus P waves are generated from an impulse from the sinus node and have a uniform shape in a single lead. In addition to being premature, PACs are generated from a focus outside of the sinus node and are shaped differently.

does not prove ventricular ectopy. This is because a PAC may be followed by such a pause (1) if the sinus node is not discharged by the PAC and (2) if the PAC discharges the sinus node and instead of resetting it, the sinus node is depressed (overdrive suppression) and delays its next expected discharge. Of course, such a depression may also result in a longer pause than expected.

A full compensatory pause is not a diagnostic clue for premature ventricular complexes (PVCs) unless the nonconducted sinus P wave can be seen; a PAC may be followed by a compensatory, noncompensatory, or more than compensatory pause.

ECG recognition

Heart rate: That of the underlying sinus rhythm.
Rhythm: Irregular because of the PACs.
P wave shape: The PAC usually has a different shape from that of the sinus P wave: different focus, different shape.
P wave location: Premature; may be hidden in the T wave.

PP interval: Irregular because of the PAC.

P′R interval: May be the same as the PR interval but is usually prolonged because of the prematurity of the P′ wave. The P′ wave may be nonconducted (followed by a pause).

QRS complex: Normal unless there is an intraventricular conduction problem. The PAC may or may not be followed by a QRS.

Pause following the PAC: May be less than, exactly, or more than fully compensatory depending on many factors.

Summary: A PAC is diagnosed because of a premature beat with a narrow QRS (a supraventricular complex) that is preceded by a P′ wave or because of a pause preceded by a distorted T wave (hidden P′ wave).

AV conduction following a PAC

Atrioventricular conduction after a PAC depends on the prematurity of the P′ wave and the health of the AV node, bundle of His, and bundle branches. The possibilities for the AV conduction of a PAC are the following:

1. Normal conduction (narrow QRS)
2. Nonconduction resulting in no QRS and a sudden pause; the block could be anywhere in the AV node or even in the His-Purkinje system.
3. Aberrant ventricular conduction (broad QRS because of bundle branch block [BBB]). The BBB is functional and is due to the sudden shortening of the cycle length rather than to any disease in the bundle branches.
4. Conducted down only one AV nodal pathway (there are two) to set up a reentry circuit within the AV node. This is the most common mechanism of symptomatic paroxysmal supraventricular tachycardia (PSVT) (discussed in Chapter 11).
5. Conducted down the AV node and up an accessory pathway to establish a circus movement tachycardia (Chapter 11). This is the second most common cause of symptomatic PSVT.

Overdrive suppression

Overdrive suppression is a property belonging to pacemaker cells in which their cycle length may be lengthened if they are depolarized from an outside source. For

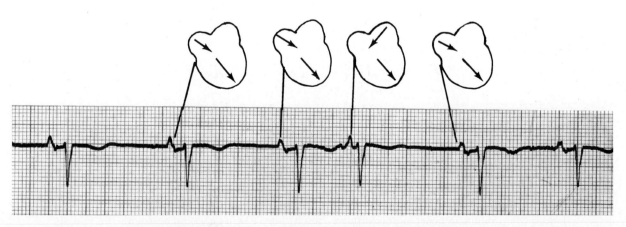

Fig. 7-2. Lead V$_1$. Sinus bradycardia with a PAC (the fourth P wave).

example, the sinus node normally exerts overdrive suppression on all subsidiary pacemakers, and a PAC may exert overdrive suppression on the sinus node.

In Fig. 7-1 you walked out the sinus rhythm and noted that the PAC had reset the sinus node, causing the pause following the PAC to be less than compensatory. In Fig. 7-2, measure the PP interval just before the PAC and then place that measurement on the P'P interval; the two are almost identical because the PAC has reset the sinus node. However, this is not usually the case. Sometimes the PAC suppresses the sinus node (overdrive suppression),[1,2] and the following sinus P wave is delayed (Figs. 7-3 and 7-4). This may result in a pause that is equal to, less than, or more than a full compensatory pause. In Fig. 7-4, *A* to *C,* the PAC has caused a long delay in the appearance of the next sinus P wave so that there is more than a full compensatory pause or at least the interval between the sinus P wave and the PAC is longer than the other PP intervals. As discussed in Chapter 12 it is possible for a PAC to be followed by a pseudo-full compensatory pause because of overdrive suppression. If ventricular conduction from such a beat is aberrant, it could simulate a premature ventricular beat.

Mechanism

The location of the ectopic focus in the atria determines the shape of the P' wave. If the focus is in the vicinity of the sinus node (as it is in the atrial tachycardia of digitalis toxicity), the resultant P' wave closely resembles the normal sinus P wave. If the ectopic focus is low in the atrium toward the septum, there will be a negative P' wave in leads II, III, and aV$_F$ because the P' vector moves away from the positive electrode of those leads. An ectopic focus in the left atrial appendage would result in a negative P' wave in lead I because the current would be moving toward the right shoulder and the position of the negative electrode for lead I. By the same token, a PAC arising from the right free wall of the atrium would produce a positive P wave in lead I.

Fig. 7-2 shows a PAC in a patient with sinus bradycardia of 48 beats/min. The PAC is the fourth P wave in the tracing. It occurs early, before the next expected sinus P wave. It is also shaped differently, being a little narrower and more pointed than the sinus P waves. The QRS configuration is the same as for the sinus-conducted beats, proving that the stimulus originated above the branching portion of the bundle of His (supraventricular).

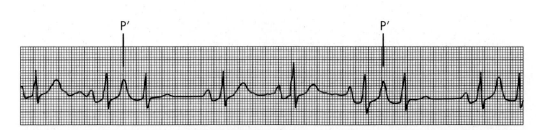

Fig. 7-3. Premature atrial complexes hidden in T waves (lead II). Notice how the T waves before the premature beats are distorted by the hidden P' waves compared with the two sinus conducted beats in the middle of the tracing.

II

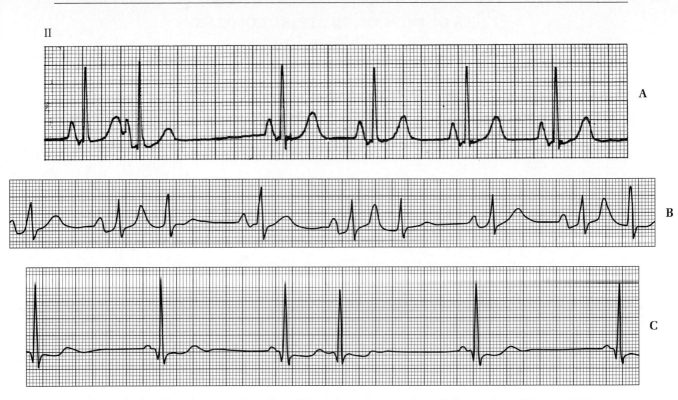

Fig. 7-4. Overdrive suppression (lead II). **A,** Note the exceptionally long pause following this premature atrial complex (PAC) (the second P wave). **B,** Atrial trigeminy. There is a PAC every third beat. The overdrive suppression is exerted on the sinus node by the PAC, causing the P′P interval to be longer than the PP interval. **C,** There is a PAC in the third T wave. The suppressant effect it has on the sinus node can be seen.

Clinical implications and causes

In normal individuals PACs may be the result of various stimuli, such as strong emotion (catecholamines), tobacco, alcohol, and caffeine[3] to name a few. Premature atrial complexes are also associated with myocardial ischemia, infection, a variety of medications, low potassium or low magnesium blood levels, and hypoxia and, because they may also result from stretch of the myocardium, are a warning signal in the development of congestive heart failure. They may also be seen when mitral stenosis or atrial septal defect causes dilated or hypertrophied atria. With critical timing a PAC may precipitate PSVT, atrial flutter, or atrial fibrillation. Rarely they may precipitate ventricular tachycardia (VT).

Treatment

Premature atrial complexes are not treated, although the cause is investigated, especially if the patient is aware of and bothered by an irregular heart beat that is due to the PACs. Some simple measures in treatment would be to improve electrolyte intake, stop drinking excessive amounts of caffeine, and stop smoking. These precautions would be especially important in the setting of WPW syndrome; in this condition it is a PAC or a PVC that initiates the PSVT.

TYPES OF PREMATURE ATRIAL COMPLEXES
PACs that hide in T waves

The PACs in Fig. 7-3 are hidden in the preceding T waves. This is a common hiding place for PACs, although they can be easily spotted as follows:
1. By noting the irregular rhythm and the narrow QRS, indicating a supraventricular mechanism
2. By comparing the shape of the T waves preceding the early QRS; the taller, peaked T waves are distorted by PACs. Three of them are found in this tracing.

Bigeminal PACs

Whenever the cardiac rhythm occurs in groups of two beats, it is called bigeminal. One of the causes of such a rhythm is a PAC following every sinus beat. In Fig. 7-5 you will note a bigeminal supraventricular rhythm. (All QRSs complexes are narrow.) If you compare the shape of the end of the T wave preceding the pause with the shape of the one following the pause, you will easily find the PACs.

Nonconducted PACs

When the PAC falls in the T wave, it may not be conducted. Fig. 7-6 illustrates the nonconducted PAC and its mechanism. The block is usually due to refractoriness in the AV node or bundle of His. The nonconducted PAC in Fig. 7-6 is not difficult to see, but in Fig. 7-7 it is more subtle. An abrupt pause is always a striking occurrence on the ECG. When this is encountered, examine the T wave preceding the pause carefully, comparing its shape with other T waves. The PAC can usually be found easily in this manner.

Bigeminal nonconducted PACs

Bigeminal nonconducted PACs can masquerade as sudden, inappropriate, profound sinus bradycardia and may be mistaken for sick sinus syndrome (SSS) because the sudden brachycardia is associated with syncope or presyncope. It should be suspected when the bradycardia is of sudden onset. In Fig. 7-8 there are two sinus conducted beats at the beginning of the tracing. The first PAC is in the third T

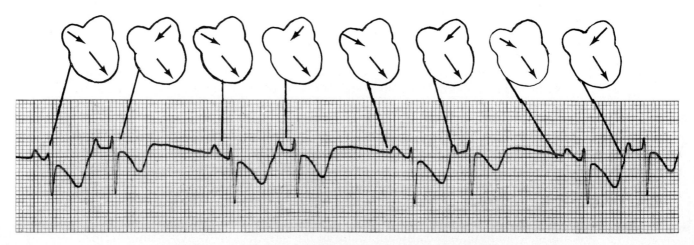

Fig. 7-5. Bigeminal premature atrial complexes in lead V$_1$.

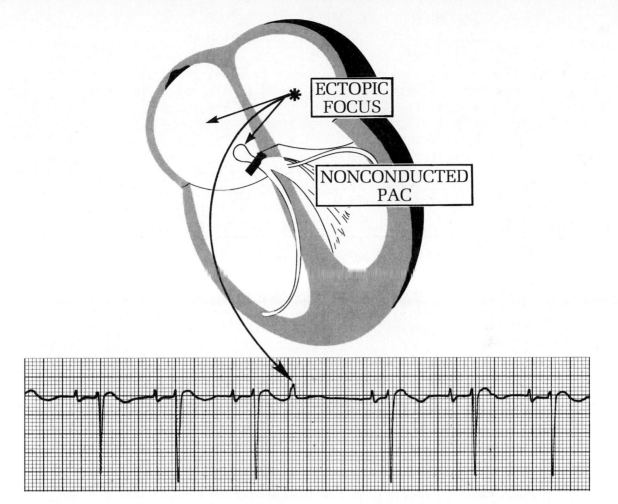

Fig. 7-6. Mechanism of the nonconducted premature atrial complex (PAC). When a PAC fires on a T wave, it may not be conducted because the AV node, bundle of His, or bundle branches are still refractory.

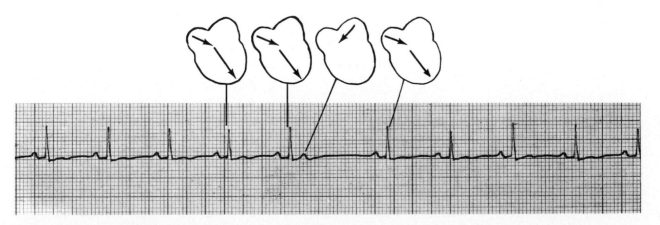
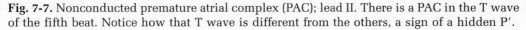

Fig. 7-7. Nonconducted premature atrial complex (PAC); lead II. There is a PAC in the T wave of the fifth beat. Notice how that T wave is different from the others, a sign of a hidden P′.

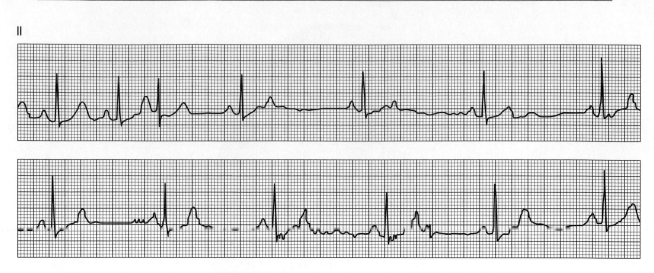

Fig 7-8 Bigeminal nonconducted premature atrial complexes (PACs) (lead II). The noncon-duction of the PAC in every other beat causes an abrupt, symptomatic bradycardia (continuous tracing).

wave, and it is conducted normally, after which there is a nonconducted P′ wave in every T wave. The failure of the PACs to conduct to the ventricles, plus some degree of overdrive suppression, causes a heart rate of less than 48 to 50 beats/min and results in loss of consciousness. In locating the P′ waves and making the diagnosis, it is helpful to note that bigeminal nonconducted PACs are a far more common cause of sudden bradycardia than sinoatrial (SA) block and that in such a case the T waves do not necessarily look abnormal, but they are different in shape from the T waves before the first PAC and they are slightly different in shape from one another. If there is a PAC in every T wave, it distorts the T wave a little differently each time because the P is not part of the T wave mechanism. Note in Fig. 7-8 that not only are the T waves before the pauses different from the two normal T waves at the beginning of the tracing, but they are also different from each other.

Fig. 7-9 provides another example of bigeminal nonconducted PACs. In Fig. 7-9, *A,* there is one nonconducted PAC. It is a sharp spike distorting the sixth T wave. In Fig. 7-9, *B,* P′ waves can be seen distorting every T wave.

Fig. 7-10 is a sinus tachycardia with two nonconducted PACs. Note that the PACs cause an irregular shape of the T waves preceding the pauses.

Differential diagnosis

Bigeminal nonconducted PACs can be mistaken for profound sinus bradycardia or SA block, and the atrial tachycardia of digitalis toxicity can be mistaken for bigeminal nonconducted PACs. In atrial tachycardia with 2:1 block that is due to digitalis toxicity there is often a shorter PP interval in the cycle that contains the QRS (ventriculophasic PP intervals), causing it to resemble bigeminal nonconducted PACs.

ATRIAL TACHYCARDIA

Atrial tachycardia may be either paroxysmal or sustained (nonparoxysmal). A paroxysmal tachycardia, by definition, is initiated by one beat and ends abruptly.

V₁

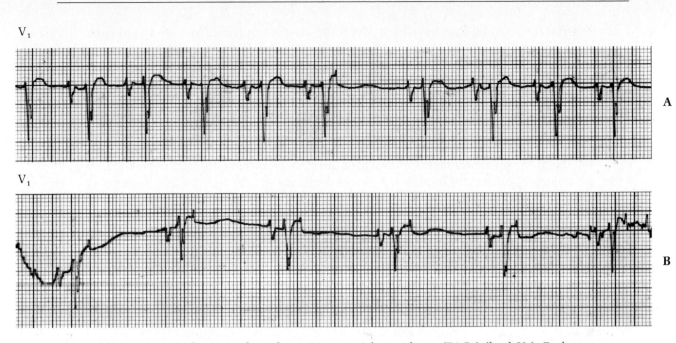

A

V₁

B

Fig. 7-9. Bigeminal nonconducted premature atrial complexes (PACs) (lead V₁). Both tracings are from the same patient. **A,** A PAC is distorting the sixth T wave. **B,** Every T has a PAC in it (nonconducted), resulting in a heart rate of 52 beats/min. Nonconducted PACs are more common than the conditions that they mimic—sinoatrial block and sinus arrest.

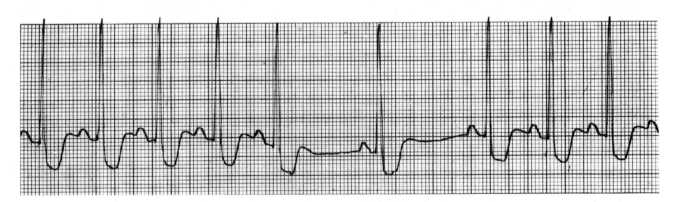

Fig. 7-10. Sinus tachycardia with two nonconducted premature atrial complexes (PACs) (lead II). The PACs distort the two T waves before the pauses; this is recognized when the T waves are compared.

The usual mechanism for paroxysmal tachycardia is reentry (80%); however, triggered activity caused by afterdepolarizations may also be a cause (20%).[4] Abnormal automaticity is thought to be the mechanism for nonparoxysmal atrial tachycardia; however, it is not easy or sometimes not possible to determine such mechanisms on the ECG.[5]

Abnormal automaticity and triggered activity are usually grouped together under "automatic atrial tachycardia," even though triggered activity may be paroxysmal and is not, strictly speaking, the same as automaticity (see Chapter 5). The types of atrial tachycardia that have been identified on electrophysiologic study are automatic atrial tachycardia and atrial tachycardia that is due to reentry.[6,7]

There is a great deal of confusion in clinical practice and in the literature about the terminology. The confusion springs from failure to understand mechanisms and to differentiate true atrial tachycardia from paroxysmal supraventricular tachycardia (PSVT) that uses the two AV nodal pathways or the AV node and an accessory pathway for the two types of PSVT reentry circuits. More confusion arises from the habitual use of the terms "PAT" and "PAT with block" (whether paroxysmal or not) for all supraventricular tachycardias, atrial and AV reciprocal, that are not atrial flutter or atrial fibrillation. Important clinical decisions are made regarding emergency and long-term therapy based on our understanding of the mechanisms. As more knowledge is gained about the ECG recognition and the mechanisms of atrial tachycardia through electrophysiologic studies and radiofrequency ablation, the terminology is bound to standardize. Then, of course, it will be a matter of education.

Pediatrics

Atrial tachycardia caused by abnormal automaticity is a more common mechanism in pediatric patients than it is in adults.[8] Some of these children have cardiac tumors or aneurysms. As in the adult, the tachycardia tends to be incessant and resistant to medical management. Children have a slower atrial rate during atrial tachycardia than adults, so that the resultant cardiomyopathy is often reversible. His bundle ablation may be necessary to prevent death if medical management fails.[9]

Automatic atrial tachycardia

Automatic atrial tachycardia exhibits prolonged or incessant episodes of a rapid atrial rhythm in which the rate becomes faster ("warm up") after onset and slows down ("cool down") before termination, a characteristic common to automaticity.[6]

Atrial rate: Less than 200 beats/min; when atrial tachycardia is caused by digitalis excess, the rate increases gradually as the digitalis is continued[7] and ranges from 130 to 250 beats/min.

Atrial rhythm: When associated with AV block, the atrial rhythm is irregular in approximately 50% of cases.[7]

P′ wave: Contour is different from that of the sinus P wave unless the atrial tachycardia is digitalis induced; in that case the P′ wave looks like a sinus P wave. This assessment is best made in lead II, where the P wave is upright and where it can be differentiated from the sawtooth pattern of atrial flutter.

P′P′: There is an isoelectric line between P′ waves seen in all leads as opposed to the sawtooth pattern of atrial flutter in the inferior leads. Although this feature helps to distinguish atrial tachycardia from atrial flutter, when the rates become rapid it may be difficult to differentiate, especially when the conduction ratio is 2:1.

P′R interval: Determined by the rate of the atrial tachycardia.

AV conduction: Block is often present; during AV block the atrial rate is not influenced.

Effect of vagal maneuvers: Atrial tachycardia continues unabated, although the maneuvers do, of course, cause AV block.[7]

Digitalis intoxication atrial tachycardia. When atrial tachycardia is caused by digitalis toxicity, the atrial rate increases and the P′R interval lengthens as the digitalis is continued.[7] Atrial tachycardia with block associated with digitalis toxicity is illustrated in Fig. 7-11. For further discussion and examples, consult Chapter 17.

II

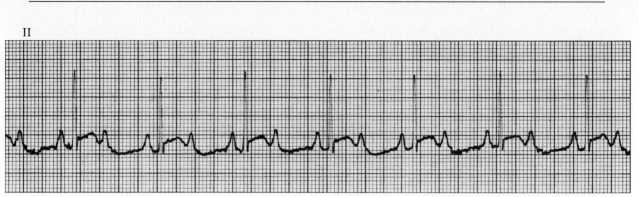

Fig. 7-11. Atrial tachycardia with a ratio 2:1 block.

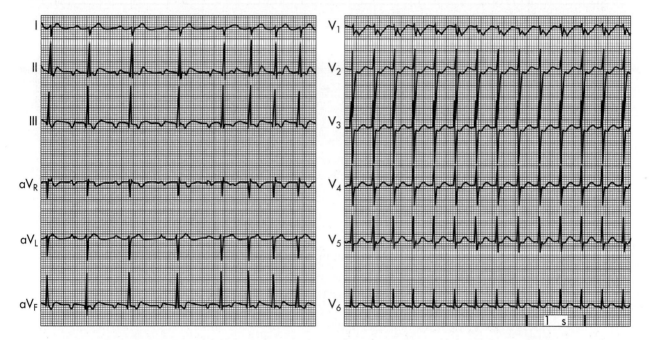

Fig. 7-12. Incessant atrial tachycardia. In the limb leads on the left there is a ratio of 2:1 followed by a ratio 1:1 AV conduction. This patient has been continuously in tachycardia for 12 years and came to medical attention with dilated cardiomyopathy. *(From Wellens HJJ. In Willerson JT, Cohn JN: Cardiovascular medicine, New York, 1995, Churchill Livingstone.)*

Incessant atrial tachycardia. In its incessant form, atrial tachycardia is present more than half the day and can result in dilated cardiomyopathy if untreated (tachycardiomyopathy).[10-13] Incessant atrial tachycardia in a patient with dilated cardiomyopathy is seen in Fig. 7-12. The left ventricular dysfunction is reversible after cure by surgery or radiofrequency ablation.[6,14]

Reentrant atrial tachycardia

Intraatrial reentry (paroxysmal atrial tachycardia) is a rare form of atrial tachycardia (Fig. 7-13) seen primarily in patients who have had previous atrial surgery, typically for the therapy of congenital heart disease.[6]

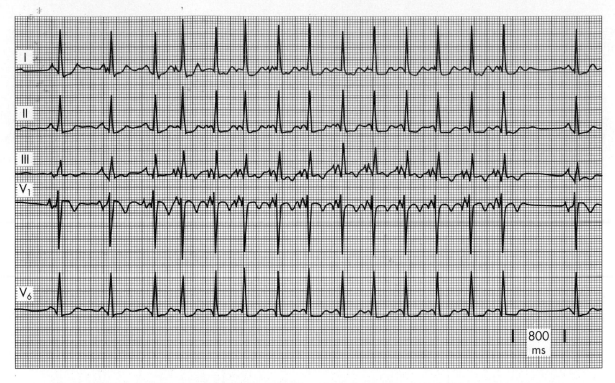

Fig. 7-13. Reentrant atrial tachycardia. The first three beats are preceded by a sinus P wave. The atrial tachycardia begins with the fourth cycle; the configuration of the P waves changes with that beat. *(From Wellens HJJ. In Willerson JT, Cohn JN: Cardiovascular medicine, New York, 1995, Churchill Livingstone.)*

ECG recognition

Atrial rate: About 130 to 180 beats/min.[15]

Rhythm: Usually regular; can be started and stopped with atrial stimulation. Spontaneous termination can be sudden, or it can be preceded by progressive slowing or long-short cycles.[7]

P′ waves: The polarity of the P′ wave is determined by the site of the ectopic focus in the atria.

P′R interval: Normal or prolonged because of digitalis, in which case there may be a gradual prolongation of the PR interval as the heart rate increases. AV dissociation may be present as a result of digitalis toxicity.

QRS complexes: Normal, unless associated with BBB.

AV conduction: Ratio may be 1:1, or there may be atrial tachycardia with block (2:1 ratio, Wenckebach [Mobitz type I]), depending on the atrial rate.

Clinical implications

Atrial tachycardia is a relatively uncommon arrhythmia and an infrequent cause of symptomatic supraventricular tachycardia (SVT). Over a period of 17 years the Wellens group in the Netherlands examined 1834 patients with ECG documentation of SVT; 7% of these patients had atrial tachycardia; one fourth of these cases were of the incessant form. Of patients with incessant atrial tachycardia, 40% came to medical attention with dilated cardiomyopathy.[14] Because incessant long-term atrial tachycardia is especially difficult to control pharmacologically, it can result in progressive cardiac dilation and congestive heart failure. These debilitating conditions are potentially reversible once the arrhythmia focus is ablated or the tachycardia controlled.[12,16-19]

In cases of atrial tachycardia with block the signs, symptoms, and prognosis are usually related to the cardiovascular status. Most of the time atrial tachycardia with block occurs in patients with heart disease (coronary artery disease or cor pulmonale) or in patients taking digitalis (a sign of intoxication), in which case hypokalemia can precipitate the atrial tachycardia.[7] Patients with inferior wall myocardial infarction accompanied by right ventricular dysfunction are more prone to have atrial rhythms than patients with preserved right ventricular function.[20]

Physical findings[7]

First heart sound: Varying intensity with varying AV block.
Jugular venous pulse: Auscultation reveals an excessive number of a waves.
Carotid sinus massage: Causes an increase in the degree of AV block and a stepwise slowing of the ventricular rate without termination of the atrial tachycardia.
In digitalis toxicity: Carotid sinus massage should not be performed (or is performed with extreme caution by an experienced physician); serious ventricular arrhythmias can result.

Treatment

In the incessant form of atrial tachycardia the focus of impulse formation is surgically isolated[12] or ablated with radiofrequency energy.[16,17,21-23] In such cases drug therapy usually fails. Clinical experience has shown that atrial tachycardia in its paroxysmal form may be treated medically with verapamil or a beta blocker.[18]

When atrial tachycardia develops in a patient taking digitalis, the assumption is made that the arrhythmia is due to digitalis toxicity[7]; failure to discontinue the drug can result in death. The mortality rate in such a clinical situation has been shown to be 100%.[24] The patient should be confined to bed, the digitalis withheld, potassium chloride administered orally or intravenously if serum potassium level is not elevated; the patient's condition should be monitored continuously (ECG and hemodynamics), and the patient protected from sympathetic stimulation (complete bed rest) because catecholamines can aggravate the triggered activity responsible for this arrhythmia. If phenytoin is used, a ventricular pacing lead should be in place and the rhythm monitored. Because of its cost, digitalis antibody is usually reserved for patients who are hemodynamically compromised.[25]

MULTIFOCAL (CHAOTIC) ATRIAL TACHYCARDIA

Multifocal or chaotic atrial tachycardia is characterized by multiple shapes of P waves and an irregular rhythm. It occurs relatively infrequently (0.36% of patients admitted to the hospital)[26] and usually in critically ill, elderly patients. Multifocal atrial tachycardia can be seen in Fig. 7-14. In this tracing of lead II at least three different shapes of P waves can be identified.

ECG recognition

Atrial rate: 100 to 130 beats/min.
Rhythm: Irregular.
P waves: Three or more different morphologic appearances in a single ECG lead.

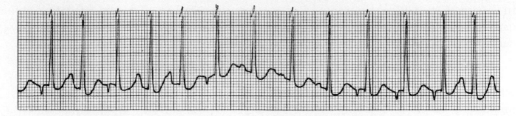

Fig. 7-14. Multifocal atrial tachycardia (lead II). Notice the different shapes of the P′ waves.

PP intervals: Varying; isoelectric PP segment.
PR intervals: Varying.
QRS complexes: Normal unless an intraventricular conduction problem exists.
AV conduction: Usually all P′ waves are conducted to the ventricles.
Summary: Multifocal atrial tachycardia is recognized because of its rapid rate and several P′ shapes, often in a patient with chronic pulmonary disease.

Mechanism

The mechanism for multifocal atrial tachycardia is thought to be triggered activity (see p. 00) because the arrhythmia responds to calcium channel blockers such as verapamil and magnesium sulfate and because the clinical conditions associated with this arrhythmia have in common the cellular potential for triggered activity.[27,28]

Clinical implications and causes

Patients with multifocal atrial tachycardia often have clinically significant pulmonary disease (60%), most commonly chronic obstructive pulmonary disease (COPD). Less commonly pulmonary infections or pulmonary embolism may be present.[26] Although this arrhythmia can occur in childhood, it is most commonly seen in older patients with COPD and may deteriorate into atrial fibrillation.

Multifocal atrial tachycardia is the result not only of the pathophysiologic features of severe pulmonary disease but also of the treatment. For example, right atrial enlargement, hypercapnia, hypoxia, acidosis, adrenergic stimulation, and drugs used for the treatment of pulmonary disease, such as isoproterenol and aminophylline, are all of themselves proarrhythmic. When the diagnosis of multifocal atrial tachycardia is first made, the clinical setting is often that of congestive heart failure. Diabetes, a common condition in patients with this arrhythmia, is present in 24% of patients.[26]

Pediatrics

In neonates and infants this arrhythmia is often mistaken for atrial flutter. It is, however, more persistent than atrial flutter and may be associated with atrial septal defect. If drug therapy is successful in slowing the ventricular rate but not that of the atria, the atria dilate, the arrhythmia is exacerbated, and congestive heart failure results.[29]

Treatment

Therapy is directed at correcting the predisposing cardiac, pulmonary, metabolic, and infectious conditions that have caused the arrhythmia.[26,27] The tachycardia may be suppressed by potassium and magnesium, improvement in oxygenation, ventilation, and the treatment of congestive heart failure.[27] Antiarrhythmic drugs are often ineffective. β-Adrenoreceptor blockers are effective if tolerated, but their use should be avoided in patients with bronchospastic pulmonary disease. Verapamil and amiodarone may also be considered.[7]

REFERENCES

1. Wit AL: Cellular electrophysiologic mechanisms of cardiac arrhythmias, *Ann NY Acad Sci* 432:1, 1986.
2. Wit AL, Rosen MR: Cellular electrophysiology of cardiac arrhythmias. In Josephson ME, Wellens HJJ, eds: *Tachycardias: mechanisms, diagnosis, treatment,* Philadelphia, 1984, Lea & Febiger.
3. Wennmalm A, Wennmalm M: Coffee, catecholamines and cardiac arrhythmia, *Clin Physiol* 9:201, 1989.
4. Wellens HJJ, Supraventricular tachycardias. In Willerson JT, Cohn JN, eds: *Cardiovascular medicine,* Boston, 1994, Churchill Livingstone.
5. Wellens HJJ, Burgada P, Vanagt E et al: New studies with triggered automaticity. In Harrison DC, ed: *Cardiac arrhythmias: a decade of progress,* Boston, 1981, GK Hall.
6. Lesh MD: Radiofrequency catheter ablation of atrial tachycardia and flutter. In Zipes DP, Jalife J, eds: *Cardiac electrophysiology from cell to bedside,* ed 2, Philadelphia, 1995, WB Saunders.
7. Zipes DP: Specific arrhythmias: diagnosis and treatment. In Braunwald E, eds: *Heart disease,* ed 4, Philadelphia, 1992, WB Saunders.
8. Ludomirsky A, Garson A Jr: Supraventricular tachycardia. In Gillette PC, Garson A Jr, eds: *Pediatric arrhythmias: electrophysiology and pacing,* Philadelphia, 1990, WB Saunders.
9. Gillette PC, Zeigler VL, Case CL: Pediatric arrhythmias: are they different? In Zipes DP, Jalife J, eds: *Cardiac electrophysiology from cell to bedside,* ed 2, Philadelphia, 1995, WB Saunders.
10. Engel TR, Bush CA, Schaal SF: Tachycardia aggravated heart disease, *Ann Intern Med* 80:384, 1974.
11. Packer DL, Bardy GH, Worly SJ et al: Tachycardia induced cardiomyopathy: a reversible form of left ventricular dysfunction, *Am J Cardiol* 57:563, 1986.
12. Prager NA, Cox JL, Lindsay BD et al: Long-term effectiveness of surgical treatment of ectopic atrial tachycardia, *J Am Coll Cardiol* 22:85, 1993.
13. Graffigna A, Vigano M, Pagani F, Salerno G: Surgical treatment for ectopic atrial tachycardia, *Ann Thorac Surg* 54:338, 1992.
14. Wellens HJJ, Rodriquez LM, Smeets JLRM et al: Tachycardiomyopathy in patients with supraventricular tachycardia with emphasis on atrial fibrillation. In Olsson SB, Allessie MA, Campbell RWF, eds: *Atrial fibrillation: mechanisms and therapeutic strategies,* Armonk, NY, 1994, Futura.
15. Haines DE, Di Marco JP: Sustained intraatrial reentrant tachycardia: clinical, electrocardiographic and electrophysiologic characteristics and long-term follow-up, *J Am Coll Cardiol* 15:1345, 1990.
16. Kay GN, Chong F, Epstein AE et al: Radiofrequency ablation for treatment of primary atrial tachycardias, *J Am Coll Cardiol* 21:901, 1993.
17. Tracy CM, Swartz JF, Fletcher RD et al: Radiofrequency catheter ablation of ectopic atrial tachycardia using paced activation sequence mapping, *J Am Coll Cardiol* 21:910, 1993.
18. Wellens HJJ: Atrial tachycardia: how important is the mechanism? *Circulation* 90:1576, 1994.
19. Packer DL, Bardy GH, Worley SJ et al: Tachycardia-induced cardiomyopathy: a reversible form of left ventricular dysfunction, *Am J Cardiol* 57:563, 1986.
20. Rechavia E, Strasberg B, Mager A et al: The incidence of atrial arrhythmias during inferior wall myocardial infarction with and without right ventricular involvement, *Am Heart J* 124:387, 1992.
21. Walsh EP, Saul P, Hulse E et al: Transcatheter ablation of ectopic atrial tachycardia in young patients using radiofrequency current, *Circulation* 86:1138, 1992.
22. Zipes DP: Arrhythmias on the endangered list, *J Am Coll Cardiol* 21:918, 1993.
23. Margolis PD, Roman CA, Moulton KP et al: Radiofrequency catheter ablation of left and right ectopic atrial tachycardia *Circulation* 82(suppl 3):718, 1990 (abstract).
24. Driefus LS, McKnight EH, Katz M et al: Digitalis intolerance, *Geriatrics* 18:494, 1963.
25. Wellens HJJ, Conover M: *The ECG in emergency decision making,* St Louis, 1992, Mosby.
26. Kastor JA: Multifocal atrial tachycardia, *N Engl J Med* 322:1713, 1990.
27. Scher DL, Arsura EL: Multifocal atrial tachycardia: mechanisms, clinical correlates, and treatment, *Am Heart J* 118:574, 1990.
28. Iseri LT, Fairshter RD, Hardemann JL, Brodsky MA: Magnesium and potassium therapy in multifocal atrial tachycardia, *Am Heart J* 110:789, 1985.
29. Gillette PC, Zeigler VL, Case CL: Pediatric arrhythmias: are they different? In Zipes DP, Jalife J, eds: *Cardiac electrophysiology from cell to bedside,* ed 2, Philadelphia, 1995, WB Saunders.

C H A P T E R
8
Atrial Fibrillation

ECG Recognition   96
Risk   98
Mechanism   98
Clinical Features   100
Ventricular Response to Atrial Fibrillation:
   "Controlled" or "Uncontrolled"   100
Concealed Conduction   101
Causes   101
Risk of Thromboembolism   101
Pediatrics   101
Symptoms   101
Physical Assessment   102
Treatment Goals and Categories   102
Treatment of Acute Atrial
   Fibrillation   102

Treatment of Subacute Atrial
   Fibrillation   105
Treatment of Chronic Atrial
   Fibrillation   105
Antithrombotic Therapy   106
Radiofrequency Ablation   106
Surgery   106
Treatment of Postoperative Atrial
   Fibrillation   106
Digitalis Toxicity in Atrial
   Fibrillation   107
Atrial Fibrillation with an Accessory
   Pathway   107
Summary   107

Atrial fibrillation is the disorganized electrical activity of the atria resulting in irregular heartbeat, hemodynamic compromise, and risk of thromboembolism. Functionally, the atria are quivering chambers connecting the great vessels with the ventricles. When atrial fibrillation occurs in the absence of any other clinical evidence to suggest a primary cardiac disorder, it is known as idiopathic or *lone atrial fibrillation.*[1]

ECG RECOGNITION

Heart rate: Ranges from 100 to 180 beats/min in uncontrolled atrial fibrillation; this rate is less when a rate control drug such as verapamil, a beta blocker, or digitalis is being taken. Paroxysmal atrial fibrillation is shown in Fig. 8-1.

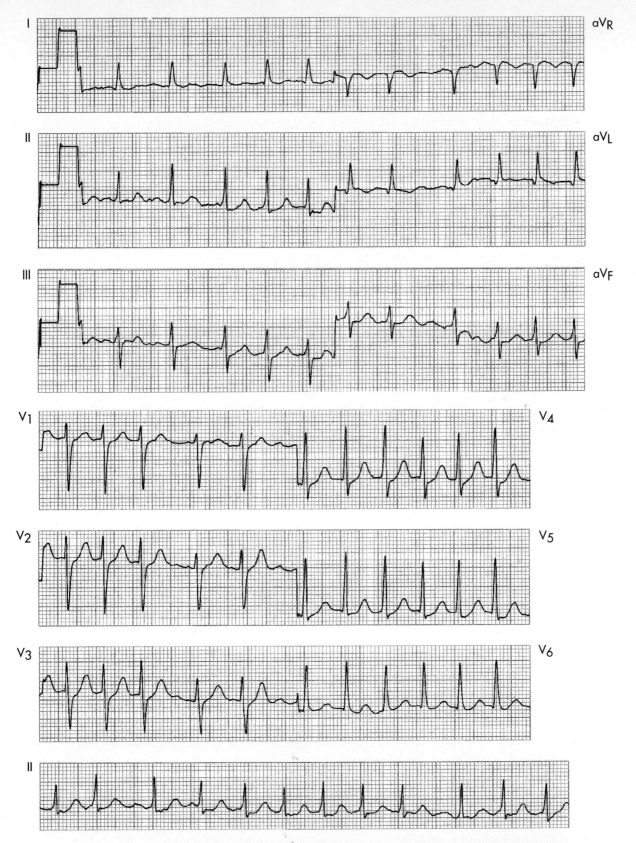

Fig. 8-1. Atrial fibrillation in a 56-year-old woman. This was the first episode for this patient of the paroxysmal type of atrial fibrillation (2 hours' duration). The patient is taking no medications. The fine fibrillatory line and the irregular ventricular response of approximately 135 to 140 beats/min are evident.

Rhythm: Irregular unless complete atrioventricular (AV) block is present or the ventricles are being dominated by a junctional or ventricular focus.

NOTE: The term "irregularly irregular" is sometimes used to differentiate random irregularity from the *group beating* ("regularly irregular") seen in one of the rhythms of atrial fibrillation resulting from digitalis toxicity (i.e., junctional tachycardia with Wenckebach exit block, described in Chapter 17). If the one were simply called "group beating," it would be unnecessary to use such burdensome and somewhat confusing terminology because the other would then simply be "irregular." The term "irregularly irregular" becomes an especially unacceptable usage *(and hazardous for the patient)* when employed by those who are unable to distinguish such a rhythm from a regularly irregular rhythm or regular irregularity.

P waves: Absent; a coarse or fine fibrillatory line is present; the fibrillatory waves ("f" waves) that characterize this rhythm represent chaotic atrial activity. If the fibrillatory line is very fine, the f waves are not seen.

QRS complexes: Narrow unless bundle branch block is also present.

Summary: Atrial fibrillation is recognized on the ECG because of absence of P waves and an irregular ventricular response (in the absence of complete AV block or digitalis toxicity).

RISK

Paroxysmal atrial fibrillation is associated with a lower stroke risk than is the chronic form.[2] In a recent study of 344 patients with chronic atrial fibrillation it was found that mortality depends on the type and severity of underlying heart disease rather than persistence of the arrhythmia.[3] In patients with no identifiable risk factors (lone atrial fibrillation) the prognosis seems generally favorable, as long as old age and other risk factors are excluded.[4]

MECHANISM

Atrial fibrillation can be generated and maintained by one or more rapidly firing ectopic foci and an irregular and fractionated type of intraatrial reentry as a basis for the continuity of impulse conduction.[5,6] These multiple waves die out at the AV ring, collide with other waves to become wavelets, or meet with refractory tissue and reverse direction by 180 degrees or a full 360 degrees to form a short-lived, closed local circuit. Fig. 8-2 diagrammatically illustrates the atrial activity of atrial fibrillation and the resulting irregular ventricular rhythm.

On the surface ECG atrial fibrillation is divided into coarse and fine fibrillation. Using a single bipolar electrogram, Waldo[7] has divided atrial fibrillation into four different types based on the type of atrial complexes and the disruptions of the electrograms between complexes. Type I has discrete complexes and a clear isoelectric baseline; type II also has discrete complexes but with a disturbed baseline; type III has no discrete atrial complexes; and type IV alternates between type III and the others.

Another group[8,9] has identified the following types based on mapping studies using 244 unipolar electrodes in 25 patients:

Type I: The right atrium is activated by broad wave fronts propagating rapidly and without significant conduction delay.

Type II: There is a higher degree of conduction delay and intraatrial block.

CONCEALED CONDUCTION

Concealed conduction is electrical activity that is not seen on the surface ECG. During atrial fibrillation the erratic, rapid atrial activity results in incomplete penetration of the AV node, so not all impulses are propagated to the ventricular myocardium. Such impulses do, however, leave the AV conduction tissue refractory, resulting in irregular RR intervals.

CAUSES

Atrial fibrillation is often seen in the following settings. Assessment of these conditions is made with the ECG, chest x-ray, thyroid profile, and patient history.

Acute MI

Long-standing hypertension

Thyrotoxicosis (10% to 20%)

Left atrial stretch that is due to mitral stenosis resulting from rheumatic heart disease or mitral regurgitation

After cardiac surgery (30%), especially in elderly patients.

Idiopathic or "lone" atrial fibrillation (absence of apparent heart disease)

Alcohol intake, chronic or acute, moderate to heavy

RISK OF THROMBOEMBOLISM

Thrombi form inside the left atrium because of a stasis of blood. When the thrombus embolizes, it may lodge in the brain, causing a "stroke," which often leaves the patient suddenly and severely disabled. Approximately 70,000 strokes per year are caused by emboli from the fibrillating left atrium, and it is estimated that about one third of all persons in atrial fibrillation will have a peripheral vascular event.[29] The risk of embolism following pharmacologic or electrical cardioversion is 1% to 5%; this risk is decreased by several weeks of anticoagulation therapy with warfarin before cardioversion.[30] Furthermore, patients with chronic or recurrent paroxysmal atrial fibrillation are exposed over a lifetime to a risk of thromboembolism that may be as high as 30% to 40%. Several studies have shown that long-term anticoagulation therapy with warfarin is effective in reducing this risk of stroke.[31-32]

PEDIATRICS

Atrial fibrillation is rare in the pediatric age-group and is characterized by rapid, chaotic atrial depolarization and a rapid ventricular response sometimes exceeding 300 beats/min. On the surface ECG there may be grossly irregular atrial fibrillatory waves, or they may not be seen.

SYMPTOMS

Symptoms range from an awareness of palpitations to hemodynamic collapse and depend on many factors, especially the cardiac status. The rate and irregularity of the ventricular rhythm, combined with the loss of AV synchrony, all contribute to the patient's hemodynamic status. Usually atrial fibrillation is tolerated well once the heart rate is controlled. However, some patients show new or exacerbated symptoms of congestive heart failure because of the reduction in cardiac output associated with the arrhythmia. Exercise intolerance may also develop.

In patients with normal or hypertrophic left ventricles (i.e., relatively small ventricular volumes) the loss of the atrial contribution to diastolic filling ("atrial kick") may result in a 25% to 30% reduction in cardiac output, whereas with moderate to severe compromises in left ventricular function the atrial kick contributes less to ventricular filling and cardiac output. In such patients the cardiac output may decrease by only 5% to 15%. The exacerbation of angina in some patients is due to increased oxygen demand, which results from the increased heart rate.

In patients with paroxysmal atrial fibrillation, as in paroxysmal supraventricular tachycardia, the tachycardia may be associated with polyuria, which may be profound enough to cause hypovolemic hypotension in the period following return to sinus rhythm. Oral fluid intake and electrolyte replacement are usually enough to correct this symptom.

PHYSICAL ASSESSMENT

Physical assessment includes checking for thromboemboli (peripheral, coronary, pulmonary, or cerebral) and looking for signs of decreased cardiac output such as hypotension, a pulse deficit, signs of heart failure, and decreased cerebral oxygen supply (presyncope or syncope). Other physical findings include varying intensity of the first heart sound, absence of *a* waves in the jugular pulse, and an irregular pulse.

When comparing the apical and radial pulses there is often a discrepancy called a pulse deficit. The irregular ventricular rhythm creates different ventricular filling volumes with each cycle, which in turn result in a variation in stroke volumes. Thus the beats following the shorter cycles are not strong enough to open the aortic valve or to transmit an arterial pressure wave that can be felt at the radial pulse, but they can be heard with the stethoscope at the apex.[34] Because of this, the heart rate is best evaluated by listening for a full minute with your stethoscope at the apex. The ECG monitor measures for a few seconds and multiplies, giving you a false reading.

The development of a regular rhythm in a patient with atrial fibrillation may be a good sign (conversion to sinus rhythm) or a bad sign (junctional or ventricular tachycardia, often resulting from digitalis toxicity). A regular rhythm may also be present in atrial flutter with a fixed conduction ratio, but uncomplicated atrial fibrillation is never regular.

TREATMENT GOALS AND CATEGORIES

Treatment of atrial fibrillation has three main goals and three categories. Treatment goals are control of the ventricular response, anticoagulation for prophylaxis of systemic thromboembolism, and return of the atria to sinus rhythm. Treatment categories are acute, subacute, and chronic atrial fibrillation.

TREATMENT OF ACUTE ATRIAL FIBRILLATION

In acute atrial fibrillation there is usually a rapid ventricular response, and there are two treatment choices: rate control with drugs or emergency direct current (DC) synchronized cardioversion.

Rate control drugs in current use are digoxin, sometimes combined with beta blockers, and calcium channel blockers (discussed later). Although these drugs are good AV nodal blocking agents, they do not convert atrial fibrillation to a normal sinus rhythm. Verapamil or diltiazem work fastest and is preferred by many physicians. Some physicians use a reduced dosage of digoxin in combination with a beta blocker or verapamil to avoid digitalis toxicity.

Antiarrhythmic drugs have an adverse effect on mortality rates[35,36] and are therefore considered with caution and only if unacceptable symptoms develop despite rate control drugs. One suggestion[37] for maintaining sinus rhythm is flecainide; if this fails, quinidine; and if this fails, amiodarone. New information suggests that flecainide, amiodarone, and sotalol may be more effective than the standard antiarrhythmic drugs.[36, 38-40]

Digoxin

When left ventricular function is impaired, digoxin remains the drug of choice for rate control. In the past, cardiac glycosides were the only agents used for rate control in acute and chronic atrial fibrillation. Digitalis increases vagal tone, which in turn reduces the calcium current in AV nodal cells, thus slowing AV conduction. During exercise digitalis may not be enough to control the ventricular rate because increased sympathetic tone and reduced vagal tone overcome the effects of digitalis; calcium channel blockers and beta blockers are logical complements.[41]

Administration. Digoxin is given intravenously in new-onset rapid atrial fibrillation. It has a half-life of 1.5 to 3 hours, achieving rate control at the AV node by dose-dependent vagal stimulation. Usually an initial dose of 0.25 to 0.50 mg is given intravenously followed by 0.25 mg intravenously every 4 to 8 hours up to 1.0 mg in the first 24 hours.

Advantages. Advantages of digoxin are that it is inexpensive, hemodynamically tolerated, and easy to administer.

Disadvantages. The two main disadvantages of digoxin are a narrow therapeutic window and the possibility of toxic effects preceding the desired therapeutic effect. Other disadvantages include the following:

1. Difficulty in acute titration of the dose to achieve a predictable heart rate
2. Significant interactions with other drugs used to treat atrial fibrillation (e.g., verapamil, quinidine, amiodarone, and procainamide)
3. Inability to control ventricular response, even with high doses, in the face of heightened sympathetic tone, such as during acute illness or stress[37,42]

The significant disadvantages just listed have led some to conclude that the emergency use of intravenous (IV) digoxin for ventricular rate control in atrial fibrillation or atrial flutter is rarely indicated, even after decades of use for this purpose.[43]

Warning. Digitalis, like calcium channel blockers, is not given for atrial fibrillation in patients with accessory pathways (Wolff-Parkinson-White [WPW] syndrome). In 30% of patients it shortens the refractory period of the accessory pathway, causing the ventricular rate to accelerate.[41,44] In addition, a prolongation of AV conduction over the AV node reduces the number of impulses entering the ventricles by that path and in turn reduces the number of impulses that, in retrograde fashion, penetrate the accessory pathway to render it refractory to some of the fibrillatory atrial activity.[45] Procainamide is the drug of choice for patients with atrial fibrillation and an accessory pathway. If procainamide is not successful, this means that the refractory period of the accessory pathway is excessively short and other antiarrhythmics will not work either. The patient should receive cardioversion immediately and be referred for radiofrequency ablation.[46] For a discussion of WPW syndrome and its arrhythmias see Chapter 23.

Beta blockers

When coronary artery disease and hypertension are present, beta blockers may be chosen for rate control in acute and chronic atrial fibrillation. Esmolol is a β_1-selective blocking agent with a half-life of 9 minutes. Heart rate control is similar to that of verapamil.[47]

Advantages. Advantages of beta blockers include swift action (IV route), lower mortality in patients with MI, and antiischemic and antihypertensive properties.

Disadvantages. Symptomatic hypotension occurs relatively frequently, necessitating the termination of the infusion. Careful observation and dose titration are indicated.[48] Beta blockers are of limited use in patients with bronchospastic lung disease or left ventricular dysfunction.[42]

Calcium channel blockers

Verapamil and diltiazem are good rate control agents when there is hypertension or angina; both have antiischemic and antihypertensive properties but lack the effect of beta blockers on mortality rates in MI. The negative inotropic effect of diltiazem is less than that of verapamil, although verapamil is a better AV blocking agent.[42]

Diltiazem has been shown to slow the ventricular response during atrial fibrillation directly by slowing AV nodal conduction in a use-dependent fashion and indirectly by increasing the potential zone of concealed conduction in the AV node in a dose-dependent fashion.[49,50] The term *use dependent* means that the drug has more effect at faster heart rates than at slower rates. Conversion to sinus rhythm is not achieved by calcium channel blockers; in fact, they may have a negative effect, since they, like digoxin, shorten the atrial action potential duration.

Administration. Diltiazem is given as a 20- to 25-mg bolus (0.25 mg/kg body weight) over 2 minutes followed by an infusion of 5 mg/hour. If the heart rate goal is not achieved, the dosage is titrated upward at approximately 3- to 4-hour intervals until the goal is reached. Reduction in heart rate during the 24-hour infusion ranges from 30% to 40%, with a low incidence of side effects.[51] The IV infusion may be used to obtain heart rate control in the acute setting and to allow time to make decisions about the need for anticoagulation and the method and means for conversion to sinus rhythm. The heart rate is evaluated with continuous ECG monitoring during the bolus and infusion. The blood pressure is monitored frequently. If furosemide is also ordered, a second IV tubing is needed, since the two drugs are incompatible in the same tubing.

Advantages. Besides the desirable effects of diltiazem on AV conduction already mentioned, it has the following advantages:
1. No known clinically important interaction with digoxin or class IA agents
2. Relatively mild negative inotropic effects (compared with verapamil)[52]

3. Well tolerated during short-term IV infusions (even in patients with conges-tive heart failure)

4. Absence of delayed drug accumulation during prolonged administration

Disadvantages. A small percentage of patients have symptomatic hypotension. The negative inotropic effect of diltiazem is considered in patients with impaired left ventricular function.

Warning. Calcium channel blockers are not given for atrial fibrillation in patients with accessory pathways. The drop in blood pressure associated with these drugs causes reflex catecholamines, which in turn shorten the refractory period of the accessory pathway, causing the ventricular rate to accelerate.[53] Procainamide is the drug of choice for this clinical setting.

Calcium channel blockers are also contraindicated in patients with second- or third-degree AV block, sick sinus syndrome without a pacemaker, severe hypotension, and cardiogenic shock and when beta blockers are a factor.

DC cardioversion

For a patient with acute hemodynamic instability, immediate synchronized electrical cardioversion is indicated; sedation is used when possible and clinically safe.[42]

In a study of 704 patients admitted to emergency departments with atrial fibrillation,[54] the most likely to convert to sinus rhythm were patients with idiopathic atrial fibrillation (93.9%), WPW syndrome (88.8%), atherosclerotic cardiovascular disease (71.6%), and thyrotoxicosis (63.2%; with antithyroid management, conversion and maintenance of sinus rhythm are expected in most cases). Patients with rheumatic heart disease and chronic obstructive pulmonary disease had the lowest percentage of successful conversion to sinus rhythm—46% and 55%, respectively.

TREATMENT OF SUBACUTE ATRIAL FIBRILLATION

Subacute atrial fibrillation is present when the ventricular rate is controlled but atrial fibrillation persists. Reversible causes are evaluated, and then cardioversion is considered. The most common reversible causes are drugs and thyroid disease.

If DC cardioversion is to be attempted, when time permits, several weeks of anticoagulation are recommended before pharmacologic or electrical cardioversion to reduce the risk of thromboembolism. The patient scheduled for DC cardioversion is receiving a rate control drug (no antiarrhythmic drugs) and is sedated.

TREATMENT OF CHRONIC ATRIAL FIBRILLATION

Chronic atrial fibrillation may be persistent or intermittent. Treatment consists of rate control, attempt at a normal sinus rhythm, and antithrombotic therapy.

Rate control

Rate control is necessary in most patients and is achieved by digoxin, beta blockers, or verapamil. Digoxin is the least expensive and the easiest to take. If this does not provide adequate rate control with exercise or increased sympathetic tone, beta blockers or verapamil is considered.

DC cardioversion

If the patient is asymptomatic and has a controlled ventricular rate and one attempt at cardioversion has failed, many physicians leave the patient in atrial fibrillation.

Direct current cardioversion is more likely to be successful if the following conditions are met:

1. Left atrial size of less than 60 mm
2. Duration of atrial fibrillation of less than 1 year
3. Normal mitral valve
4. Absence of major pulmonary dysfunction
5. Absence of major left ventricular dysfunction

Contraindications to DC cardioversion are digoxin toxicity, untreated hyperthyroidism, sick sinus syndrome, hypokalemia, and prior history of recurrent atrial fibrillation after successful cardioversion.

The only major risk of DC cardioversion is embolism; lesser risks are chest wall burns, hypotension (3% to 4%), and sinus node dysfunction or ventricular arrhythmias. Patients who have been in atrial fibrillation for more than 2 days are started on warfarin therapy for 3 to 4 weeks before attempted cardioversion.

ANTITHROMBOTIC THERAPY

Antithrombotic studies all show the following:

1. There is significant reduction in strokes with anticoagulation.[31,55,56]
2. There is low risk of hemorrhage if warfarin therapy is monitored carefully by experienced nurses (less than 2% risk of major hemorrhage per year)[57,58]
3. In young people (under 50 to 60 years of age) with no associated heart disease the risk of strokes is very low, even without antithrombotic therapy.
4. One study[59] suggests that aspirin (325 mg daily) is as effective as warfarin in most patients with atrial fibrillation, but perhaps not in patients who are over 75 years of age.

RADIOFREQUENCY ABLATION

Occasionally rate control cannot be accomplished by drug therapy. In such patients complete heart block may be accomplished by transvenous radiofrequency ablation of the AV junction; an implanted pacemaker is generally required following this procedure.[60-62]

SURGERY

Surgical treatment of atrial fibrillation is controversial. There are two procedures, the Maze procedure[63,64] and "the corridor operation."[65,66]

TREATMENT OF POSTOPERATIVE ATRIAL FIBRILLATION

Given an adequate ventricular function, IV beta blockers or verapamil are used to slow the ventricular rate. The therapeutic index for digitalis in postoperative patients is especially narrow given the high circulating catecholamine level. Some surgeons postpone DC cardioversion until 7 to 10 days after surgery, when the risk of the arrhythmia returning is less. Anticoagulation therapy is usually not initiated in the early postoperative period because of the risk of bleeding from the surgical wounds.[17]

DIGITALIS TOXICITY IN ATRIAL FIBRILLATION

The ECG signs of digitalis toxicity in patients with atrial fibrillation include regularization or group beating of the ventricular rhythm. The mortality rate with such rhythms is 100%. The mechanism, ECG recognition, clinical implications, and emergency treatment of digitalis toxicity are illustrated and discussed in detail in Chapter 17.

ATRIAL FIBRILLATION WITH AN ACCESSORY PATHWAY

Atrial fibrillation with conduction over an accessory pathway is recognized because of a broad QRS tachycardia that is irregular. It is the second most common arrhythmia in patients with WPW syndrome. Without knowledgeable emergency intervention, such an event may be terminal as a result of the very rapid heart rate that results. The mechanism, ECG recognition, emergency treatment, and cure of this life-threatening arrhythmia are covered in Chapter 23.

SUMMARY

Atrial fibrillation is recognized on the ECG because of absence of P waves and an irregular ventricular response, resulting in a drop in cardiac output up to 20%, a tendency to develop thromboembolism, and an increased mortality rate. This condition may be acute with a rapid, uncontrolled ventricular response; subacute with a controlled ventricular rate but persistent atrial fibrillation; or chronic. Treatment involves antithrombotic therapy, ventricular rate control, and attempts to convert to normal sinus rhythm.

Rate control drugs in current use are digoxin, beta blockers, and calcium channel blockers. If digoxin is used, it is usually combined with a beta blocker or verapamil to avoid digitalis toxicity. Antiarrhythmic drugs are avoided because of high mortality rates associated with their use. DC cardioversion is indicated when there is acute hemodynamic instability; in chronic asymptomatic individuals usually one attempt is made to achieve sinus rhythm.

REFERENCES

1. Evans W, Swann P: Lone auricular fibrillation, *Br Heart J* 16:189, 1954.
2. Kannel WB, Abbott RD, Savage DD, McNamara PM: Coronary heart disease and atrial fibrillation: the Framingham Study, *Am Heart J* 106:389, 1983.
3. Van Gelder IC, Hilege HL, Gosselink M, Crijns HJ: Mortality in patients with atrial fibrillation is related to the underlying heart disease and not to the arrhythmia, *Circulation* 90:I-541, (abstract 2914) 1994.
4. Ruffy R: Atrial fibrillation. In Zipes DP, Jalife J, eds: *Cardiac electrophysiology from cell to bedside,* ed 2, Philadelphia, 1995, WB Saunders.
5. Allessie MA, Lammers WJEP, Bonke FIM, Hollen J: Experimental evaluation of Moe's multiple wavelet hypothesis of atrial fibrillation. In Zipes DP, Jalife J, eds: *Cardiac arrhythmias,* New York, 1985, Grune & Stratton.

6. Falk RH, Podrid PJ: *Atrial fibrillation: mechanism and management,* New York, 1991, Raven Press.

7. Waldo AL: Atrial fibrillation following open heart surgery. In Olsson SB, Allessie MA, Campbell RWF, eds: *Atrial fibrillation: mechanisms and therapeutic strategies,* Mount Kisco, NY, 1994, Futura.

8. Konings KTS, Kirchhof CJHJ, Smeets JRLM et al: High density mapping of electrically induced atrial fibrillation in man, *Circulation* 89:1665, 1994.

9. Allessie MA: Reentrant machanisms underlying atrial fibrillation. In Zipes DP, Jalife J, eds: *Cardiac electrophysiology from cell to bedside,* ed 2, Philadelphia, 1995, WD Saunders.

10. Gosselink ATM, Crijns HJGM, Hamer HPM et al: Changes in left and right atrial size after cardioversion of atrial fibrillation: role of mitral valve disease, *J Am Coll Cardiol* 22:1666, 1993.

11. Sanfilippo AJ, Abascal VM, Sheenan M et al: Atrial enlargement as a consequence of atrial fibrillation, *Circulation* 82:792, 1990.

12. Hod H, Lew AS, Keltai M et al: Early atrial fibrillation during evolving myocardial infarction: a consequence of impaired left atrial perfusion, *Circulation* 75:146, 1987.

13. Sugiura T, Iwasaka T, Takahashi N et al: Atrial fibrillation in inferior wall Q-wave acute myocardial infarction, *Am J Cardiol* 67:1135, 1991.

14. Sugiura T, Iwasaka T, Takahashi N et al: Factors associated with atrial fibrillation in Q wave anterior myocardial infarction, *Am Heart J* 121:1409, 1991.

15. The National Heart, Lung and Blood Institute Working Group on Atrial Fibrillation: Atrial fibrillation: current understandings and research imperatives, *J Am Coll Cardiol* 22:1830, 1993.

16. Albers GW, Atwood JE, Hirsch J et al: Stroke prevention in nonvalvular atrial fibrillation, *Ann Intern Med* 115:727, 1991.

17. Antman EM: Medical management of the patient undergoing cardiac surgery. In Braunwald E, ed: *Heart disease,* ed 4, Philadelphia, 1992, WB Saunders.

18. Coumel P, Attuel P, Leclercq JF: Arhythmies auriculaires d'origine vagale ou catécholergique: effects comparés du traitement bêtabloqueur et phénomènes d'échappement, *Arch Mal Coeur Vaiss* 75:373, 1982.

19. Rothberger CJ, Winterberg H: Vorhofflimmern und Arhythmia perpetua, *Wien Klin Wochenschr* 22:839, 1909.

20. Moe, GK, Abildskov, JA: Observations on the ventricular dysrhythmia associated with atrial fibrillation in the dog heart, *Circ Res* 14:447, 1964.

21. Langendorf R, Pick A, Katz LN: Ventricular response in atrial fibrillation: role of concealed conduction in the AV junction, *Circulation* 32:69, 1965.

22. Moore EN: Observations on concealed conduction in atrial fibrillation, *Circ Res* 21:201, 1967.

23. Yamada K, Okajima M, Hori K et al: On the genesis of the absolute ventricular arrhythmia associated with atrial fibrillation, *Circ Res* 22:707, 1968.

24. Kirsh JA, Sahakian AV, Baerman JM, Swiryn S: Ventricular response to atrial fibrillation: role of atrioventricular conduction pathways, *J Am Coll Cardiol* 12:1265, 1988.

25. Zipes DP, Mendez C, Moe GK: Evidence for summation and voltage dependency in rabbit atrioventricular nodal fibers, *Circ Res* 32:170, 1973.

26. Mazgalef T, Dreifus LS, Bianchi J, Michelson EL: Atrioventricular nodal conduction during atrial fibrillation in rabbit heart, *Am J Physiol* 243:H754, 1982.

27. Levy MN, Martin P: Parasympathetic control of the heart. In Randall WC, ed: *Nervous control of cardiovascular function,* New York, 1984, Oxford University.

28. Rawles JM: What is meant by "controlled" ventricular rate in atrial fibrillation? *Br Heart J* 63:157, 1990.

29. Halperin JL, Hart RG: Atrial fibrillation and stroke: New ideas, persisting dilemmas, *Stroke* 19:937, 1988.

30. Bjerkelund CJ, Ornigh OM: The efficacy of anticoagulant therapy in preventing embolism related to D.C. electrical conversion of atrial fibrillation, *Am J Cardiol* 23:208, 1969.

31. Peterson P, Boysen G, Godtfredsen J et al: Placebo-controlled, randomized trial of warfarin and aspirin for prevention of thromboembolic complications in chronic atrial fibrillation: the Copenhagen AFASAK Study, *Lancet* 1:175, 1989.

32. Stroke Prevention in Atrial Fibrillation Study Group Investigators: Preliminary report of the stroke prevention in atrial fibrillation study: special report, *N Engl J Med* 322:863, 1990.

33. Boston Area Anticoagulation Trial for Atrial Fibrillation Investigators: The effect of low-dose warfarin on the risk of stroke in patients with nonrheumatic atrial fibrillation, *N Engl J Med* 33:1505, 1990.

34. Zipes DP: Specific arhythmias: diagnosis and treatment. In Braunwald E, ed: *Heart disease,* ed 4, Philadelphia, 1992, WB Saunders.

35. Karlson BW, Herlitz J, Edvardsson N, Olsson SB: Prophylactic treatment after electroconversion of atrial fibrillation, *Clin Cardiol* 13:279, 1990.

36. Coplen SE, Antman EM, Berlin JA et al: Efficacy and safety of quinidine therapy for maintenance of sinus rhythm after cardioversion: a meta-analysis of randomized control trials *Circulation* 82:1106, 1990 (published erratum appears in *Circulation* 83:714, 1991).
37. McAnulty JH: Treatment of atrial fibrillations. American Heart Assoc Maine Affiliate 44th Annual Scientific Session, Portland, Maine, Jan 29-30, 1994.
38. Crijns HJ, Van Gelden IC, Van Gilst WH et al: Serial antiarrhythmic drug treatment to maintain sinus rhythm after electrical cardioversion for chronic atrial fibrillation or atrial flutter, *Am J Cardiol* 68:335, 1991.
39. Flaker GC, Blacksheer JL, McBride R et al and SPAF Investigators: Antiarrhythmic drug therapy and cardiac mortality in atrial fibrillation, *J Am Coll Cardiol* 20:527, 1992.
40. Gosselink AM, Crijns HJ, Van Gelden IC et al: Low dose amiodarone for maintenance of sinus rhythm after cardioversion of atrial fibrillation, *JAMA* 246:3289, 1992.
41. Rosen MR, Strauss HC, Janse MJ: The classification of antiarrhythmic drugs. In Zipes DP, Jalife J, eds: *Cardiac electrophysiology from cell to bedside,* ed 2, Philadelphia, 1995, WB Saunders.
42. Blazing MA, Morris JJ Jr: Atrial fibrillation: conventional wisdom reappraised, *Heart Dis Stroke,* March, April:78, 1992.
43. Ewy GA: Urgent parenteral digoxin: a requiem, *J Am Coll Cardiol* 15:1248, 1990.
44. Wellens HJJ, Currer F: Effect of digitalis on atrioventricular conduction and circus movement tachycardia in patients with Wolff-Parkinson-White syndrome, *Circulation* 47:1229, 1973.
45. Falk RH: Proarrhythmic responses to atrial antiarrhythmic therapy. In Falk RH, Podrid PJ, eds: *Atrial fibrillation: mechanisms and management,* New York, 1992, Raven Press.
46. Wellens HJJ, Conover M: *The ECG in emergency decision making,* Philadelphia, 1992, WB Saunders.
47. Platia EV, Michelson EL, Porterfield JD, Das G: Esmolol versus verapamil in the acute treatment of atrial fibrillation or atrial flutter, *Am J Cardiol* 63:925, 1989.
48. Greet GS, Ramirez NM, Fananapazir L et al: Bolus esmolol in the treatment of supraventricular tachycardias, *Circulation* 76(suppl 4):IV-67, 1987.
49. Ellenbogen KA, German LD, O'Callaghan WG et al: Frequency-dependent effects of verapamil on atrioventricular nodal conduction in man, *Circulation* 72:344, 1985.
50. Talajic M, Nayebpour M, Jing W, Nattel S: Frequency-dependent effects of diltiazem on the atrioventricular node during experimental atrial fibrillation, *Circulation* 80:380, 1989.
51. Ellenbogen KA, Dias VC, Plumb VJ et al: A multicenter placebo controlled trial of continuous intravenous diltiazem infusion (IV FILT) for twenty-four hour rate control during atrial flutter/fibrillation, *J Am Coll Cardiol* 15(2):40A, 1990.
52. Bohm M, Schwinger RGH, Erdman E: Different cardiopressant potency of various calcium antagonists in human myocardium, *Am J Cardiol* 65:1039, 1990.
53. Wellens HJJ, Brugada P, Roy D et al: Effects of isoproterenol on the antegrade refractory period of the accessory pathway in patients with the Wolff-Parkinson-White syndrome, *Am J Cardiol* 50:180, 1982.
54. Davidson E, Weinberger I, Rotenberg Z et al: Atrial fibrillation: cause and time of onset, *Arch Intern Med* 149(2):457, 1989.
55. Preliminary Report of the Stroke Prevention in Atrial Fibrillation: Stroke prevention in atrial fibrillation investigators, *N Engl J Med* 322(12):863, 1990.
56. Connolly SJ, Laupacis A, Gent M et al and CAFA Study Coinvestigators: Canadian Atrial Fibrillation Anticoagulation Study, *J Am Coll Cardiol* 18:349, 1991.
57. Ezedowitz MD, Bridgers SL, James KE et al for the Veterans Affairs SPINAF Investigators: Warfarin in the prevention of stroke associated with nonrheumatic atrial fibrillation, *N Engl J Med* 327:1406, 1992.
58. The Boston Area Anticoagulation Trial for Atrial Fibrillation Investigators: The effect of low-dose warfarin on the risk of stroke in patients with nonrheumatic atrial fibrillation, *N Engl J Med* 323(22): 1505, 1990.
59. Stroke Prevention in Atrial Fibrillation Investigators: Predictors of thromboembolism in atrial fibrillation: clinical features in patients at risk, *Ann Intern Med* 1:1, 1992.
60. Huang SK: Radio-frequency catheter ablation of cardiac arrhythmias: appraisal of an evolving therapeutic modality, *Am Heart J* 118(6):1317, 1989.
61. Bharati S, Lev M: Histopathologic changes in the heart including the conduction system after catheter ablation, *PACE Pacing Clin Electrophysiol* 12(1, pt 2):159, 1989.
62. Langberg JJ, Chin MC, Rosenquist M et al: Catheter ablation of the atrioventricular junction with radiofrequency energy, *Circulation* 80:1527, 1989.
63. Ferguson TB Jr, Cox JL: Successful surgical treatment for atrial fibrillation, *Prim Cardiol,* 18:15, 1992.
64. Cheng TO: Atrial fibrillation, stroke, and antithrombotic treatment, *Am Heart J* 127:961, 1994.

4

65. Guiraudon GM: Early clinical results of corridor surgery for treatment of chronic atrial fibrillation, *J Am Coll Cardiol* 2(2):111A, 1988 (abstract).

66. Guiraudon GM, Klein GJ, Sharma AD, Yee R: Surgical alternatives for supraventricular tachycardias. In Touboul P, Waldo AL, eds: *Atrial arrhythmias: current concepts and management,* St Louis, 1990, Mosby.

67. Puech P, Gallay P, Grolleau R: Mechanism of atrial flutter in humans. In Touboul P, Waldo AL, eds: *Atrial arrhythmias: current concepts and management,* St Louis, 1990, Mosby.

9

Atrial Flutter

Terminology *111*
ECG Recognition *111*
Differential Diagnosis *114*
Mechanism *114*
F-Wave Morphology *115*
Atrioventricular Conduction *117*
Clinical Setting and Incidence *119*

Pediatrics *120*
Physical Signs *120*
Emergency Treatment *120*
Long-Term Treatment *120*
Flutter-Fibrillation (Impure Flutter) *121*
Summary *121*

Atrial flutter is a rapid, regular atrial rhythm with a rate that is around 300 beats/min and a typical sawtooth pattern in the inferior leads. In 1979 Wells et al.[1] described type I (common or classical) and type II (uncommon) atrial flutter according to the atrial rate and response to treatment.[2]

TERMINOLOGY

entrainment The ability to capture the reentry circuit with atrial pacing.[3]
excitable gap A cyclic area of nonrefractory tissue within the pathway of a reentry circuit.
F wave An atrial flutter wave.

ECG RECOGNITION

Atrial flutter is characterized by uniformity in its rate, configuration of the F waves, and beat-to-beat cycle length.[4] Figs. 9-1 and 9-2 show the two types of atrial flutter.

Ventricular rate: Depends on atrioventricular (AV) conduction ratio; usually 150 to 170 beats/min because of a 2:1 AV conduction ratio.

Atrial rate in type I: Ranges from 240 to 340 beats/min (long, excitable gap). The rate may be slower (e.g., in right atrial enlargement).

Atrial rate in type II: Ranges from 340 to 433 beats/min (short, excitable gap) with some overlap between the two types.[1,5]

Atrial rhythm: Regular, although slight shortening of the cycle length may occur following ventricular contraction. This *ventriculophasic* phenomenon is

II

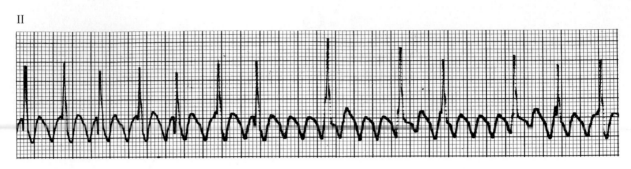

Fig. 9-1. Atrial flutter, type I. The atrial rate is 300 beats/min with a 2:1 conduction ratio at the beginning of the tracing, changing to a 4:1 AV conduction ratio because of carotid sinus massage.

V₁

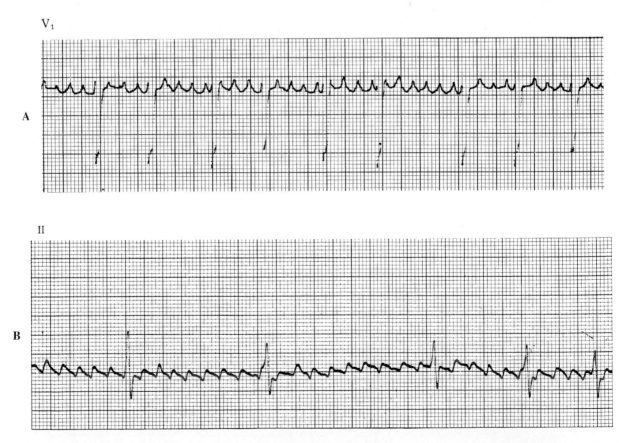

Fig. 9-2. Atrial flutter, type II. **A,** The atrial rate is 380 beats/min with a variable conduction ratio. **B,** The atrial rate is 345 beats/min with high-grade AV block.

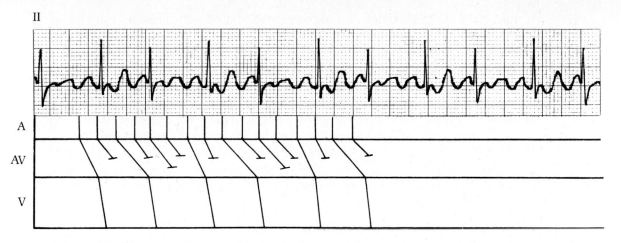

Fig. 9-3. Atrial flutter with group beating in the ventricles. The laddergram demonstrates the mechanism. The atrial tier *(A)* shows a relatively regular atrial flutter. There are two levels in the AV tier. In the upper level there is a 2:1 conduction ratio. In the lower AV node there is a 3:2 Wenckebach conduction ratio. This results in group beating and alternating fixed relationships of the flutter waves to the R waves.

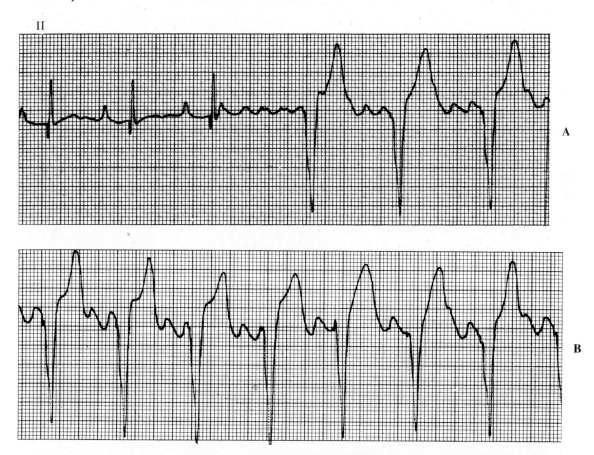

Fig. 9-4. Atrial flutter with AV dissociation. **A,** A prolonged PR interval and a premature atrial complex in the third T wave. This results in atrial flutter. The pause in ventricular response following the premature atrial complex unmasks an accelerated idioventricular rhythm. **B,** The signs of atrial flutter with AV dissociation are nicely evident. Note the changing F-R relationship indicates no conduction when the ventricular rhythm is regular.

the result of atrial stretch, which shortens atrial refractoriness and the travel time for the intraatrial reentry circuit.[1,6]

Ventricular rhythm: Regular if there is a fixed conduction ratio; group beating if there is Wenckebach conduction, as seen in Fig. 9-3.

F-R relationship: The relationship between the F wave and the R wave that follows should be fixed *if the ventricular rhythm is regular.* This F-R relationship alternates *if there is group beating* (Fig. 9-3). However, if the F-R relationship is not fixed, despite a regular ventricular rhythm, there is AV dissociation, which is the result of complete AV block or an accelerated junctional or ventricular rhythm. Fig. 9-4 shows the onset of atrial flutter, along with the development of an accelerated idioventricular rhythm (Fig. 9-4, *A*) that is, the atria are in flutter, and the ventricles are under the control of a ventricular focus. The AV dissociation can be nicely seen in changing F-R relationships in Fig. 9-4, *B.*

Effect of carotid sinus massage: Temporary slowing of the ventricular rate because of AV block or no effect.

DIFFERENTIAL DIAGNOSIS

Chronic monomorphic atrial tachycardia may be difficult to distinguish from atrial flutter with a slow atrial rate (e.g., 200 beats/min), or in other cases of atrial flutter (especially type II) the typical sawtooth pattern may not be seen because concealment of part of atrial depolarization on the surface ECG produces an isoelectric line between F waves. The atrial rhythm can be of help in distinguishing between the two supraventricular tachycardias (SVTs) on the surface ECG. In atrial flutter the rhythm is regular; in chronic atrial tachycardia the atrial rate changes in response to variations of the autonomic nervous system.[7]

Even when the typical sawtooth pattern is present, atrial flutter can be missed when the conduction ratio is 2:1. This diagnostic error can be avoided if you use a vagal manuver to rule out atrial flutter in SVTs in the rate range of 150 to 170 beats/min.

MECHANISM

Atrial flutter is due to a reentrant mechanism, seemingly a single stable reentrant circuit located in the right atrium.[5] A predisposing factor for its development is prolonged atrial conduction time.

Type I atrial flutter

Studies in humans have demonstrated that type I atrial flutter is due to a reentry circuit that uses the right atrial anatomic structure and fiber orientation for its pathway; the left atrium is a bystander.[7-15] Within this reentry circuit there is a 30- to 50-ms gap of excitable tissue ("excitable gap"), which has been demonstrated by "transient entrainment" of the tachycardia, that is, the ability to capture the reentry circuit with atrial pacing.[3] Within the circuit is an area of slow conduction located in the low posteroseptal right atrium.[13]

Type II atrial flutter

The mechanism of type II atrial flutter remains speculative because transient entrainment, a proof of reentry, has not yet been shown.[3] Only a few cases have been mapped during intraatrial studies, and the results cannot yet be generalized.[7] The reentry circuit was reported to proceed in a clockwise direction, descending the interatrial septum and left posterior paraseptal portion of the atria and crossing the inferior right atrium in the opposite direction to type I atrial flutter.

F-WAVE MORPHOLOGY
Type I atrial flutter

Although atrial flutter is generated by a reentry circuit in the right atrium, the F-wave polarity on the ECG is determined primarily by the sequence of activation in the left atrium in both types of atrial flutter. In type I the reentry circuit spreads in a counterclockwise direction, ascending from the lower left right atrium to its upper right section and descending the anterolateral atrial wall (Fig. 9-5).[7]

Fig. 9-6 shows type I atrial flutter in lead II with AV block and an absent junctional or ventricular escape mechanism. This tracing offers an opportunity to study a long section of undistorted F waves; Fig. 9-7 shows atrial flutter in all 12 leads. The negative portion of the F wave in leads II, III, aV_F, and V_6 reflects activation of the atrial septum and the left atrium (inferior to superior); the positive portion reflects activation of the right atrial free wall.[7] In lead V_1 the F waves of type I atrial flutter are positive peaks.

Type II atrial flutter

The morphologic appearance of the F waves in the uncommon form of atrial flutter (type II) differs from that in type I; the waves are positive in both the frontal

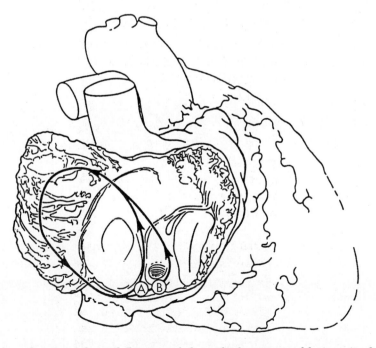

Fig. 9-5. The mechanism of atrial flutter and the radiofrequency ablation site for atrial flutter. This schematic cut-away view of the right atrium shows the direction of activation during atrial flutter. *A* and *B*, The two locations where radiofrequency ablation was shown to terminate atrial flutter. *(Redrawn from Feld GK, Fleck RP, Chen PS et al: Circulation 86:1233, 1992.)*

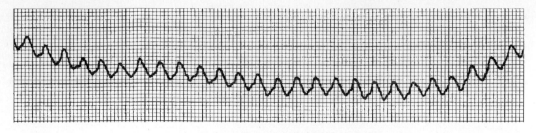

Fig. 9-6. Atrial flutter with complete AV block and failure of junctional or ventricular escape mechanisms. The typical features of atrial flutter are easily demonstrated. The regular sawtooth pattern with a rate of 300/min is evident. This tracing and the ones in Fig. 9-4 are from the same patient; this tracing was made after the administration of lidocaine.

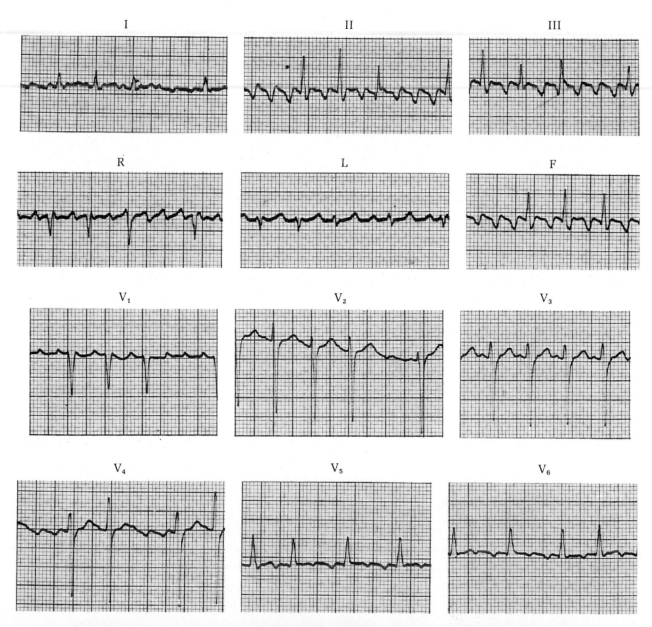

Fig. 9-7. Common form of atrial flutter in all 12 leads. The typical sawtooth pattern in the inferior leads, II, III, and aV$_F$ and the positive peaks in lead V$_1$ are evident.

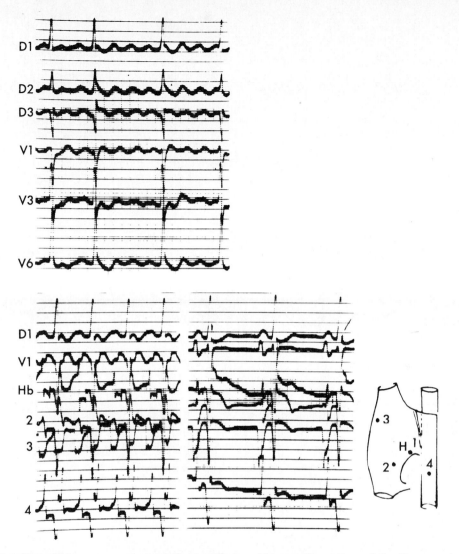

Fig. 9-8. Type II (uncommon) atrial flutter. The positive configuration of the F waves is evident in both the frontal plane *(D1* to *D3)* and the precordial leads. *(From Puech P, Gallay P, Grolleau R. In Touboul P, Waldo AL, eds: Atrial arrhythmias: current concepts and management, St Louis, 1990, Mosby.)*

plane and the precordial leads, as seen in Fig. 9-8. The positive component of the F wave reflects the descending limb of the reentry circuit in the intraatrial septum and left atrium, the chamber that determines the morphologic appearance of the F wave. The ascending limb of the reentry circuit is not reflected on the surface ECG.

ATRIOVENTRICULAR CONDUCTION

During atrial flutter a normal AV node there is usually a physiologic AV block with a 2:1 conduction ratio. Higher degrees of AV block can occur in patients with AV nodal disease or increased vagal tone or when drugs that cause AV block are in use. In fact, vagal maneuvers may be used to compound the AV block so that the

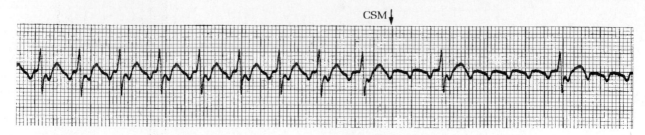

Fig. 9-9. Atrial flutter with a 2:1 AV conduction ratio that changes to 4:1 and 6:1 because of carotid sinus massage (CSM).

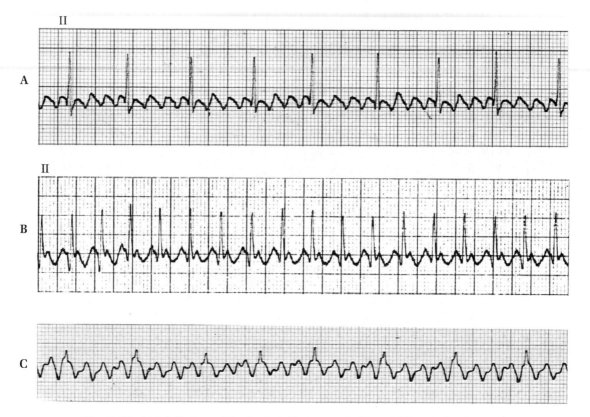

Fig. 9-10. Atrial flutter with, **A,** 4:1, **B,** 2:1, and, **C,** variable conduction ratios.

typical sawtooth pattern can be seen; such a case is shown in Fig. 9-9. If atrial flutter occurs in a patient with Wolff-Parkinson-White (WPF) syndrome, there may be a 1:1 or 2:1 conduction ratio. This rhythm is indistinguishable from ventricular tachycardia (see Chapter 23). In this situation the patient is usually seriously compromised hemodynamically and requires immediate electrical cardioversion. In both type I and type II atrial flutter the following principles govern AV conduction:

1. Conduction ratios are usually even (e.g., 2:1, 4:1, and 6:1).[16,17]
2. Wenckebach conduction often causes an apparently irregular ventricular rhythm (i.e., group beating).[18]
3. Atrial impulses that appear to be completely blocked actually penetrate into

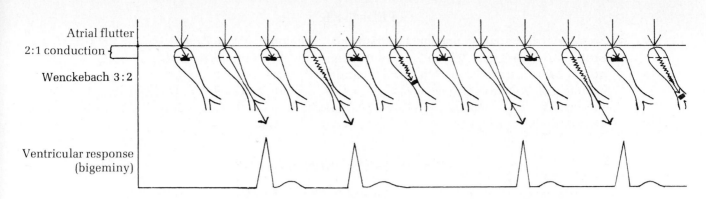

Fig. 9-11. A common mechanism for AV conduction during atrial flutter: 2:1 conduction ratio at the top of the AV node and Wenckebach conduction at the lower AV node. Atrial flutter is illustrated by the regularly spaced vertical arrows. At the top of the olive-shaped AV node is a 2:1 conduction ratio. The beats that pass through the node are conducted with a 3:2 Wenckebach ratio; that is, for every three beats that pass through, only two are conducted to the ventricles, causing the ventricular group beating. The slowing of conduction between the first and second conducted beats is illustrated.

different levels of the AV junction (concealed conduction),[19] with 2:1 block at the upper level and Wenckebach conduction of the beats that reach the lower level of the AV node.

Fig. 9-10 shows 4:1, 2:1, and variable conduction ratios. In Fig. 9-10, *A,* there is a 4:1 ratio; in Fig. 9-10, *B,* 2:1; and in Fig. 9-10, *C,* both 4:1 and 3:1.

Mechanism of Wenckebach conduction in atrial flutter

In Fig. 9-11 three levels of activity are shown: atrial, AV nodal, and His bundle. At the atrial level the vertical arrows represent atrial flutter. Within the AV node there is 2:1 block. Thus every other impulse arrives at the His bundle. From the His bundle into the ventricle conduction becomes slower and then blocks, creating group beating, as previously shown in Fig. 9-3.

CLINICAL SETTING AND INCIDENCE

Acute or transient atrial flutter is one of the atrial tachyrhythmias that is a typical complication following open heart surgery. Supraventricular tachycardia occurs in 30% of cases; one third of these SVTs are atrial flutter, which may convert to atrial fibrillation and back again, especially immediately following the surgery.[2] In this clinical setting atrial flutter is probably caused by the diffuse sterile pericarditis and atrial inflammation associated with the surgical procedure.[20] Atrial flutter may also be seen during the acute phase of myocardial infarction and in patients with pulmonary embolism with or without preexisting cardiac disease.[21] Chronic atrial flutter is most often seen in persons over 40 years of age and is commonly associated with organic heart disease, making termination and prevention of the arrhythmia important.[15]

Patients with accessory pathways who have atrial flutter are particularly at risk because of the high ratio of ventricular response, sometimes 1:1. In such cases, the first line of treatment is radiofrequency ablation of the accessory pathway.

PEDIATRICS

Atrial flutter is a common mechanism in the neonate; atrial rates usually approach 400 beats/min with a 2:1 conduction ratio.[22] In the newborn this arrhythmia is usually associated with normal cardiac structure. It can be treated by transesophageal overdrive pacing or external synchronized cardioversion. Once treated, in some patients it may never return. Most infants outgrow this arrhythmia by 12 to 18 months of age.[23,24]

PHYSICAL SIGNS

Rapid flutter waves may be seen in the jugular venous pulse. The first heart sound has a constant intensity if the F-R relationship remains constant. It is possible on occasion to auscultate the sounds of the atrial contractions.[25]

EMERGENCY TREATMENT

Emergency treatment depends on the clinical setting[5]: direct current (DC) cardioversion (<50 joules) or rapid atrial pacing is a preferred choice; antiarrhythmic drug therapy may be initiated before either treatment, to accomplish the following:
1. Slow the ventricular response (beta blockers or calcium channel blockers)
2. Enhance the effect of rapid atrial pacing (Class IA drugs)
3. Maintain sinus rhythm once converted (Class IA, IC, or III)

If the patient has chronic obstructive pulmonary disease or has taken a meal recently, this factor determines the choice between DC cardioversion or atrial pacing. (An anesthetic is required for DC cardioversion.) In such cases rapid atrial pacing or antiarrhythmic drugs to slow the ventricular response are preferred to DC cardioversion. In postoperative patients who have an epicardial wire, rapid atrial pacing is performed to convert the atrial flutter.

LONG-TERM TREATMENT

1. **Drugs.** Antiarrhythmic drugs may be used, but may not be completely effective. New drugs are being investigated in animal models and hold some promise.[26]
2. **Implanted antitachycardia pacemaker.** Such therapy is considered for the treatment of recurrent atrial flutter.[5]
3. **Radiofrequency ablation.** Currently radiofrequency catheter ablation is used to create a high degree of AV block at the His bundle (usually third degree). This therapy is, of course, combined with the installation of a permanent pacemaker.

   Radiofrequency ablation of the area of slow conduction within the reentry circuit supporting the atrial flutter is still being developed. Studies involving a small series of patients have shown that radiofrequency ablation of a relatively small area of endocardium terminates and prevents recurrence of type I atrial flutter.[27,28] Recent data indicate that type II atrial flutter can also be cured with radiofrequency ablation.[29,30] For the ablation procedure, atrial flutter is induced and the sequence of atrial activation mapped; the area of slow conduction is identified and destroyed. Fig. 9-5 demonstrates the locations in the inferior right atrium where radiofrequency ablation has been applied for this purpose.
4. **Anticoagulation therapy.** There is no clear consensus regarding anticoagulants in patients with atrial flutter. Data from 85 consecutive patients undergoing cardioversion for atrial flutter suggest that clinically apparent thromboemboli may

occur in chronic atrial flutter and that anticoagulation therapy is recommended awaiting further studies.[31] Waldo[5] suggests that aspirin therapy should be considered in patients younger than 75 years old and warfarin therapy should be considered on an individual basis.

FLUTTER-FIBRILLATION (IMPURE FLUTTER)

Flutter-fibrillation is a term sometimes applied to a dysrhythmia in which the baseline resembles atrial flutter with a sawtooth pattern and yet is not regular enough and seems to lose a defined form. The ventricular response is irregular. Flutter-fibrillation is often a transitional stage from fibrillation to pure atrial flutter when the patient is taking class I antiarrhythmic drugs.[67]

SUMMARY

Atrial flutter is a rapid, regular atrial rhythm with a rate of approximately 300 beats/min and a unique ECG pattern. Two types have been described: type I atrial flutter has a rate of 250 to 320 beats/min and can be interrupted with rapid atrial pacing. Type II atrial flutter has a rate of more than 320 beats/min, and it is difficult to accomplish cardioversion or even to slow the rapid ventricular rate with pharmacologic agents. A cure is available in the form of radiofrequency ablation of the slow arm of the intraatrial reentry circuit.

REFERENCES

1. Wells JL, MacLean WAH, James TN, Waldo AL: Characterization of atrial flutter: studies in man after open heart surgery using fixed atrial electrodes, *Circulation* 60:665, 1979.
2. Waldo AL, MacLean WAH: *Diagnosis and treatment of cardiac arrhythmias following open heart surgery,* Mount Kisco, NY, 1980, Futura.
3. Waldo AL, Carlson MD, Biblo LA, Henthorn RW: The role of transient entrainment in atrial flutter. In Touboul P, Waldo AL, eds: *Atrial arrhythmias: current concepts and management,* St Louis, 1990, Mosby.
4. Waldo AL: Atrial flutter: new directions in management and mechanism, *Circulation* 81:1142, 1990.
5. Waldo AL: Atrial flutter: mechanisms, clinical features, and management. In Zipes DP, Jalife J, eds: *Cardiac electrophysiology from cell to bedside,* ed 2, Philadelphia, 1995, WB Saunders.
6. Ravelli F, Disertori M, Cozzi F et al: Ventricular beats induce variations in cycle length of rapid (type II) atrial flutter in humans: evidence of leading circle reentry, *Circulation,* 89:2017, 1994.
7. Puech P, Gallay P, Grolleau R: Mechanism of atrial flutter in humans. In Touboul P, Waldo AL, eds: *Atrial arrhythmias: current concepts and management,* St Louis, 1990, Mosby.

8. Waldo AL: Mechanisms of atrial fibrillation, atrial flutter, and ectopic atrial tachycardia: a brief review, *Circulation* 75:37, 1987.
9. Disertori M, Inama G, Vergara G et al: Evidence of a reentry circuit in the common type of atrial flutter in man, *Circulation* 67:434, 1983.
10. Klein, GJ, Guiradon GM, Sharma AD, Milstein S: Demonstration of macroreentry and feasibility of operative therapy in the common type of atrial flutter, *Am J Cardiol* 57:587, 1986.
11. Olshansky B, Okumura K, Henthorn R et al: Atrial mapping of human atrial flutter demonstrates reentry in the right atrium, *J Am Coll Cardiol* 7:194A, 1988 (abstract).
12. Cosio FG, Arribas F, Barbero JM et al: Validation of double-spike electrograms as markers of conduction delay or block in atrial flutter, *Am J Cardiol* 61:775, 1988.
13. Olshansky B, Okumura K, Hess PG, Waldo AL: Demonstration of an area of slow conduction in human atrial flutter, *J Am Coll Cardiol* 16:1639, 1990.
14. Schoels W, Offner B, Brachmann J et al: Circus movement atrial flutter in the canine sterile pericarditis model: relation of characteristics of the surface electrocardiogram and conduction properties of the reentrant pathway, *J Am Coll Cardiol* 23:799, 1994.
15. Wellens HJJ: Atrial flutter: progress, but no final answer, *J Am Coll Cardiol* 17:1235, 1991 (editorial comment).

16. Ashman R, Hull E: *Essentials of electrocardiography,* ed 2, New York, 1941, Macmillan.
17. Katz LN: *Electrocardiography,* ed 2, Philadelphia, 1946, Lea & Febiger.
18. Lewis T: *The mechanism and graphic registration of the heart beat,* ed 3, London, 1925, Shaw & Sons.
19. Langendorf R: Concealed A-V conduction: the effect of blocked impulses on the formation and conduction of subsequent impulses, *Am Heart J* 35:542, 1948.
20. Page PL, Plumb VJ, Okumura K, Waldo AL: A new animal model of atrial flutter, *J Am Coll Cardiol* 8:872, 1986.
21. Brugada P, Gorgels AP, Wellens HJJ: The electrocardiogram in pulmonary embolism. In Wellens HJJ, Kulbertus HE, eds: *What's new in electrocardiography,* The Hague, 1981, Martinus Nijhoff.
22. Porter CJ: Premature atrial contractions and atrial tachyarrhythmias. In Gillette PC, Garson A Jr, eds: *Pediatric arrhythmias: electrophysiology and pacing,* Philadelphia, 1990, WB Saunders.
23. Dunnigan A, Benson DW Jr, Benditt DG: Atrial flutter in infancy: diagnosis, clinical features, and treatment, *Pediatrics* 75:725, 1985.
24. Gillette PC, Ziegler VL, Case CL: Pediatric arrhythmias: are they different? In Zipes DP, Jalife J, eds: *Cardiac electrophysiology from cell to bedside,* ed 2, Philadelphia, 1995, WB Saunders.
25. Zipes DP: Specific arrhythmias: diagnosis and treatment. In Braunwald E, ed: *Heart disease,* ed 4, Philadelphia, 1992, WB Saunders.
26. Restivo M, Hegazy M, Caref EB et al: Termination and prevention of circus movement atrial flutter in the sterile pericarditis model by a novel type III agent, azimilide (NE-10064), *Circulation* 90:I-413, abstract 2214, 1994.
27. Feld GK, Fleck RP, Chen PS et al: Radiofrequency catheter ablation for the treatment of human type 1 atrial flutter, *Circulation* 86:1233, 1992.
28. Saoudi N, Atallah G, Deschamps D et al: The role of transient entrainment in atrial flutter. In Touboul P, Waldo AL, eds: *Atrial arrhythmias: current concepts and management,* St Louis, 1990, Mosby.
29. Kirkorian G, Moncada E, Defeo M et al: Radiofrequency ablation of atrial tissue is also effective in atypical atrial flutter, *Circulation* 90:I-337, abstract 1802, 1994.
30. Satake S, Okishiga K, Azegami K et al: Radiofrequency catheter ablation of uncommon type atrial flutter, *Circulation* 90:I-594, abstract 3201, 1994.
31. Pagadala P, Gummadi SS, Olshansky B: Thromboembolic risk of chronic atrial flutter: is the risk underestimated? *Circulation* 90:I-398, abstract 2141, 1994.

C H A P T E R

10

Junctional Beats and Rhythms

Terminology *123*

AV Junction *124*

Premature Junctional Complex *125*

Nonparoxysmal Junctional

Tachycardia *126*

Junctional Escape Beats and

Rhythms *129*

Summary *130*

TERMINOLOGY

nonparoxysmal   Of gradual onset and termination.

accelerated junctional rhythm   When the junctional rate is more than 60 beats/min and less than 100 beats/min.

accelerated idiojunctional rhythm   "Idio-" added to the word junctional implies independent beating of the ventricles (atrioventricular [AV] dissociation).

junctional tachycardia   The term "junctional tachycardia," in its strict sense, is used when the junctional rate is 100 beats/min or more. Junctional tachycardias with rates of less than 100 beats/min are, strictly speaking, *accelerated idiojunctional rhythms.* Whether the rate is 70 beats/min, 99.8 beats/min, or 100 beats/min, the mechanism is the same, so it seems less cumbersome to simply refer to any junctional rhythm with a rate greater than 60 beats/min as junctional tachycardia. This term makes dialogue easier and acknowledges that any rate over 60 beats/min is too fast to qualify as junctional escape.

retrograde conduction   This term implies that a junctional or ventricular focus was conducted up the AV node to activate the atria inferiorly to superiorly. Whether retrograde conduction to the atria occurs depends on the physiologic properties of the individual AV node (up to 15% of normal individuals do not have ventriculoatrial [VA] conduction[1]) and the effect of drugs on AV nodal conduction. When retrograde conduction does occur, the retrograde P′ wave that results is negative in the inferior leads (II, III, and aV$_F$) and isoelectric in lead I. This is because the current proceeds from an inferior position to the top of the heart (away from the positive electrodes of the inferior leads). Because the AV node is located more or less equidistant between the right and left atria, the mean current proceeds straight up, crossing the axis of lead I at right angles and resulting in an isoelectric P′ wave. The location of the P′ wave relative to the QRS, of course, depends on the speed of retrograde AV nodal conduction.

AV dissociation   AV dissociation is the independent beating of atria and ventricles (see Chapter 20). If retrograde conduction from a junctional or ventricular pace-

maker is blocked, the atria are under the control of the sinus node or an atrial
ectopic focus and the ventricles are under the control of the junctional or ventricular focus.

AV JUNCTION

The AV junction consists of the AV node and the bundle of His down to where
it begins to branch. The different regions of the AV junction are divided according to the various cell types: atrionodal (AN), nodal (N), nodal-His (NH), and
His bundle. Fig. 10-1 is an artist's conception of the divisions of the AV junction.

Atrionodal (AN) region

The AN region is a transitional zone where the atrial fibers gradually merge
with the compact AV node. The best-known AV nodal fibers are found posteriorly
(the slow pathway) and anteriorly (the fast pathway). These pathways are responsible for the maintenance of the AV nodal reentry mechanism, one of the most common causes of paroxysmal supraventricular tachycardia (see Chapter 11).

Nodal (N) region

The N region is the compact AV node, especially the midnodal region. It is
noted for the virtual absence of junctional beats along with an increase in the electrical resistance at the coupling of the cells. In the N region the normal and rate-
related conduction delay occurs.[2] The newly described atrial fibers emanating from
the compact mode are illustrated in Chapter 11 (see Fig. 11-1).

Nodal-His (NH) region

The NH region is the merging of fibers from the lower AV node with those of
the His bundle. Some investigators have defined this region as the primary focus
for the junctional escape rhythm.[3]

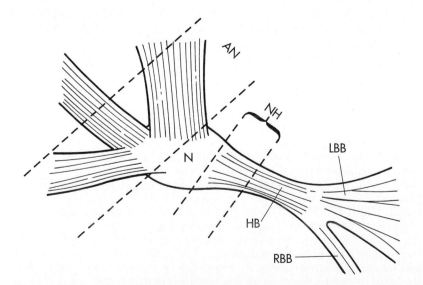

Fig. 10-1. The divisions of the AV junction. *AV*, Atrionodal; *N*, compact *AV* node; *NH*, nodal-
His; *HB*, His bundle; *LBB*, left bundle branch; *RBB*, right bundle branch.

Junctional rhythm

The distinguishing feature of a junctional rhythm is a QRS complex that is supraventricular in shape and has a regular rhythm with a rate of 70 to 140 beats/min. Atrioventricular dissociation may be present.

PREMATURE JUNCTIONAL COMPLEX

A premature junctional complex (PJC) originates in the AV junction, usually in the NH region. It discharges before the next expected sinus impulse and activates the ventricles through the His bundle and bundle branches in the normal manner. In fact, it is recognized because its shape does not differ from that of the normal sinus-conducted beat. There may be retrograde conduction to the atria from this focus. This depends on the ability of the AV node to conduct in a retrograde fashion. For example, in cases of digitalis toxicity there is some degree of AV block, impairing conduction in both directions across the AV node.

If retrograde conduction does take place, the resulting P′ wave is negative in the inferior leads II, III, and aV$_F$. The location of the retrograde P′ wave relative to the QRS depends on the speed of conduction up into the atria compared with the conduction speed down to the ventricles. Thus the P′ wave may occur before, during, or after the QRS. Fig. 10-2 illustrates the possibilities for P′ wave location in PJCs. It is also possible for a junctional focus to discharge and fail to conduct an-

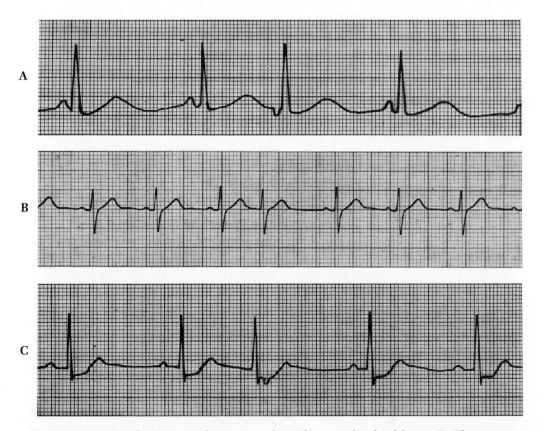

Fig. 10-2. Junctional premature beats. **A** and **C,** They are the third beats. **B,** The premature junctional complex is the fourth complex.

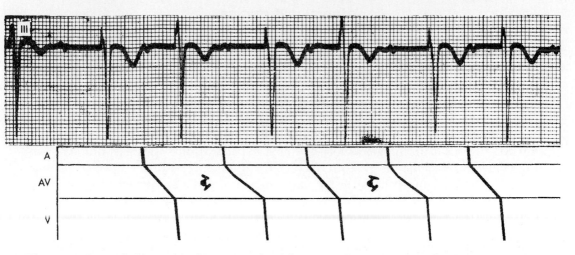

Fig. 10-3. Concealed junctional extrasystoles (shown in the atrioventricular *(AV)* tier of the laddergram) produce alternating PR and RR intervals. The mechanism is suspected because of the unexplained PR lengthening. (It is obviously not a Wenckebach period because there are no dropped beats.) *(From Marriott HJL, Conover M: Advanced concepts in arrhythmias, ed 2, St Louis, 1992, Mosby.)*

terogradly or retrogradly. Such an occurrence is called a *concealed junctional extrasystole;* it is recognized because of the effect it has on the subsequent cycle. For example, there may be unexplained lengthening of the PR interval, as seen in Fig. 10-3, or an unexplained type II AV block.[4]

ECG recognition

Heart rate: That of the underlying rhythm.

Rhythm: Irregular because of the PJC.

P′ wave: If a P′ wave occurs, it is negative in leads II, III, and aV$_F$ and may occur before, during, or after the QRS.

P′R interval: If the P′ wave occurs before the QRS, the P′R interval is less than 0.12 sec.

QRS complex: Normal in shape and duration unless there is an intraventricular conduction abnormality.

Treatment

Premature junctional complexes are not usually treated. If they initiate a more serious arrhythmia (for example, ventricular tachycardia [VT]), therapy is directed at the VT.[5]

NONPAROXYSMAL JUNCTIONAL TACHYCARDIA

Nonparoxysmal junctional tachycardia is a narrow QRS tachycardia with gradual onset and termination that originates within AV junctional fibers (AV node–His bundle).

ECG recognition

Heart rate: Ranges from 70 to 140 beats/min (may be seen between 60 beats/min and 70 beats/min if there is sinus bradycardia or sinoatrial [SA] block). As with atrial tachycardia resulting from digitalis toxicity, the rate of the junctional tachycardia gradually increases as more digitalis is given.[5]

Rhythm: Nonparoxysmal; appears to be regular but may slowly increase its rate.

P waves: Retrograde P′ waves before, during, or after the QRS. If there is AV dissociation (junctional tachycardia with retrograde AV block), there will be normal sinus P waves.

P′R interval: Less than 0.12 sec if the P′ wave occurs before the QRS.

QRS complex: Normal in duration and shape; this is the distinguishing feature of the junctional rhythm.

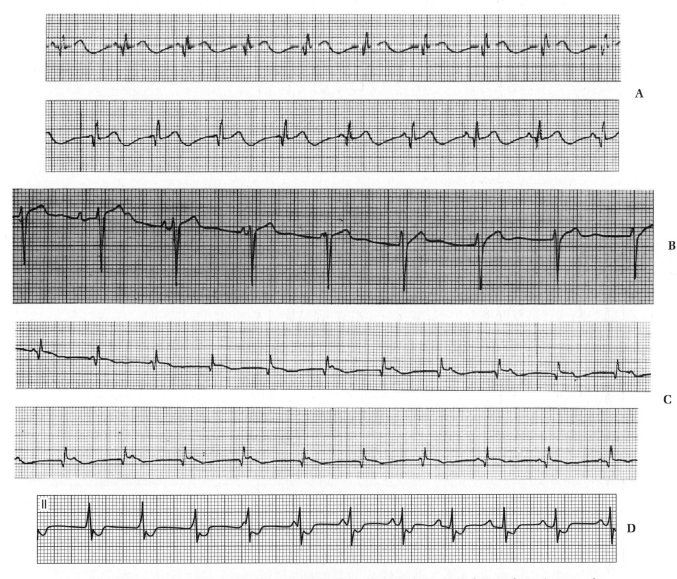

Fig. 10-4. Junctional tachycardia with rates of, **A,** 70 beats/min; **B** and **C,** 74 beats/min; and, **D,** 96 beats/min. There is AV dissociation in all tracings. **D** is from a 16-year-old boy who attempted suicide with an overdose of digitalis *(**D** courtesy of William P. Nelson M.D.)*

Response to carotid sinus massage: No response. (This is not a reentry mechanism like that of paroxysmal supraventricular tachycardia [PSVT].)

AV dissociation: The atria and the ventricles usually beat independently in the presence of junctional tachycardia. The ventricles are under the control of the junctional focus, and the atria are in sinus rhythm or their own ectopic rhythm. It is even possible to have a second junctional focus controlling the atria.

There is AV dissociation in all of the tracings in Fig. 10-4. For further discussion of AV dissociation see Chapter 20. Of course, retrograde activation of the atria is possible and does occur, with the retrograde P′ wave (negative in the inferior leads) falling before, during, or after the QRS.

Mechanism

Because the ectopic focus of junctional tachycardia is pacemaker tissue, it is possible for the mechanism to be enhanced normal automaticity in the His bundle; of course, abnormal automaticity or triggered activity is also a possibility.[6,7]

Causes

Probably the most important cause of nonparoxysmal junctional tachycardia is digitalis toxicity[8]; in such cases the mortality rate can be very high when the condition is not treated properly.[9]

Other causes include the following:

Inferior myocardial infarction

Myocarditis, often a result of acute rheumatic fever

After open heart surgery

Idiopathic

Pediatrics

Postoperative junctional tachycardia often occurs in infants following complex open heart surgery[10] and abates after 48 to 72 hours. The junctional rate is responsive to temperature, catecholamines, and decreased vagal tone and can be controlled by cooling, electrolyte replacement, enhancement of vagal tone, and reduction in sympathetic stimulation. If medical management fails, His bundle ablation may be lifesaving.[11] In congenital nonparoxysmal junctional tachycardia the infant mortality rate is relatively high.[12]

Physical signs

The physical signs of nonparoxysmal AV junctional tachycardia, as in other arrhythmias, are determined by the ventricular rate, the atrial rate, the relationship of the P wave to the QRS complex, ventricular function, and the absence or presence of underlying heart disease.[5]

First heart sound: Varies in intensity if AV dissociation is present; is of constant intensity if AV dissociation is not present (i.e., there is retrograde conduction to the atria).

Jugular venous pulse: Irregular cannon *a* waves appear if AV dissociation is present (in the absence of coexisting atrial fibrillation).

Treatment

If the junctional tachycardia is due to digitalis toxicity, it is usually sufficient to discontinue the drug. However, if there is hemodynamic compromise, digitalis antibody may be lifesaving.

JUNCTIONAL ESCAPE BEATS AND RHYTHMS

Junctional escape beats and rhythms are protective mechanisms that are normally prevented from pacing the heart because they are discharged by the sinus rhythm. Junctional cells have an inherent rate of 35 to 60 beats/min. When they are not discharged in a timely fashion by the impulse from the sinus node, they reach threshold and discharge themselves. Thus AV junctional cells can normally assume the passive role of pacemaker only when the sinus node defaults, for example, in marked sinus bradycardia and SA block, during the pause caused by a nonconducted PAC, or when there is AV block.

ECG recognition

Heart rate: Bradycardia (35 to 60 beats/min).

Rhythm: Regular for junctional escape rhythms, although at its onset the rate increases ("warm-up" phenomena characteristic of automatic fibers).

P′ waves: May or may not be linked to the junctional complex.

QRS complex: Normal or the same shape as the sinus conducted beats.

Summary: Junctional escape beats and rhythms are recognized because of an underlying bradycardia or pauses that are terminated by the appearance of a normal QRS complex with or without a retrograde P′ wave. Figs. 10-5 to 10-8 show junctional escape beats and rhythms.

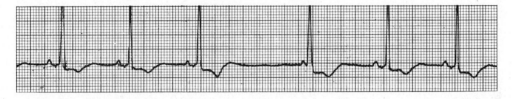

Fig. 10-5. Junctional escape beat following a pause created by a nonconducted premature atrial complex (distorting the third T wave). The premature atrial complex is not conducted because it is very early; a pause results and is terminated by a junctional escape beat (fourth complex). The sinus P wave immediately in front of the escape beat is too close to have been conducted.

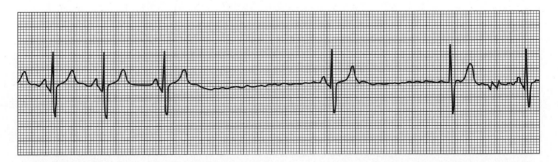

Fig. 10-6. Sinoatrial block and sinus arrest with a 2.4-sec pause. A junctional escape beat *(asterisk)* terminates the second pause. This beat resembles the sinus conducted ones, missing only the initial q wave. There is artifact in the tracing following the junctional escape beat. This patient had presyncope as a result of these pauses. *(From Angeli SJ: Am Heart J 120:433, 1990.)*

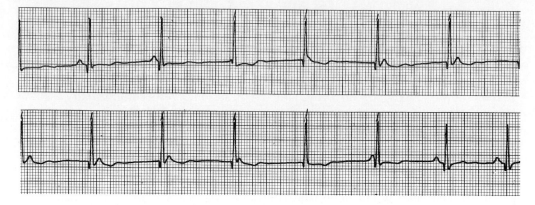

Fig. 10-7. Sinus bradycardia with a junctional escape rhythm of 58 beats/min, resulting in AV dissociation (continuous tracing). If you mark off the first two P waves, they can be "walked out" through the tracing when they distort the QRS in front and in back or are completely hidden within the QRS. The first P wave in the tracing may conduct to the ventricles. (The PR interval is 0.12 sec.) Because the RR intervals are exactly the same across the tracing, the first QRS is probably a junctional beat as well.

II   Retrograde P′

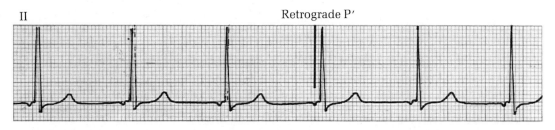

Fig. 10-8. Junctional escape rhythm (60 beats/min) without AV dissociation. There is retrograde conduction to the atria. The retrograde P′ wave (negative in lead II) is evident.

Treatment

Frequently no treatment is necessary. At times, consideration may be given to increasing the rate of the sinus node to improve cardiac output by restoring AV synchrony.[5]

SUMMARY

Junctional beats and rhythms are recognized because the QRS is narrow and the P wave either is not associated with the QRS (AV dissociation) or is retrograde (negative in leads II, III, and aV$_F$). When the rate of a junctional rhythm exceeds that expected of a junctional focus (approximately 60 beats/min), this is an abnormal acceleration and the cause should be identified and treated. Junctional rates up to 140 beats/min may be seen with digitalis toxicity. When the junctional rhythm is less than 60 beats/min, it is a protective escape mechanism, usually in the setting of sinus bradycardia or complete AV nodal block.

REFERENCES

1. Reiffel JA: Clinical electrophysiology of the sinus node in man, *Prog Clin Biol Res* 275:239, 1988.
2. Meijler FL, Janse MJ: Morphology and electrophysiology of the mammalian atrioventricular node, *Physiol Rev* 68(2):608, 1988.
3. Sherf L, James TN, Woods T: Function of the atrioventricular node considered on the basis of observed histology and fine structure, *J Am Coll Cardiol* 5:770, 1985.
4. Marriott HJJ, Conover M: *Advanced concepts in arrhythmias,* ed 2, St Louis, 1989, Mosby.
5. Zipes DP: Specific arrhythmias: diagnosis and treatment. In Braunwald E, ed: *Heart disease,* ed 4, Philadelphia, 1992, WB Saunders.
6. Vos MA, Gorgels APM, de Wit B et al: Premature escape beats: a model for triggered activity in the intact heart? *Circulation* 82:213, 1990.
7. Viamonte VAM, Rosen MR: Premature escape beats induced by overdrive pacing in canine Purkinje fibers: evidence for the role of normal automaticity as an underlying cellular mechanism, *Circulation* 82:234, 1990.
8. Naccarelli GV, Shih HT, Jalal S: Sinus node reentry and atrial tachycardias. In Zipes DP, Jalife J, eds: *Cardiac electrophysiology from cell to bedside,* ed 2, Philadelphia, 1995, WB Saunders.
9. Akhtar M: Supraventricular tachycardias, electrophysiologic mechanisms, diagnosis, and pharmacologic therapy. In Josephson ME, Wellens HJJ, eds: *Tachycardias: mechanisms, diagnosis, treatment,* Philadelphia, 1984, Lea & Febiger.
10. Gillette PC: Diagnosis and management of postoperative junctional ectopic tachycardia, *Am Heart J* 118:192, 1989 (editorial).
11. Gillette PC, Zeigler VL, Case CL: Pediatric arrhythmias: are they different? In Zipes DP, Jalife J, eds: *Cardiac electrophysiology from cell to bedside,* ed 2, Philadelphia, 1995, WB Saunders.
12. Villain E, Vetter VL, Garcia JM et al: Evolving concepts in the management of congenital junctional ectopic tachycardia, *Circulation* 81:1544, 1990.

11

Paroxysmal Supraventricular Tachycardia

Terminology   *132*
Atrioventricular Nodal Reentry
   Tachycardia   *133*
Circus Movement Tachycardia
   (Atrioventricular Reciprocating
   Tachycardia)   *137*
Circus Movement with a Slowly
   Conducting Acessory Pathway   *143*
Emergency Response to Paroxysmal
   Supraventricular Tachycardia   *144*
Rationale of Emergency Response   *144*

Mechanism and Methods of Vagal
   Stimulation   *147*
Carotid Sinus Massage   *148*
Symptoms of Paroxysmal Supraventricular
   Tachycardia   *150*
Physical Signs of Paroxysmal
   Supraventricular Tachycardia   *151*
Pediatrics: Paroxysmal Supraventricular
   Tachycardia in the Fetus and
   Neonate[31]   *152*
Summary   *152*

The two most common mechanisms for paroxysmal supraventricular tachycardia (PSVT) in symptomatic patients seeking medical attention have been shown to be atrioventricular nodal reentry tachycardia (AVNRT) and orthodromic circus movement tachycardia (CMT), also called AV reciprocating tachycardia. Of cases of symptomatic PSVT, AVNRT accounts for half and CMT for 40%.[1] Intra-atrial reentry or a reentry circuit involving the sinoatrial (SA) node are less common causes of PSVT. This chapter deals with the differential diagnosis between these two most common causes of PSVT.

TERMINOLOGY

orthodromic: In the same direction as the normal current through the AV node; "-dromic" refers to conduction.

antidromic: In the opposite direction of the normal current through the AV node.

reciprocating: The return of an impulse to its place of origin; for example, in AV reciprocating tachycardia the supraventricular impulse enters the ventricles via one AV pathway and then returns to the atria via another pathway.

circus movement: A reentry circuit; commonly used to refer to the AV reentry circuit using an accessory pathway and the AV node.

paroxysmal: Begins and ends abruptly; for example, a rapid rhythm of sudden onset that changes from sinus rhythm to a tachycardia in one beat.

ATRIOVENTRICULAR NODAL REENTRY TACHYCARDIA

Atrioventricular nodal reentry tachycardia is a PSVT caused by a reentry circuit using the slow and fast AV nodal pathways for entrance into the ventricles and return to the atria. In its common form the impulse enters the ventricles via the slow pathway and returns to the atria via the fast pathway; in its uncommon form the circuit moves in the opposite direction. The following properties of the AV node make it particularly vulnerable for dissociation of its pathways and the establishment of a reentry circuit:

- The possibility for retrograde conduction through the AV node exists in many individuals. In most cases the impulse is conducted up the fast AV nodal fibers to the atria. In fact, half of all ventricular rhythms are conducted retrogradely into the atria.
- There are two distinctly different conduction pathways connecting the atria to the body of the AV node. One is inferior (a slow pathway), and the other is superior (a fast pathway).[2]
- Not only do the conduction velocities in the two pathways differ, so do their refractory periods; for example, the slower pathway has the shorter refractory period.

Location of the fast and slow atrioventricular nodal pathways

Recent data[3] suggest that the fibers of the fast and slow pathways run along opposite edges of the compact AV node into the atrium in a fanlike fashion. Fig. 11-1 shows the compact AV node and its atrial fibers. The fast fibers are located

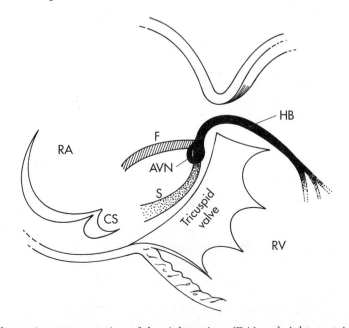

Fig. 11-1. A schematic representation of the right atrium (RA) and right ventricle (RV) opened to reveal the compact atrioventricular node (AVN) and its atrial fibers. The fast fibers are superior; the slow fibers are inferior, arising near the os of the coronary sinus (CS). *(Adapted from Kiem S, Werner P, Jazayeri M et al: Circulation, 86:919, 1992.)*

superiorly along the compact node and exit into the atrial septum near the tendon of Todaro. The slow fibers arise near the coronary sinus os and are directed inferiorly along the tricuspid annulus toward the compact AV node. Block in the slow pathway has no impact on the PR interval during sinus rhythm.

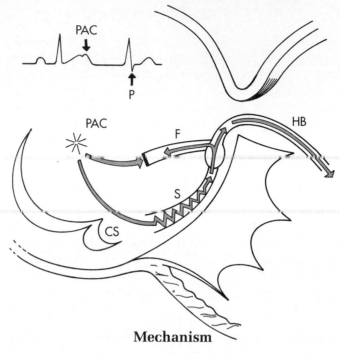

Mechanism

An early premature atrial complex (PAC) finds the fast AV nodal pathway refractory and proceeds to enter the body of the AV node via the slow AV nodal pathway, (producing a significantly long P′R interval, about 0.38 sec). Within the AV node the impulse travels in two directions, up to the atria and down the His bundle to the ventricles.

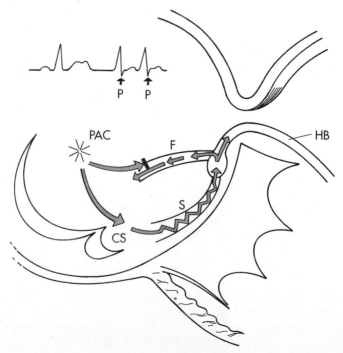

An AV nodal reentry circuit is thus established. This is the common form of AV nodal reentry with anterograde conduction in the slow AV nodal pathway and retrograde conduction in the fast AV nodal pathway. In this way the atria and ventricles are activated simultaneously, placing the P' wave within the QRS.[3,4] The P' wave may be completely hidden, or it may distort the end of the QRS (pseudo s wave in the inferior leads and/or pseudo r' wave in lead V_1; arrows in figure below).

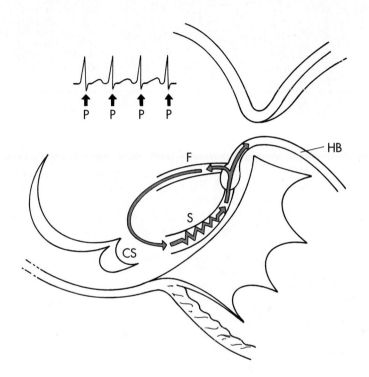

Although the mechanism of AVNRT is not difficult to understand and in the drawings it is perfectly clear why the P' waves are completely or partially hidden, in clinical practice the differential diagnosis can be difficult. Fig. 11-2 shows AVNRT. Examine the tracings for the ECG signs that confirm the diagnosis. Keep in mind that this mechanism is the cause of 50% of symptomatic PSVT. Without an understanding of the statistics and the mechanism the examiner would be looking *in front of* the QRS for the P wave instead of looking for a distorted terminal QRS (AVNRT) or for a P' wave immediately after the QRS (circus movement tachycardia [CMT]).

ECG recognition

Heart rate: 170 to 250 beats/min.

Rhythm: May be regular or irregular because of varying conduction through the AV node.

Initiating P'R interval: Approximately 0.38 sec because of anterograde conduction down the slow AV nodal fibers.

Location of the P' waves: Buried within the QRS and not seen at all or distorting the end of the QRS, looking like terminal QRS forces.

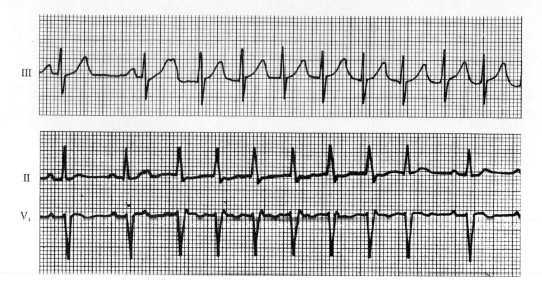

Fig. 11-2. The two most common patterns in atrioventricular nodal reentry tachycardia (AVNRT). At the onset of these tachycardias are premature atrial complexes (PACs) with critically prolonged P'R interval (0.36 sec in both cases.) **A,** The P' wave is completely hidden within the QRS. The QRS of the tachycardia is identical to that of the sinus beat. **B,** The P' wave is distorting the end of the QRS. Compare the QRS of the tachycardia with that of the sinus beat: you will note that the P' wave looks like an S wave in lead II and like r' in lead V_1.

Polarity of the P' waves: Negative in leads II, III, and aVF. This is because atrial activation originates inferiorly in the right atrium. Therefore if the P' wave can be seen in the inferior leads, it will appear in the QRS as a *pseudo s wave.* It will not be seen in lead I, since in this lead it is isoelectric because the atrial impulse originates at the AV node and travels more or less straight up (perpendicular to the axis of lead I). If the P' wave can be seen in lead V_1, it will look like an r' wave (described by Wellens as a *"pseudo right bundle branch block [RBBB] pattern"*).

QRS complex: Normal if the P' is completely hidden, as it is in Fig. 11-2, *A.* However, the QRS is often distorted by the P' wave, causing a pseudo s wave in the inferior leads and/or a pseudo r' in lead V_1, as seen in Fig. 11-2, *B.*[5] QRS alternans (alternating heights of the R wave or depths of the S wave) is rare in AVNRT.

Conduction ratio: The conduction ratio is usually 1:1; that is, every time the ventricles are activated, so are the atria. It is rare to see AVNRT with 2:1 AV conduction; it has been described in the literature.

Aberrant ventricular conduction: Uncommon. This is because in the common form of AVNRT the impulse reaches the ventricles by way of the slow AV nodal pathway, giving the bundle branches time to repolarize. Aberrant ventricular conduction is discussed in Chapter 14.

Distinguishing features: AV nodal reentry tachycardia is recognized because of a paroxysmal, narrow QRS tachycardia that is either identical in shape to the normal sinus-conducted beats in all leads (hidden P' waves) or distorted by the P' wave (pseudo s wave in leads II, III, and aV_F and/or pseudo r' in lead V_1).

Clinical implications

Atrioventricular nodal reentry tachycardia is usually benign and self-limiting or easily terminated by a vagal maneuver. However, patient education is indicated because prolonged runs of PSVT may result in atrial fibrillation or atrial flutter.

Patient education. The patient should understand that such a tachycardia is usually initiated by a PAC. Therefore the preventable arrhythmogenic practices in a patient's lifestyle should be eliminated or controlled (such as too much caffeine, cigarette smoking, stress, or poor nutrition). The patient should be shown several vagal maneuvers and instructed to terminate the tachycardia as soon as it is perceived.

Emergency treatment

Emergency treatment for AVNRT and CMT is exactly the same, that of PSVT; long-term treatment differs. Please turn to p. 144 for a discussion of emergency response to PSVT.

Treatment with radiofrequency ablation

In a significant number of cases the ANVRT can be recurrent, symptomatic, and refractory to digitalis, calcium channel blockers, and beta blockers. For such patients radiofrequency ablation has been shown to be safer than class IA drugs. Such patients are candidates for selective ablation or modification of the slow posterior pathway with radiofrequency energy and should be referred to centers skilled in this procedure.[4,6-17]

In ablating the posterior slow pathway there is some risk of causing complete AV block. Great care is taken and the amount of radiofrequency energy used is sometimes not enough to completely ablate the pathway; a repeat porcedure on another day is often necessary. In some centers, exceptionally skilled physicians are choosing radiofrequency ablation over a lifetime on prophylactic drugs.

Uncommon form

In the uncommon form of ANVRT the impulse enters the ventricles via the fast pathway and returns to the atrium via the slow pathway. Thus the P' wave follows the QRS as in CMT (discussed in the next section). The differential diagnosis is made with electrophysiologic studies.

CIRCUS MOVEMENT TACHYCARDIA (ATRIOVENTRICULAR RECIPROCATING TACHYCARDIA)

Circus movement tachycardia is a PSVT caused by a reentry circuit using the normal AV nodal pathway for entrance into the ventricles (narrow QRS) and an accessory pathway for return to the atria. Because anterograde conduction proceeds normally down the AV node, this type of CMT is called *orthodromic*. There are two less common forms of CMT, *incessant CMT* and *antidromic CMT*, which are discussed in more detail in Chapter 23.

Location of the accessory pathways

Accessory pathways may be located at almost any point around the annulus fibrosus, although the two most common locations are the left free wall (58%) and the posteroseptum (24%).

Mechanism

Circus movement tachycardia may be initiated by a critically timed PAC or premature ventricular complex (PVC), an accelerated sinus rhythm in the young, and a junctional escape beat with retrograde block.[18]

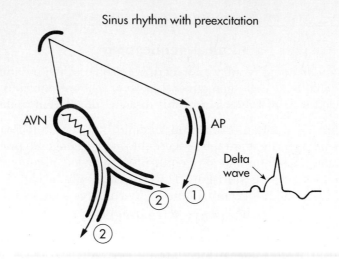

In overt Wolff-Parkinson-White (WPW) syndrome the normal sinus rhythm is conducted initially down the accessory pathway (AP), *1*, causing preexcitation, which is reflected by a delta wave on the ECG. Activation of the ventricles may also occur via the AV node (AVN) and bundle of His, *2*, producing a fusion beat (delta force fuses with normal). In some cases the impulse enters the ventricle via the accessory pathway so early that there is no contribution via the AV node; at other times the impulse may be delayed entering the ventricles via the accessory pathway.

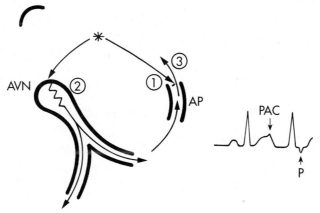

A PAC is blocked, *1*, in the accessory pathway, travels down the AV node, *2*, into the ventricles to produce a narrow QRS complex, and reenters the atrium via the accessory pathway, *3*, to produce a separate P′ wave.

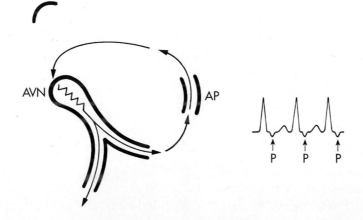

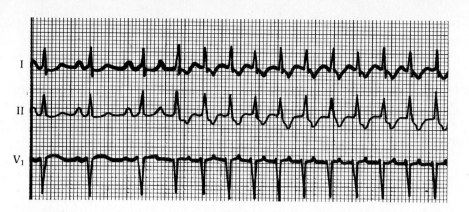

Fig. 11-3. Orthodromic circus movement tachycardia (CMT). The initiating PAC is distorting the third 'T' wave. Note that the initiating P'R interval is normal. (In AVNRT it would be prolonged.) During the tachycardia the P' waves are nicely seen in all three leads; an additional helpful clue is the QRS alternans in lead I.

The impulse then returns to the ventricles via the AV node, and a reentry circuit is established. The most essential point to note is that the reentry circuit of CMT activates the ventricles and atria in sequence, not simultaneously as in AVNRT. The ECG pattern is distinctive, with the P' wave separate from and immediately following the QRS, as seen in all three leads in Fig. 11-3. In the common form of CMT, conduction up the accessory pathway is rapid, placing the P' wave close to the preceding QRS.

ECG recognition

Heart rate: 170 to 250 beats/min.

Rhythm: Regular but may be irregular because of changing conduction through the AV node.

Initiating P'R interval: Not prolonged, because anterograde conduction uses the fast AV nodal pathway.

Location of the P' waves: Always separate from the QRS.

Polarity of the P' waves: Depends on the atrial insertion of the accessory pathway. A left free-wall location would cause the P' wave to be negative in lead I; this is a diagnostic sign for CMT.

QRS complex: Normal unless there is aberrant ventricular conduction (Chapter 14).

Conduction ratio: Always 1:1.

Aberrant ventricular conduction: Common. Fig. 11-4 shows a right bundle branch block aberration in a patient with a right-sided accessory pathway.

Heart rate during aberrancy: When the accessory pathway is on the same side as the bundle branch block, the heart rate is slower during the aberrancy than it is without, as shown in Fig. 11-4. When this is seen, it is diagnostic. The mechanism is demonstrated and explained in Fig. 11-5.

QRS alternans: Alternating heights or depths of the QRS are common in CMT. This is remarkable in all leads except V_4 of Fig. 11-6. QRS alternans is a phenomenon that is present 25% to 30% of the time during CMT but is rarely seen in AVNRT. QRS alternans may be seen with and without aberrant ventricular conduction and is seen especially in right bundle branch block aberration, but not if there is preexisting bundle branch block. QRS alternans may also be seen in ventricular tachycardia but not usually in more than four leads. The presence or absence of this sign is evaluated only after the first 5 to 6 seconds of the tachycardia because AVNRT may also have QRS alternans at its onset.[19,20]

Distinguishing features: Circus movement tachycardia is recognized because of a paroxysmal narrow QRS tachycardia with a P′ wave separate from and following the QRS. Circus movement tachycardia is frequently associated with QRS alternans and aberrant ventricular conduction.

Circus movement tachycardia initiated by a premature ventricular complex

When PSVT is initiated by a PVC, the mechanism is usually CMT. This is because the ventricular impulse easily enters the atria via the rapidly conducting accessory pathway, whereas retrograde penetration of the AV node occurs more slowly than it would through the accessory pathway, if it occurs at all. Having activated

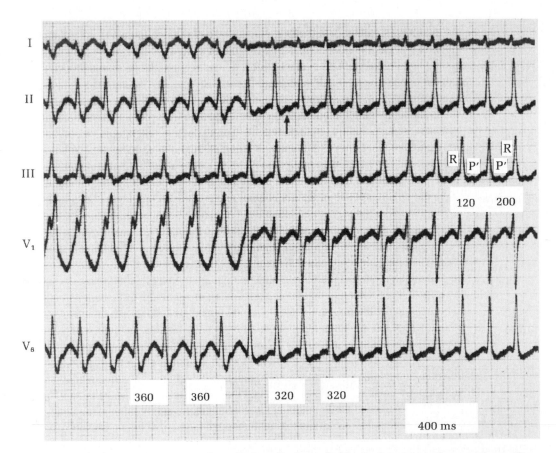

Fig. 11-4. Orthodromic CMT with right bundle branch block aberration that resolves after seven beats. In this tracing there are four signs that support or are diagnostic of CMT: (1) the aberration itself, (2) the slower heart rate during aberration, (3) the QRS alternans, and (4) a P′ wave separate from and following the QRS *(arrow)*. *(Courtesy Hein JJ Wellens, MD, Maastricht, The Netherlands.)*

the atria, the impulse passes down the AV node to the ventricles and a reentry circuit is established with the two AV structures (node and accessory pathway) being out of synchronization with each other. This lack of synchronization perpetuates the reentry circuit in all forms of reentry.

ECG signs negating the possibility of circus movement tachycardia

AV dissociation: Because the atria and ventricles are activated in sequence during CMT, AV dissociation is not possible.

Second or third degree AV block: Because second- or third-degree AV block eliminates the ventricles from the reentry circuit, neither condition is possible in CMT.

No visible P waves: Absence of P waves during the tachycardia after all leads have been carefully searched implies simultaneous activation of atria and ventricles and rules out CMT.

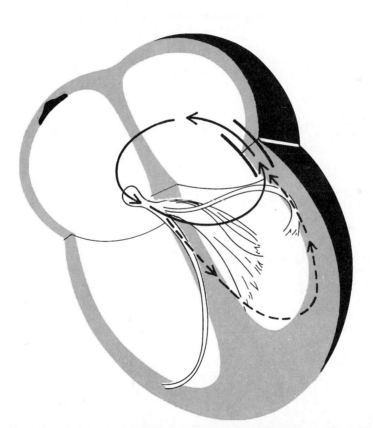

Fig. 11-5. The mechanism for the phenomenon of a slower heart rate during aberrancy than without aberrancy. Note that after entering the ventricles through the AV node and bundle of His the impulse must take the long way around to complete the reentry loop back into the atria via the left-sided accessory pathway. Of course, if the accessory pathway were on the right side and the aberration that of left bundle branch block, there would be no change in heart rate with or without aberration. This phenomenon occurs only when the accessory pathway is on the same side as the aberration (i.e., right bundle branch block and right-sided accessory pathway or left bundle branch block and left-sided accessory pathway).

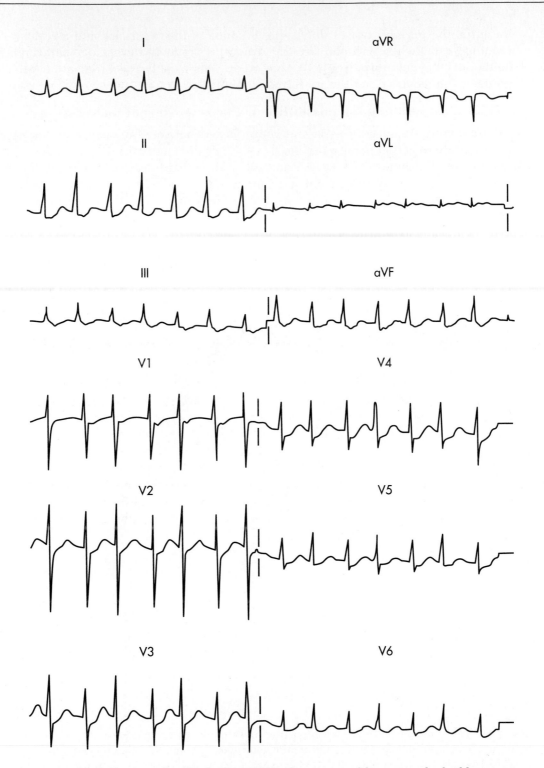

Fig. 11-6. Orthodromic CMT. This is the tracing of a 41-year-old woman who had been symptomatic for 5 years. Note the QRS alternans and the small P' wave closely following the QRS, best seen in leads III, aV$_F$, and V$_1$. A nursing diagnosis was made because of this emergency tracing, and the patient was referred to a physician for successful ablation of her accessory pathway with radiofrequency energy. *(Courtesy Teresita Harrison, RN, Calgary, Alberta, Canada.)*

Clinical implications

A patient who is symptomatic with CMT is in danger of developing atrial fibrillation, in which case the ventricular response is over 200 beats/min and often as fast as 300 beats/min. Thus it is important for clinicians who evaluate ECGs to be skilled in the recognition of this arrhythmia.

Emergency treatment

Emergency treatment for AVNRT and CMT is the same (that of PSVT). Please turn to p. 144 for this discussion.

Treatment (cure) with radiofrequency ablation

Long-term treatment for symptomatic CMT is transvenous radiofrequency ablation of the accessory pathway; this cures the patient of PSVT and eliminates the threat of sudden death should atrial fibrillation develop (see Chapter 23).

The ablation electrode is positioned where the accessory pathway potential is recorded under the AV valves or on top of the AV ring, or it is positioned at the location of the shortest ventriculoatrial interval during CMT.

CIRCUS MOVEMENT TACHYCARDIA WITH A SLOWLY CONDUCTING ACCESSORY PATHWAY

When CMT is supported by a slowly conducting accessory pathway, the RP interval is longer than the PR interval and the tachycardia usually occupies more than 12 hours of the patient's day. "Incessant," "persistent," and "permanent" are all terms given to this relatively rare and extremely debilitating type of CMT. The persistent nature of this tachycardia leads to atrial damage and congestive heart failure. The reentry circuit consists of conduction into the ventricles via the AV node (thus the narrow QRS) and retrograde conduction to the atria via a slowly conducting accessory pathway, placing the P′ wave well beyond the QRS (RP > PR). Remember that during CMT using a rapidly conducting accessory pathway the P′ wave

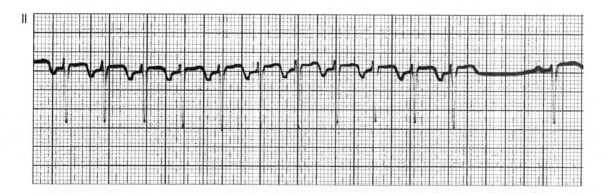

Fig. 11-7. Persistent CMT (incessant junctional tachycardia). This condition is recognized because of the persistent nature of the tachycardia (more than 12 hours per day) and the ECG (RP longer than PR). A slowly conducting accessory pathway is inserted into the coronary sinus os, accounting for the negative P′ wave in lead II. In this tracing there are two sinus beats in the middle of the strip.

is located close to but separate from the preceding QRS (RP < PR). Fig. 11-7 shows a persistent CMT ("incessant junctional tachycardia"). Such a tachycardia can be cured with radiofrequency ablation, after which the tachycardia related cardiomyopathy resolves considerably.

EMERGENCY RESPONSE TO PAROXYSMAL SUPRAVENTRICULAR TACHYCARDIA
Hemodynamically stable patient

- **Record** the tachycardia in at least five leads (I,II,III,V_1, and V_6).
- **Terminate** the tachycardia.[21]
    1. Vagal maneuver; if unsuccessful:
    2. Adenosine 6 mg intravenous (IV), rapidly; if it is unsuccessful, the dosage is increased to 12 mg; this may be repeated once. If it is unsuccessful:
    3. Procainamide 10 mg/kg body weight IV over 5 min; if it is unsuccessful:
    4. Electrical cardioversion.
- **Record** the sinus rhythm in the same leads.
- **Stabilize** the patient and take a history.
- **Diagnose** by close examination of the tracings with and without the tachycardia.
- **Refer** for radiofrequency ablation if CMT or refractory AVNRT is diagnosed.

Hemodynamically unstable patient

If the patient is hemodynamically unstable, record the rhythm in at least five leads and terminate the tachycardia with synchronized direct-current cardioversion. Once the patient is stabilized, the ECG tracings should be carefully examined and a differential diagnosis made. This symptomatic patient should be referred for evaluation to a center experienced in the use of radiofrequency ablation.

RATIONALE OF EMERGENCY RESPONSE
Why multiple lead recordings?

In PSVT, unlike ventricular tachycardia (VT), it is not necessary to make the differential diagnosis before terminating the tachycardia. In hemodynamically stable patients the primary consideration is to record the tachycardia in as many leads as possible. Obtaining a record in at least five leads (I, II, III, V_1, and V_6) is considered a minimal requirement. For patients with PSVT this is extremely important, since such patients have often had symptoms of palpitations and even presyncope for many years without seeking medical attention. The PSVT may be a fleeting experience for the patient, so the opportunity to record it is fortunate and the responsibility to do so should be taken very seriously.

Such tachycardias in patients with WPW syndrome may be harbingers of a more life-threatening arrhythmia. If delta waves are not present during sinus rhythm, as would be the case with latent or concealed WPW syndrome, short of invasive studies the diagnosis can only be made during the tachycardia by observing the presence and position of P′ waves. Thus the responsibility of the emergency department, critical care unit, or telemetry unit personnel to record the tachycardia in multiple leads cannot be overemphasized. Even if the admitting professional is not skilled in making the differential diagnosis of PSVT, a strict protocol should be followed so that the cardiologist has the opportunity to evaluate the tachycardia in enough leads to make the diagnosis and proper recommendations.

When the symptomatic patient is evaluated by cardiac catheterization, arrhythmias that are not clinically significant can be elicited by the intracardiac catheter. It is of great help to the examining physician to have a record of the clinical arrhythmia, another compelling reason to record multiple leads during the tachycardia.

Interrupting the reentry circuit

Treatment of the hemodynamically stable patient is initially aimed at lengthening the refractory period in the AV node with the vagal maneuver, adenosine, or verapamil. If this fails, procainamide is used. It blocks the retrograde fast AV nodal pathway and thus terminates AVNRT, and it blocks an accessory pathway should it be part of the reentry circuit and thus terminates CMT. The action of drugs on the slow and fast pathways of the AV node and on the accessory pathway is illustrated in Figs. 11-8 and 11-9. If the tachycardia continues after these three approaches, electrical cardioversion is indicated.

Vagal maneuver

Once the tachycardia has been recorded, a vagal maneuver can be used to terminate it. The mechanism of the vagal maneuver and the different types are de-

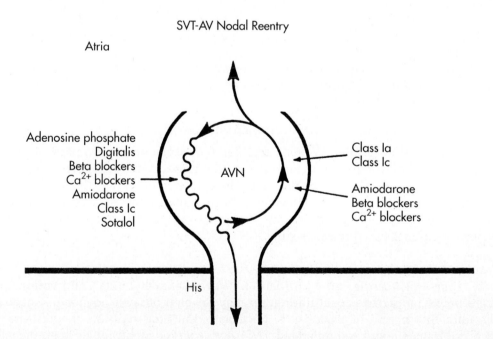

Fig. 11-8. Site of drug effects in AVNRT. The common form of AV nodal reentry is depicted, in which anterograde conduction is via the slow AV nodal pathway and retrograde conduction is via the fast AV nodal pathway. Although the main action of calcium channel blockers is along the slow AV nodal pathway, on occasion the retrograde fast AV nodal pathway is remarkably suppressed. Class IA is quinidine, procainamide, and disopyramide; class IC is flecainide propafenone and encainide. *(From Akhtar M, Tchou P, Jazayeri M: Circulation 80[suppl 4]:31, 1989.)*

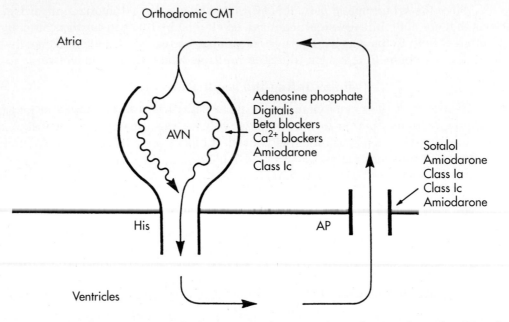

Fig. 11-9. Site of drug action in orthodromic CMT (anterograde conduction down the AV node [AVN] and retrograde conduction up the accessory pathway [AP]). Calcium channel blockers act primarily on the AV nodal component of the circuit, whereas class I drugs exert a more pronounced effect on the retrograde component (the accessory pathway). *(From Akhtar M, Tchou P, Jazayeri M: Circulation 80[suppl 4]:31, 1989.)*

scribed later in this chapter. If carotid sinus massage fails to terminate the tachycardia, it may be that the rhythm has been established for so long that the sympathetic nervous system is dominating.

Adenosine (Adenocard)

Adenosine blocks the AV node and has the tremendous advantage of an extremely short half-life (0.6 to 10 sec). Because of its short half-life, correct administration procedure is critical. The drug must be delivered quickly to the heart by very rapid IV push followed by a saline flush in the antecubital fossa or another vein close to the heart. The arm is then raised and the vein milked down to the axilla to ensure as rapid a delivery as possible.

Adverse effects. Adverse effects include flushing, dyspnea, headache, cough, chest pain, sinus bradycardia, atrial fibrillation, ventricular arrhythmias, and various degrees of AV block. The atrial fibrillation may develop because adenosine shortens the refractory period of atrial fibers. Because of the short half-life, the adverse effects are transient and well tolerated. Unlike verapamil, adenosine does not usually cause a fall in blood pressure, and it has replaced verapamil in the emergency setting of PSVT.[13,22] Adenosine is also given as a central IV bolus for termination of PSVT. The initial dose is 3 mg.[23]

Adenosine is not used in the differential diagnosis of broad QRS tachycardia or in the "diagnosis of SVT" because of two important pitfalls. First, although noted for its blocking action on the AV node, adenosine is also capable of terminating certain types of VT ("adenosine-sensitive VT")[24] and incapable of terminating certain types of SVT (those with atrial fibrillation or atrial flutter and accessory pathways). Thus an idiopathic VT (adenosine-sensitive) would be assumed to be SVT, unless, of course, the informed practitioner was aware of this action of adenosine and suspected this type of VT from the QRS morphologic appearance, QRS axis, and history (see p. 178). Second, atrial fibrillation or atrial flutter with an accessory pathway may be misdiagnosed (VT). Both cases can be cured by radiofrequency ablation, and a misdiagnosis deprives such patients of a correct diagnosis, referral, and cure.

Verapamil

If verapamil is used instead of adenosine, it is given IV 10 mg over 3 min. If the patient is taking a beta blocker or is hypotensive, the dose is reduced to 5 mg.[21]

Procainamide (Pronestyl)

Procainamide has the advantages of lengthening the refractory period in retrograde fast AV nodal pathways, which interrupts AVNRT, and lengthening the refractory period in accessory pathways, which interrupts CMT.

Cardioversion

If vagal maneuvers, including carotid sinus massage (performed by the physician), and drugs have not converted the PSVT to sinus rhythm, electrical cardioversion should now be used; as little as 10 J is frequently effective; 100 J is almost always successful.

Recording the sinus rhythm

After converting the patient to a sinus rhythm, a 12-lead ECG is taken. At the very least, the sinus rhythm should be recorded in the same leads that recorded the tachycardia (I,II,III,V_1, and V_6). The purpose of this is not only to look for delta waves or other abnormalities during sinus rhythm, but also that P′ waves can be more easily located by comparing the shape of the ST segment during sinus rhythm with that during the tachycardia. The P′ wave will not necessarily be seen clearly in all leads, so comparison with the shape of the J point (the point where the QRS ends and the ST segment begins), ST segment, and T wave is very helpful in locating a P′ in hiding.

Taking a history

The history may reveal the occurrence of previous incidences of tachycardia. The patient should be queried about polyuria associated with the tachycardia. Such a finding is present in 20% to 50% of patients with PSVT or atrial fibrillation[25] and is thought to be related to the changes in atrial pressure and rhythm, which induce the cardiac secretion of atrial natriuretic factor. This hormone is thought to cause the polyuria and hypovolemic hypotension sometimes associated with PSVT.[26]

MECHANISM AND METHODS OF VAGAL STIMULATION

Stimulation of the vagal nerve causes a release of acetylcholine, which in turn lengthens the refractory period of the AV node and thus terminates PSVT; the maneuver, however, may also have no effect on the tachycardia. The reentry circuits responsible for both CMT and AVNRT use the AV node as one arm of the reentry circuit, or a microreentry circuit is confined to the compact AV node and its atrial pathways. The AV block produced by the vagal maneuver upsets the delicate balance between anterograde and retrograde currents supporting the reentry circuit. Of course, because the AV and sinus nodes are closely related and are both supplied by the vagus nerve, automaticity of the sinus node is also suppressed. With strong vagal stimulation the sinus node may cease to beat.

Coughing is an excellent prehospital vagal maneuver. The patient may also be instructed to lie on the floor with legs elevated against the wall or perform Valsalva's maneuver, such as blowing against a closed glottis, gagging, or squatting. In the hospital setting, carotid sinus massage (described in the next section) and immersion of the face in cold water (the dive reflex) are excellent and strong vagal maneuvers. Caution: Never use eyeball pressure. Such a maneuver is extremely dangerous: it may cause retinal detachment. It is unpleasant for the patient and usually ineffective.

CAROTID SINUS MASSAGE

The carotid sinus is located at the bifurcation of the carotid artery at the angle of the jaw (not in the neck). The location of the carotid body is illustrated in Fig. 11-10. In the hands of the informed physician carotid sinus stimulation is an excellent diagnostic and therapeutic vagotonic maneuver. Massage of this area creates an elevation of blood pressure in the carotid sinus so that there will be reflex slowing of AV conduction.

Carotid sinus massage may be either diagnostic or therapeutic. It is diagnostic when it causes a transient block in AV conduction and unmasks atrial flutter (Fig. 11-11, *A*) or atrial tachycardia or when it causes temporary sinus slowing during sinus tachycardia. It is therapeutic when it terminates the tachycardia (Fig. 11-11, *B*). The abrupt termination of the tachycardia means only that the AV node was part of the reentry circuit; the decision regarding mechanism must still be made by

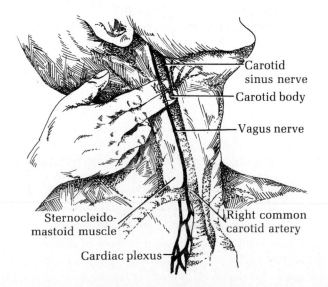

Fig. 11-10. The carotid sinus (carotid body) is located at the bifurcation of the carotid artery at the angle of the jaw.

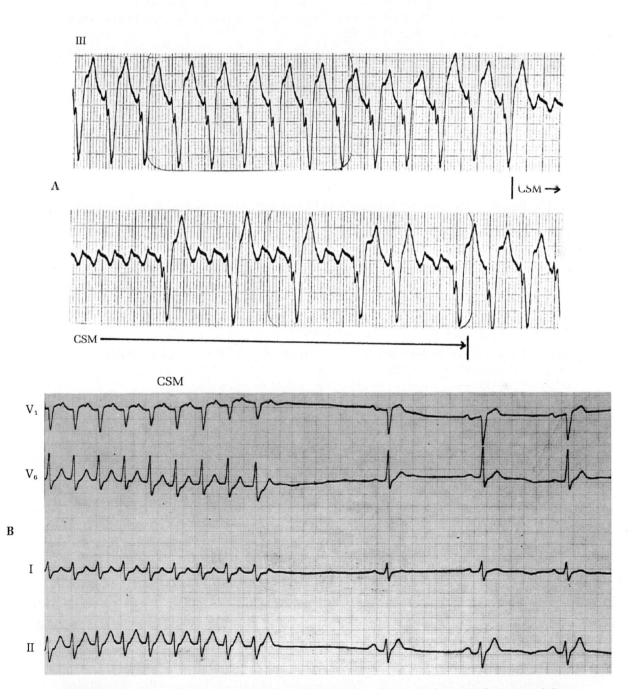

Fig. 11-11. A, Carotid sinus massage causes AV block and reveals the underlying atrial flutter. **B,** The AV block caused by carotid sinus massage in this patient terminated the CMT. During the tachycardia, the P′ waves can be seen in lead V₁, separate from the QRS. *(A from Stein E:* The electrocardiogram, *Philadelphia, 1976, WB Saunders; **B,** courtesy Hein JJ Wellens, MD, Maastricht, The Netherlands.)*

closely examining the ECG during the tachycardia and noting the position and polarity of the P' waves.

Effect of carotid sinus massage on supraventricular tachycardia[27]

1. *Sinus tachycardia:* Gradual and temporary slowing of the heart rate.
2. *Atrial tachycardia:* When, because of reentry, there is cessation of the tachycardia or the maneuver has no effect.
3. *Atrial fibrillation* or *persistent atrial tachycardia* (also called "incessant" atrial tachycardia): Temporary slowing of the ventricular rate, AV block, or the maneuver has no effect.
4. *Atrial flutter:* Temporary slowing of ventricular rate, AV block, conversion into atrial fibrillation, or the maneuver has no effect.
5. *PSVT:* Termination of the tachycardia or no effect.

Caution

1. Do not use carotid sinus massage on patients with a history of transient ischemic attacks, the findings of carotid artery stenosis on palpation, or carotid bruits.
2. Do not apply pressure for longer than 5 sec.
3. Do not use carotid sinus massage on patients over 65 years of age; sinus pauses of 3 to 7 sec have been reported under such circumstances. With aging there is a normal development of the parasympathetic nervous system, which is exacerbated by carotid sinus massage.

Procedure

1. Place the patient in a supine position with a small pillow or your arm under the patient's shoulders to extend the neck.
2. Turn the patient's head away from the side to be massaged.
3. Locate the bifurcation of the carotid artery just below the angle of the jaw (Fig. 11-10).
4. If the patient is not hypersensitive (begin with slight pressure): press the carotid sinus against the lateral processes of the cervical vertebrae with a massaging action for no more than 5 sec.
5. Monitor the effect of carotid sinus massage on the ECG; if an ECG monitor is not available, listen to the heart with the stethoscope as you massage the carotid sinus.

SYMPTOMS OF PAROXYSMAL SUPRAVENTRICULAR TACHYCARDIA

Symptoms depend on the duration and rate of the tachycardia and the presence of structural heart disease. (There is usually none.) Symptoms include feelings of palpitations, nervousness, polyuria, anxiety, angina, heart failure, syncope, or shock, depending on the duration and rate of the tachycardia and whether there is structural heart disease.

Syncope may be caused by the tachycardia itself (fall in cardiac output and reduced cerebral circulation) or by the overdrive suppression following the termination of the tachycardia (automaticity of the sinus node is suppressed by the tachycardia.) The prognosis for patients without heart disease is usually good.[28]

PHYSICAL SIGNS OF PAROXYSMAL SUPRAVENTRICULAR TACHYCARDIA
The neck veins

"Frog sign." Even before the ECG electrodes are applied, observation of the neck veins often helps to rapidly distinguish between SVT and VT. During PSVT the atria contract against closed AV valves, causing a reflux of blood up the jugular veins. This results in a rapid, regular expansion of the neck veins resembling the rhythmic puffing motion of a frog. Wellens[21] refer to this physical finding as the "frog sign." The patient usually reports a history of palpitations and seeks medical attention when the palpitations are associated with lightheadedness, shortness of breath, or anxiety. When questioned, the patient or family may have noticed the frog sign.

Other tachycardias. The pulsations in the neck veins often reveal the mechanism of other tachycardias as well.[27] Sinus tachycardia and atrial tachycardia are the only two SVTs that do not result in abnormal pulsations in the neck veins. In atrial flutter there are flutter waves, and in atrial fibrillation, irregular pulsations in the neck veins. In VT with AV dissociation these pulsations are irregular because of the occasional simultaneous beating of atria and ventricles.

Pulse, blood pressure, and heart sounds

In all types of regular SVT, the pulse is regular and the blood pressure and the loudness of the first heart sound constant. On the other hand, these parameters vary when there are changing RR intervals and AV conduction varies, as in atrial fibrillation and atrial flutter with variable conduction ratios. The jugular venous pressure may be elevated, but the waveform generally remains constant.[28]

Polyuria

In a significant number of patients (20% to 50%) PSVT is associated with polyuria. This response typically occurs with heart rates greater than 120 beats per min and a duration of 10 to 30 min. Polyuria has also been noted during episodes of atrial fibrillation, atrial flutter, and VT.[25] Factors responsible are changes in atrial rhythm and pressure, resulting in the release of the atrial natriuretic factor, a hormone that causes diuresis and may also play a role in the post-tachycardia, hypovolemic hypotension sometimes associated with PSVT.[26,29]

Syncope

The syncope that frequently occurs in upright PSVT is thought to be caused by a particular hemodynamic response to the stress of tachycardia and does not imply a more malignant or rapid tachycardia. The sequence is thought to be as follows[30]:
1. Paroxysmal supraventricular tachycardia causes a short diastolic filling time and ineffective timing of atrial and ventricular contraction, reducing left ventricular filling.
2. An increase in sympathetic tone occurs at the onset of the tachycardia.
3. The upright position also causes reduced left ventricular volume and increased sympathetic tone.
4. This in turn may precipitate inappropriate stimulation of left ventricular stretch receptors, causing an inadequate hemodynamic response to the tachycardia and syncope. The mechanism is similar to that postulated for vasovagal syncope.

5. During the tachycardia, syncope can occur because the rapid ventricular rate fails to provide adequate cerebral circulation; following the tachyarrhythmia syncope can occur because of overdrive suppression of the sinus node by the tachycardia.

PEDIATRICS: PAROXYSMAL SUPRAVENTRICULAR TACHYCARDIA IN THE FETUS AND NEONATE[31]

Circus movement tachycardia is the most common arrhythmia in the neonate[32] and accounts for most of the PSVTs that occur in infants. Wolff-Parkinson-White syndrome is overt in 50% of cases and concealed in the other half (Chapter 23).[31] Although 30% of the children with overt WPW syndrome lose the delta wave in the first year of life and 50% of them no longer have their PSVT after that time, the PSVT returns by the time they are 20 years of age.[33] Until then, no treatment is required.[31]

Heart rate. The usual rate of SVT in an infant is 300 beats/min.

Mechanisms. The two common mechanisms for SVT in the fetus are intraatrial reentry and atrioventricular reentry.

Diagnosis. During random fetal heart rate monitoring the tachycardia is noted; rarely, the mother reports a decrease in fetal movements. The mechanism is diagnosed by visualizing on echocardiography the atrial and ventricular contractions or the movement of the AV valves, or both. For example, if the atrial contractions outnumber the ventricular ones, intraatrial reentry is diagnosed. Because of the AV block, it is assumed that the AV junction is not part of the reentry circuit. This type of PSVT is present in many fetuses. However, should there be a one-to-one relationship between the atria and the ventricle, an AV reciprocating tachycardia is assumed. This, of course, produces a faster ventricular rate than the SVT with AV block.

Clinical implications. In the infant up to the age of 1 year a rate of 300 beats/min is generally well tolerated for several hours. In the fetus, such a heart rate is not well tolerated and results in hydrops fetalis in just a few hours.

SUMMARY

Table 11-1 is a summary of the ECG differences between CMT and AVNRT. The distinction between the two mechanisms is made because of the position of the P' wave in the cardiac cycle. In AVNRT the P' wave is buried within the QRS; in CMT the P' wave is separate from the QRS. In addition, QRS alternans and aberrant ventricular conduction are more common in CMT than in AVNRT; a slowing of the rate

Table 11-1. Differential diagnosis in paroxysmal supraventricular tachycardia

ECG sign	Atrioventricular nodal reentry tachycardia	Circus movement tachycardia
QRS alternans	Rare	Common
Initial P'R interval	Prolonged	Normal
P'-wave location	Hidden in the QRS or may look like terminal QRS forces	Separate from QRS
P' polarity	Negative in inferior leads (pseudo s wave); may be positive in lead V_1 (pseudo r')	Varies with accessory pathway location
Aberrancy	Rare	Common
AV conduction	Usually 1:1	Always 1:1

during aberration as compared with the rate without aberration is diagnostic of CMT; and when a PVC initiates PSVT, the mechanism is usually CMT.

Once PSVT has been recorded in multiple leads, it should be terminated and time can then be spent locating P′ waves and making a studied, accurate diagnosis. Termination of the tachycardia is usually accomplished with a vagal maneuver. If this is unsuccessful, adenosine or verapamil is used as an AV nodal blocker, and if that is also unsuccessful, procainamide is used because it blocks both the retrograde fast AV nodal pathway and accessory pathway. Each of these drugs is capable of terminating both mechanisms of PSVT. If the tachycardia persists after this, cardioversion is attempted.

REFERENCES

1. Josephson ME, Wellens HJJ: Differential diagnosis of supraventricular tachycardia, *Cardiol Clin* 8:411, 1990.
2. McGuire MA, Bourke JP, Robotin MC et al: High resolution mapping of Koch's triangle using sixty electrodes in humans with atrioventricular junctional (AV nodal) reentrant tachycardia, *Circulation* 88(pt 1):2315, 1993.
3. Keim S, Werner P, Jazayeri M et al: Localization of the fast and slow pathways in atrioventricular nodal reentrant tachycardia by intraoperative ice mapping, *Circulation* 86:919, 1992.
4. Mitrani RD, Klein LS, Hackett FK et al: Radiofrequency ablation for atrioventricular node reentrant tachycardia: comparison between fast (anterior) and slow (posterior) pathway ablation, *J Am Coll Cardiol* 21:432, 1993.
5. Farré J, Wellens HJJ: The value of the electrocardiogram in diagnosing site of origin and mechanism of supraventricular tachycardia. In Wellens HJJ, Kulbertus JE, eds: *What's new in electrocardiography,* The Hague, 1981, Martinus Nijhoff.
6. Moultin K: Radiofrequency catheter ablation for AV nodal reentry: a technique for rapid transection of the slow AV nodal pathway, *PACE Pacing Clin Electrophysiol* 16:760, 1993.
7. Li HG, Klein GJ, Stites HW et al: Elimination of slow pathway conduction: an accurate indicator of clinical success after radiofrequency atrioventricular node modification, *J Am Coll Cardiol* 22:1849, 1993.
8. Moulton L, Grant J, Miller, Moulton K: Radiofrequency catheter ablation for supraventricular tachycardia, *Heart Lung* 22:3, 1993.
9. Scheinman MM: Atrioventricular reentry: lessons learned from radiofrequency modification of the node, *Circulation* 85:1619, 1992.
10. Chen SA, Chiang CE, Tsanf WP et al: Selective radiofrequency catheter ablation of fast and slow pathways in 100 patients with atrioventricular nodal reentrant tachycardia, *Am Heart J* 125:1, 1993.
11. Lindsay BD, Chung MK, Gamache MC et al: Therapeutic end points for the treatment of atrioventricular node reentrant tachycardia by catheter-guided radiofrequency current, *J Am Coll Cardiol* 22:733, 1993.
12. Jackman WM, Beckman KJ, McClelland JH et al: Treatment of supraventricular tachycardia due to atrioventricular nodal reentry by radiofrequency catheter ablation of slow-pathway conduction, *N Engl J Med* 327:313, 1992.
13. Haissaguerre M, Gaita F, Fischer B et al: Elimination of atrioventricular nodal reentrant tachycardia using discrete slow potentials to guide application of radiofrequency energy, *Circulation* 85:2162, 1992.
14. Kay GN, Epstein AE, Dailey SM, Plumb VJ: Selective radiofrequency ablation of the slow pathway for the treatment of atrioventricular nodal reentrant tachycardia: evidence for involvement of perinodal myocardium within the reentrant circuit, *Circulation* 85:1675, 1992.
15. Jazayeri MR, Hempe SL, Sra JS et al: Selective transcatheter ablation of the fast and slow pathways using radiofrequency energy in patients with atrioventricular nodal reentrant tachycardia, *Circulation* 85:1318, 1992.
16. Lee MA, Morady F, Kadish A et al: Catheter modification of the atrioventricular junction with radiofrequency energy for control of atrioventricular nodal reentry tachycardia, *Circulation* 83:827, 1991.
17. Metzger JT, Cheriex EC, Smeets JLRM et al: Safety of radiofrequency catheter ablation of accessory atrioventricular pathways, *Am Heart J* 127:1533, 1994
18. Durrer D et al: The role of premature beats in the initiation and termination of supraventricular tachycardia in the Wolff-Parkinson-White syndrome, *Circulation* 36:644, 1967.
19. Green M, Heddle B, Kassen W et al: Value of QRS alternation in determining the site of origin of narrow QRS supraventricular tachycardia, *Circulation* 68:368, 1983.
20. Bar FW, Brugada P, Dassen WRM, Wellens HJJ: Differential diagnosis of tachycardia with narrow QRS complex (shorter than 0.12 second), *Am J Cardiol* 54:555, 1984.
21. Wellens HJJ, Conover M: *The ECG in emergency decision making,* Philadelphia, 1992, WB Saunders.

22. Parker RB, McCollam PL: Adenosine in the episodic treatment of paroxysmal supraventricular tachycardia, *Clin Pharm* 9(4):261, 1990.

23. McIntosh-Yellin NL, Drew BJ, Scheinman MM: Safety and efficacy of central intravenous bolus administration of adenosine for termination of supraventricular tachycardia, *J Am Coll Cardiol* 22:741, 1993.

24. Wilber DJ, Baerman J, Olshansky B et al: Adenosine-sensitive ventricular tachycardia: clinical characteristics and response to catheter ablation, *Circulation* 87:126, 1993.

25. Nicklas JM, DiCarlo LA, Koller PT et al: Plasma levels of immunoreactive atrial natriuretic factor increase during supraventricular tachycardia, *Am Heart J* 112:923, 1986.

26. Roy D, Paillard F, Cassidy D et al: Atrial natriuretic factor during atrial fibrillation and supraventricular tachycardia, *J Am Coll Cardiol* 9:509, 1987.

27. Wellens HJJ, Brugada P, Bar F: Diagnosis and treatment of the regular tachycardia with a narrow QRS complex. In Kulbertus HE, eds: *Medical management of cardiac arrhythmias,* Edinburgh, 1986, Churchill Livingstone.

28. Zipes DP: Specific arrhythmias: diagnosis and treatment. In Braunwald E, ed: *Heart disease,* ed 4, Philadelphia, 1992, WB Saunders.

29. Kojima S, Fujii T, Ohe T et al: Physiologic changes during supraventricular tachycardia and release of atrial natriuretic peptide, *Am J Cardiol* 62:576, 1988.

30. Leitch JW, Klein GJ, Yee R et al: Syncope associated with supraventricular tachycardia: an expression of tachycardia rate or vasomotor response? *Circulation* 85:1064, 1992.

31. Gillette PC, Zeigler VL, Case CL: Pediatric arrhythmias: are they different? In Zipes DP, Jalife J, eds: *Cardiac electrophysiology from cell to bedside,* ed 2, Philadelphia, 1995, WB Saunders.

32. Ludomirsky A, Garson A Jr: Supraventricular tachycardia. In Gillette PC, Garson A Jr, eds: *Pediatric arrhythmias: electrophysiology and pacing,* Philadelphia, 1990, WB Saunders.

33. Gillette PC, Blair HL, Crawford FA: Preexcitation syndromes. In Gillette PC, Garson A Jr, eds: *Pediatric arrhythmias: electrophysiology and pacing,* Philadelphia, 1990, WB Saunders.

C H A P T E R

12

Premature Ventricular Complexes

ECG Recognition *155*
Mechanism *156*
QRS Width *157*
QRS Shape *157*
Increased Amplitude *158*
T Wave of Opposite Polarity *158*
The Full Compensatory Pause *158*
Overdrive Suppression *160*

Types of Premature Ventricular
  Complexes *161*
Rule of Bigeminy *169*
Pediatrics *170*
Physical Signs *170*
Clinical Implications *170*
Treatment *171*
Summary *171*

A premature ventricular complex (PVC) is a single beat or a pair of ventricular ectopic beats that occurs before the expected sinus-conducted QRS. Other terms used are ventricular premature beat (VPB) or ventricular premature complex (VPC). A PVC is recognized on the ECG because of its prematurity and its shape.

ECG RECOGNITION

Heart rate: Underlying rate may be normal or abnormal. Premature ventricular complexes are more likely to appear during bradycardia, when there is more time for them to emerge.

Rhythm: Irregular because of the PVC.

P wave: The PVC does not have a related P wave unless there is retrograde conduction, and then the P′ wave follows the PVC or is buried in its T wave.

PP intervals: Can be "walked out" across the PVC approximately 50% of the time (AV dissociation).

QRS complex: That of the PVC is broad and premature and has increased amplitude. The shape of the PVC can be diagnostic. This is discussed later.

Full compensatory pause: Present approximately 50% of the time.

T wave: The T wave of the PVC is opposite in polarity to the terminal QRS.

Distinguishing features: A PVC is usually recognized because it is broad and premature and has an increased amplitude and a T wave of opposite polarity to the QRS. Fig. 12-1 illustrates a single PVC in a patient with acute myocardial infarc-

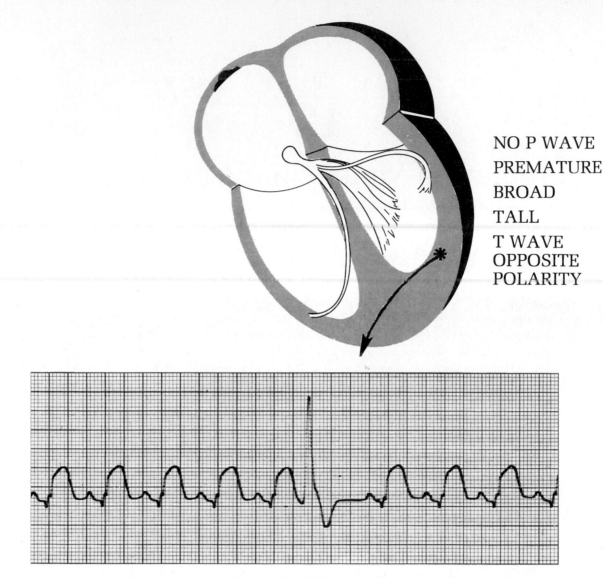

NO P WAVE

PREMATURE

BROAD

TALL

T WAVE
OPPOSITE
POLARITY

Fig. 12-1. A premature ventricular complex (PVC) is initially suspected because of its prematurity and its width.

tion. The prematurity of the PVCs in Fig. 12-2 is not quite so obvious. PVCs that occur at the end of diastole may be only slightly premature, and they may be fusion beats.

MECHANISM

A PVC may be the result of enhanced normal automaticity in the His-Purkinje system (catecholamines); abnormal automaticity anywhere in the ventricles (ischemia, electrolyte imbalance, or injury); reentry through slowly conducting tissue within the ventricles (ischemia or injury); or triggered activity occurring within the His-Purkinje system (digitalis excess or catecholamines) or within the ventricular myocardium (e.g., class 1A or 1C drugs).

V₁

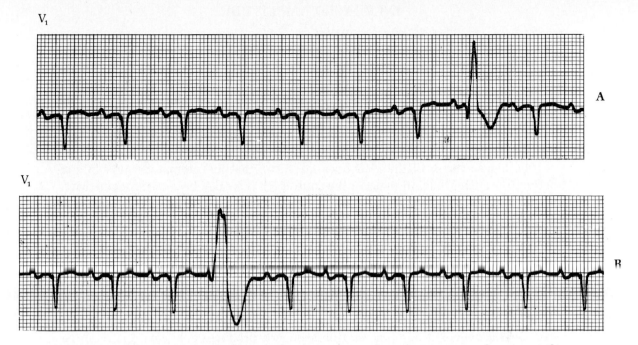

Fig. 12-2. A, Premature ventricular complex is premature by only 0.08 sec and occurs at the end of diastole ("end-diastolic" PVC); it is preceded by a P wave, which has time to conduct and partially activate the ventricles at the same time as the PVC (a fusion beat). **B,** Tracing from the same patient. This end-diastolic PVC is too early to be a fusion beat, i.e., the ventricles have already been activated by the ectopic focus. The sinus P wave can be seen distorting the beginning of the PVC, but its shape is purely that of the PVC. The PVC in **A** is narrower than the one in **B** (the hallmark of a fusion beat).

QRS WIDTH

The excessive width of the PVC is due to ventricular activation that begins outside the conduction system and therefore does not have the advantage of speedy, organized delivery to the myocardium. A width of 0.14 sec or more is one of the distinguishing features of the ventricular ectopic beat or rhythm. Exceptions are ventricular fascicular beats (see Chapter 17) and fusion beats (see Chapter 21). Premature ventricular complexes may also appear to be narrow in certain leads when initial or terminal forces are isoelectric; this is easily recognized by looking at the questionable beat in other leads (where the PVC is broad).

QRS SHAPE

The shape of the QRS can be diagnostic of ventricular ectopy. To make this judgment, lead V₁ must be available; sometimes leads V₂ and V₆ are also necessary. If V₁ is positive, look for a monophasic or biphasic complex to indicate a PVC; two peaks with the first peak higher is also diagnostic for a PVC. If the complex in V₁ is negative, any one of the following signs indicates ventricular ectopy: R wave broader than 0.03 sec, a slurred S downstroke, delayed S nadir in V₁ or V₂, or q in V₆.

INCREASED AMPLITUDE

The greater amplitude of the PVC is caused by a stronger vector. Normally the right and left ventricles are activated simultaneously from endocardium to epicardium, with the currents activating the right ventricle being canceled out by the stronger ones in the left ventricle. With a ventricular ectopic beat the sequence of activation is such that most currents are traveling in one direction (e.g., from the left to the right ventricle) without the canceling-out effect of the normal activation sequence. The resultant stronger vector is reflected in the ECG tracing by a complex of higher amplitude than that of the dominant sinus rhythm.

The bigger vector of the PVC does not mean that the premature muscle contraction is stronger than normal. On the contrary, it is weaker because it occurs early, not allowing for complete ventricular filling, and because the contraction resulting from a PVC is not uniform. In fact, it is the conducted sinus beat following the PVC that is stronger than other sinus beats. This is because the pause following the PVC allows for more ventricular filling.

T WAVE OF OPPOSITE POLARITY

Whenever the process of depolarization is abnormal, as it is with a PVC or bundle branch block, the repolarization sequence produces a T wave that is opposite in polarity to the terminal part of the QRS. This is called a *secondary T wave change* and is expected in these conditions. The normal repolarization process produces a T wave that is the same polarity as the QRS. After a PVC the repolarization process is reversed, producing a T wave that is opposite in polarity to the QRS.

THE FULL COMPENSATORY PAUSE

A full compensatory pause is the pause that follows a PVC and is caused by nonconduction of a normal sinus beat. The sinus beat fails to conduct to the ventricles because the PVC has left them refractory. Thus a full compensatory pause is found only when the sinus rhythm is uninterrupted by the PVC and when one sinus P wave is not conducted. True full compensatory pauses are seen after only about half of the PVCs (the ones with retrograde block to the atria); the other half have retrograde conduction to the atria, which resets the sinus rhythm and negates the possibility for a true full compensatory pause. In Fig. 12-3 the sinus rhythm can be "walked out" across the PVC. The sinus P wave can actually be seen within the T wave of the PVC. To measure for the presence of a full compensatory pause, place a piece of paper under the tracing and mark precisely three P waves. Then move the paper so that the first mark is on the conducted beat before the PVC; the third mark should fall exactly on the P wave following the pause. A caliper can also be used to walk out the sinus rhythm; the P waves will be on time, despite the interruption by the PVC; one P wave is not conducted, causing the "pause."

It is possible to have a PVC with less or more than a full compensatory pause because of retrograde conduction to the atria from the PVC or because of a sinus arrhythmia. In the case of retrograde conduction to the atria the sinus node is either discharged early or delayed because of overdrive suppression (explained later). A delay of the sinus discharge can cause the P wave following the pause to be right on time (chance), late, or late but earlier than the next expected P. Thus it is that the full compensatory pause, as Dr. Marriott would say, is a "broken reed." You can

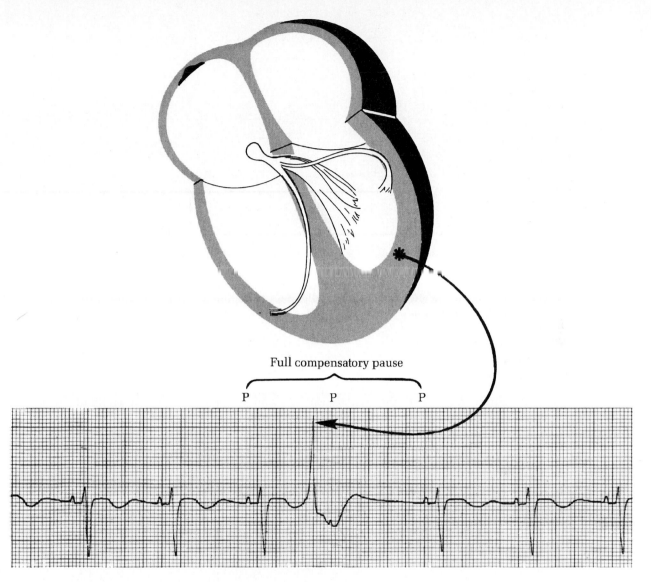

Fig. 12-3. The full compensatory pause is the result of an uninterrupted sinus rhythm and a sinus P wave that is not conducted to the ventricles. The sinus P wave that is not conducted in this tracing is seen in the T wave of the PVC; note that it is right on time with the other PP intervals.

count on it as a diagnostic sign of a PVC only if the nonconducted sinus P wave can actually be seen (as in Fig. 12-3).

In Fig. 12-4 there is retrograde conduction to the atria, causing the sinus node to be discharged early and the next sinus P wave to be early. Thus, although this is a PVC, there is not a full compensatory pause. More weight is placed on the morphologic appearance of the PVC in lead V_1 than on the presence of a full compensatory pause. For example, the broad beat in Fig. 12-5 is followed by a full compensatory pause. However, the sinus P wave occurring during the broad beat cannot be seen, placing the accuracy of such a pause in doubt. The monophasic R wave in V_1

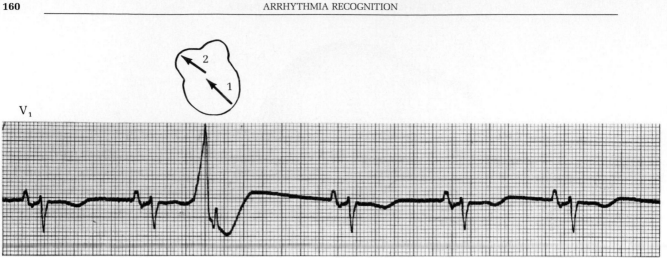

Fig. 12-4. Premature ventricular complex has retrograde conduction to the atria. Note that the retrograde P′ wave is distorting the T of the PVC. When you attempt to "walk out" this rhythm, the retrograde P′ is premature and disturbs the regular beating of the sinus node. In this case it suppresses the sinus node, causing the next expected sinus beat to be later than expected (overdrive suppression).

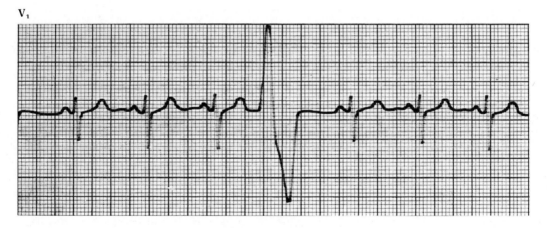

Fig. 12-5. An apparently full compensatory pause follows this PVC. However, the nonconducted sinus P wave cannot be seen, leaving some doubt. The morphologic appearance of the broad complex in V_1 identifies it as a PVC (monophasic R).

plus the excessive width of the QRS (0.16 sec) and its prematurity identify it as a PVC.

OVERDRIVE SUPPRESSION

Overdrive suppression is a property belonging to all pacemaker cells by which their premature discharge causes their cycle to lengthen. For example, the sinus node sometimes is delayed in reaching threshold potential if it is discharged early by retrograde conduction to the atria or by any other early beat (e.g., PAC). This can

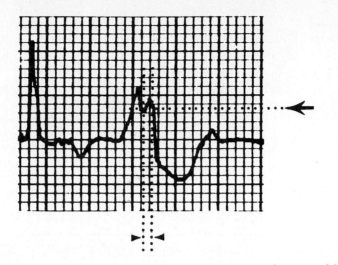

Fig. 12-6 Method of measuring the notch in the PVC. (1) Draw a horizontal line at the level of the lowest point in the notch (its nadir). (2) Make vertical lines at the two peaks. *(From Moulton KP, Medcalf T, Lazzara R: Circulation 81:1245, 1990.)*

be seen in the length of the P'P interval (the distance from the ectopic P to the next sinus P). This distance is longer than the PP intervals of the dominant rhythm.

TYPES OF PREMATURE VENTRICULAR COMPLEXES

Premature ventricular complexes (PVC) may occur at any time during the cardiac cycle from one, two, or many foci and may occur in certain shapes and sets. The many different types of PVC are illustrated in the following section.

The "ugly" premature ventricular complex

Clinical implications may be derived from the shape of the PVC.[1] The "ugly PVC" (broad and notched) has been shown to indicate a dilated and globally hypokinetic left ventricle in a nonspecifically diseased heart, whereas the smooth, narrower PVC reflects normal heart size and normal or near-normal systolic function, despite the presence of underlying disease.[1] Fig. 12-6 demonstrates the method of measuring ugliness (i.e., the notch). In Fig. 12-7, ugly PVCs are compared with smooth PVCs and the clinical implications are explained.

Unifocal premature ventricular complexes

Unifocal PVCs are illustrated in Fig. 12-8. They are identical in form because they originate from the same focus. Every time the ectopic focus fires, currents pass through the ventricular myocardium, taking the same route as before so that the complex is identical in shape each time, as long as the ECG lead remains the same.

Multifocal premature ventricular complexes

Multifocal or multiform PVCs are ventricular extrasystoles from different foci; other terms are *multiform* or *polymorphic*. Note in Fig. 12-9 that the PVCs have two different shapes.

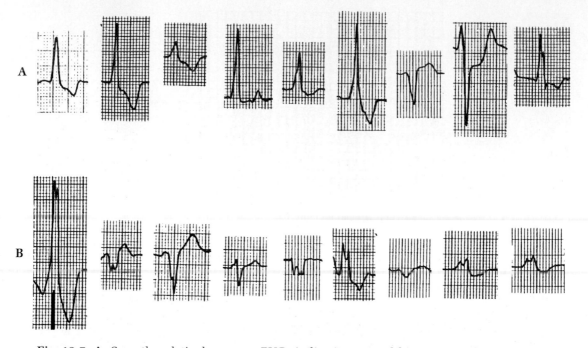

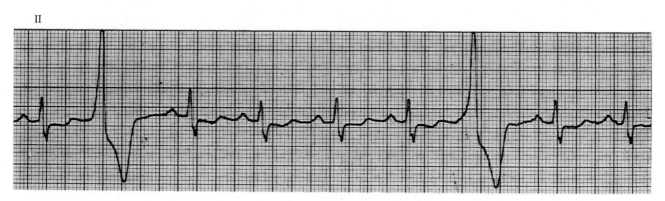

Fig. 12-7. A, Smooth, relatively narrow PVCs indicating normal heart size and normal systolic function, despite presence of underlying disease. **B,** "Ugly PVCs" are broad (>0.16 sec) with a notch of 0.04 sec or more, indicating a dilated and globally hypokinetic left ventricle in a nonspecifically diseased heart. *(From Moulton KP, Medcalf T, Lazzara R: Circulation 81:1245, 1990.)*

Fig. 12-8. Unifocal PVCs originate in the same focus, take the same route of conduction, and are identical in shape.

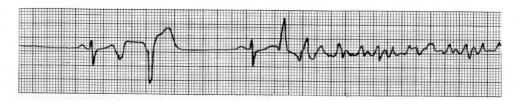

Fig. 12-9. Multifocal or multiform PVCs have different foci. These PVCs are occurring on the T wave in a patient with ischemic heart disease and result in ventricular fibrillation.

Bigeminy, trigeminy, quadrigeminy, and pairs

A bigeminal rhythm consists of pairs. In ventricular bigeminy, every other beat is a PVC. Note in Fig. 12-10 that each PVC is also precisely coupled to the preceding normal complex. The most common cause of this precise coupling is coronary artery disease. In that case the mechanism is reentry resulting from slow conduction in one area of the myocardium; ventricular bigeminy is sometimes seen in digitalis toxicity, in which case the mechanism is probably triggered activity. A trigeminal rhythm is made up of groups of three (Fig. 12-11, *A*). Fig. 12-11, *B*, is an ex-

V_1

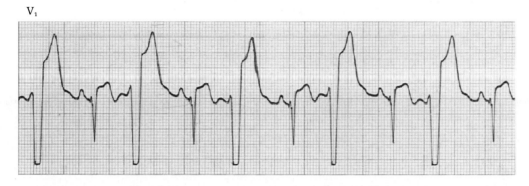

Fig. 12-10. Ventricular bigeminy with fixed coupling. Fixed coupling means that the interval between the sinus beat and the PVC is the same each time, implying a cause-and-effect relationship.

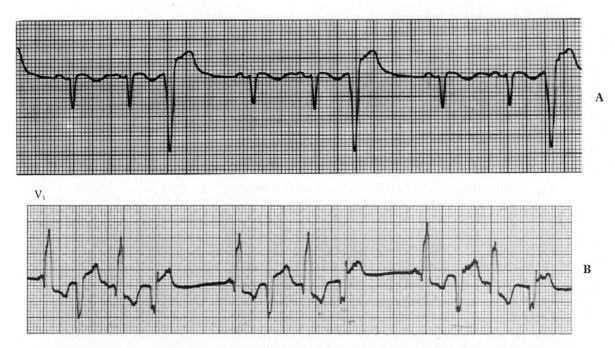

V_1

Fig. 12-11. A, Ventricular trigeminy—two normal complexes and one PVC. **B,** Ventricular quadrigeminy—groups of four.

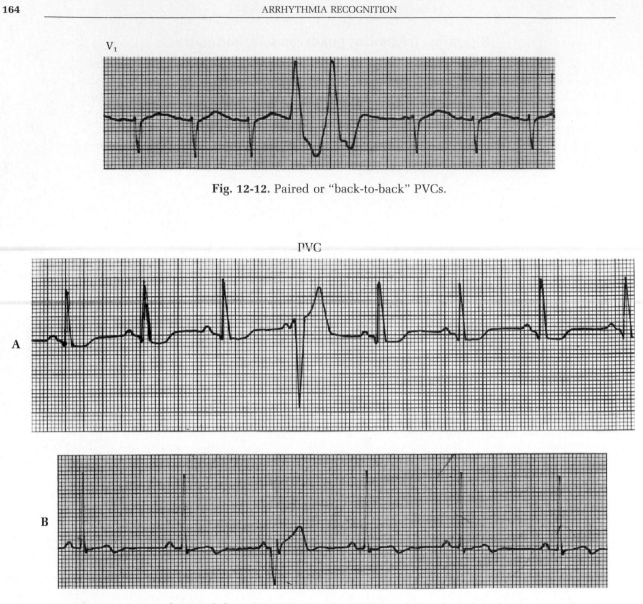

V_1

Fig. 12-12. Paired or "back-to-back" PVCs.

PVC

A

B

Fig. 12-13. A and B, End-diastolic PVCs. B, The PVC is a fusion beat (conduction into the ventricle from both the sinus beat and the ventricular ectopic focus).

ample of quadrigeminy. Fig. 12-12 illustrates PVCs that occur in pairs or back to back. When there are three or more ventricular ectopic beats, the rhythm is called ventricular tachycardia.

End-diastolic premature ventricular complexes

The end-diastolic PVC occurs late in the cardiac cycle before the ventricles can be activated or partially activated by the sinus beat. In Fig. 12-13, A, there is a P wave immediately preceding but unrelated to an end-diastolic PVC. The PR interval preceding the end-diastolic PVC may be shorter than the dominant one. In Fig. 12-13, B, the end-diastolic PVC is a fusion beat because it was late enough to permit the sinus impulse entrance into the ventricles at the same time as ectopic activation. An end-diastolic PVC may be the occasional manifestation of an accelerated

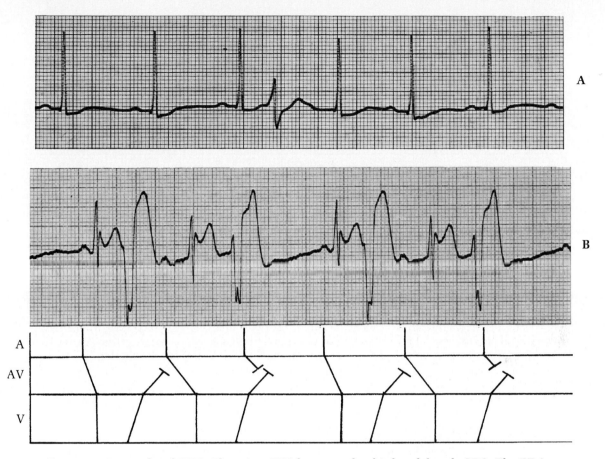

Fig. 12-14. Interpolated PVC. There is a PVC between the third and fourth QRS. The PR interval following the PVC is longer than the others. (The P wave can be found distorting the T wave of the ectopic beat.)

idioventricular rhythm trying to surface or, if such PVCs occur frequently, in the setting of acute myocardial infarction they may be a sign of congestive heart failure. It is known that enhanced automaticity may result when myocardial fibers are stretched. Such would be the case with the elevated left-ventricular end-diastolic pressure that results from heart failure.

Interpolated premature ventricular complexes

An interpolated PVC is a premature ectopic beat sandwiched between two normal sinus-conducted beats; therefore it does not have a full compensatory pause. In fact, there is no pause at all in the sinus rhythm and ventricular response. Many times there is retrograde concealed conduction into the fast pathway of the atrioventricular (AV) node, causing the P wave following the PVC to be conducted into the ventricles via the slow AV nodal pathway. Thus the PR interval following the PVC is often longer than normal. Such is the case in Fig. 12-14: the sinus rate is 65 beats/min. Notice the long PR interval of the sinus beat after the PVC. In Fig. 12-15 interpolated PVCs create groups of four. The laddergram below this tracing helps to demonstrate the mechanism of concealed conduction, explained in the legend of that figure.

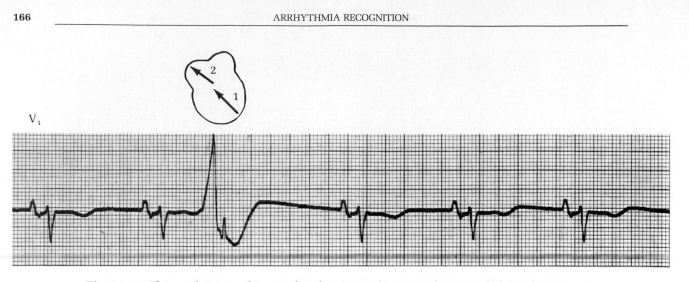

Fig. 12-15. The mechanism of interpolated PVCs with retrograde concealed conduction into the AV node is demonstrated with a laddergram. There is an interpolated PVC following the first beat of each group of four. The PVCs are actually bigeminal, but because one is interpolated, it creates an interesting quadrigeminal pattern. The laddergram below this tracing consists of three tiers representing atrial *(A)*, AV nodal *(AV)* and ventricular (V) activity. In the A tier (atrial activity) the sinus P waves are right on time. The first and second P waves are conducted to the ventricles with lengthening conduction time (represented in the AV tier). In the AV tier one can show how the PVC (second line in the V tier) caused the longer PR of the second sinus beat. . . concealed conduction into the AV node.

Fascicular premature ventricular complexes

Premature ventricular complexes originating in the fascicles of the intraventricular conduction system are narrower than other PVCs and have morphologic appearances identical to left or right bundle branch block aberration. The relative narrowness (approximately 0.13 sec) of the QRS results because the impulse is within the intraventricular conduction system rather than in ventricular myocardium where conduction is slower.

Anterior fascicular beats have right axis deviation (Fig. 12-16), and posterior fascicular beats, left axis deviation (Fig. 12-17); both have an RBBB configuration in lead V_1 and a relatively narrow QRS (<0.14 sec). Axis deviation occurs whenever there is an ectopic focus in the fascicles of the left bundle branch or when there is a block in one of these fascicles. The RBBB pattern occurs because the impulse originates within the left ventricular fascicles and the right ventricle is the last to be activated. The complexes are narrower than other ventricular ectopic beats because they originate within the conduction system and the impulse is therefore delivered to both ventricles very rapidly.

R-on-T phenomenon

The term "R on T" is used to indicate that an R wave (PVC) has occurred at the peak of the T wave—the vulnerable period of the ECG. During the first 4 hours after the onset of symptoms of myocardial infarction, primary ventricular fibrillation (VF) and R-on-T ventricular ectopics are frequent, decreasing rapidly with time.

Fig. 12-18 shows tracings from a patient in the emergency department who had shortly before sustained an inferior wall myocardial infarction. At the slower heart

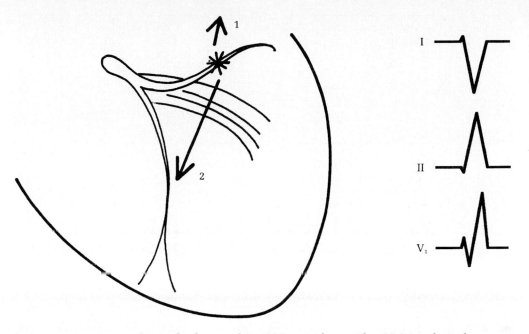

Fig. 12-16. An anterior fascicular beat and its ECG complexes. The QRS is relatively narrow (<0.14 sec) because of an origin within the conduction system. There is right axis deviation and a right bundle branch block pattern. The indicated 1-2 conduction sequence explain the right axis deviation and the QRS shape in the limb leads.

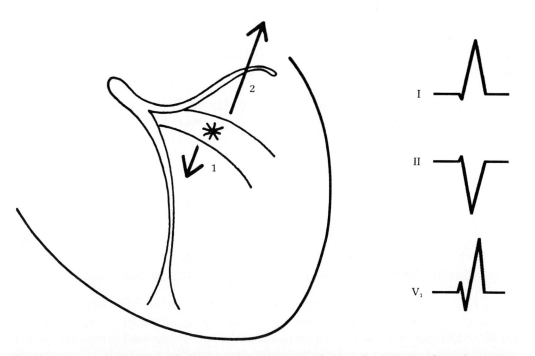

Fig. 12-17. A posterior fascicular beat and its ECG complexes. The QRS is relatively narrow (<0.14 sec) because of an origin within the conduction system. There is left axis deviation and a right bundle branch block pattern. The indicated 1-2 conduction sequence explain the left axis deviation and the QRS shape in the limb leads.

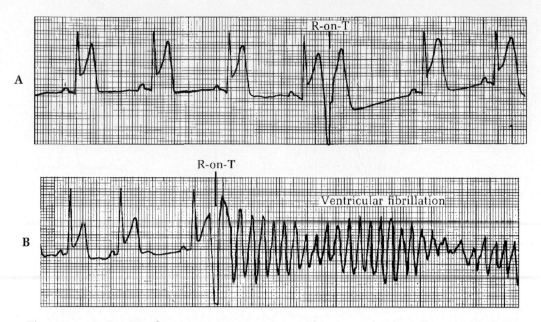

Fig. 12-18. **A,** R-on-T phenomenon in a patient with acute inferior wall myocardial infarction. **B,** In the same patient, R on T later causes ventricular fibrillation.

rate (Fig. 12-18, *A*) the R on T did not result in ventricular tachycardia or fibrillation. However, Fig. 12-18, *B,* shows the increase in heart rate and the pause before the R on T resulted in VF. The increase in sympathetic drive (increased heart rate) and the pause in rhythm are factors that have been identified by Coumel et al.[2] and Leclerck et al.[3] as two main determinants of sudden death in a study of 45 Holter monitor tapes of VF recorded during ambulatory monitoring.

The mechanism of the R-on-T phenomenon is thought to be the early afterdepolarizations.[4,5] One of the characteristics of this mechanism is a short coupling interval. (Ectopic firing occurs at the beginning of phase 3 of the action potential.) This would coincide with the apex of the T wave, the vulnerable period of the ECG. Simultaneously present during the T wave are a dispersion of repolarization, excitability, and conduction velocity. A stimulus applied in such an environment can provoke fibrillation. In fact, the early afterdepolarization is the only mechanism that is capable of producing an extrasystole that arises during the T wave; an extrasystole caused by reentry would come after the T wave, and one caused by a delayed afterdepolarization tends to appear in early diastole or mid diastole.[7] The R-on-T phenomenon is clearly a cause for concern when it appears in adults with a history of ischemic heart disease.[5-8]

As early as 1928 Louis Katz[9] emphasized the danger of PVCs falling on the T wave. The term *R-on-T phenomenon* was first used by Smirk[10] in 1949, who found that many patients showed the R-on-T phenomenon and that they were subject to lethal ventricular tachycardia (VT) and sudden death. Some Holter monitor recordings during the onset of cardiac arrest have demonstrated the R-on-T phenomenon just before the lethal arrhythmia.[11,12] This phenomenon appears to reflect unstable myocardium and transient vulnerability to potentially lethal arrhythmias rather than a sign of long-term high risk.[6,13,14]

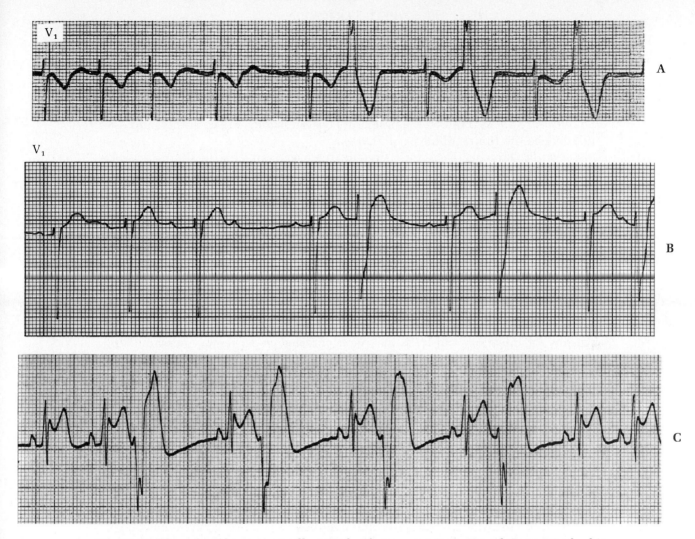

Fig. 12-19. The rule of bigeminy is illustrated. After a pause in **A, B,** and **C,** ventricular bigeminy is initiated. The underlying rhythm in **A** is atrial fibrillation (note absence of P waves); in **B** the underlying rhythm is AV Wenckebach. In **C** a PVC creates a pause that initiates ventricular bigeminy. At the end of this tracing the sinus rate increases, shortening the pause and eliminating the ventricular bigeminy.

RULE OF BIGEMINY

The rule of bigeminy says that a long cycle tends to precipitate a PVC after the next supraventricular beat.[15] This is illustrated in Fig. 12-19. In Fig. 12-19, *A* and *B,* there were no PVCs until a long cycle appeared, following which there was a PVC after every normal beat. In Fig. 12-19, *C,* the pause following one PVC perpetuated a bigeminal rhythm until the pause after the fourth PVC shortened, terminating the bigeminal rhythm. The implication is that the long cycle causes a longer refractory period and perhaps inhomogeneity of refractoriness. Thus the bigeminal rhythm perpetuates itself, since there is usually a pause after every PVC.

PEDIATRICS

Premature ventricular complexes may occur in children (especially pubertal or prepubertal) with no detectable heart disease and are considered benign.

PHYSICAL SIGNS

Compensatory pause: Follows the premature beat; it is longer than normal and does not change the timing of the basic rhythm.

Heart sounds: Often decreased intensity; the first heart sound can be sharp and snapping, and the second heart sound can be abnormally split, depending on the origin of the ventricular complex.

Peripheral pulse: decreased or absent.[16] The signs of AV dissociation are present about half the time.

CLINICAL IMPLICATIONS

Premature ventricular complexes are a common occurrence, even without heart disease, and increase in number with age. The incidence of PVCs is greater with acute myocardial infarction and ventricular scarring resulting from infarction, hypertrophy, or infection, and PVCs may be aggravated by ischemia, increased sympathetic activity, and increased or reduced heart rate.[17] Other causes include fever, volume depletion, infection, drug excesses of all types, hypokalemia, hypercalcemia, and excess or even moderate alcohol intake in certain individuals.[18]

Nonsymptomatic patient with no structural heart disease

In this setting PVCs are considered benign and are not treated; they have no impact on longevity, nor do they require restricted activity. A symptomatic patient is reassured.[16]

Apparently healthy middle-age men

Premature ventricular complexes and complex ventricular arrhythmias may be markers of heart disease but have not been shown to play a role in sudden death, nor has antiarrhythmic therapy been shown to reduce the incidence of sudden death in such patients.[16]

Acute myocardial infarction

The presence of PVCs following myocardial infarction identifies a patient at greater risk for sudden cardiac death. The role of PVC in initiating sustained VT is less clear. Although PVCs of any type have not been shown to be prognostically helpful in the setting of acute myocardial infarction, certain types of PVCs have been regarded as "malignant" or likely to result in VF; they are PVCs of more than five or six per minute, paired, multiform, or occurring on the T wave ("R on T"). In half of the patients with myocardial infarction who have these types of PVCs, VF does not develop, and of those patients in whom VF does develop, approximately half had not manifested such PVCs before the VF. Electrophysiologic testing to identify patients at risk of developing VT or sudden cardiac death after myocardial infarction is controversial.[16,19,20]

A study[21] involving 3290 patients defined the risk factors after myocardial infarction as follows:

1. Prior myocardial infarction

2. ST depression on resting ECG
3. Chest x-ray cardiothoracic ratio of more than 50% (indicative of cardiac enlargement)
4. Complex ventricular ectopic activity (more than 10 PVCs per hour, paired or multiform PVCs or VT)

Patients who have had myocardial infarction with two of the first three risk factors plus complex ventricular ectopic activity (factor no. 4) had a 25-month mortality rate of 21%. Patients with all four risk factors had a mortality rate in that same period of 41%.

TREATMENT

When PVCs are provoked by fast or slow heart rates, they can often be abolished by correcting the heart rate. For slow rates atropine, isoproterenol, or pacing can be used.[16]

Although ventricular arrhythmias in patients with left ventricular systolic dysfunction can be suppressed by type I antiarrhythmic drugs (blocking sodium channels), a study confined to patients who had sustained a prior myocardial infarction showed that these same drugs produced an increased mortality in most, if not all, subsets of patients with ischemic heart disease. The unexpected and dramatic results of the Cardiac Arrhythmia Suppression Trial (CAST I) became available in 1989.[22] Thus prophylactic use of lidocaine is no longer routinely indicated for patients with acute myocardial infarction, and it is rarely indicated for patients without symptomatic arrhythmias or sustained VT or VF.[23,24]

For further discussion of treatment of ventricular ectopy see Chapter 13.

SUMMARY

A PVC is noticed first because of its prematurity, excessive width, increased amplitude, and T wave of opposite polarity. If the sinus rhythm can be seen to be uninterrupted by the premature beat (full compensatory pause), this is a helpful sign in identifying a PVC. The morphologic appearance of the premature beat is often diagnostic.

REFERENCES

1. Moulton KP, Medcalf T, Lazzara R: Premature ventricular complex morphology: a marker for left ventricular structure and function, *Circulation* 81:1245, 1990.
2. Coumel P, Leclerck J, Qimmerman M, Funck-Brentano J: Antiarrhythmic therapy: noninvasive guided strategy versus empirical or invasive strategies. In Brugada P, Wellens HJJ, eds: *Cardiac arrhythmias: where to go from here?* Mount Kisco, NY, 1987, Futura.
3. Leclerck JF, Coumel P, Maisonblanch P et al: Mechanisms determining sudden death: a cooperative study of 69 cases recorded during the Holter method, *Arch Mal Coeur Vaiss* 79:1420, 1986.
4. Cranefield PF, Aronson RS: *Cardiac arrhythmias: the role of triggered activity and other mechanisms,* Mount Kisco, NY, 1988, Futura.
5. El-Sherif N: The ventricular premature complex: mechanisms and significance—an update. In Mandel W, ed: *Cardiac arrhythmias: their mechanisms, diagnosis, and management,* ed 2, Philadelphia, 1987, JB Lippincott.
6. Campbell RWF, Murray A, Julian DG: Ventricular arrhythmias in the first 12 hours of acute myocardial infarction, *Br Heart J* 46:351, 1981.
7. Adgey AAJ, Devlin JE, Webb SW, Mulholland HC: Initiation of ventricular fibrillation outside hospital in patients with acute ischemic heart disease, *Br Heart J* 47:55, 1982.
8. Bigger JT, Coromilas J: Ventricular tachyarrhythmias in the various stages of ischemic heart disease. In Surawicz B, Reddy CP, Prystowsky EN, eds: *Tachycardias,* Boston, 1984, Martinus Nijhoff.
9. Katz LN: The significance of the T wave in the

electrogram and the electrocardiogram, *Physiol Rev* 8:447, 1928.

10. Smirk FH: R waves interrupting T waves, *Br Heart J* 11:23, 1949.

11. Hinkle LE, Argyros DC, Hayes JC et al: Pathogenesis of an unexpected sudden death: role of early cycle ventricular premature contractions, *Am J Cardiol* 39:873, 1977.

12. Nikolic G, Bishop RL, Singh JB: Sudden death recorded during Holter monitoring, *Circulation* 66:218, 1982.

13. Campbell RWF: Treatment and prophylaxis of ventricular arrhythmias in acute myocardial infarction, *Am J Cardiol* 52:55C, 1983.

14. El-Sherif N, Myerburg RJ, Scherlag BJ et al: Electrocardiographic antecedents of primary ventricular fibrillation, *Br Heart J* 38:415, 1976.

15. Langerdorf R, Pick A, Winternitz M: Mechanisms of intermittent bigeminy. I. Appearance of ectopic beats dependent upon the length of the ventricular cycle: the "rule of bigeminy," *Circulation* 11:422, 1955.

16. Zipes DP: Specific arrhythmias: diagnosis and treatment. In Braunwald E, ed: *Heart disease* ed 4, Philadelphia, 1992, WB Saunders.

17. Bigger JT Jr: Definition of benign versus malignant ventricular arrhythmias: targets for treatment, *Am J Cardiol* 52:47C, 1983.

18. Naccarelli GV, Willerson JT, Blomquist CG: Recognition and physiologic treatment of cardiac arrhythmias and conduction disturbances. In Willerson JT, Choh JN, eds: *Cardiovascular medicine,* New York, 1995, Churchill Livingstone.

19. Zipes DP, Akhtar M, Denes P et al: ACC/AHA guidelines for clinical intracardiac electrophysiologic studies, *J Am Coll Cardiol* 14:1827, 1989.

20. Wellens HJJ: The approach to nonsustained ventricular tachycardia after myocardial infarction, *Circulation* 82:633, 1990.

21. Kostis JB, Byington R, Friedman LM et al: Prognostic significance of ventricular ectopic activity in survivors of acute myocardial infarction, *J Am Coll Cardiol* 10:231, 1987.

22. The Cardiac Arrhythmia Suppression Trial (CAST) Investigators: Preliminary report: effect of encainide and flecainide on mortality in a randomized trial of arrhythmia suppression after myocardial infarction, *N Engl J Med* 321:406, 1989.

23. Singh BN: Do anti-arrhythmic drugs work? some reflections on the implications of the Cardiac Arrhythmia Suppression Trial, *Clin Cardiol* 13:725, 1990.

24. Singh BN: Routine prophylactic lidocaine administration in acute myocardial infarction: an idea whose time is all but gone? *Circulation* 86:1033, 1992.

Monomorphic Ventricular Tachycardia

Terminology   *173*

Diagnosis   *174*

Mechanisms   *175*

Incidence   *176*

Prognosis and Clinical Implications   *176*

Pediatrics   *177*

Management of Sustained Broad-QRS
  Tachycardia Without Hemodynamic
  Decompensation   *177*

When in Doubt   *178*

Looks Like Ventricular Tachycardia,
  Rhythm Irregular, Rate Over 200
  Beats/min?   *178*

If Supraventricular Tachycardia with
  Aberrancy is Suspected   *178*

Idiopathic Ventricular Tachycardia   *178*

Bundle Branch Reentrant Ventricular
  Tachycardia   *183*

Radiofrequency Ablation for Ventricular
  Tachycardia   *186*

Treatment of Drug-Related Ventricular
  Tachycardia   *187*

Signal-Averaged ECG in Patients with
  Sustained Ventricular Tachycardia   *188*

Ventricular Flutter and Ventricular
  Fibrillation   *188*

V entricular tachycardia (VT) consists of at least three consecutive ventricular complexes with a rate of more than 100 beats/min. The focus is distal to the branching portion of the His bundle. Monomorphic VT is usually regular and has a uniform beat-to-beat QRS morphologic appearance.

TERMINOLOGY

fascicular ventricular tachycardia: Ventricular tachycardia with the focus usually in the anterior or posterior fascicle of the left bundle branch (LBB) or in the right bundle branch (RBB). When originating in the fascicles of the LBB, it results in a typical ECG pattern (right bundle branch block [RBBB]), right or left axis deviation, and QRS duration of less than 0.12 sec (see p. 253).

idiopathic ventricular tachycardia: Ventricular tachycardia in patients who have no clinical manifestation of structural heart disease.

nonsustained ventricular tachycardia: Ventricular tachycardia that terminates spontaneously within 30 sec and does not lead to hemodynamic collapse.

polymorphic ventricular tachycardia: Ventricular tachycardia with constantly changing, sometimes subtle, beat-to-beat QRS configurations (see Chapter 15).

primary ventricular tachycardia or **ventricular fibrillation:** Ventricular tachycardia or ventricular fibrillation (VF) that is not secondary to end-stage heart failure or shock.

proarrhythmic effect: Drug-induced worsening of an arrhythmia or the development of a new arrhythmia. The term generally, but not exclusively, refers to ventricular arrhythmias.

sustained ventricular tachycardia: Ventricular tachycardia that lasts more than 30 sec or, if less than 30 sec, requires intervention because of hemodynamic collapse.

DIAGNOSIS

Figs. 13-1 and 13-2 show nonsustained and sustained monomorphic VT. Note the uniform beat-to-beat appearance of the broad ventricular complexes. Evaluation of the QRS morphologic appearance is helpful in differentiating VT from supraventricular tachycardia (SVT) with aberrant ventricular conduction and in determining the type of VT. However, when applying morphologic rules, it is important to also consider information from the history and physical examination. As you will see, some VTs have the QRS width and morphologic appearance of SVT with aberration on the ECG, for example, idiopathic VT, bundle branch reentry VT, and fascicular VT; some SVTs are identical in QRS morphologic appearance to VT, that is, the SVTs that use an accessory pathway for entry into the ventricles. The ECG recognition of VT and its differential diagnosis are discussed in detail in Chapter 14.

If the diagnosis cannot be made with the ECG, careful history taking, and physical examination, other noninvasive tests are the following:

1. A 24-hour ambulatory recording that documents the tachycardia and correlates it with the patient's symptoms.
2. Provocation of the tachycardia with exercise testing.
3. The upright tilt test to provoke symptoms in patients with unexplained syncope.

II

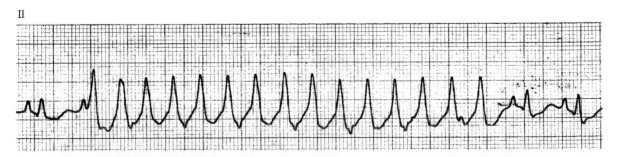

Fig. 13-1. Nonsustained monomorphic ventricular tachycardia (VT). Note the identical morphologic appearance of the ventricular complexes and the 2:1 retrograde conduction ratio, recognized when the P′ wave is negative in lead II. A negative distortion can be seen in this tracing in every other T wave.

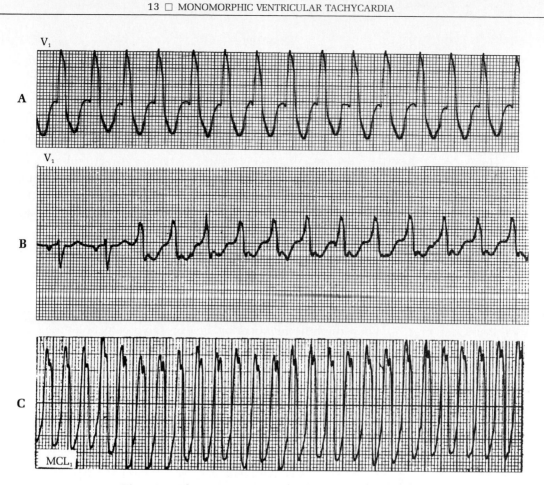

Fig. 13-2. Three cases of sustained monomorphic VT.

4. Signal-averaged ECG for risk stratification in patients with myocardial infarction (MI) (Chapter 30). Patients with malignant ventricular arrhythmias are referred for cardiac catheterization.
5. Other useful tests in assessing the state of the myocardium are echocardiography, thallium exercise testing, and testing for ejection fraction.
6. Electrophysiologic study with programed stimulation is recommended when symptoms are thought to be caused by arrhythmias but the physician is unable to diagnose or treat them.

MECHANISMS

Arrhythmogenic mechanisms are discussed in more detail in Chapter 5 and mentioned briefly here. In the setting of myocardial ischemia or infarction, it is probable that all of the known mechanisms of arrhythmias have a role; there may be only one mechanism involved, or mechanisms may act in combination. Hence abnormal impulse generation (automatic or triggered) may initiate a reentry mechanism, or a reentry arrhythmia may induce delayed afterdepolarizations, which in turn cause triggered activity.[1]

Reentry

Most instances of chronic sustained VT associated with coronary artery disease, MI, and dilated cardiomyopathy arise as a result of reentry.[2] As shown in Chapter 5, reentry circuits arising after MI are complex and include slow conduction zones as well as normal bystander tissue.[3]

Abnormal automaticity

In the postinfarction period the ischemia itself has both a direct and an indirect arrhythmogenic effect. The direct effect is the development of abnormal automaticity; this can occur in any ischemic fibers, even those that did not have the capability of automaticity in health. The indirect effect is slow conduction through the depressed tissue and reentry arrhythmias.

Triggered activity

A less common mechanism is triggered activity caused by either delayed or early afterdepolarizations. When class IA drugs are being used, triggered activity caused by long QT intervals and early afterdepolarizations may cause polymorphic VT (see Chapter 15). When digitalis intoxication or excessive catecholamines are factors, triggered activity caused by delayed afterdepolarizations with foci in the His-Purkinje system is the suspected mechanism (see Chapter 17). Ischemia can cause afterdepolarizations and triggered activity in experimental preparations, but reentry is the commonly accepted mechanism of ventricular tachycardia that follows MI. Some of the reperfusion ventricular arrhythmias are thought to be caused by triggered activity or possibly by accelerating automaticity.

INCIDENCE

There are two major phases of ventricular arrhythmias following acute MI, early and late. During the early phase (first 4 hours after the onset of symptoms) all types of ventricular arrhythmias are frequent, including primary VF and R-on-T phenomenon; the incidence of R-on-T phenomenon decreases rapidly with time. Primary VF is rare after 12 hours. In the late phase there is an increase in the incidence of VT and PVCs (back-to-back and isolated). Short runs of VT have been detected in 73% of patients within the first 24 hours of the appearance of symptoms and longer runs of 10 or more beats in 27% of patients. Sustained VT or cardiac arrest occurs in 2% to 4% of patients after acute MI.[4,5]

PROGNOSIS AND CLINICAL IMPLICATIONS
Nonsustained ventricular tachycardia

Patients with and without heart disease may have nonsustained VT, which may be associated with symptoms such as palpitations or recurrent syncope. In postinfarction patients nonsustained VT is definitely a risk factor for sudden cardiac death. When the episodes of nonsustained VT are frequent, rapid, and more prolonged and occur in the second week after anterior infarction, they may be warning signs of VF and may require aggressive evaluation and treatment.[4]

Sustained ventricular tachycardia

Sustained monomorphic VT is most commonly seen in adults with prior MI or chronic coronary artery disease. It is also seen in patients with dilated cardiomyopathy and in those with no apparent structural heart disease (idiopathic VT).[6] Typically the patient with sustained VT has a history of MI with extensive muscle necrosis and an ejection fraction of less than 40%, marked wall motion abnormality, aneurysm (70%), and acute complications within the first 48 hours after the infarction (80%). These complications include BBB (in anterior wall MI), congestive heart failure, primary VF, and hypotension requiring pressor support.[7] After MI 60% of patients have their first episode of VT within the first year.[8] The VT in patients with dilated cardiomyopathy usually appears the same as that seen in patients with prior MI. The mechanism for this type of VT produces very rapid heart rates with serious hemodynamic deterioration, including cardiac arrest.[6]

PEDIATRICS

Ventricular tachycardia is seen in many clinical situations in children. The most common origin or cause in children under 5 years of age is the hamartoma.*[9] In older children the most common cause is surgery.[10] The mechanism of VT in children is almost never ischemic heart disease. Other causes include long QT syndrome, myocarditis, cardiomyopathy, arrhythmogenic right ventricular dysplasia, and coronary artery anomalies.[11] Surgery for tetralogy of Fallot or more complex congenital defects carries with it a risk of ventricular arrhythmias and sudden death, especially if repair was late and the results were not optimal.[10]

MANAGEMENT OF SUSTAINED BROAD-QRS TACHYCARDIA WITH HEMODYNAMIC DECOMPENSATION

1. Obtain a 12-lead ECG.
2. Perform prompt direct-current (DC) cardioversion; very low energies can terminate VT. Begin with a synchronized shock of 10 to 50 watt-seconds.[12]
3. Digitalis-induced VT is treated by pharmacologic means.[12]
4. Obtain a history.
5. Examine ECGs before and after cardioversion to determine the origin of the arrhythmia.

MANAGEMENT OF SUSTAINED BROAD-QRS TACHYCARDIA WITHOUT HEMODYNAMIC DECOMPENSATION

1. Obtain a 12-lead ECG, and systematically evaluate it to confirm the diagnosis.
2. Examine the patient for signs of atrioventricular (AV) dissociation to confirm the diagnosis of VT (see Chapter 14).
3. Obtain a history.
4. In cases of sustained VT most physicians give intravenous (IV) procainamide 6 to 13 mg/kg at 0.2 to 0.5 mg/kg per min (14 to 35 mg/min).[13]
5. If IV procainamide is not successful, DC cardioversion is used (synchronized 10 to 50 watt-seconds).[12]

---

*A hamartoma is a benign, tumorlike nodule that occurs because of an acceleration of growth in a circumscribed area. The nodule is composed of mature cells that are normally present in the surrounding tissue.

Procainamide versus lidocaine

Although use of IV procainamide is a departure from the recommended approach to VT made in 1992,[14] studies have questioned the use of lidocaine as initial therapy in VT,[15,16] and one study has shown the superiority of procainamide over lidocaine in patients with nonischemic VT. In a randomized study involving 56 episodes of sustained VT that occurred outside an episode of acute ischemia, Gorgels et al.[17] found procainamide to be clearly superior to lidocaine in terminating VT. In this study patients were randomly assigned to receive either IV lidocaine 1.5 mg/kg in 3 min or IV procainamide 10 mg/kg in 5 min. When one drug failed to convert the VT, the other drug was used after 20 min. Lidocaine terminated only 4 of 22 episodes of VT, whereas procainamide terminated 24 of 32 episodes. Of course, in hypotensive patients procainamide is contraindicated; even in normotensive patients the dosage of procainamide is decreased because the blood pressure dips.

Precordial thump

The precordial thump can sometimes terminate VT[18] and was first applied in 1919 in a woman with asystole.[19] However, if the blow to the chest happens to fall during the vulnerable period, it may precipitate VF or cause the rate of the VT to increase.

WHEN IN DOUBT

If there is any doubt about the mechanism of the tachycardia (SVT vs. VT) *do not give verapamil; give procainamide.*[20] Procainamide, of course, is not given if there is a possibility of torsades de pointes (see Chapter 15).

LOOKS LIKE VENTRICULAR TACHYCARDIA, RHYTHM IRREGULAR, RATE OVER 200 BEATS/MIN?

Give procainamide; do not give verapamil or digitalis.[21]

In such a case atrial fibrillation with conduction over an accessory pathway is highly suspect, and blocking the AV node with verapamil or digitalis is of no help and may cause the rate to accelerate and VF to develop. If procainamide does not slow this rhythm, perform cardioversion immediately. In any case, the patient is referred to a center experienced in the treatment of patients with Wolff-Parkinson-White syndrome.

IF SUPRAVENTRICULAR TACHYCARDIA WITH ABERRANCY IS SUSPECTED

If the patient's condition is relatively stable, vagal maneuvers can be tried at any time (carotid sinus massage or Valsalva's maneuver). If these are unsuccessful, adenosine may be used. The effect is transient and should not make VT worse.[22]

IDIOPATHIC VENTRICULAR TACHYCARDIA

Idiopathic VT is diagnosed when the only abnormality is the arrhythmia, as determined by current diagnostic techniques, including a careful history and physical examination and a careful examination of the 12-lead ECG, signal-averaged ECG (see Chapter 30) during sinus rhythm, chest x-ray, and echocardiogram. No abnormalities are visible during cardiac catheterization. For more information on a complete workup of this patient please see the reference noted. Of 706 patients with VT who were studied in the electrophysiology laboratory at one institution, 75 were found to have idiopathic VT.[23] Figs. 13-3 to 13-5 show idiopathic VT.

History

Paroxysmal VT in young, healthy hearts was first described by Gallavardin[24] in 1922 and was known as "right ventricular outflow tract tachycardia." It was described again in 1953 by Froment et al.[25] In 1979 Zipes et al.[26] described the ECG characteristics of idiopathic VT with a focus in the left ventricle, that is, QRS duration of less than 0.12 sec and RBBB-like pattern with left axis deviation. The tachycardia could be induced by exercise, atrial or ventricular pacing, and premature atrial complexes (PACs) or PVCs. In 1980 Wellens et al.[27] reported that this type of VT may be terminated by verapamil, an observation proved in a later series.[28] The focus is thought to be in the posterior fascicle of the LBB.[57,00,00]

Types of idiopathic ventricular tachycardia

Two main types of idiopathic ventricular tachycardia have been identified, one with a LBBB-shaped pattern and a focus in the right ventricular outflow tract and the other with an RBBB-shaped pattern. This RBBB pattern itself appears to have two distinct groups,[57] group A with a focus in the posterior fascicle of the LBB and group B with a focus in the inferoapical left ventricle.

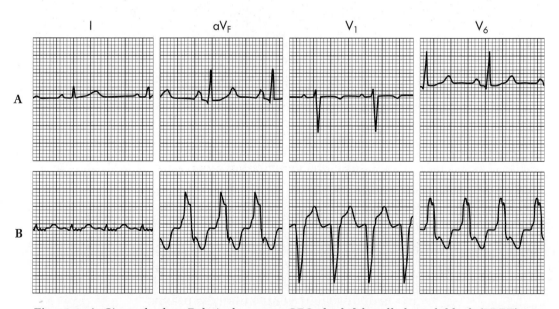

Fig. 13-3. A, Sinus rhythm. Relatively narrow QRS, the left bundle branch block (LBBB) pattern in V_1 and V_6, and the inferior axis (aVF positive) are evident. **B,** Idiopathic right VT at a rate of 145 beats/min (focus in the right ventricular outflow tract). *(From Bhadha K, Marchlinski FE, Iskandrian AS: Am Heart J 126:1194, 1993.)*

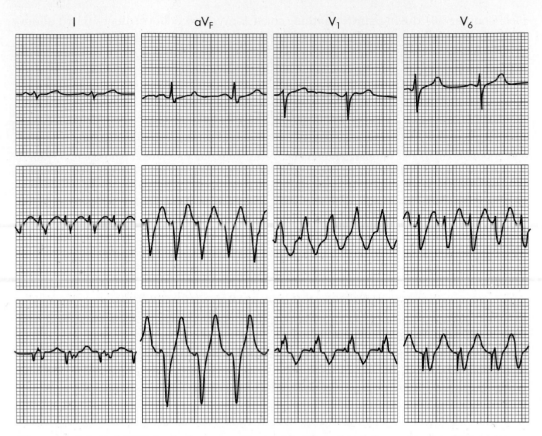

Fig. 13-4. Selected ECG leads from a patient with idiopathic left ventricular (LV) tachycardia. Top panel shows baseline ECG; middle panel shows idiopathic LV tachycardia. Lower panel shows ventricular pacing from the LV. *(From Bhadha K, Marchlinski FE, Iskandrian AS: Am Heart J 126:1194, 1993.)*

ECG recognition of LBBB-shaped idiopathic ventricular tachycardia as compared with ischemic ventricular tachycardia or the ventricular tachycardia of right ventricular dysplasia[23,31]

QRS width: Relatively narrow.
QRS axis: Inferior, usually, absence of left axis deviation.
QRS morphologic appearance in lead aVL: QS.
Height of R wave in limb leads: More than 40 mm.

ECG recognition of RBBB-shaped idiopathic ventricular tachycardia as compared with ischemic ventricular tachycardia or the ventricular tachycardia of right ventricular dysplasia[23]

QRS width: Group A, approximately 0.12 sec; Group B, approximately 0.15 sec.
QRS axis: Group A, left axis deviation ($-64 \pm 11°$); Group B, northwest ("no man's land," $-105 \pm 5°$).

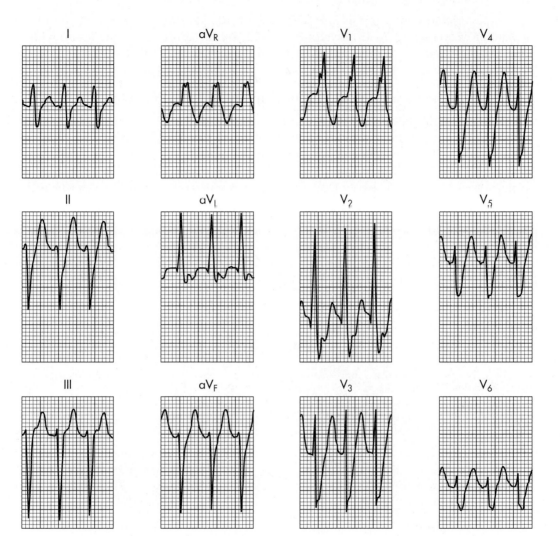

Fig. 13-5. An emergency department tracing from a 27-year-old man with idiopathic VT. The RBBB pattern in V_1 and superior axis are evident. *(Courtesy Ara Tilkian, MD, Van Nuys, Calif.)*

Clinical implications

Most patients with VT but without structural heart disease have an excellent prognosis.[32] Sudden cardiac death is rare, as opposed to the very high mortality rate associated with postischemic recurrent VT. Frequent episodes of VT may result in cardiomyopathy and would render the decision for radiofrequency ablation of the focus more imperative.

Symptoms

Palpitations or episodes of syncope are possible.[33]

Emergency treatment of idiopathic ventricular tachycardia

Zipes recommends that idiopathic VT be managed like other VTs. Unless the physician is an expert electrophysiologist, verapamil is contraindicated for all wide-QRS tachycardias. Adenosine can be used and is effective for some of the right ventricular outflow tract VTs.[34]

Long-term treatment of idiopathic ventricular tachycardia

Symptomatic patients receive treatment, especially if the tachycardia has resulted in cardiomyopathy. Radiofrequency ablation has been shown to be successful and safe in treating (curing) symptomatic idiopathic VT.[23,27,29,30,35-41] Fig. 13-6 shows ablation sites in the right ventricular outflow tract. Adenosine-sensitive VT appears to arise from relatively discrete sites predominantly located in the free wall of the pulmonary infundibulum. The localized nature of this tachycardia renders it

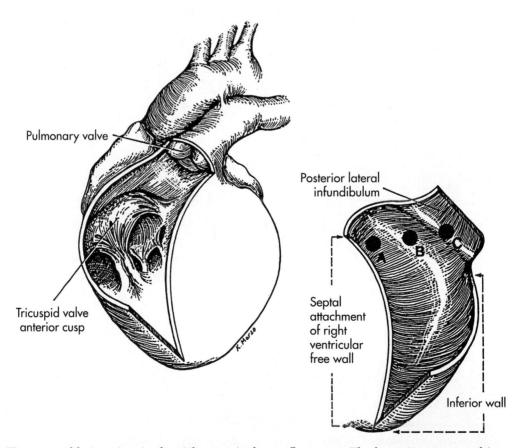

Fig. 13-6. Ablation sites in the right ventricular outflow tract. The heart is represented in an angulated left anterior oblique projection. The right ventricle is opened with the endocardial surface of the free wall depicted on the segment to the right. **A, B,** and **C,** The sites in the right ventricular outflow tract that, during pace mapping, produced QRS complexes identical to the VT. Radiofrequency ablation was successfully performed at these sites in seven patients. *(Redrawn from Wilbur DJ, Baerman J, Olshansky B et al: Circulation 87:126, 1993.)*

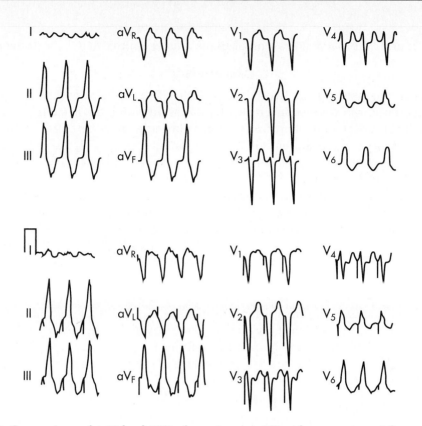

Fig. 13-7. Comparison of a 12-lead ECG of spontaneous VT and a pace map at the successful ablation site in the posteroseptal region of the left ventricle. The very close match of both R/S ratio and fine notching in all leads is evident. *(From Coggins DL, Lee RJ, Sweeney J et al: J Am Coll Cardiol 23:1333, 1994.*

amenable to cure by catheter ablation techniques.[34] Pacing is performed in the right ventricular outflow tract, and the complexes are analyzed with respect to R/S ratio and fine notching in each lead until the paced complexes match the spontaneous QRS patterns during tachycardia. This site becomes the site of ablation. Fig. 13-7 shows a representative pacing map from a successful ablation site.[42]

BUNDLE BRANCH REENTRANT VENTRICULAR TACHYCARDIA

Sustained bundle branch reentrant VT (BBR-VT) is a highly malignant form of monomorphic VT that frequently becomes evident with syncope, palpitations, or sudden cardiac death. It is important to recognize BBR-VT because it can be cured with radiofrequency ablation although the structural heart disease associated with this type of VT remains.[43]

ECG recognition

QRS morphologic appearance
During sinus rhythm: Incomplete LBBB consistent with His-Purkinje system disease.
During the VT: Right or left BBB, depending on the bundle branch that is used for anterograde propagation.

Axis

With an LBBB pattern the frontal plane axis is approximately +30 degrees.

Mechanism

The mechanisms of the two forms of BBR-VT are illustrated in Fig. 13-8. The mechanism is a well-defined macroreentry circuit in which the His bundle, the right and left bundle branches, and transseptal ventricular muscle conduction are the components of the reentrant circuit.[44,45] An absolute prerequisite for such a reentry loop is conduction delay in the His-Purkinje system[46]; note the slow conduction depicted within the LBB.

There is an LBBB pattern when the ventricles are activated via the RBB and an RBBB pattern when the ventricles are activated via the LBB. During the tachycardia an LBBB pattern is the most common. Because the mechanism of this tachycardia uses the His-Purkinje system, the resultant QRS morphologic appearance will be that of *SVT with aberration*. Fig. 13-9 shows BBR-VT with anterograde conduction down the RBB. Note that the negative complex in lead V$_1$ has none of the signs of VT described on p. 211. This is because the mechanism is being sustained by a reentry loop that uses the His-Purkinje system. In Fig. 13-10 a less common form of BBR-VT is shown, in which the ventricles are activated with anterograde conduction down the LBB, resulting in an RBBB pattern.

When the patient is not in VT, he or she is either in atrial fibrillation or in sinus rhythm; in such a case the QRS contour reflects intraventricular conduction delay with an LBBB pattern. If there is sinus rhythm, the PR interval is prolonged.[43]

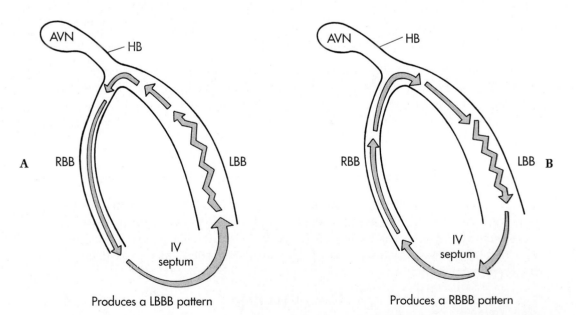

Fig. 13-8. The mechanism of bundle branch reentry VT is schematically depicted. **A,** Its most common form, with anterograde conduction in the RBB to produce an LBBB pattern; The required delay of conduction is evident in the ascending limb of the circuit. **B,** The least common form, with anterograde conduction in the LBBB to produce an RBBB pattern.

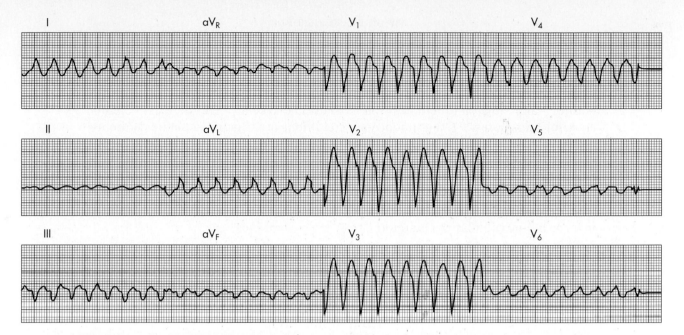

Fig. 13-9. A bundle branch reentrant tachycardia with an LBBB pattern and left axis deviation at a rate of 215 beats/min. Because ventricular activation occurs by way of the right bundle branch, the QRS is relatively narrow and its configuration suggests supraventricular tachycardia with LBBB aberrant ventricular conduction. *(From Blanck Z, Sra J, Dhala A et al. In Zipes DP, Jalife J, eds: Cardiac electrophysiology from cell to bedside, ed 2, Philadelphia, 1995, WB Saunders.)*

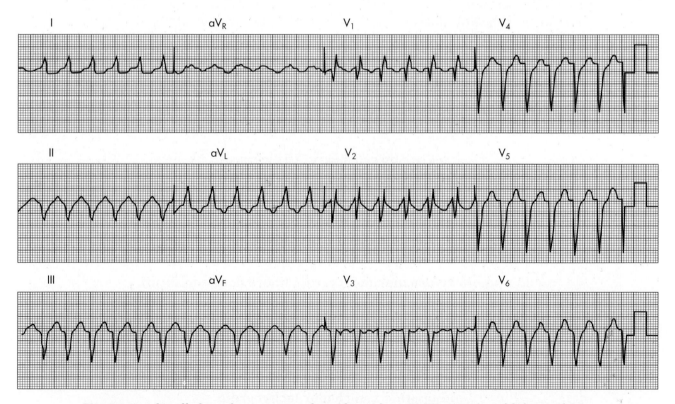

Fig. 13-10. A bundle branch reentrant tachycardia with an RBBB pattern and left axis deviation at a rate of 150 beats/min. Because ventricular activation occurs by way of the left bundle branch, the QRS is relatively narrow and its configuration suggests supraventricular tachycardia with RBBB aberrant ventricular conduction. *(From Blanck Z, Sra J, Dhala A et al. In Zipes DP, Jalife J, eds: Cardiac electrophysiology from cell to bedside, ed 2, Philadelphia, 1995, WB Saunders.)*

Pathophysiology

Bundle branch reentrant ventricular tachycardia usually occurs in individuals with significant structural heart disease; dilated cardiomyopathy (usually idiopathic)[47] and slow conduction in the His-Purkinje system[47] are the most common anatomic substrates.[46] Other underlying conditions are dilated ischemic cardiomyopathy and nonspecific intraventricular conduction abnormalities. Bundle branch reentrant ventricular tachycardia may also occur in the setting of dilated ventricles resulting from coronary or significant valvular heart disease.[6] Three cases have been reported of BBR-VT in patients who have conduction abnormalities on the surface ECG suggestive of His-Purkinje system disease but who have no manifestation of myocardial or valvular dysfunction.[48]

Emergency treatment

For the patient in unstable condition cardioversion is the treatment of choice; for the patient in stable condition procainamide or lidocaine may be used.

Long-term treatment (cure)

If electrophysiologic studies establish that the mechanism of the VT is bundle branch reentry, as is often the case in dilated cardiomyopathy, catheter ablation of the RBB eliminates the possibility of reentry and is a permanent cure of the reentrant tachycardia and the treatment of choice.[49-51] Because of the availability of such a cure, recognition of this condition through electrophysiologic studies avoids therapy with the automatic implantable defibrillator or antiarrhythmic drugs.[45] After ablation, long-term follow-up of 48 patients did not document bundle branch reentry, but congestive heart failure was a common cause of death.[46]

Prognosis

The prognosis is generally poor, and some patients with the combination of BBR-VT and dilated cardiomyopathy may be considered for cardiac transplantation.[6]

RADIOFREQUENCY ABLATION
FOR VENTRICULAR TACHYCARDIA

Radiofrequency ablation is established as a highly successful therapy for certain types of SVT. The experience with using this procedure for certain types of VT is rapidly accumulating. The characteristics of these types of VT and the indications and efficacy of radiofrequency ablation are summarized in this section.[52]

Idiopathic ventricular tachycardia (more common form)

Mechanism: Focal lesion, right ventricular outflow tract.
QRS morphologic appearance: LBBB.
QRS axis: Inferior.
Clinical characteristic: Often exercise induced.
Radiofrequency ablation: Highly successful with low risk.

Idiopathic ventricular tachycardia

Mechanism: Focal lesion, left ventricle; perhaps posterior fascicle or inferoapical left ventricle.

QRS morphologic appearance: RBBB.

Axis: Superior.

Clinical characteristic: Most commonly exercise induced; often terminated by IV verapamil, falsely suggesting SVT with aberrancy.

Radiofrequency ablation: Successful, but number of patient studies is small.

Bundle-branch reentry ventricular tachycardia

Mechanism: Macroreentry involving both bundle branches, the intraventricular septum, and the bundle of His.

QRS morphologic appearance: RBBB or LBBB during the VT; LBBB during sinus rhythm.

Axis: Normal quadrant.

Clinical characteristics: Cardiomyopathy or valvular disease; rapid palpitations, syncope, or sudden death.

Radiofrequency ablation: Highly successful.

Ventricular tachycardia late after myocardial infarction

Mechanism: Large reentry circuit within ischemic and scarred regions that may be epicardial, intramural, or endocardial in location.

QRS morphologic appearance: That of VT.

Axis: Normal or abnormal, depending on area of reentry.

Clinical characteristics: Palpitations, syncope, or sudden death.

Radiofrequency ablation: Difficult but successful in 20% to 60% of selected patients; experience relatively limited; risks not well defined.

TREATMENT OF DRUG-RELATED VENTRICULAR TACHYCARDIA

Patients with sustained VT associated with severe left ventricular dysfunction are particularly vulnerable to the proarrhythmic effects of antiarrhythmic drugs.

Well-known arrhythmias caused by antiarrhythmic drugs are torsades de pointes (quinidine, procainamide, and disopyramide) and sustained monomorphic VT (classes IA and IC drugs). An approach to their treatment is briefly outlined here.

Torsades de pointes (see Chapter 15)

1. Stop the offending drug.
2. Give magnesium chloride or magnesium sulfate 1 to 2 g IV bolus over 5 mins; infusion: 1 to 2 g/hr for 4 to 6 hours.
3. If IV magnesium is unsuccessful, increase heart rate by using isoproterenol or pacing.

Sustained (incessant) monomorphic ventricular tachycardia induced by antiarrhythmic drugs

1. Stop the offending drug.
2. In case of hemodynamic compromise, give inotropic support by using dopamine (Intropin) or dobutamine (Dobutrex) and, occasionally, aortic counterpulsation. Sometimes a sodium load is used (sodium bicarbonate or sodium lactate).
3. If VT persists and is poorly tolerated, the atrium is paced at the rate of the VT using an AV interval that provides maximal contribution of atrial contraction to ventricular filling.

SIGNAL-AVERAGED ECG IN PATIENTS WITH SUSTAINED
VENTRICULAR TACHYCARDIA

The signal-averaged ECG is explained and illustrated in Chapter 30. Briefly, signal averaging is the amplification, averaging, and filtering of the ECG signal that is recorded on the body surface by orthogonal leads. The recording detects low-amplitude cardiac electrical signals in the last part of the QRS and in the ST segment. Such late potentials may represent delayed activation of abnormal myocardium, an arrhythmogenic substrate. In patients who have had MI and those with chronic coronary artery disease, a combination of clinical and investigative variables, including the signal-averaged ECG, best identifies patients at highest risk.[53]

VENTRICULAR FLUTTER AND VENTRICULAR FIBRILLATION

Ventricular flutter and ventricular fibrillation are severe derangements of the electrical rhythm of the heart. They are associated with hemodynamic collapse and without prompt intervention usually result in death within 3 to 5 minutes.

ECG recognition

In ventricular flutter the QRS and T waves form a regular, large, zigzag, oscillating pattern (sinusoidal morphologic appearance). The rate is usually approximately 200 beats/min but ranges from 150 to 300 beats/min (Fig. 13-11).

In ventricular fibrillation electrical activation in the ventricles is fractionated, resulting in an ECG of irregular undulations (Fig. 13-12) without clearcut ventricular complexes. Fibrillatory waves with amplitudes of less than 0.2 mV identify a patient with a poor survival rate. Such a pattern develops when termination of ventricular fibrillation has been delayed.[12]

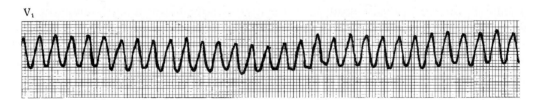

Fig. 13-11. Ventricular flutter. The rate of almost 300 beats/min and the sine wave configuration can be seen.

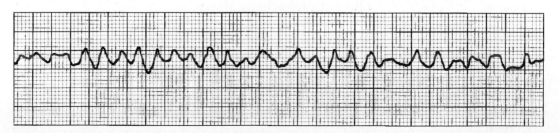

Fig. 13-12. Ventricular fibrillation.

Mechanisms

The most common setting for the development of ventricular fibrillation is coronary artery disease. Other clinical settings include hypertension, hyperlipidemia, cigarette smoking, obesity, impaired glucose tolerance, left ventricular hypertrophy during antiarrhythmic drug administration, hypoxia, ischemia, atrial fibrillation in patients with accessory pathways, and the period after cardioversion.[54]

Prognosis

Cardiac arrest survivors who do not sustain MI are at greater risk of sustaining another event than those who do have an infarct. In fact, if cardiac arrest occurs during acute MI, the recurrence rate at 1 year is less than 2%, whereas in the setting of chronic ischemic heart disease without infarction the recurrence rate is 30% or more at 1 year.[55]

Symptoms

Often no warning.
Faintness and loss of consciousness.
Blood pressure and pulse cannot be obtained.
Heart sounds are usually absent.
Cyanosis
In response to the lack of oxygen to the brain there are seizures, apnea, and finally death if the fibrillation is not terminated.

Treatment: immediate electrical shock

- Direct-current defibrillation (200 to 400 J); the earlier the better, since fewer joules are required if administered early.[56]
- Do not waste precious time; cardiopulmonary resuscitation is used only until the defibrillator is readied.
- If the patient is not being monitored, do not waste seconds waiting for an ECG; administer *immediate* electrical shock. It may terminate ventricular fibrillation, and it may start the asystolic heart.
- If return to sinus rhythm with markedly inadequate circulation: cardiopulmonary resuscitation as needed (use of anesthesia judged by patient's condition).
- Following conversion, monitor continuously.

REFERENCES

1. Binah O, Rosen MR: Mechanisms of ventricular arrhythmias, *Circulation* 85(suppl 1):1, 1992.
2. Josephson ME, Gottlieb CD: Ventricular tachycardias associated with coronary artery disease. In Zipes DP, Jalife J, eds: *Cardiac electrophysiology,* Philadelphia, 1990, WB Saunders.
3. Akhtar M: Clinical spectrum of ventricular tachycardia, *Circulation* 75:41, 1987.
4. Josephson ME: Treatment of ventricular arrhythmias after myocardial infarction, *Circulation* 74:653, 1986.
5. Campbell RWF: Treatment and prophylaxis of ventricular arrhythmias in acute myocardial infarction, *Am J Cardiol* 52:55C, 1983.
6. Akhtar M: The Clinical spectrum of ventricular tachycardia, *Circulation* 82:1561, 1990.
7. Marchlinski FE: Ventricular tachycardia: clinical presentation, course and therapy. In Zipes DP, Jalife J, eds: *Cardiac electrophysiology,* Philadelphia, 1990, WB Saunders.
8. Marchlinski FE: Ventricular tachycardia associated with coronary artery disease. In Zipes DP, Rowlands DJ, eds: *Progress in cardiology,* Philadelphia, 1988, Lea & Febiger.
9. Zeigler VL, Gillette PC, Crawford FA et al: New approaches to treatment of incessant ventricular tachycardia in the very young, *J Am Coll Cardiol* 16:681, 1990.
10. Garson A Jr: Chronic postoperative arrhythmia. In Gillette PC, Garson A Jr, eds: *Pediatric arrhythmias: electrophysiology and pacing,* Philadelphia, 1990, WB Saunders.
11. Gillette PC, Zeigler VL, Case CL: Pediatric arrhythmias: are they different? In Zipes DP, Jalife J, eds: *Cardiac electrophysiology from*

cell to bedside, ed 2, Philadelphia, 1995, WB Saunders.

12. Zipes DP: Specific arrhythmias: diagnosis and treatment. In Braunwald E, ed: *Heart disease,* ed 4, Philadelphia, 1992, WB Saunders.

13. Zipes DP: Management of cardiac arrhythmias: pharmacological, electrical, and surgical techniques. In Braunwald E, ed: *Heart disease,* ed 4, Philadelphia, 1992, WB Saunders.

14. Emergency Cardiac Care Committee and Subcommittees, American Heart Association: Guidelines for cardiopulmonary resuscitation and emergency cardiac care, *JAMA* 268:2171, 1992.

15. Armengol RE, Graff J, Baerman MJ, Swirn S: Lack of effectiveness of lidocaine for sustained, wide QRS complex tachycardia, *Ann Emerg Med* 18:254, 1989.

16. Wesley RC, Resh W, Zimmerman D: Reconsiderations of the routine and preferential use of lidocaine in the emergent treatment of ventricular arrhythmias, *Crit Care Med* 19:1439, 1991.

17. Gorgels AP van den Dool A, Hof A et al: Procainamide is superior to lidocaine in terminating sustained ventricular tachycardia, *Circulation* 80:2590, 1989.

18. Gertsch M, Hottinger S, Mettler D et al: Conversion of induced ventricular tachycardia by single and serial chest thumps: a study in domestic pigs 1 week after experimental myocardial infarction, *Am Heart J* 118:248, 1989.

19. Schott E: Ueber Ventrikelstillstand (Adams-Stokes'sche Anfälle) nebst Bemerkungen über andersartige Arrhythmien passagerer Natur, *Dtsch Arch Klin Med* 131:211, 1919.

20. Wellens HJJ: The wide QRS tachycardia, *Ann Intern Med* 104:879, 1986.

21. Wellens HJJ, Conover M: *The ECG in emergency decision making,* Philadelphia, 1992, WB Saunders.

22. Zipes DP: Personal communication, February, 1995.

23. Wellens HJJ, Rodriquez LM, Smeets JL: Ventricular tachycardia in structurally normal hearts. In Zipes DP, Jalife J, eds: *Cardiac electrophysiology from cell to bedside,* ed 2, Philadelphia, 1995, WB Saunders.

24. Gallavardin L: Extrasystolie ventriculaire a paroxysmes tachycardiques prolonges, *Arch Mal Coeur Vaiss* 15:298, 1922.

25. Froment R, Gallavardin L, Cahen P: Paroxysmal ventricular tachycardia: a clinical classification, *Br Heart J* 15:172, 1953.

26. Zipes DP, Foster PR, Troup PJ, Pedersen DH: Atrial induction of ventricular tachycardia: reentry versus triggered automaticity, *Am J Cardiol* 44:1, 1979.

27. Wellens HJJ, Farré J, Bär FW: The significance of the slow response in ventricular arrhythmias. In Zipes D, Bailey J, Elmarrar V, eds: *The slow inward current,* The Hague, 1980, Martinus Nijhoff.

28. Belhassen B, Rotmensch HH, Laniado S: Response of recurrent sustained ventricular tachycardia to verapamil, *Br Heart J* 16:679, 1981.

29. Nakagawa H, Beckman KJ, McClelland JH et al: Radiofrequency catheter ablation of idiopathic left ventricular tachycardia guided by a Purkinje potential, *Circulation* 88:2607, 1993.

30. Wellens HJJ, Smeets JLRM: Idiopathic left ventricular tachycardia: cure by radiofrequency ablation, *Circulation* 88:2978, 1993 (editorial).

31. Coumel P, Leclercq JF, Attuel P, Slama R: The QRS morphology in post-myocardial infarction ventricular tachycardia: a study in 100 tracings compared with 70 cases of idiopathic ventricular tachycardia, *Eur Heart J* 5:792, 1984.

32. Bhadha K, Marchlinski FE, Iskandrian AS: Ventricular tachycardia in patients without structural heart disease, *Am Heart J* 126:1104, 1993.

33. Buston AE, Waxman HL, Marchlinski FE et al: Right ventricular tachycardia; clinical and electrophysiological characteristics, *Circulation* 68:917, 1983.

34. Wilber IDJ, Baerman J, Olshansky B et al: Adenosine-sensitive ventricular tachycardia: clinical characteristics and response to catheter ablation, *Circulation* 87:126, 1993.

35. Aizawa Y, Chinushi M, Naitoh N et al: Catheter ablation with radiofrequency current of ventricular tachycardia originating from the right ventricle, *Am Heart J* 125:1269, 1993.

36. Klein SL, Shih HT, Hackett K et al: Radiofrequency catheter ablation of ventricular tachycardia in patients without structural heart disease, *Circulation* 85:1666, 1992.

37. Smeets JLRM, Rodriquez LM, Metzger J et al: Can ventricular tachycardia in the absence of structural heart disease be cured by radiofrequency catheter ablation? *Eur Heart J* 14(suppl II):256, 1993.

38. Yoshifusa A, Chinushe M, Naitoh N et al: Catheter ablation with radiofrequency current of ventricular tachycardia originating from the right ventricle, *Am Heart J* 125:1269, 1993.

39. Morady F, Kadish AH, DiCarlo L et al: Long-term results of catheter ablation of idiopathic right ventricular tachycardia, *Circulation* 82:2093, 1990.

40. Breithardt G, Borggrefe M, Wichter T: Catheter ablation of idiopathic right ventricular tachycardia, *Circulation* 82:2273, 1990 (editorial).

41. Wen MS, Yeh SJ, Wang CC et al: Radiofrequency ablation therapy in idiopathic left ventricular tachycardia with no obvious structural heart disease, *Circulation* 89:1690, 1994.

42. Coggins DL, Lee RJ, Sweeney J et al: Radiofrequency catheter ablation as a cure for idiopathic tachycardia of both left and right ventricular origin, *J Am Coll Cardiol* 23:1333, 1994.

43. Blanck Z, Sra J, Dhala A et al: Bundle branch reentry: mechanisms, diagnosis, and treatment. In Zipes DP, Jalife J, eds: *Cardiac electrophysiology from cell to bedside,* ed 2, Philadelphia, 1995, WB Saunders.
44. Akhtar M, Damato AN, Batsford WP et al: Demonstration of reentry within the His-Purkinje system in man, *Circulation* 50:1150, 1974.
45. Blanck Z, Dhala A, Deshpande S et al: Bundle branch reentrant ventricular tachycardia: cumulative experience in 48 patients, *J Cardiovasc Electrophysiol* 4:253, 1993.
46. Blanck Z, Akhtar M: Ventricular tachycardia due to sustained bundle branch reentry: diagnostic and therapeutic considerations, *Clin Cardiol* 16:619, 1993.
47. Caceres J, Jazayeri M, McKinnie J et al: Sustained bundle branch reentry as a mechanism of clinical tachycardia, *Circulation* 79.250, 1989.
48. Blanck Z, Jazayeri M, Dhala A et al: Bundle branch reentry: a mechanism of ventricular tachycardia in the absence of myocardial or valvular dysfunction, *J Am Coll Cardiol* 22:1718, 1993.
49. Tchou P, Jazayeri M, Denker S, Dongas J: Transcatheter electrical ablation of the right bundle branch: a method of treating macroreentrant ventricular tachycardia due to bundle branch reentry, *Circulation* 78:246, 1988.
50. Langberg JJ, Desai J, Dullet N, Scheinman MM: Treatment of macroreentrant ventricular tachycardia with radiofrequency ablation of the right bundle branch, *Am J Cardiol* 62:220, 1989.
51. Gallay P: Ventricular tachycardia caused by bundle branch reentry, *Arch Mal Coeur Vaiss* 85:77, 1992.
52. Stevenson WG: Ventricular tachycardia catheter ablation: what is its real role? New developments in arrhythmia management: the changing perspectives, presented for *UCLA School of Medicine,* Dallas, November 13, 1994.
53. McClements BM, Adgey AAJ: Value of signal-averaged electrocardiography, radionuclide ventriculography, Holter monitoring and clinical variables for prediction of arrhythmic events in survivors of acute myocardial infarction in the thrombolytic era, *J Am Coll Cardiol* 21:1419, 1993.
54. Epstein AE, Ideker RE: Ventricular fibrillation. In Zipes DP, Jalife J, eds. *Cardiac electrophysiology from cell to bedside,* ed 2, Philadelphia, 1995, WB Saunders.
55. Epstein AE, Ideker RE: Ventricular fibrillation. In Zipes DP, Jalife J, eds: *Cardiac electrophysiology from cell to bedside,* ed 2, Philadelphia, 1995, WB Saunders.
56. Winkle RA, Mead HR, Ruder MA: Effect of duration of ventricular fibrillation on defibrillation efficacy in humans, *Circulation* 81:1477, 1990.
57. Rodriquez LM, Smeets JLRM, Lokhandwala Y et al: New observations in idiopathic left ventricular tachycardia, *Circulation* (Special Issue) 188A: 745-753, 1995.

CHAPTER

14

Aberration Versus Ectopy

Aberrant Ventricular Conduction   *192*

Phase 3 Block   *192*

Retrograde Concealed Conduction   *193*

Importance of Differentiating Among
Broad QRS Tachycardias   *194*

Importance of Taking a History   *195*

Atrioventricular Dissociation   *195*

Finding P Waves in the Broad QRS
Tachycardia   *196*

Retrograde Conduction to the Atria During
Ventricular Tachycardia   *199*

ECG Diagnosis of Broad QRS
Tachycardia   *200*

QRS Width   *200*

Axis   *200*

Capture Beats and Fusion Beats   *201*

Concordant Pattern   *201*

QRS Morphologic Appearance   *202*

Value of a Baseline 12-Lead ECG   *212*

When in Doubt   *213*

Summary   *214*

ABERRANT VENTRICULAR CONDUCTION

Aberrant ventricular conduction (also called functional or physiologic bundle branch block [BBB]) is defined as abnormal conduction through the ventricles. It is usually caused by shortening of the cycle length (phase 3 aberration is its common mechanism) or less commonly by excessively prolonged cycle lengths (phase 4 aberration). This chapter deals with phase 3 aberration. Retrograde concealed conduction is a mechanism for the maintenance of the BBB caused by phase 3 aberration.

PHASE 3 BLOCK

Phase 3 block is the type with which we are most familiar in the clinical setting. It is the result of stimulation of the bundle branches while one bundle branch is still refractory (phase 3 of the action potential). Because the right bundle branch (RBB) repolarizes slightly later than the left bundle branch (LBB) it is the more susceptible to block or at least to delay in conduction when confronted with an early impulse, although BBB aberration is common in circus movement tachycardia (CMT). In fact, aberration itself is more common in CMT using an accessory pathway than it is in atrioventricular (AV) nodal reentry tachycardia.

Fig. 14-1 illustrates phase 3 aberration following premature atrial complexes (PACs). Note the classic triphasic rSR' pattern following the PACs in all three tracings. Even in lead II (Fig. 14-2), when the shape of the ventricular complex is not useful, the presence of aberrant ventricular conduction can be recognized when the PAC is seen in front of the wide QRS complex. In addition, in Fig. 14-2 the QRS of the premature beat is narrower than 0.14 sec, and there is a less-than-full compensatory pause (discussed on p. 81). Both are signs of aberrancy.

RETROGRADE CONCEALED CONDUCTION

Although phase 3 block is the mechanism of aberrant ventricular conduction, retrograde conduction into the blocked bundle may be the sustaining mechanism

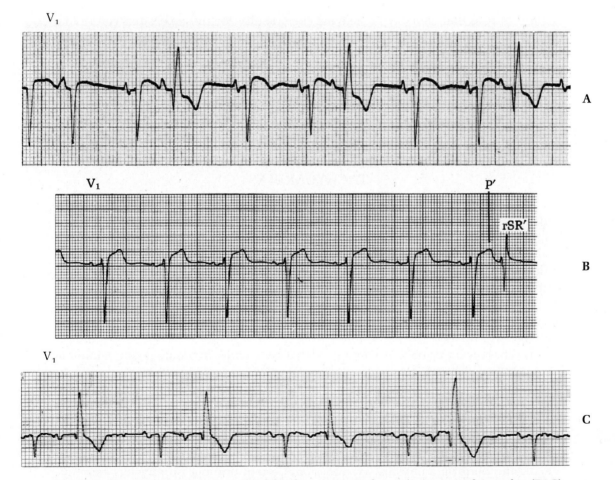

Fig. 14-1. Phase 3 aberration. In each of the three tracings the premature atrial complex (PAC) occurs early (in the T wave), finds the right bundle branch still refractory, and is therefore conducted with right bundle branch block (RBBB) aberration. **A,** The first P wave in the tracing is a PAC. It is followed by a sinus beat with normal conduction. There are three more PACs; all are conducted with RBBB aberration (rSR' pattern in V_1). **B,** There is one PAC (P') followed by RBBB aberration. **C,** Bigeminal PACs are conducted with RBBB aberration (the upright complexes).

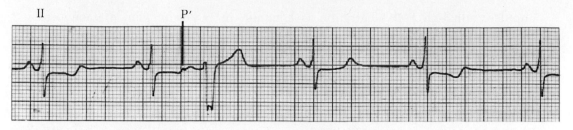

Fig. 14-2. An early PAC (P′) is conducted with aberrant ventricular conduction. Although this is lead II, where the shape of the QRS is not helpful, aberration is easily recognized because the P′ wave is easily visible and there is less than a full compensatory pause.

For example, if there is functional LBBB at the initiation of supraventricular tachycardia (SVT), it is possible for the blocked left bundle to be activated in retrograde fashion during that same cycle, leaving it refractory for the next supraventricular beat. So it is that the initial mechanism of aberrancy (phase 3 block) creates a setting allowing that same bundle branch to be activated in retrograde fashion, guaranteeing that the next supraventricular beat will also be blocked in that bundle—a self-propagating mechanism. Although the affected bundle may be capable of shortening its refractory period in response to the tachycardia, it continues to be unable to conduct in anterograde fashion because of the retrograde penetration.[1]

IMPORTANCE OF DIFFERENTIATING AMONG BROAD QRS TACHYCARDIAS

Misdiagnosis of ventricular tachycardia (VT) may result in immediate hemodynamic collapse in the acute stage of therapy, or if the patient survives this and his or her condition is still misdiagnosed, subsequent mismanagement may result in death. Akhtar et al.[2] analyzed the data obtained from 150 consecutive patients with wide QRS tachycardia and found that 122 patients had VT, 21 had SVT with aberration, and 7 had accessory pathway conduction. One of the findings of this study was that only 39 of the 122 patients with VT received a correct diagnosis in the acute setting. Reasons for this shocking discovery were unclear, but the following were suggested:

1. There is an erroneous perception that SVT with aberrancy is as common as VT.
2. In most patients who come to medical attention with wide-complex tachycardia and hemodynamic stability, the clinician wrongly assumes that VT is unlikely.
3. The emergency nature of the clinical setting motivates the clinician to judge quickly rather than to thoroughly analyze the 12-lead ECG, take a history, and perform a physical examination. Certain findings on physical examination and on the ECG often swiftly provide a correct diagnosis.

Not only is it important to recognize VT because of the dire consequences that result from mistreatment and subsequent mismanagement of such patients, but also it is important to recognize SVT, especially when an accessory pathway is involved. Although a given emergency treatment may terminate both VT and SVT (e.g., procainamide), if an incorrect diagnosis is made, the patient is denied a safe and permanent cure. For example, a patient arrives at the emergency department with a broad QRS tachycardia and a history of palpitations. The emergency room physician incorrectly judges the rhythm to be nonischemic VT and gives intravenous (IV) procainamide. (Lidocaine may have been tried first with no success.) The procainamide immediately converts the rhythm to normal sinus rhythm. The patient is relieved, and those involved in the emergency care of the patient feel a sense of accomplishment. In reality, the rhythm treated was paroxysmal supraventricular tachycardia (PSVT) with LBBB aberration; the mechanism of the tachycardia could have been AV reentry (circus movement) using an accessory pathway. Procainamide blocked the accessory pathway and therefore converted the tachycardia to normal sinus rhythm. However, the patient is now denied a cure (radiofrequency ablation) and exposed to potential life-threatening arrhythmias. Although the arrhythmia was successfully treated, an incorrect diagnosis was made; in this case the mistake may eventually lead to recurrences and could also be lethal.

IMPORTANCE OF TAKING A HISTORY

The history is helpful in making a correct diagnosis. One study[3] found that a history of structural heart disease suggested VT in 112 (95%) of 118 patients, and a history of myocardial infarction (MI) was associated with a high incidence of VT as the mechanism of wide-complex tachycardia in 87 (98%) of 89 patients.

ATRIOVENTRICULAR DISSOCIATION

Atrioventricular dissociation is the independent beating of atria and ventricles and is present in approximately 50% of ventricular tachycardias. The finding of AV dissociation is the most reliable criterion for a correct diagnosis of VT. Its most reliable indicators are its physical signs.

Physical signs

1. Irregular cannon A waves in the jugular pulse
2. Varying intensity of the first heart sound
3. Beat-to-beat changes in systolic blood pressure

Any one of the preceding clues indicates AV dissociation, although the absence of clues does not rule out VT, nor does it rule out AV dissociation. For example, in atrial fibrillation with VT there is AV dissociation without its usual physical or ECG signs.

Jugular pulse. During AV dissociation the atria and the ventricles are beating independently; this beating occasionally coincides, so that the atria contract against closed AV valves, causing a reflux of blood up the jugular veins. Such irregular, unpredictable expansions in the pulsation of the jugular pulse are called *cannon A waves.*

Varying intensity of the first heart sound. The first heart sound is caused by the closing of the AV valves. During sinus rhythm it has a fixed intensity because the position of the leaflets of the AV valves is the same for every ventricular systole. During AV dissociation this position differs from beat to beat, causing a varying intensity of the first heart sound. Other conditions in which this would occur are complete heart block, AV Wenckebach, and atrial fibrillation.

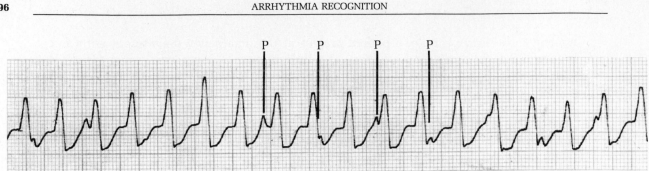

Fig. 14-3. Atrioventricular (AV) dissociation. The regular, independent sinus P waves during the tachycardia can be seen. The P waves are easily found when a distortion is seen in the ST-T segment of one cycle that is not seen in another. In this tracing P waves distorting the QRS can also be identified. There are three QRS complexes in this tracing that are distorted by P waves, making them look like rR' complexes; they are the third, eleventh, and second to last.

Changes in systolic blood pressure. Atrioventricular dissociation can be identified at the bedside by using the sphygmomanometer and blood pressure cuff. During AV dissociation there are beat-to-beat changes in systolic blood pressure because the lapse of time between atrial and ventricular contraction is different with each cycle, resulting in varying ventricular filling times.

ECG signs of atrioventricular dissociation

Atrioventricular dissociation is often missed on the surface ECG. In one study[2] involving 150 patients with wide QRS tachycardia, AV dissociation was present in 67 patients (45%) but could be detected by the surface ECG in only 38 of those patients. The greatest danger is that the clinician may mistake T waves for P waves, a mistake that leads to an incorrect diagnosis and possibly lethal consequences. During the broad QRS tachycardia P waves can best be found by looking for a distortion in one cycle that cannot be found in another. For example, in Fig. 14-3 independent P waves can be seen throughout the tracing; four of them are marked. These P waves are found because they distort the ECG cycle differently each time; that is, following the first QRS there is a little nubbin that cannot be seen in the same place following the next QRS. Therefore this little nubbin cannot be part of the QRS or the T wave. It is undeniably a P wave.

FINDING P WAVES IN THE BROAD QRS TACHYCARDIA
Exercise 1

Wrong approach. The most common error is to look for P waves as a consistent finding in every cycle; this leads to the costly error of mistaking T waves for P waves. For example, when examining the 12 leads seen in Fig. 14-4, the examiner looked in leads V_3 and V_4 among other leads and decided that there were P waves in front of every QRS and that this was SVT. Because of this uninformed and rash judgment on the part of the clinician, the patient received verapamil with devastating consequences.

Right approach. This time, look for P waves in Fig. 14-4 (the same Figure) by searching for distortions in one cycle that are not seen in another. Such distortions are

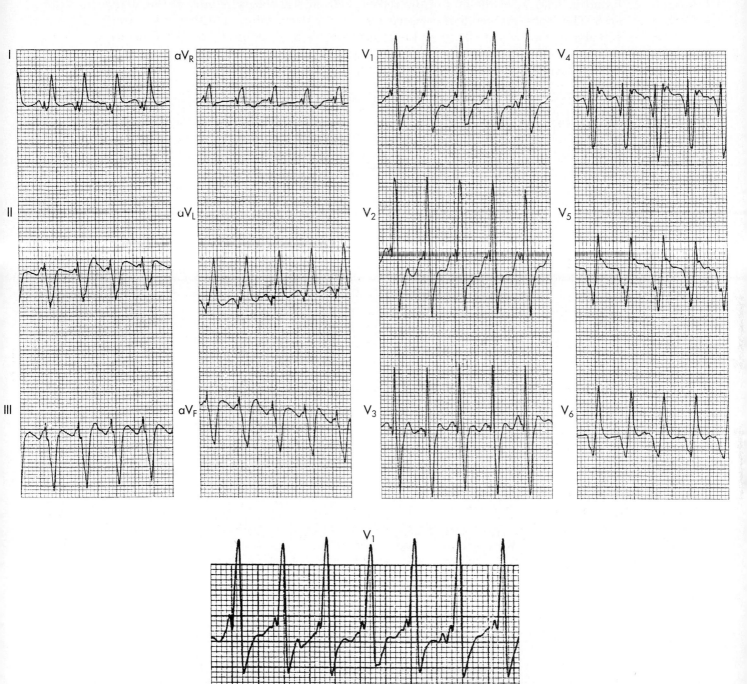

Fig. 14-4. Exercise 1. Find the sinus P waves in this ventricular tachycardia (VT). They are best found by looking in each lead for a distortion in one cycle that is not found in another. This is nicely seen in leads V_1 and V_2, where there is a small positive deflection following the second QRS that is not seen in neighboring cycles. Another such distortion is in front of the sixth QRS.

found in lead V_1 at the end of the second QRS and at the beginning of the sixth QRS. These are independent P waves; there is AV dissociation and this is VT. You can also see a P wave distorting the fourth T wave in leads II and III. This distortion is identified as a P wave because the same distortion is not found in the neighboring T waves.

Exercise 2

Wrong approach. When evaluating Fig. 14-5, an uninformed clinician may look first for beat-to-beat deflections that look like P waves and, of course, easily finds round, little P-like nubbins in lead V_1! If the decision to treat is made on this finding, the consequence to the patient may be loss of life.

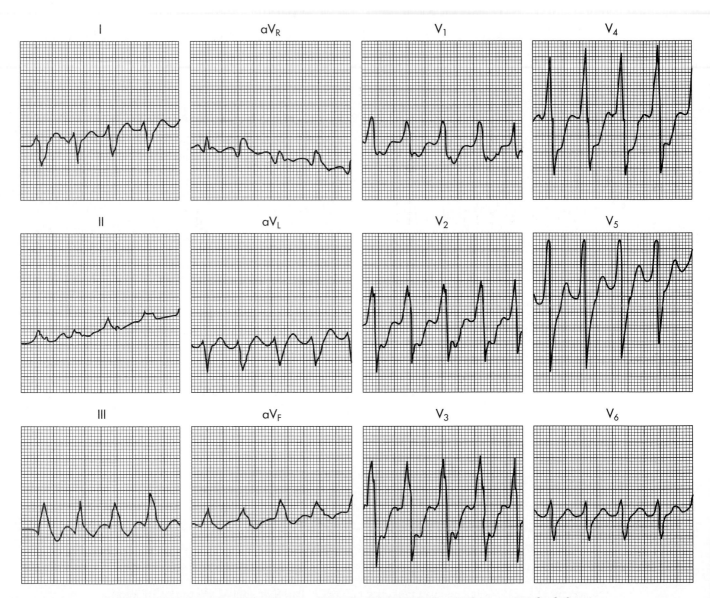

Fig. 14-5. Exercise 2. In an attempt to discover AV dissociation and prove VT, look for sinus P waves (seen in lead II). There is a P wave between the first and second QRS complexes and one distorting the fourth QRS complex.

Right approach. In assessing for AV dissociation, the informed examiner evaluates all leads in Fig. 14-5, looking for a distortion in one cycle that is not seen in another. This is found in lead II. There is a sinus P wave before the second QRS and one distorting the third QRS. The P waves are independent; therefore this is AV dissociation and the patient has VT.

RETROGRADE CONDUCTION TO THE ATRIA DURING VENTRICULAR TACHYCARDIA

Fifty percent of the time there is some form of retrograde conduction to the atria during VT. (The P′ waves are negative in leads II, III, and aV$_F$ and positive in

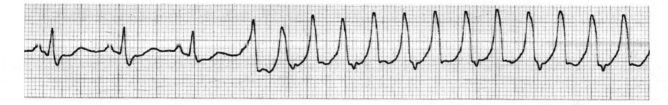

Fig. 14-6. Ventricular tachycardia with 2:1 retrograde conduction ratio. The retrograde P′ waves (negative in lead II) in every other T wave are diagnostic of VT. In approximately 50% of cases VT has some form of retrograde conduction to the atria.

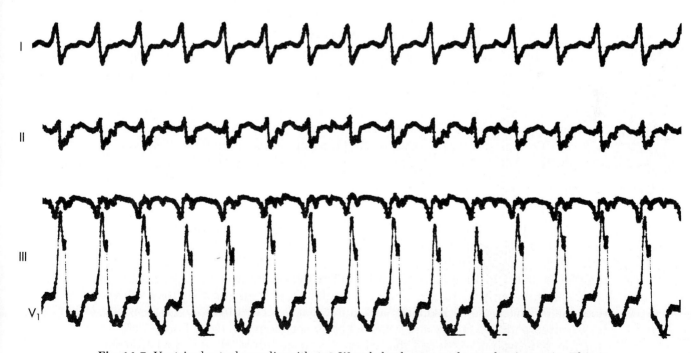

Fig. 14-7. Ventricular tachycardia with 4:3 Wenckebach retrograde conduction ratio. This is best seen in lead III. Start by looking between the third and fourth QRS complexes. The P wave seen there is not in the same place in the next cycle. You will now easily see the P′ waves distorting the first and second T waves and then note that there is no P′ wave at all in or near the fourth T wave. This sequence then repeats itself, with the RP′ becoming longer until ventriculoatrial (VA) conduction fails. *(From Wellens HJJ et al. In Josephson ME, ed: Ventricular tachycardia: mechanisms and management, Mount Kisco, NY, 1982, Futura.)*

lead aV_R.) To visualize this on the ECG, however, ventriculoatrial (VA) conduction must be sufficiently long so that the P' waves occur outside the QRS complex. Ventriculoatrial conduction with a 1:1 ratio is present in one fourth to one third of patients with VT at heart rates of less than 180 beats/min (without drugs). When the heart rate is more than 200 beats/min, this condition is uncommon.[2]

Fig. 14-6 is VT with 2:1 retrograde conduction. Note the negative P' waves in every other T wave. Fig. 14-7 is VT with 4:3 retrograde Wenckebach conduction. In Fig. 14-7 the P' waves are best seen in leads II and III. Find the P' wave between the third and fourth QRS; it is easy to spot because it is separate from the T wave. After identification of the P' and the T in that cycle, it becomes evident that the preceding two T waves are distorted by P' waves and that the cycle following the fourth QRS has no T wave at all. This Wenckebach sequence of lengthening RP' intervals and then nonconduction is repeated. Other signs that support a diagnosis of VT in Fig. 14-7 are the left axis deviation, the QRS width of more than 0.14 sec, and the "rabbit ear" sign in lead V_1 (discussed later in this chapter).

ECG DIAGNOSIS OF BROAD QRS TACHYCARDIA

1. Look for signs of AV dissociation in all 12 leads; look for a distortion in one cycle (a P wave) that is not seen in another.
2. Measure QRS width.
3. Determine QRS axis.
4. Evaluate QRS morphologic appearance.

QRS WIDTH

In the broad QRS tachycardia, a QRS duration of more than 0.14 sec is highly suggestive of VT. Wellens[4] has shown in a study of 100 cases of SVT with aberration that a QRS width less than or equal to 0.14 sec was present in all patients. He and his associates also studied 100 cases of VT and found that 59% had a QRS duration of more than 0.14 sec. Akhtar et al.[2] found "excellent" diagnostic accuracy for VT when they used a criterion for QRS duration of more than 0.14 sec with a V_1-positive pattern and more than 0.16 sec with a V_1-negative pattern.

AXIS

The most helpful axis observation in the broad QRS tachycardia is that of −90 degrees to ±180 degrees (sometimes called "no man's land", indeterminant, or the northwest quadrant). Such an axis does not occur in SVT; it is an apical focus and therefore reliably distinguishes VT from SVT with aberration or accessory pathway conduction. When V_1 is negative and the frontal plane leads show right axis deviation, the diagnosis is VT. Akhtar et al.[2] found that this combination was seen only in VT (nine patients), a fact also reported by Rosenbaum[5] in 1969. Furthermore, a study by Kindwall et al.[6] found that when V_1 was negative, left axis deviation was not useful, being common to both VT and SVT with aberration.

Clinical correlations[4]

Previous myocardial infarction. When VT occurs in such patients, the QRS axis in the frontal plane is usually abnormal. This is especially true when V_1 is positive. In such cases the axis is often superior (left or no man's land; negative in aV_F).

Idiopathic ventricular tachycardia. In the normal heart VT can have a normal axis, but most commonly there is a marked right axis deviation or the axis is directed superiorly.

Preexisting bundle branch block. A markedly abnormal axis may occur in patients with preexisting BBB who have SVT.

Accessory pathways. Marked left axis deviation (left of −30 degrees) may be seen in SVT with conduction over a right-sided or posteroseptal accessory pathway, and marked right axis deviation may be seen in SVT with conduction over a left lateral accessory pathway.

Class IC drugs. Patients taking class IC drugs can have SVT with an axis to the left of −30 degrees.

Summary of axis

In the wide-complex tachycardia

1. A QRS axis in no man's land (−90 degrees to ±180 degrees) reliably indicates VT.
2. When lead V_1 is negative, a right axis indicates VT.
3. When lead V_1 is negative, a left axis is not helpful.
4. When lead V_1 is positive, axis is not helpful.

CAPTURE BEATS AND FUSION BEATS

Capture beats and fusion beats are rarely seen and therefore have limited value. They occur during VT when a sinus impulse is conducted into the ventricle and either entirely captures the ventricle or collides with the ventricular ectopic impulse (fusion), which is discharging at approximately the same time. Either case results in a narrow beat. Fig. 14-8 shows ventricular fusion during VT. A fusion beat is a strong sign of VT.

CONCORDANT PATTERN

The term *concordant pattern* refers to entirely positive or entirely negative QRS complexes in the precordial leads during the tachycardia. Negative precordial concordance (Fig. 14-9) usually reflects a focus in the anteroapical left ventricle. Positive precordial concordance results when ventricular activation originates in the posterobasal left ventricle. Thus such a pattern can result both from VT with a focus in that region (Fig. 14-10) and from SVT with an accessory pathway located in

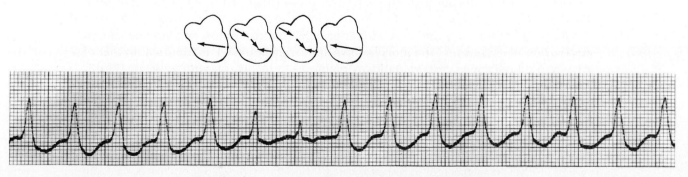

Fig. 14-8. Ventricular tachycardia with fusion beats.

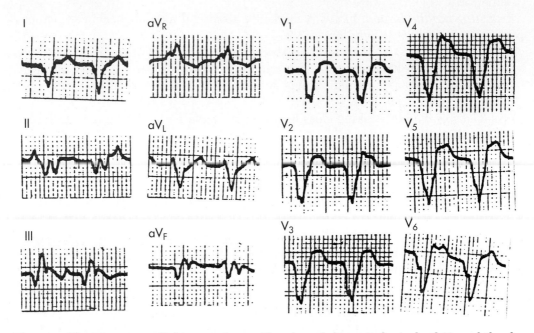

Fig. 14-9. Negative precordial concordance. The slurred downstroke in lead V_1 and the delayed S nadir in leads V_1 and V_2 (discussed on p. 211) are also evident.

that region (Fig. 14-11). However, because positive precordial concordance caused by SVT is rare, this finding should raise the level of suspicion for VT.

QRS MORPHOLOGIC APPEARANCE

There are two sets of morphologic rules that help to differentiate aberrancy from ectopy. One set of rules applies to the V_1-positive wide-complex tachycardia and uses leads V_1 and, sometimes, V_6. The other set of rules applies to the V_1-negative wide-complex tachycardia* and uses leads V_1, V_2, and V_6. It is important not to switch the rules, especially when evaluating lead V_6. If the broad QRS tachycardia is approached systematically (history, physical examination, QRS axis, AV dissociation, and QRS morphologic appearance), these rules provide greater than 90% accuracy.[7]

Be aware that in some clinical settings QRS morphologic appearance can be misleading. For example, the morphologic appearance of SVT is identical to that of VT when there is an accessory pathway connecting the atrium and ventricle (Wolff-Parkinson-White syndrome) and when the patient is taking drugs that slow intraventricular conduction. Likewise, VT can be mistaken for SVT in cases of digitalis

*In the medical literature the V_1-positive broad QRS complex is referred to as "RBBB" or "RBBB-like", and the V_1-negative broad QRS complex as "LBBB" or "LBBB-like". These terms do not imply mechanism or precise QRS morphologic appearance, merely the polarity of the QRS in V_1; that is, the RBBB pattern is positive in V_1 and the LBBB pattern is negative.

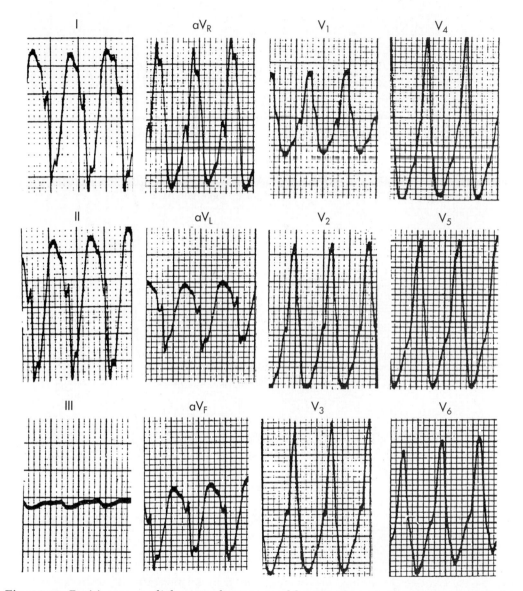

Fig. 14-10. Positive precordial concordance caused by VT. The axis from −90 to ±180 degrees ("no man's land") can also be seen.

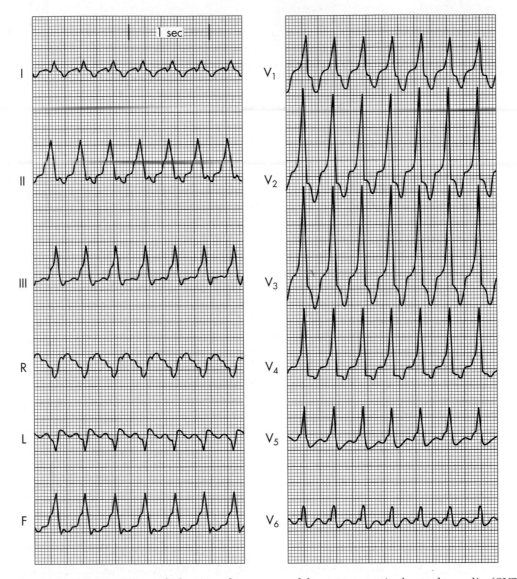

Fig. 14-11. Positive precordial concordance caused by supraventricular tachycardia (SVT) (atrial flutter with 2:1 conduction ratio over a left-sided accessory pathway). *(From Wellens HJJ, Conover M: The ECG in emergency decision making, Philadelphia, 1992, WB Saunders.)*

Table 14-1. Classification of broad QRS tachycardias

Type (clinical setting)	ECG (morphologic appearance)	Emergency treatment	Cure	Chapter no. for reference
VT THAT LOOKS LIKE VT				
Torsades de pointes (using class IA or class III drugs such as sotalol; hypolakemia)	Multiform	Discontinue class 1A drugs; give magnesium sulfate or magnesium chloride; potassium		15
Polymorphous VT (ischemia-related)	Multiform	Beta blocker (esmolol); lidocaine; cardioversion		15
Broad QRS	Negative precordial concordance	Lidocaine or procainamide (if symptomatic)		14
V$_1$-negative, broad QRS	Right axis deviation; in V$_1$ and/or V$_2$: broad R, slurred S downstroke, delayed S nadir; in V$_6$: any Q	Lidocaine or procainamide (if symptomatic)		14
Broad QRS	Axis from −90 to ±180 degrees	Lidocaine or procainamide (if symptomatic)		14
V$_1$-positive, broad QRS	Rr′ in V$_1$ (rabbit ear sign); monophasic or biphasic	Lidocaine or procainamide (if symptomatic)		14
VT THAT LOOKS LIKE SVT				
Idiopathic VT (normal heart)	LBBB with inferior axis; RBBB with superior axis	Lidocaine or procainamide unless experienced electrophysiologist	Radiofrequency ablation	13
Fascicular VT (using digoxin)	RBBB; axis deviation	Discontinue digitalis; bed rest; if unstable: digitalis antibodies or phenytoin (with pacing lead in place)		17
Bundle-branch reentry VT (cardiomyopathy)	Usually LBBB	Cardioversion	Radiofrequency ablation	13
SVT THAT LOOKS LIKE VT (MAY HAVE A HISTORY OF PALPITATIONS)				
Atrial fibrillation with AP conduction	That of VT (irregular)	Procainamide	Radiofrequency ablation	23
Atrial flutter with AP conduction	That of VT	Procainamide	Radiofrequency ablation	23
Antidromic CMT (AV reentry using anterograde AP and retrograde AV node	That of VT	Vagal maneuver; adenosine; procainamide; cardioversion	Radiofrequency ablation	23

NOTE: The terms *RBBB* and *LBBB* indicate QRS patterns of physiologic or functional bundle branch block, not merely the polarity of the complex in lead V$_1$.

AP, Accessory pathway; *AV,* atrioventricular; *CMT,* circus movement tachycardia; *ECG,* electrocardiogram; *LBBB,* left bundle branch block; *RBBB,* right bundle branch block; *SVT,* supraventricular tachycardia; *VT,* ventricular tachycardia.

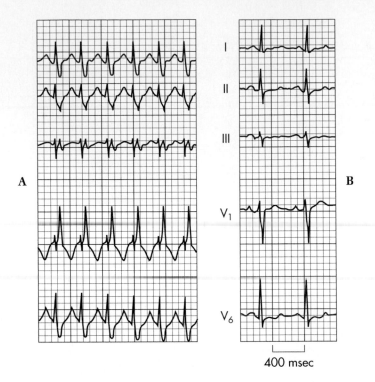

Fig. 14-12. A, Supraventricular tachycardia with RBBB aberration with, **B,** sinus rhythm from the same patient. *(From Wellens HJJ. In Willerson JT, Cohn JN, eds: Cardiovascular medicine, New York, 1995, Churchill Livingstone.)*

toxicity (fascicular VT), idiopathic VT, and bundle branch reentry VT. Please refer to Table 14-1 for types of broad QRS tachycardia, possible causes, emergency treatment, and cures (chapter references).

When lead V_1 is positive

ECG signs supporting a diagnosis of supraventricular tachycardia

1. Triphasic pattern of RBBB (rSR′ in V_1 and qRs in V_6). This pattern (Fig. 14-12) occurs more often in SVT than in VT.[8,9] In V_1 during the tachycardia the small r wave reflects septal activation, the S wave reflects left ventricular activation, and the terminal R wave reflects late activation of the right ventricle.
2. QRS of less than 0.14 sec.
3. R:S ratio in V_6 greater than 1 (R greater than S).

NOTE: Certain types of VT may also have this triphasic pattern in V_1 and the relatively narrow QRS (i.e., fascicular VT, left ventricular idiopathic VT, and bundle branch reentry VT).

ECG signs supporting a diagnosis of ventricular tachycardia

1. A monophasic (Fig. 14-13) or biphasic complex (R, qR, or RS) in lead V_1 (more common in VT). It is possible for such a pattern to also occur in SVT, which

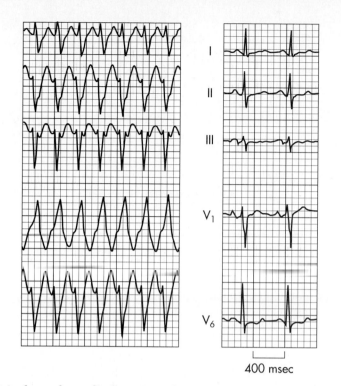

I

II

III

V₁

V₆

400 msec

Fig. 14-13. Ventricular tachycardia in patient shown in Fig. 14-12. The monophasic R wave in lead V₁, the superior axis, and the R/S ratio of less than 1 in lead V₆ are evident. *(From Wellens HJJ. In Willerson JT, Cohn JN, eds: Cardiovascular medicine, New York, 1995, Churchill Livingstone.)*

emphasizes the systematic approach to the patient with all factors being evaluated.[7]

2. The rabbit ear sign in V₁ (Rr'). Such a rabbit ear pattern has two positive peaks in V₁; the initial peak is taller. *Note:* It is not uncommon to see the Rr' pattern in sinus rhythm with RBBB, especially in the face of right axis deviation. Figs. 14-14 and 14-15 compare the patterns of VT and SVT with aberration when V₁ is positive. The opposite rabbit ear configuration with the initial peak shorter (Fig. 14-16) is seen equally in both VT and SVT and therefore is not useful in diagnosis. When such a pattern is seen, it is necessary to evaluate the R/S ratio in lead V₆. Because of the influence of the QRS axis on the shape of the QRS complex in V₆, the R/S ratio in that lead is helpful if the frontal plane axis is left; that is, in such a case an R/S ratio of less than 1 supports a diagnosis of VT. This finding is of no value if the axis is inferior (normal or right).[7]

Pitfalls

It must be emphasized that in applying these criteria, especially in V₁-positive tachycardias, an understanding of the clinical setting (drugs being taken, history of myocardial infarction [MI], cardiomyopathy, presence of heart disease, and so forth) is critical. In the setting of broad QRS tachycardia this information is not always available, which limits the value of the criteria.[2]

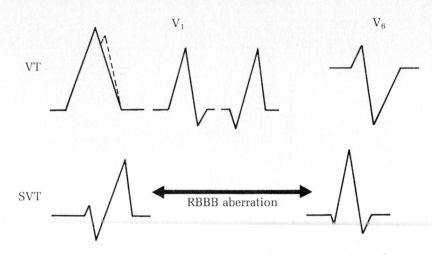

Fig. 14-14. Morphologic appearance in V_1-positive wide-complex tachycardia. A monophasic or biphasic complex indicates VT. A triphasic (rSR′) pattern indicates SVT. The "rabbit ear" clue (Rr′) in V_1 (initial peak taller) indicates VT. When the two peaks are reversed (rR′), a deep S (R/S ratio of less than 1) indicates VT.

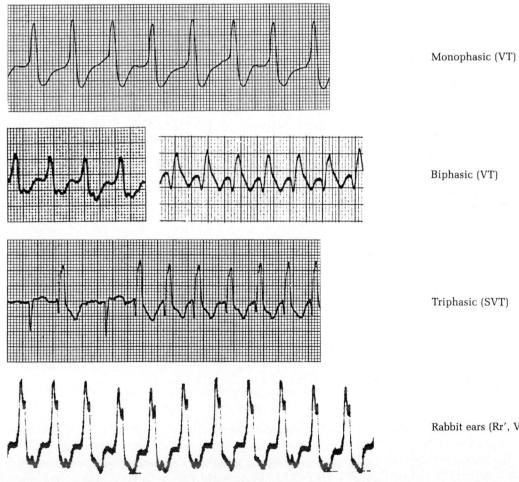

Monophasic (VT)

Biphasic (VT)

Triphasic (SVT)

Rabbit ears (Rr′, VT)

Fig. 14-15. Tachycardias with a V_1-positive configuration.

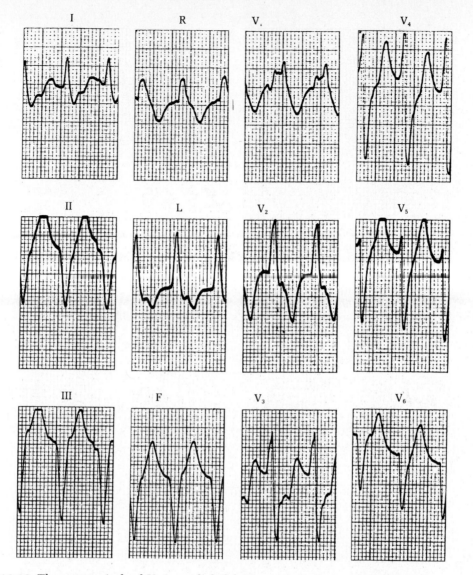

Fig. 14-16. The pattern in lead V_1 is not helpful. However, in that same lead a P wave is seen in front of the first QRS but not in front of the next one. This is a sign of AV dissociation and diagnostic of VT. Another helpful clue is the R/S ratio in V_6. When the axis is left, as it is here, such a ratio supports a diagnosis of VT.

When lead V_1 is negative

ECG signs supporting a diagnosis of supraventricular tachycardia

1. If there is an R wave in V_1 or V_2, or both, during LBBB aberration, it is narrow and sharp with a low amplitude.
2. The S downstroke is swift and clean in V_1 and V_2, reflecting conduction in the His-Purkinje system.
3. The nadir of the S wave is early (≤ 0.06 sec) in V_1 and V_2.

The patterns of V_1-negative VT and LBBB aberration are compared in tracings in Fig. 14-17. It is important to realize that these signs apply to leads V_1 and V_2. If V_1

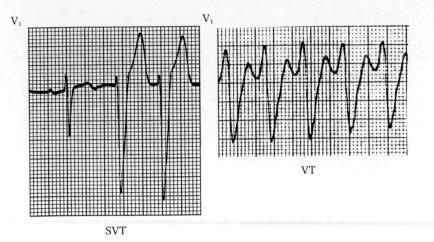

Fig. 14-17. V_1-negative wide-complex tachycardias compared. Indicators of VT are a broad R, slurred S downstroke, and a delayed S nadir in V_1 or V_2. Supraventricular tachycardia has a narrow, sharp R wave in V_1 or V_2 and a fast S downstroke. In SVT the R wave of the tachycardia is smaller than that of the sinus beat, another indicator of SVT; VT supported by a bundle-branch reentry mechanism could also look like this LBBB pattern.

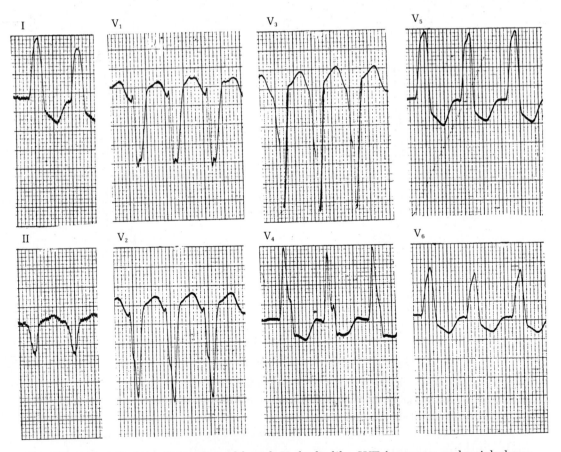

Fig. 14-18. Ventricular tachycardia. Although V_1 looks like SVT (narrow r and quick downstroke), lead V_2 shows a slurred downstroke, V_6 has a small q wave, V_4 shows signs of AV dissociation (the distortion in the QRS of the second beat is a P wave), and the QRS is 0.16 sec wide.

looks like SVT, it is necessary to check out V_2 before making that judgment. Fig. 14-18 illustrates this fact. In V_1 the narrow r and clean, swift downstroke are both signs of SVT. However, when V_2 is checked, the slurred downstroke that 1 identifies this rhythm as VT is immediately apparent. Other signs of VT in Fig. 14-17 are the small q wave in lead V_6 and signs of AV dissociation in V_4. (Note the P wave distorting the middle complex.)

ECG signs supporting a diagnosis of ventricular tachycardia
1. *Wide R (V_1 and/or V_2):* Seen in more than 90% of VTs associated with inferior infarction and in only 25% of tachycardias associated with anterior infarction; in the latter a QS complex is more common.[7]
2. *Slurred S downstroke (V_1 and/or V_2):* Sensitivity of only 36%, and usually occurs in anterior infarction.
3. *Delayed S nadir (V_1 and/or V_2):* The distance from the onset of the QRS to the lowest point of the S wave (its nadir) is more than 0.06 sec. This finding is seen in two thirds of patients who have V_1-negative VT.
4. *Q in V_6:* Confirms VT.

All four signs of VT are diagramatically illustrated in Fig. 14-19 and are compared with the pattern of LBBB aberration. In Figs. 14-20 and 14-21 three of these signs are seen in V_1 and V_2, that is, broad R, slurred S downstroke, and delayed S nadir. In Fig. 14-21 the right axis deviation contributes to the certainty that this condition is VT; remember that when V_1 is negative, left axis deviation is not helpful. The absence of all four of the previously listed signs is highly suggestive of SVT.[6] Even in the setting of preexisting BBB, the broad R and notched downstroke are characteristic of VT.[10,11] In the V_1-negative wide-complex tachycardia there is usually a

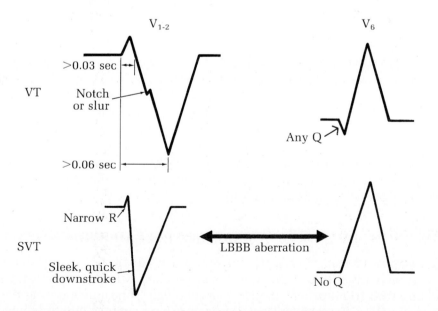

Fig. 14-19. Morphologic appearance in V_1-negative wide-complex tachycardia. In V_1 and V_2 a wide R, slurred S downstroke, or delayed nadir indicates VT. In lead V_6 any Q wave indicates VT. In SVT the R in leads V_1 and V_2 is narrow and the S downstroke quick and sleek. In SVT there is no Q in V_6 when V_1 is negative.

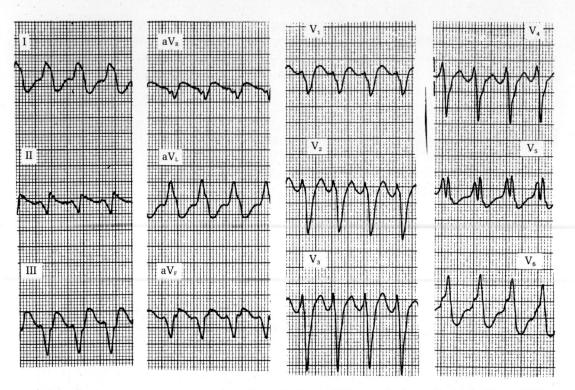

Fig. 14-20. In the V_1-negative pattern three features of VT can be seen. In leads V_1 and V_2 there is a broad R wave, a slurred S downstroke (V_1 only), and a delay from the beginning of the ventricular complex to the lowest point of the S wave (its nadir). The left axis deviation is not a helpful sign.

monophasic R wave in lead V_6 during SVT.[6,12] A Q wave in this lead suggests VT and is almost always present when the tachycardia originates from the anterior septum.[7]

In 1991 Brugada et al.[17] pointed out that a duration from the onset of R to the nadir of the S wave in the precordial leads of more than 100 ms is an indication of VT. However, this criterion has limited usefulness because such a duration may also occur in SVT with the following conditions: conduction over an accessory pathway, administration of drugs that slow intraventricular conduction, and preexisting BBB (most especially, preexisting LBBB).[4]

VALUE OF A BASELINE 12-LEAD ECG

A baseline 12-lead ECG is, of course, always advantageous, especially when there is preexisting BBB or ECG evidence of previous MI. In patients with VT and preexisting BBB (right or left) the QRS morphologic appearance during the tachycardia is clearly different from that recorded during sinus rhythm.[2,13] whereas in SVT the morphologic appearance is usually identical to that of the sinus rhythm (Fig. 14-22).

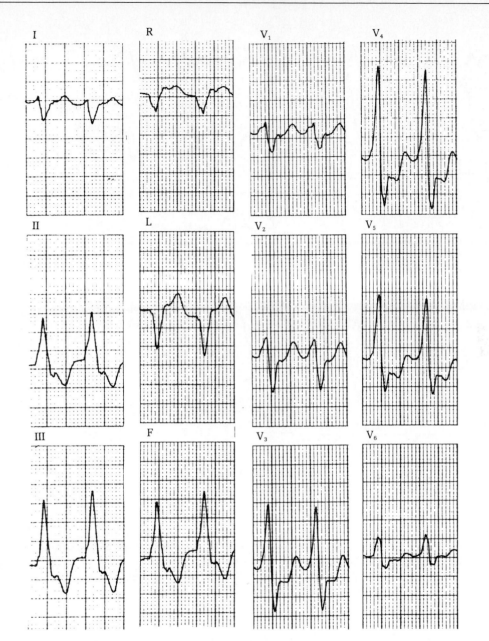

Fig. 14-21. Ventricular tachycardia. The slurred S downstroke in lead V_1, the broad R wave in V_2, and the delayed S nadir in both leads can be seen. When V_1 is negative, right axis deviation is diagnostic of VT.

WHEN IN DOUBT

When the diagnosis in wide-complex tachycardia remains uncertain after applying the rules described in this chapter, application of the following rules protects your patient from receiving the wrong drugs:

1. Do not give verapamil; give procainamide, unless there is a possibility that you are dealing with torsades de pointes.

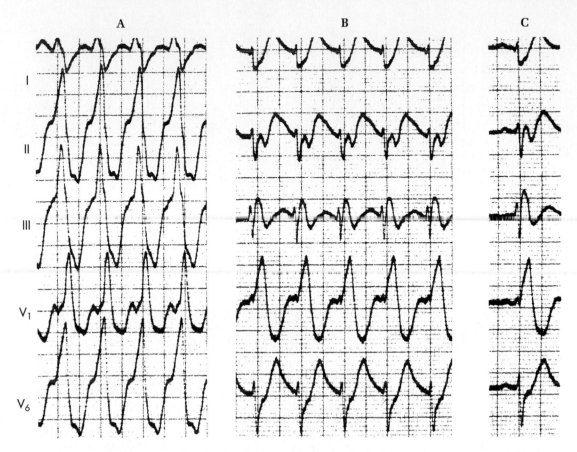

Fig. 14-22. Electrocardiograms from a 15-year-old boy who had complete correction of Fallot's tetralogy. **A** and **B,** A tachycardia with a wide QRS complex; **C,** sinus rhythm with RBBB and left axis deviation. During programed stimulation the tachycardia in **A** was found to be ventricular and the one in **B** originated in the AV node (SVT). The shape of the QRS, **B,** is identical to the shape of the sinus rhythm, **C.** These ECGs demonstrate that if a patient is admitted in tachycardia showing the recording of **B,** the clinician probably would make the incorrect diagnosis of VT. They demonstrate the necessity of careful comparison with the ECG during sinus rhythm in patients with wide QRS during tachycardia. *(C, from Wellens HJJ et al. In Josephson ME, ed: Ventricular tachycardia: mechanisms and management, Mount Kisco, NY, 1982, Futura.)*

   2. When confronted with a wide QRS tachycardia that is greater than 200 beats/min and irregular, do not give digitalis or verapamil; give procainamide.[1]

Although both verapamil and procainamide have negative inotropic effects, procainamide causes the rate of the VT to slow,[14] partially compensating for the fall in blood pressure.[14] Procainamide also blocks conduction in accessory pathways to interrupt AV reentry using an accessory pathway, blocks the retrograde fast pathway in the AV node to terminate PSVT caused by AV nodal reentry, and terminates nonischemic VT.[16]

SUMMARY

   When differentiating between aberrant ventricular conduction and ventricular ectopy it is important to keep in mind the following:

1. Ventricular tachycardia is more common than SVT with aberration.
2. Ventricular tachycardia is frequently associated with structural heart disease and previous MI.
3. The use of IV verapamil should be avoided in the treatment of patients with wide QRS tachycardia.
4. A correct diagnosis can generally be made from the surface ECG when all criteria are applied.
5. Highly reliable ECG criteria for VT are as follows:
   Atrioventricular dissociation
   QRS duration greater than 0.14 sec in V_1-positive patterns
   QRS duration greater than 0.16 sec in V_1-negative patterns
   Negative precordial QRS concordance
   Axis of -90 degrees to ±180 degrees
   V_1-negative patterns associated with right axis deviation
   In patients with underlying BBB a QRS pattern that is different during the tachycardia
   In V_1-negative patterns a broad R, slurred S downstroke, and delayed S nadir in V_1 or V_2, or both, or a Q wave in V_6
   In V_1-positive patterns a monophasic R, biphasic pattern, or rabbit ear sign in V_1

REFERENCES

1. Wellens HJJ, Conover M: *The ECG in emergency decision making,* Philadelphia, 1992, WB Saunders.
2. Akhtar M, Shenasa M, Jazayeri M et al: Wide QRS complex tachycardia: reappraisal of a common clinical problem, *Ann Intern Med* 109:905, 1988.
3. Tchou P, Young P, Mahmud R et al: Useful clinical criteria for the diagnosis of ventricular tachycardia, *Am J Med* 84:53, 1988.
4. Wellens HJJ: Wide QRS tachycardia. In Willerson JT, Cohn JN, eds: *Cardiovascular medicine,* New York, 1995, Churchill Livingstone.
5. Rosenbaum MB: Classification of ventricular extrasystoles according to form, *J Electrocardiol* 2:289, 1969.
6. Kindwall KE, Brown J, Josephson ME: Electrocardiographic criteria for ventricular tachycardia in wide complex left bundle branch block morphology tachycardia, *Am J Cardiol* 61:1279, 1988.
7. Josephson ME, Wellens HJJ: Differential diagnosis of supraventricular tachycardia, *Cardiol Clin* 8:411, 1990.
8. Sandler JA, Marriott HJL: The differential morphology of anomalous V_1 ventricular complexes of RBBB type in lead V_1: ventricular ectopy versus aberration, *Circulation* 31:551, 1965.
9. Marriott HJL, Sandler JA: Criteria, old and new, for differentiation between ectopic ventricular beats and aberrant ventricular conduction in the presence of atrial fibrillation, *Prog Cardiovasc Dis* 9:18, 1966.
10. Josephson ME Horowitz LN, Waxman HL, Cain ME: Sustained ventricular tachycardia: role of the 12-lead electrocardiogram in localizing site of origin, *Circulation* 64:257, 1981.
11. Miller JM, Marchlinski FE, Buxton AE, Josephson ME: Relationship between the 12-lead electrocardiogram during ventricular tachycardia and endocardial site of origin in patients with coronary artery disease, *Circulation* 77:759, 1988.
12. Wellens HJJ, Bär FWHM, Lie K: The value of the electrocardiogram in the differential diagnosis of a tachycardia with a widened QRS complex, *Am J Med* 64:27, 1978.
13. Wellens HJJ, Bär FWHM, Brugada P: Ventricular tachycardia: the clinical problem. In Josephson ME, ed: *Ventricular tachycardia: mechanism and management,* Mount Kisco, NY, 1982, Futura.
14. Marchlinski FE, Buxton AE, Vassallo JA et al: Comparative electrophysiologic effects of intravenous and oral procainamide in patients with sustained ventricular arrhythmias, *J Am Coll Cardiol* 4:1247, 1984.
15. Wellens HJJ: The wide QRS tachycardia, *Ann Intern Med* 104:879, 1986.
16. Gorgels AP, van den Dool A, Hofs A et al: Procainamide is superior to lidocaine in terminating sustained ventricular tachycardia, *Circulation* 80:2590, 1989.
17. Brugada P, Brugada J, Mont L et al: A new approach to the differential diagnosis of a regular tachycardia with a wide QRS complex, *Circulation* 83:1649, 1991.

15

Torsades de Pointes and Polymorphic Ventricular Tachycardia

Torsades de Pointes or Polymorphic
  Ventricular Tachycardia? The Difference
  is Important 216
Torsade de Pointes 217

Polymorphic Ventricular Tachycardia
  (Without QT Prolongation) 225
Summary 229

TORSADES DE POINTES OR POLYMORPHIC VENTRICULAR TACHYCARDIA? THE DIFFERENCE IS IMPORTANT

The correct identification of torsades de pointes (TdP) is critical; misdiagnosis may have fatal consequences if the wrong treatment is chosen.

Torsades de pointes

Torsades de pointes is associated with a prolonged QT interval, is initiated by a pause (long-short), and has a typical undulating pattern in which the QRS peaks first appear to be up and then to be down. Recognition of this life-threatening arrhythmia is important because it is not treated like other VTs and can be exacerbated by the administration of class IA drugs, some class IC drugs, and sotalol[1] but responds to intravenous magnesium and possibly class IB drugs.[2]

Torsades de pointes is divided into two major groups: *acquired* and *congenital* (or idiopathic) *long QT syndrome (LQTS).* The acquired form is usually iatrogenic, whereas the congenital form is inherited. Three forms of the congenital type have been named; two are hereditary, one with and one without deafness, and one is sporadic. Although uncommon, the familial form of LQTS is a potentially treatable cause of sudden cardiac death.

Polymorphic ventricular tachycardia

Polymorphic ventricular tachycardia (VT) has a similar morphologic appearance to that of TdP but usually *does not have a prolonged QT interval,* nor is it related to sinus bradycardia, preceding sinus pauses, or electrolyte abnormalities as is TdP.[3] It is important to distinguish between the two because they have different mechanisms and treatments. Standard antiarrhythmic drugs are given for normal QT polymorphic VT.[2]

TORSADE DE POINTES
Torsade or torsades?

The term *torsade de pointes* is a French expression meaning "twisting of the points" that was applied by Dessertene in 1966[4] to describe a different form of VT in the setting of complete atrioventricular (AV) block. Philippe Coumel has enlightened us regarding the use of the singular and plural forms. The singular form, *torsade de pointes,* is used to refer to several (5 to 10) "pointes". The plural form, *torsades de pointes,* is used when referring to more than one episode or to a prolonged attack.[4] Since its first description this arrhythmia was given many names, which caused confusion in clinical practice. Now most investigators agree that the term *torsades de pointes* (or its plural) should be used to describe a particular form of VT that occurs in the setting of *markedly prolonged repolarization.*[5-7]

ECG diagnosis

Since torsade de pointes was originally described, it has become apparent that the simple ECG criterion of a QRS that appears to twist around the isoelectric line is insufficient for accurate diagnosis in borderline cases. Thus TdP is recognized not only because of the undulating pattern of the QRS during the tachycardia but also because of the prolonged QT interval and its onset (pause dependent). These features of the long QT syndrome are shown in Fig. 15-1.

Warning signs

QT prolongation: Marked; usually more than 0.50 sec in the sinus beats preceding the tachycardia. This is the hallmark of TdP and an important way to differentiate it from ischemia-related polymorphic VT. The precise degree of QT prolongation that predicts TdP is not known. In quinidine-induced TdP the QT intervals have exceeded 0.60 sec and most patients with drug-induced TdP have a QTc of more than 0.44 sec. In contrast, in patients with LQTS the QT interval seems to be more variable and may even be normal.[8] In Fig. 15-2 QT prolongation can be seen; A PVC appears during the T wave.

In nonsymptomatic members of a family with congenital LQTS, measurement of the corrected QT (QTc) interval may not be diagnostic, since there may be an overlap in the range of QTc values between normal individuals and those with congenital LQTS.[9] In addition, it has been shown that correcting the QT interval for heart rate may mask repolarization abnormalities in high-risk patients. The shape of the T wave may be an additional helpful diagnostic clue.[10]

T waves: T-wave alternans or bizarre T-wave aberration following a postextrasystolic pause is a specific early warning sign. In congenital LQTS, recent data suggest that T-wave distortions ("humps"), along with measurement of the QT interval, represent a phoentypic marker of the inherited form of the long QT syndrome and may be useful in identifying asymptomatic family members.[11] This marker may be an especially valuable diagnostic tool in light of the limitations of QT measurements and correction for heart rate. Specifically the T wave may be biphasic, bifid, or notched, particularly in the precordial leads. Fig. 15-3 depicts

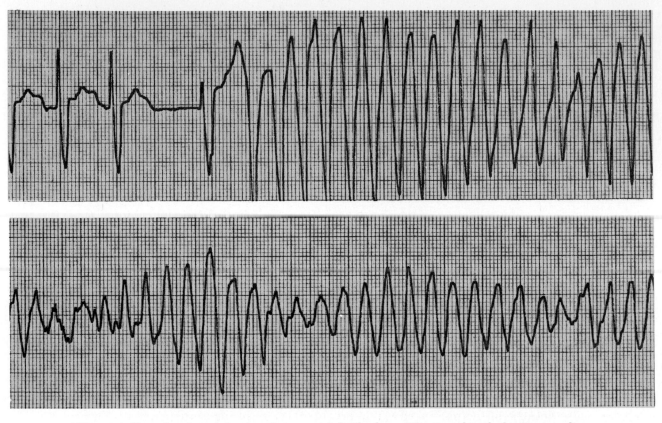

Fig. 15-1. Torsades de pointes (continuous strip). The long QT interval with the U wave distorting it, the pause before the onset of the tachycardia, and the typical undulating, spindle appearance of the pattern are evident. *(From the late Dr. Alan Lindsay collection, Salt Lake City, Utah.)*

such a T-wave hump (T2), between the initial T wave (T1) and the U wave. Fig. 15-4 illustrates three grades of T-wave humps collected from a study of 13 families with congenital LQTS.[12] Grade I, although subtle, does demonstrate a distinct bulge in the downslope of the T wave that is unusual when compared with the usually brisk, normal T descent. In grades II and III the T humps are more distinct.

Prominent U wave: May appear in the conducted sinus beats.

Initiation

Long-short cycle: Commonly precedes the onset of TdP; that is, the initiation of torsade de pointes is pause dependent.

Short-long-short sequence. The paroxysm of VT is usually initiated by a short-long-short cycle sequence,[13] causing the beat following the long cycle to have an even more prolonged QT interval. Clark et al.[14] found a characteristic short-long-short ventricular cycle length as the initiating sequence in 41 of 44 episodes of TdP. For example, in Fig. 15-1 there is an unexplained pause at the beginning of the tracing, causing the ventricular complex after the pause to prolong its QT interval even more.

II

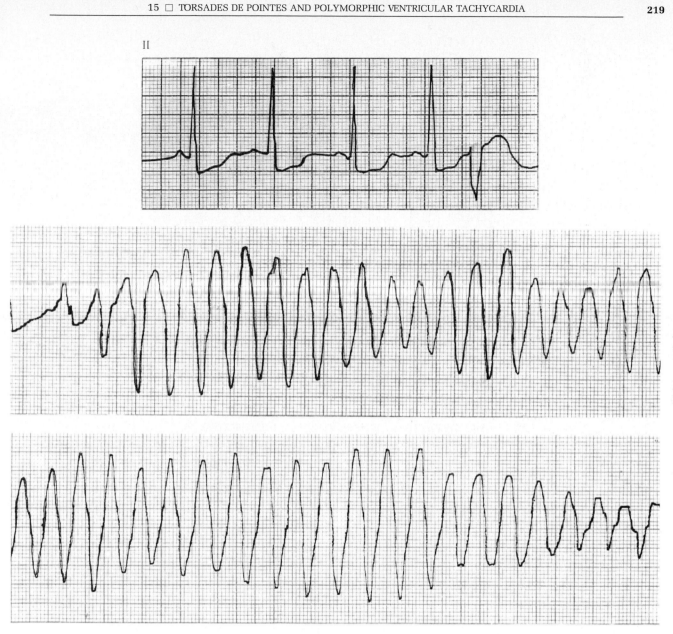

Fig. 15-2. Warning signs and the development of torsade de pointes in a patient receiving oral procainamide 500 mg four times a day. **A,** The prolonged QT interval and the PVC are occurring on the T wave. **B** and **C,** The typical pattern of torsade de pointes has developed.

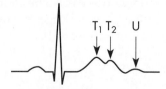

Fig. 15-3. Schematic depiction of an ECG complex showing the primary T wave (T1), a T-wave hump (T2), and the U wave. *(From Lehmann MH, Suzuki F, Fromm BS et al: J Am Coll Cardiol 24:746, 1994.)*

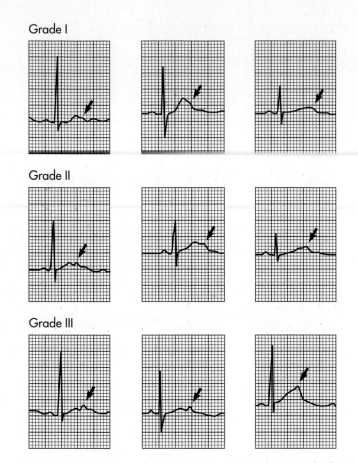

Fig. 15-4. A grading for T-wave humps in patients with congenital long QT syndrome. In grade I there is a slight bulge on the downslope of the T wave. The distortions in grades II and III are more obvious. *(From Lehmann MH, Suzuki F, Fromm BS et al: J Am Coll Cardiol 24:746, 1994.)*

The tachycardia typically arises after the peak of the T wave in the cycle following the pause. In Fig. 15-5 the typical onset of TdP can be seen in a patient with bradycardia (caused by complete heart block) and frequent PVCs. The PVC causes a short cycle, and a long cycle follows the PVC. The junctional beat that terminates the pause is then followed by TdP Fig. 15-6 shows the onset of TdP. In Fig. 15-6 a U wave is prominent, making the QT seem even longer. In Fig. 15-6, *A,* intermittent PVCs begin to appear on the T wave. In Fig. 15-6, *B,* there is a short run of VT. Torsades de pointes ensues in Fig. 15-6, *C.*

The tachycardia itself
QRS heights: Undulate.
Heart rate: 200 to 250 beats/min.

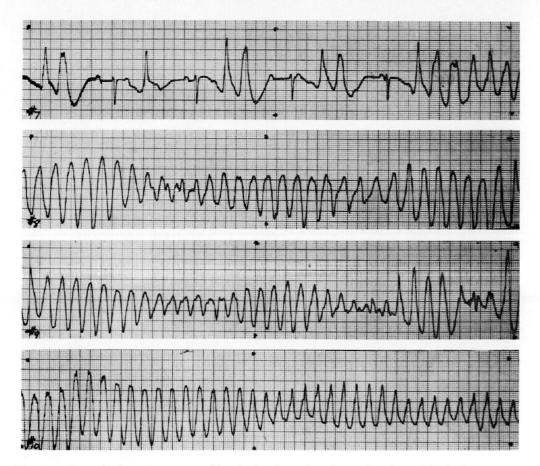

Fig. 15-5. Torsade de pointes caused by the bradycardia of complete heart block. *(From Manion WC, Nelson WP, Hall RJ et al: Am Heart J 83:535, 1972.)*

Characteristic features of quinidine-related torsades de pointes

The following characteristic features of quinidine-related TdP have been described by Roden et al.[15]:

1. Low quinidine plasma concentrations
2. Absence of marked QRS prolongation
3. Hypokalemia (potassium level less than 4 mEq/L)
4. Almost invariably, abrupt slowing of the heart rate just before the initiation of torsade de pointes

Mechanism

The mechanism of TdP is not yet known; triggered activity, reentry, and "spiral wave activity" have all been suggested, but without final proof. Most investigators favor triggered activity resulting from early afterdepolarizations.[8,16-20] Reentry resulting from dispersion of repolarization has been suggested to account for the bizarre patterns seen in TdP. Recently a spiral wave activity has been proposed to be the mechanism.[21] Schwartz et al.[22] have suggested that more than one mechanism may be involved, one for the initiation of TdP (e.g., early afterdepolarization) and another for its maintenance (reentry). The two mechanisms may also be inter

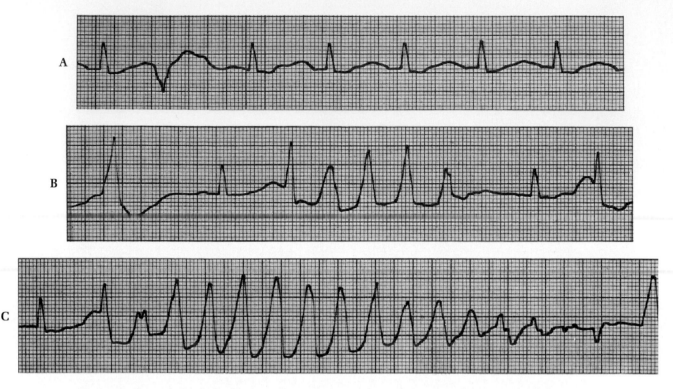

Fig. 15-6. The onset of torsade de pointes. **A,** A prolonged QT-U and a PVC. **B,** There is a short run of VT, which develops into torsade de pointes, **C.**

linked; the prolonged action potential duration that is responsible for the early afterdepolarizations may also be responsible for critically slow conduction that contributes to the development of reentry.

Causes of acquired torsade de pointes

Acquired TdP is usually associated with therapeutic drug doses that lengthen the QT interval (quinidine, procainamide, N-acetylprocainamide, sotalol, amiodarone, disopyramide, phenothiazines, nonsedating antihistamines such as terfenadine (Seldane), antibiotics (such as erythromycin),[23,24] and antidepressants such as thioridazine (Mellaril).[8] It may occur in the setting of other conditions that prolong the QT interval, such as severe bradyarrhythmias, hypokalemia, hypomagnesemia, liquid protein diet, starvation, central nervous system lesions, cardiac ganglionitis, and mitral valve prolapse. In a study involving 65 patients with 74 episodes of TdP the most common cause was therapy with diuretics (30 episodes); second place was shared by d,1-sotalol and hypokalemia of less than 3.6 mEq/L (23 episodes each); quinidine was the third most common cause with 18 episodes.[7] One study has shown that quinidine and disopyramide, although both class IA drugs, have significantly different effects on repolarization after a pause, possibly accounting for the greater frequency of TdP with quinidine.[25]

Causes of congenital (idiopathic) torsades de pointes (long QT syndrome)

Idiopathic long QT syndrome includes the Jervell and Lange-Nielsen syndrome (autosomal recessive) and the Romano-Ward syndrome (autosomal dominant), which become evident with a familial pattern in children and young adults. The Jervell and Lange-Nielsen syndrome can be associated with sensorineural deafness. A nonfamilial form has also been identified and is called the sporadic form. In these syndromes the tachycardia typically occurs in the setting of increased adrenergic tone (fright or exertion).[7]

Symptoms

Often the patient is not aware of palpitations, but if the attack is prolonged, there are episodes of dizziness, syncope, and rarely, sudden death, probably from a deterioration of TdP into ventricular fibrillation.[2] When syncope is the presenting symptom, patients are sometimes misdiagnosed as epileptic.[26] Before we were aware of the mechanism and ECG identification of TdP, the term "quinidine syncope" was used to describe these symptoms.

Possible outcomes

1. Slowing and then spontaneous conversion
2. Conversion and then a new attack
3. Ventricular standstill
4. Ventricular fibrillation

Patients with idiopathic LQTS who are at increased risk for sudden death are those who have a family member who died suddenly at an early age and those who have had syncope.

Prevention

After initiation of drugs that prolong the QT interval do the following:[27]
1. Monitor the QT interval.
2. Modify the dosage of the drug if the QT interval reaches 0.56 to 0.60 sec.
3. Discontinue the drug and hospitalize the patient immediately if the patient complains of lightheadedness or syncope or if there are increased frequency and complexity of PVCs.
4. Congenital TdP can be screened with stress testing and Valsalva's maneuver, which can prolong the QT, produce T wave alternans, and cause TdP in afflicted patients. Acquired TdP, on the other hand, is usually manifested during bradycardia or long pauses in the ventricular rhythm.
5. When an individual is discovered to be symptomatic with TdP, all family members should have prolonged ECG recording during subjection to various stresses (auditory stimuli, psychologic stress, cold pressor stimulation, and exercise).

Emergency treatment of torsades de pointes in the setting of acquired long QT syndrome

The following measures are taken for the emergency treatment of TdP[7,28]:
1. The patient is monitored continuously; ascertain that you are truly dealing with a long QT segment or U wave, or both, in the basic rhythm.
2. All agents that may be potentially responsible for TdP and QT prolongation are immediately discontinued.
3. Intravenous (IV) potassium is given to correct the electrolyte abnormalities. Blood samples are drawn for later evaluation and confirmation of deficiencies and drug levels.

4. Intravenous magnesium is regarded as the treatment of choice for TdP[29] and is suggested even in normomagnesemia.[30]
5. If IV magnesium is unsuccessful, overdrive ventricular pacing or isoproterenol may be necessary as a means to increase the basic heart rate and thus shorten the QT interval. Temporary ventricular or atrial pacing suppresses the VT, and it may remain abated after pacing is discontinued.[5]
6. Direct-current cardioversion is usually transiently effective in terminating TdP. When the arrhythmia is caused by high doses of class IA agents, repeated cardioversions may be necessary.

The class IA (quinidine, procainamide, and disopyramide) drug-induced torsade de pointes usually appears soon after the initial administration of the drug, while the patient is still in the hospital. In this setting the problem is recognized early, and treatment is straightforward.

Emergency treatment of torsades de pointes in the setting of congenital long QT syndrome

For a full discussion of the therapy and many ramifications of TdP caused by congenital LQTS the reader is referred to the excellent chapter written by Schwartz et al.[31]

Sympathetic activity usually triggers the TdP of congenital LQTS; therefore patients may benefit from beta blockers, as both short-term and long-term therapy. In the emergency setting high doses of a beta blocker may be necessary. Intravenous magnesium may be effective. Unlike in acquired LQTS, isoproterenol and atropine may be hazardous. If the tachycardia is related to episodes of bradycardia, cardiac pacing may be helpful, although data from Garson et al.[32] do not support the use of pacing when beta blockers have failed.

Suggested dosage regimens for magnesium chloride or Magnesium sulfate

An intravenous bolus of magnesium chloride (MgCl) or magnesium sulfate (MgSO$_4$) 1 to 2 g over 5 min, followed by IV infusion of MgCl or MgSO$_4$ 1 to 2 g/hr for 4 to 6 hours, is suggested.

The following IV dosage regimen is advised by Iseri, Allen, and Brodsky[33]: 10 to 15 ml 20% MgSO$_4$ over 1 min, followed by infusion of 500 ml 2% MgSO$_4$ over 5 hours. A second infusion of 500 ml over 10 hours may be necessary.

If the serum potassium level is at or falls below 4 mEq/L, 20 to 40 mEq/L potassium chloride should be added. Magnesium deficiency can be confirmed by a low serum level or by greater than 50% retention of administered magnesium.

Contraindications for magnesium

The continued use of magnesium is contraindicated in the following:
1. Renal failure
2. Disappearance of deep tendon reflex
3. Rise in serum magnesium level above 5 mEq/L
4. Drop in systolic blood pressure below 80 mm of mercury
5. Drop in pulse below 60 beats/min

Advantages of magnesium for torsade de pointes

Studies have shown that prompt suppression of this arrhythmia in acquired and in the congenital (idiopathic)[34] LQTS can be achieved with IV magnesium.[27]

Magnesium has the advantage of safety and simplicity of administration. When the diagnosis of TdP is uncertain, magnesium does not aggravate the VT that is not TdP, as would isoproterenol.

Magnesium plays an essential role in maintaining the cellular resting membrane potential. It is a necessary intracellular ingredient for the phosphorylation of adenosine triphosphatase (ATP) and sodium in the sodium pump.[35,36]

Isoproterenol or cardiac pacing is sometimes used to shorten the QT interval by a rate increase. Although effective, both have disadvantages. Isoproterenol is contraindicated in patients with hypertension or ischemic heart disease, and cardiac pacing requires skilled personnel and fluoroscopy.

Latent long QT syndrome

Identification of patients at risk for torsade de pointes involves computing the QTc interval during rest and after a stress test. Kadish et al.[37] have shown that although patients may have a normal QTc interval during rest, if they demonstrate a prolonged QTc with exercise, they are at risk for torsades de pointes when given type IA antiarrhythmic agents.

In the preceding study 10 of 11 patients with newly documented drug-related torsades de pointes had an abnormal repolarization response to exercise, compared with 11 control patients. The patients with torsades de pointes, when drug free, had a normal QTc at rest but a long QTc with exercise, although the uncorrected QT actually shortened with exercise.

Corrected QT interval

The QTc is computed by dividing the square root of the RR interval into the QT interval (measurements are in seconds). The QTc is 0.39 sec ± 0.04 sec at any heart rate. The upper limit for the normal QT interval corrected for heart rate is said to be 0.44 sec. However, the normal QTc interval may be longer, 0.46 sec for men and 0.47 sec for women, with a normal range ±15% of the mean value.

A heart rate of 60 beats/min is the only one in which the QTc is the same as the measured normal QT (i.e., 0.39 sec). Some computer readouts give the QTc interval; in such cases it is necessary only to know the normal value (0.39 ± 0.4 sec) to evaluate QT prolongation.

The QT interval shortens with tachycardia and lengthens with bradycardia because of respective shortening and lengthening of the refractory period and ventricular repolarization. Usually the QT interval is not more than 0.39 sec when the heart rate is between 60 and 80 beats/min. A rule of thumb is that at heart rates of 60 to 100 beats/min the QT normally does not exceed half the RR interval.[38]

POLYMORPHIC VENTRICULAR TACHYCARDIA (WITHOUT QT PROLONGATION)

Most of the patients with polymorphic VT without QT prolongation have coronary artery disease. Akhtar[39] described two subgroups, one associated with chronic coronary artery disease and the other with acute myocardial ischemia caused by critical coronary artery stenosis.

Chronic coronary artery disease

Fig. 15-7 shows a polymorphic VT without QT prolongation with stable coronary artery disease and prior myocardial damage but with no evidence of acute isch-

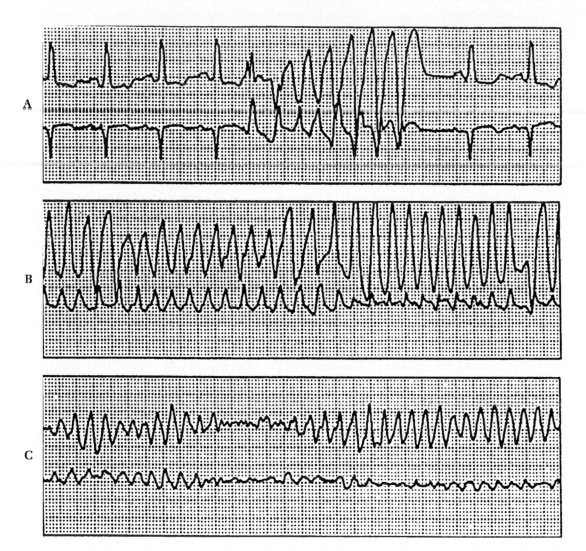

Fig. 15-7. Polymorphic ventricular tachycardia (VT) with a normal QT interval in a patient with chronic coronary artery disease. **A,** Spontaneous episode of polymorphic VT. **B,** Sustained episode leading to ventricular fibrillation. **C,** Patient had coronary artery disease but continued to have such episodes after myocardial revascularization and beta blockade. Class I agents readily controlled this arrhythmia. *(From Akhtar M: Circulation 82:1561, 1990.)*

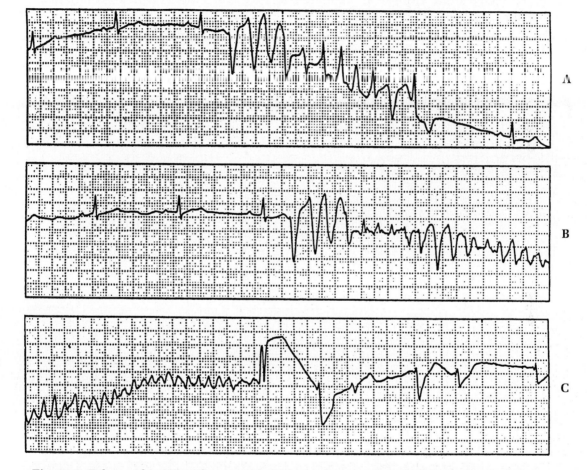

Fig. 15-8. Polymorphic VT with a normal QT interval in a patient with acute myocardial ischemia. **A,** Nonsustained polymorphic VT. **B,** Another episode that leads to rapid degenera-
tion into ventricular fibrillation. *(From Akhtar M: Circulation 82:1561, 1990.)*

emia. Treatment options are similar to those for sustained monomorphic VT in association with chronic coronary artery disease.[39]

Acute myocardial ischemia

Fig. 15-8 shows a polymorphic VT in a patient and acute ischemia caused by an occluding bypass graft. This type of VT is often, but not always, accompanied or preceded by angina or ischemic ECG changes, and it responds well to beta blockers and myocardial revascularization.

Figs. 15-9 and 15-10 are tracings from patients who had symptoms of angina or ST segment deviation, or both, immediately before the initiation of the polymorphous tachycardia. Wolfe et al.[3] found the following in patients with polymorphous VT after myocardial infarction:

1. Although the QT interval and the QTc interval were normal or mildly prolonged, the arrhythmia failed to respond to class I antiarrhythmics.
2. Intravenous amiodarone appeared to be effective in suppressing the VT.
3. The tachycardia was associated with symptoms or ECG evidence of recurrent ischemia.

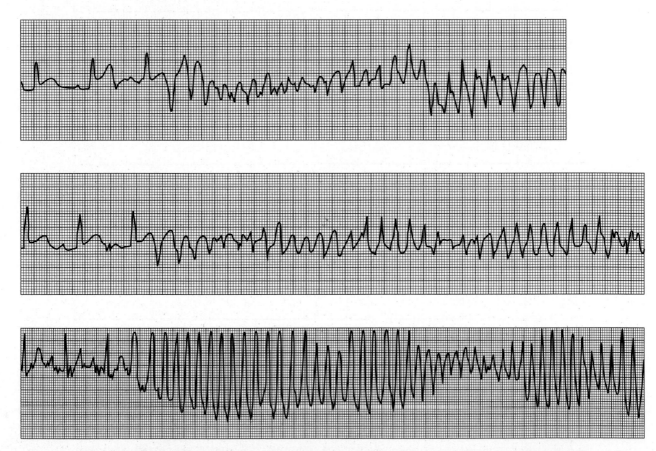

Fig. 15-9. Recordings of three episodes of polymorphous VT in a patient on day 5 after an acute inferior myocardial infarction. The first two episodes were preceded by ST-segment elevation on the ECG. The normal QT interval and the absence of bradycardia or a sinus pause immediately before the initiation of polymorphous VT are evident. *(From Wolfe CL et al: Circulation 84:1543, 1991.)*

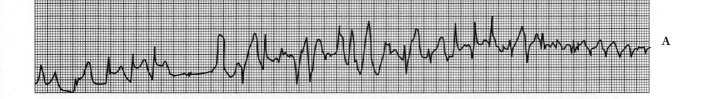

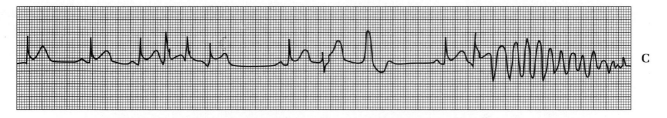

Fig. 15-10. Recordings from recurrent episodes of polymorphous VT in a patient who had received intravenous tissue-type plasminogen activator for treatment of an acute anterior myocardial infarction. All three tracings show ST-segment elevation before the onset of the tachycardia. **A** and **C,** A pause immediately precedes the onset of the tachycardia. **B,** An episode of VT that is not preceded by a sinus pause. **A** and **B,** Tracings are continuous. *(From Wolfe CL et al: Circulation 84:1543, 1991.)*

SUMMARY

Torsades de pointes and polymorphic VT are separate entities. Although the tachycardia of both may have the same undulating pattern, the clinical settings and treatments differ substantially. Torsades de pointes is associated with a prolonged QT interval and is initiated by a pause (long-short). Polymorphic VT usually does not have a prolonged QT interval, nor is it related to sinus bradycardia, preceding sinus pauses, or electrolyte abnormalities as is TdP. It is important to distinguish between the two because they have different mechanisms and treatments. TdP is either acquired or congenital (idiopathic). The acquired form is usually iatrogenic, whereas the congenital form is inherited. Polymorphic VT is seen in the setting of chronic coronary artery disease, in ischemic conditions, or in conditions after myocardial infarction.

REFERENCES

1. Arstall MA, Hii JT, Lehman RG, Horowitz JD: Sotalol-induced torsade de pointes: managment with magnesium infusion, *Postgrad Med J* 68:289, 1992.
2. Zipes DP: Specific arrhythmias: diagnosis and treatment. In Braunwald E, ed: *Heart disease,* ed 4, Philadelphia, 1992, WB Saunders.
3. Wolfe CL, Nibley C, Bhandari A et al: Polymorphous ventricular tachycardia associated with acute myocardial infarction, *Circulation* 84: 1543, 1991.

4. Coumel P, Leclercq JF, Dessertenne F: Torsades de pointes. In Josephson ME, Wellens HJJ, eds: *Tachycardias: mechanisms, diagnosis, treatment,* Philadelphia, 1984, Lea & Febiger.

5. Jackman WM, Friday KJ, Anderson JL et al: The long QT syndromes: a critical review, new clinical observations and a unifying hypothesis, *Prog Cardiovasc Dis* 31:115, 1988.

6. Tzivoni D, Keren A, Banai S, Stern S: Terminology of torsade de pointes, *Cardiovasc Drugs Ther* 5:505, 1991.

7. Haverkamp W, Shenasa M, Borggrefe M, Breithardt G: Torsades de pointes. In Zipes DP, Jalife J, eds: *Cardiac electrophysiology from cell to bedside,* ed 2, Philadelphia, 1995, WB Saunders.

8. Roden DM: Torsade de pointes, *Clin Cardiol* 16:683, 1993.

9. Vincern GM, Timothy KW, Leppert M, Keating M: The spectrum of symptoms and IQT intervals in carriers of the gene for the long QT syndrome, *N Engl J Med* 327:846, 1992.

10. Fei L, Statters DJ, Anderson MH et al: Is there an abnormal QT interval in sudden cardiac death survivors with a "normal" QTc? *Am Heart J* 128:73, 1994.

11. Malfatto G, Beria G, Sala S et al: Quantitative analysis of T wave abnormalities and their prognostic implications in the idiopathic long QT syndrome, *J Am Coll Cardiol* 23:296, 1994.

12. Lehman MH, Suzuki F, Fromm BS et al: T wave "humps" as a potential electrocardiographic marker of the long QT syndrome, *J Am Coll Cardiol* 24:746, 1994.

13. Cranefield PF, Aronson RS: Torsade de pointes and other pause-induced ventricular tachycardias: the short-long-short sequence and early afterdepolarizations, *PACE Pacing Clin Electrophysiol* 11(6, pt 1):6708, 1988.

14. Kay GN, Plumb VJ, Arciniegas JG et al: Torsade de pointes: the long-short initiating sequences and other clinical features: observations in 32 patients. *J Amer Coll Cardiol* 2:806, 1983.

15. Roden DM, Thompson KA, Hoffman BF, Woosley RL: Clinical features and basic mechanisms of quinidine-induced arrhythmias, *J Am Coll Cardiol* 8(1, suppl A):73A, 1986.

16. Vos MA, Verduyn SC, Gorgels APM et al: Reproducible induction of early afterdepolarizations and torsade de pointes arrhythmias by d-Sotalol and pacing in dogs with chronic atrioventricular block, *Circulation* 91:864-872, 1995.

17. Miyazaki T, Pride HP, Zipes DP: Prostaglandin modulation of early afterdepolarizations and ventricular tachyarrhythmias induced by cesium chloride combined with efferent cardiac sympathetic stimulation in dogs, *J Am Coll Cardiol* 16:1287, 1990.

18. Kaseda S, Zipes DP: Effects of alpha adrenoceptor stimulation and blockade on early afterdepolarizations and triggered activity induced by cesium in canine cardiac Purkinje fibers, *J Cardiovasc Electrophysiol* 1:31, 1990.

19. Jackman WM, Szabo B, Friday KJ et al: Ventricular tachyarrhythmias related to early afterdepolarizations and triggered firings: relationship to QT interval prolongation and potential therapeutic role for calcium channel blocking agents, *J Cardiovasc Electrophysiol* 1:170, 1990.

20. El-Sherif N, Craelius W, Boutjdir M, Gough WB: Early afterdepolarizations and arrhythmogenesis, *J Cardiovasc Electrophysiol* 1:145, 1990.

21. Davidenko JM: Spiral wave activity: a possible common mechanism for polymorphic and monomorphic ventricular tachycardias, *Cardiovasc Electrophysiol* 4:730, 1993.

22. Schwartz PJ, Locati EH, Napolitano C, Priori SG: The long QT syndrome. In Zipes DP, Jalife J, eds: *Cellular electrophysiology from cell to bedside,* Philadelphia, 1992, WB Saunders.

23. Rezkalla MA, Pochop C: Erythromycin induced torsades de pointes: case report and review of the literature, *SD J Med* 47:161, 1994.

24. Brandriss MW, Richardson WS, Barold SS: Erythromycin-induced QT prolongation and polymorphic ventricular tachycardia (torsades de pointes): case report and review, *Clin Infect Dis* 18:995, 1994.

25. Bursill JA, Qyse KR, Campbell TJ: Quinidine but not disopyramide prolongs cardiac Purkinje fiber action potentials after a pause, *J Cardiovasc Pharmacol* 23:833, 1994.

26. Gospe SM Jr, Choy M: Hereditary long Q-T syndrome presenting as epilepsy: electroencephalography laboratory diagnosis, *Ann Neurol* 25:514, 1989.

27. Keren A, Tzivoni D: Torsades de pointes: prevention and therapy, *Cardiovasc Drugs Ther* 5:509, 1991.

28. Wellens HJJ, Conover M: *The ECG in emergency decision making,* Philadelphia, 1992, WB Saunders.

29. Banai S, Tzivoni D: Drug therapy for torsade de pointes, *J Cardiovasc Electrophysiol* 4:206, 1993.

30. Iseri LT, Chung P, Tobis J: Magnesium therapy for intractable ventricular tachyarrhythmias in normomagnesemic patients, *West J Med* 138:823, 1983.

31. Schwartz PJ, Locati EH, Napolitano C, Priori G: The long QT syndrome. In Zipes DP, Jalife J, eds: *Cellular electrophysiology from cell to bedside,* ed 2, Philadelphia, 1995, WB Saunders.

32. Garson A Jr, MacDonald D II, Fournier A et al: The long QT syndrome in children: an international study of 287 patients, *Circulation* 87:1866, 1993.

33. Iseri LT, Allen BJ, Brodsky MA: Magnesium therapy of cardiac arrhythmias in critical-care medicine, *Magnes Res* 8(5-6):299, 1989.

34. Igawa O, Fujimoto Y, Kotake H, Mashiba H: Treatment of torsade de pointes with intravenous magnesium in idiopathic long QT syndrome, *Jpn Circ J* 55:1057, 1991.
35. Tzivoni D, Keren A: Suppression of ventricular arrhythmias by magnesium, *Am J Cardiol* 65:1397, 1990.
36. Gadsby DC: The Na/K pump of cardiac myocytes. In Zipes DP, Jalife J. eds: *Cardiac electrophysiology*, Philadelphia, 1990, WB Saunders.
37. Kadish AH, Weisman HF, Veltri EP et al: Paradoxical effects of exercise on the QT interval in patients with polymorphic ventricular tachycardia receiving type IA antiarrhythmic agents, *Circulation* 81:14, 1990.
38. Marriott HJL: *Practical electrocardiography*, Baltimore, 1983, Williams & Wilkins.
39. Akhtar M: The clinical spectrum of ventricular tachycardia, *Circulation* 82:1561, 1990.

16

Accelerated Idioventricular Rhythm and Ventricular Escape

Accelerated Idioventricular Rhythm   *232*   Ventricular Escape   *237*

The accelerated idioventricular rhythm (AIVR) was first described in 1950 by Harris[1] as "a ventricular focus with a frequency of impulse formation almost equal to that of the sinoatrial node was alternating gaining and losing dominance of the cardiac rhythm." Harris also noted that the rhythm was benign. The rhythm was known by several names until 1966, when Marriott and Menendez[2] gave us the descriptive term by which it is now known.

Definition of accelerated idioventricular rhythm

An *accelerated idioventricular rhythm* consists of three or more successive ventricular beats with a rate between 60 and 110 beats/min that begins with a long coupling interval. Because its rate is so similar to that of the sinus node, there are fusion beats at its beginning and end (Figs. 16-1 and 16-2) or even throughout its duration (Fig. 16-3) as the two pacemakers (sinus and ventricular) compete for dominance. The ventricular rhythm achieves dominance when it accelerates or when the sinus node slows its rate. Sinus rhythm is finally victorious when the sinus rhythm increases its rate or the ventricular rhythm decreases its rate. The fusion beats, of course, are proof of the ventricular origin of the ectopic rhythm. In the reperfusion phase of acute myocardial infarction the AIVR is a sign of reperfusion. Sometimes an AIVR is unmasked because of a pause. For example, in Fig. 16-4 the AIVR emerges during the pauses following a nonconducted PAC and the initiation of atrial flutter; in Fig. 16-5, during a sinus pause; and in Fig. 16-6, during the pause after a premature ventricular complex (PVC).

ECG recognition of accelerated idioventricular rhythm during reperfusion

Rhythm: Transient and intermittent; lasting for three or more successive beats to 1 minute; may be regular or irregular.

Rate: Faster than the intrinsic escape rate of the ventricles (30 to 40 beats/min) but slower than VT; usually between 60 and 110 beats/min.

Onset: Gradual (nonparoxysmal), beginning with a long coupling interval, often with a ventricular fusion beat.

Termination: Gradual, often ending in ventricular fusion beats.

Atrioventricular dissociation: Common, often isorhythmic sinus and ventricular rhythms maintain the same rate.

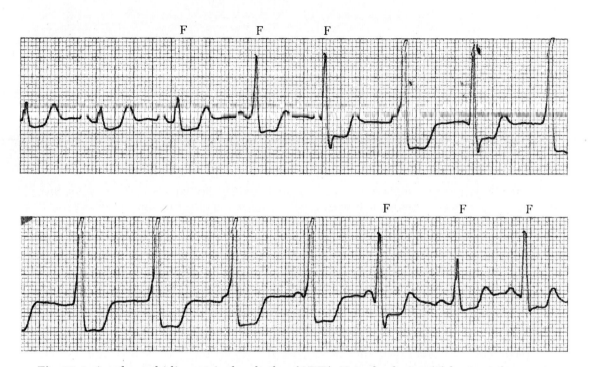

Fig. 16-1. Accelerated idioventricular rhythm (AIVR). Note the fusion (F) beats at the onset of the tachycardia and at the end of this continuous tracing. The rate of the tachycardia is approximately that of the sinus rhythm, which explains the fusion beats at the onset and at the end.

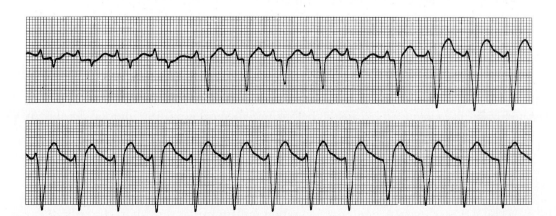

Fig. 16-2. Accelerated idioventricular rhythm (continuous tracing). The tracing begins with four sinus-conducted beats followed by at least six fusion beats at the onset of the AIVR.

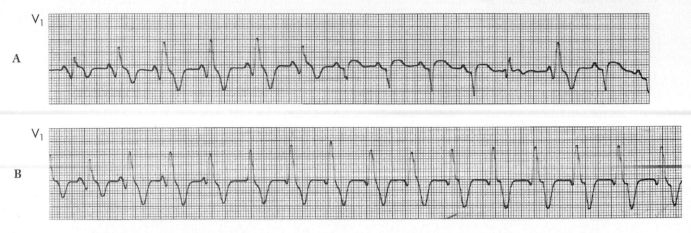

Fig. 16-3. A, An AIVR composed mostly of fusion beats. The last complex (the only one that is not fusion) has a PR interval of 0.16 sec, slightly longer than the two similar-looking beats. **B,** The tracing shows the dominance of the AIVR with a rate of 96 beats/min.

ECG identification of the area of reperfusion

The QRS configuration and the axis of the AIVR may help in identifying or at least in ruling out the occluded vessel.

Left anterior descending coronary artery reperfusion: Multiple QRS configurations during the AIVR and a relatively narrow QRS.

Circumflex reperfusion: Ruled out when lead V_1 is negative.

Right coronary artery reperfusion: Ruled out when the electrical axis is inferior between 0 and 180 degrees.[3]

ECG recognition of accelerated idioventricular rhythm *not* related to reperfusion

The AIVR that occurs during the first 24 hours of infarction but after the reperfusion phase should be distinguished from that which occurs during reperfusion. The former is recognized because it begins with a short coupling interval, as shown in Fig. 16-7. Obviously then, because the onset is more premature, it does not begin with fusion beats, as does the reperfusion-related AIVR, although it may end with them. This type of AIVR is sometimes called "slow VT."[3,4]

Clinical implications

The AIVR is usually benign (even when multiform) and of short duration (lasting seconds to a minute), is well tolerated in hemodynamic terms, and does not seriously affect the clinical course or prognosis. The AIVR is usually associated with

II

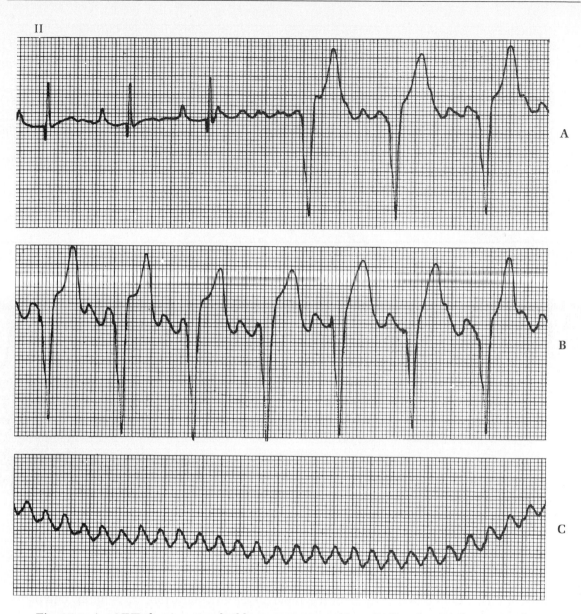

Fig. 16-4. An AIVR that is unmasked by a pause caused by a PAC and atrial flutter. **A,** There is first-degree atrioventricular (AV) block that is complicated by the appearance of a very early PAC (in the third ST segment). Atrial flutter ensues, compounding the AV block. An AIVR emerges because of the pause. Its initial rate is 64 beats/min, and, **B,** it "warms up" to 78 beats/min. When lidocaine was given, **C,** the AIVR was completely suppressed, leaving the patient with nothing but atrial flutter and complete AV block.

heart disease of some type, especially *acute myocardial infarction* (occurring at the moment of reperfusion) or *digitalis toxicity*.[5,6] It can also be seen in cocaine intoxication and normal hearts of adults and children.

A reperfusion arrhythmia. Accelerated idioventricular rhythm indicates both reperfusion (spontaneous or following thrombolytic therapy) and myocardial necrosis. Ap-

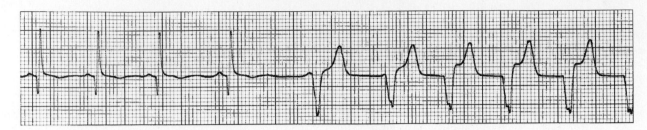

Fig. 16-5. An AIVR (92 beats/min) that is unmasked by a sinus pause.

PVC   ⊢→AIVR

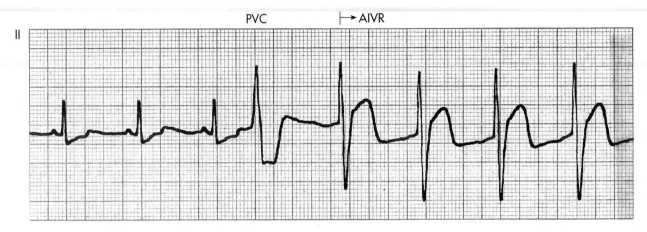

Fig. 16-6. An AIVR (72 beats/min) that is unmasked by the pause following a premature ventricular complex.

proximately 50% of patients with reperfusion after myocardial infarction have this arrhythmia. It has a high specificity (>80%) for reperfusion; that is, its presence strongly favors reperfusion. However, the sensitivity is only moderate (50% or less); that is, its absence does not preclude reperfusion). In addition, there is an equal distribution of AIVR in inferior and anterior myocardial infarction, and the appearance of AIVR does not depend on infarct size.[3,4] Thus when coronary angiography is not available, this sign may be helpful in recognizing reperfusion.[7] Other ECG signs of reperfusion are normalization of the ST segment, development of terminal T wave inversion, and a two-fold increase in PVCs.[7a]

Mechanisms

The mechanism of the AIVR is not known. Its ECG characteristics are suggestive of abnormal automaticity,[8,9] and its response to verapamil[10] is suggestive that triggered activity may be the mechanism. Ferrier et al.[11] have shown in studies of isolated ventricular tissue preparations that the reperfusion type of AIVR depends on the duration of exposure to ischemic conditions. When reperfusion follows 40 minutes of ischemic conditions, arrhythmias consist of late premature beats and coupled activity characteristic of delayed afterdepolarizations. When reperfusion follows a short ischemic period, arrhythmias have the characteristics of reentry (ear-

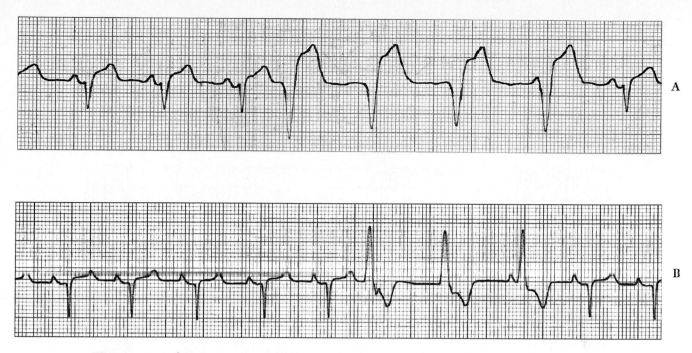

Fig. 16-7. A and **B,** Two cases of AIVR not caused by reperfusion. Both cases occurred within the first 24 hours of infarction but after reperfusion. The short initial coupling interval and the fusion beats are evident.

ly premature beats and rapid, sustained VT), whereas when following a longer ischemic period, they have the characteristics of triggered activity caused by delayed afterdepolarizations (late premature beats and coupling).

Treatment

Reperfusion arrhythmia: An AIVR requires no treatment other than the care of the underlying problem.[6] Reperfusion arrhythmias have not been associated with an increased incidence of ventricular fibrillation or in-hospital mortality.[12]

Digitalis toxicity: When digitalis is the cause, the drug should be discontinued.

Hemodynamic symptoms: When associated with hemodynamic impairment, the sinus rate may be increased with atropine or atrial pacing. This is usually sufficient to suppress the AIVR. Such hemodynamic symptoms are caused either by the atrioventricular dissociation (loss of "atrial kick") or by the ventricular rate being too fast.[5,6]

Other conditions when therapy (same as for VT) is considered[5]

When double tachycardia (AIVR and a more rapid VT) occurs

When AIVR begins with an R-on-T phenomenon

When ventricular fibrillation is a consequence

VENTRICULAR ESCAPE

If the ventricles are not being activated from the sinus node, an atrial ectopic pacemaker, or a junctional pacemaker, a focus in the bundle branches escapes and paces the ventricles. Fig. 16-8, *A,* illustrates a single ventricular escape beat. There

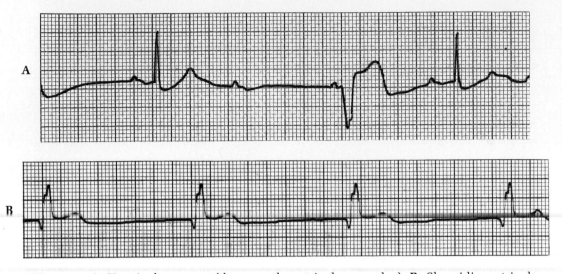

Fig. 16-8. A, Ventricular escape (the second ventricular complex). **B,** Slow idioventricular rhythm.

is atrioventricular block in which not every sinus P wave results in a ventricular complex, nor are there junctional escape beats to terminate the long pause. In Fig. 16-8, *B,* the ventricular rate is 37 beats/min and the QRS complexes are broad (0.20 sec), giving evidence of a pacemaker that is low in the conductive system. No P waves are apparent. They may be seen in another lead, or they may be truly absent; if absent, there is atrial standstill with a slow ventricular escape rhythm.

REFERENCES

1. Harris AS: Delayed development of ventricular ectopic rhythms following experimental coronary occlusion, *Circulation* 1:1318, 1950.
2. Marriott HJL, Menendez MM: A-V dissociation revisited, *Prog Cardiovasc Dis* 8:522, 1966.
3. Gorgels APM, Vos MA, Letsch IS et al: Usefulness of the accelerated idioventricular rhythm as a marker for myocardial necrosis and reperfusion during thrombolytic therapy in acute myocardial infarction, *Am J Cardiol* 61:231, 1988.
4. Goldberg S, Greenspon AJ, Urban PL et al: Reperfusion arrhythmia: a marker of restoration of anterograde flow during intracoronary thrombolysis for acute myocardial infarction, *Am Heart J* 105:26, 1983.
5. Zipes DP: Specific arrhythmias: diagnosis and treatment. In Braunwald E, ed: *Heart disease,* ed 4, Philadelphia, 1992, WB Saunders.
6. Grimm W, Marchlinski FE: Accelerated idioventricular rhythm: bidirectional ventricular tachycardia. In Zipes DP, Jalife J, eds: *Cardiac electrophysiology from cell to bedside,* ed 2, Philadelphia, 1995, WB Saunders.
7. Wellens HJJ, Conover M: *The ECG in emergency decision making,* Philadelphia, 1992, WB Saunders.
7a. Doevendans PA, Gorgels AP, van der Zee R et al: Electrocardiographic diagnosis of reperfusion during thrombolytic therapy in acute myocardial infarction, *Amer J Cardiol* 75:1206, 1995.
8. Wit AL, Janese MJ: Relationship of experimental delayed ventricular arrhythmias to clinical arrhythmias. In Wit AL, Janese MJ, eds: *The ventricular arrhythmias of ischemia and infarction: electrophysiological mechanisms,* New York, 1993, Futura.
9. Lerman BB, Wasley RC, DiMarco JP Jr et al: Antiadrenergic effects of adenosine on His-Purkinje automaticity: evidence for accentuated antagonism, *J Clin Invest* 82:2127, 1988.
10. Sclarovsky S, Strasberg B, Fuchs J et al: Multiform accelerated idioventricular rhythm in acute myocardial infarction: electrocardiographic characteristics and response to verapamil, *Am J Cardiol* 52:43, 1983.
11. Ferrier GR, Guyette CM, Li GR: Cellular mechanisms of reperfusion arrhythmias: studies in isolated ventricular tissue preparations. In Zipes DP, Jalife J, eds: *Cardiac electrophysiology,* Philadelphia, 1990, WB Saunders.
12. Opie LH: Reperfusion injury and its pharmacologic modification, *Circulation* 80:1049, 1989.

C H A P T E R

17

Digitalis-Induced Dysrhythmias

Acute Myocardial Uptake of
  Digoxin *240*
Mechanisms of Digitalis-Induced
  Tachyarrhythmias *240*
Systematic Approach *242*
Factors that Affect Digitalis Dosage
  Requirements *242*
Alerting Features of the Arrhythmias
  in Digitalis Intoxication *242*
Bigeminal Rhythms *243*
Sinus Bradycardia *243*
Sinoatrial Block *243*
Atrioventricular Block *245*

Atrial Tachycardia with Block *246*
Nonparosysmal Junctional
  Tachycardia *249*
Fascicular Ventricular Tachycardia *253*
Bifascicular Ventricular
  Tachycardia *254*
Double Tachycardias *255*
Noncardiac Signs of Digitalis
  Toxicity *257*
Treatment *257*
Emergency Approach *258*
Summary *258*

Digitalis is a cardiotonic steroid and a specific inhibitor of the sodium-potassium pump, which is responsible for establishing and maintaining the intracellular milieu that is vital to normal cardiac cellular function.[1] Thus it is easy to appreciate why there are often lethal consequences associated with chronic overdose and acute administration of high doses of digitalis.

With the possible exception of fascicular ventricular tachycardia (VT), the arrhythmias resulting from digitalis intoxication are learned in basic ECG courses. They are sinus bradycardia, atrioventricular (AV) block, sinoatrial (SA) block, premature ventricular complexes (PVCs), atrial tachycardia, and junctional tachycardia. In practice, however, there may be more than one arrhythmia at a time, presenting a confusing picture. For example, blocks may appear in combination with a tachycardia or bradycardia and an escape rhythm, or there may be double tachycardias. In addition, because the arrhythmias are nonparoxysmal, they may not be recognized for what they are—potentially lethal.

In clinical practice the toxic manifestations of digitalis continue to persist as "common adverse drug reactions."[2,3] In this chapter the mechanism of and emergency response to the arrhythmias of digitalis intoxication are discussed, and a systematic approach to ECG recognition is suggested.

ACUTE MYOCARDIAL UPTAKE OF DIGOXIN

Powell et al.[4] have demonstrated that following intravenous (IV) injection of digoxin, human myocardial uptake is prolonged and extensive. Peak myocardial digoxin content of the injected digoxin dose was 4.1%. This same study confirmed that digoxin induces significant increases in myocardial contractility, prolongation of the PR interval, and increased mean arterial pressure. A significant effect on myocardial contractility occurs 3 min after drug injection with maximal effect after 27 min (18.5% increase). Maximal PR interval prolongation was observed 12 min after digoxin administration. Because the effects of digoxin on AV conduction reflect predominantly parasympathetic stimulation there is a disparity between myocardial drug content and AV conduction. Digoxin is excreted primarily in the urine in unchanged form, although a variety of metabolites have been identified. In patients with renal failure there is an accumulation of digoxin metabolites, and tests of serum digoxin levels may measure not only the unchanged digoxin but also the inactive metabolites.[5]

MECHANISMS OF DIGITALIS-INDUCED TACHYARRHYTHMIAS

It appears that delayed afterdepolarizations and triggered activity are important in the genesis of many digitalis-induced tachycardias. This mechanism may occur by itself or along with reentry or abnormal automaticity. An important feature of delayed afterdepolarizations is that they can be exacerbated by a shortening of the cycle length and by catecholamines. In fact, the tachycardias of digitalis intoxication occur more readily at faster intrinsic heart rates. As the heart rate increases, so does the amplitude of the delayed afterdepolarization. Finally it reaches threshold potential and induces ectopic action potentials. In addition, the rate of the tachycardia is faster if the prior heart rate was rapid.[6]

Other factors that influence the production of delayed afterdepolarizations are hypokalemia, hypercalcemia, hypomagnesemia, diuretics, ischemia, reperfusion, increased ventricular wall tension, and heart failure. All, of themselves, are capable of producing triggered activity caused by delayed afterdepolarizations. Catecholamines induce intracellular calcium overload, one of the factors in the production of delayed afterdepolarizations.[7]

Delayed afterdepolarizations are oscillations in transmembrane potential that follow full repolarization of the membrane.[8] Such oscillations are the result of the poisoning of the sodium-potassium pump (Na^+-K^+ adenosine triphosphatase [ATPase]) by digitalis. The sequence of events that occur is as follows:

1. Digitalis competes with potassium for its binding site on the membrane (Fig. 17-1), disabling the Na^+-K^+ ATPase pump.
2. Sodium accumulates within the cell, and the exchange between sodium and calcium across the cell membrane is altered, as is the release of calcium from sarcoplasmic reticulum and other intracellular stores.
3. Calcium accumulates within the cell.
4. When the cell repolarizes, there is still free calcium within the cell.
5. This elicits a transient inward sodium current. It is precisely this inward sodium current that causes the oscillation following the action potential.

Fig. 17-2 is a drawing of a normal action potential followed by a delayed afterdepolarization *(solid line)*. If this abnormal oscillation reaches threshold potential, an action potential results *(dotted line)*. This is a "triggered" beat, since it is dependent on the preceding action potential. The mechanism differs from the other ar-

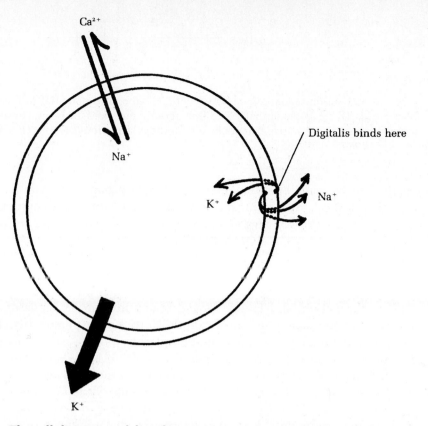

Fig. 17-1. The cellular action of digitalis. It competes with potassium (K$^+$) for a binding site on the membrane, poisoning the sodium-potassium (Na$^+$-K$^+$) pump and ultimately causing an increase in intracellular calcium (Ca^{2+}).

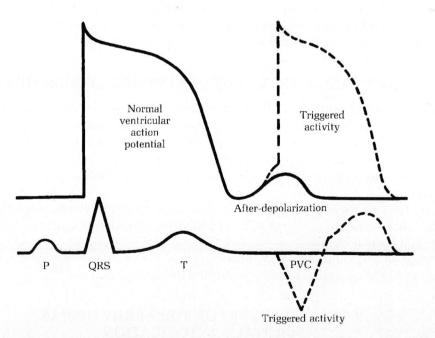

Fig. 17-2. An action potential and afterdepolarization as it relates to the surface ECG. The dotted lines represent the sequence of events that result when an afterdepolarization reaches threshold potential. The solid line represents cellular and ECG activity when the afterdepolarization does not reach threshold potential.

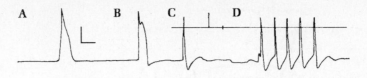

Fig. 17-3. A, Normal action potential compared with, **C,** an action potential followed by an afterdepolarization. **D,** Triggered activity. The first action potential is driven. Those that follow are triggered (that is, they arise from delayed afterdepolarizations). *(From Cranefield PF: Circ Res 41:415, 1977.)*

rhythmogenic mechanisms of automaticity or reentry (Chapter 3). The normal action potential (Fig. 17-3, *A*) is compared with one followed by an afterdepolarization (Fig. 17-3, *B*) and a run of triggered activity (Fig. 17-3, *C*) that occurs when the afterdepolarization reaches threshold potential.

SYSTEMATIC APPROACH

1. Talk to the patient and family regarding any noncardiac signs of digitalis intoxication (especially red/green color distortions and personality changes), dosage, additional medication, and complaints.
2. Evaluate the atrial rhythm. Are there P waves? If so, what is the rate, the rhythm (regular or irregular), and the polarity of the P waves in leads II and aV_F? The P waves will be positive if atrial tachycardia is caused by digitalis.
3. Is there AV conduction? If so, what type (2:1 or AV Wenckebach)?
4. If there is no AV conduction, are the ventricular beats junctional or fascicular in origin? This is evaluated in lead V_1 or MCL_1 (see p. 8).
5. If atrial fibrillation is present, is the rhythm appropriately irregular and not too slow? Or is there regularity or group beating? If the rhythm is regular, what is the morphologic appearance of the QRS in V_1?

FACTORS THAT AFFECT DIGITALIS DOSAGE REQUIREMENTS

The frequently prescribed cardioactive drugs that interact with digitalis to cause an increase in serum digoxin concentration are quinidine, amiodarone, verapamil, and diltiazem. Other factors that require a decrease in dosage of digoxin are renal disease, old age, hypothyroidism, small stature, chronic pulmonary disease, hypokalemia, hypomagnesemia, congestive heart failure, myocardial ischemia, and hypercalcemia.

Factors that require an increase in digoxin are malabsorption, antacids, neomycin, cholestyramine, colestipol, hyperthyroidism, hyperkalemia, reserpine, youth, and hypocalcemia.[9]

Drugs that do not appear to affect digoxin concentration are procainamide, disopyramide, mexiletine, flecainide, moricizine, and nifedipine.[10]

ALERTING FEATURES OF THE ARRHYTHMIAS
IN DIGITALIS INTOXICATION

Watch for the following:
Bradycardia

Sinoatrial block
    Atrioventricular block
Tachycardia
    Atrial tachycardia with block
    Junctional tachycardia
    Fascicular VT
Regularity in atrial fibrillation
    Junctional tachycardia
    Atrioventricular block with junctional escape
Group beating in atrial fibrillation: junctional tachycardia with Wenckebach exit block
Group beating in sinus rhythm
    Ventricular bigeminy
    Sinoatrial Wenckebach
    Atrioventricular Wenckebach
Atrial flutter with the following
    AV dissociation
    High-degree AV block (bradycardia)

BIGEMINAL RHYTHMS

A bigeminal rhythm is the most characteristic form of the delayed afterdepolarization. The coupling interval remains fixed as long as the basic cycle length does not change. As the cycle length shortens, so do the coupling intervals. At a critical cycle length there may be sequences of tachycardia. Fig. 17-4 shows a bigeminal rhythm in a case of accidental digitalis overdose. As in most cases of advanced digitalis intoxication, the rhythms are complicated. You will note that, apart from the obvious ventricular bigeminy, only the first P wave is conducted. After that the PR intervals become progressively shorter as an accelerated idioventricular rhythm takes over at a rate of 64 beats/min.

SINUS BRADYCARDIA

Slowing of the sinus node rate by digitalis is mediated by the vagus nerve and by the direct effect of digitalis. Sinus bradycardia is often accompanied by a junctional escape rhythm (Fig. 17-5).

SINOATRIAL BLOCK

Digitalis, even in therapeutic doses,[2] can impair the conduction of the sinus impulse to the atrial tissue. Such a block can be of the Wenckebach type. Sinoatrial Wenckebach is recognized because of the following:
Sinus rhythm
Group beating
Shortening PP intervals
Pauses less than twice the shortest PP cycle
In the case of a 36-year-old woman with SA Wenckebach who was taking digitalis (Fig. 17-6) there were two levels of block, SA and AV. There is, first, an obvious 3:2 and 4:3 SA Wenckebach. (Notice the missing P wave coincidental with the pause.) The groups of two reflect 3:2 SA conduction. That is, there are three sinus

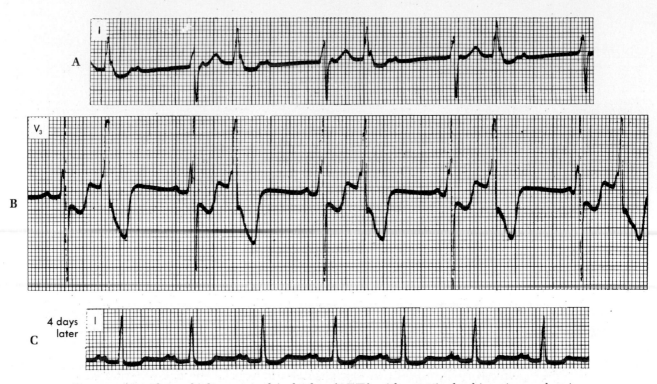

Fig. 17-4. Accelerated idioventricular rhythm (AIVR) with ventricular bigeminy and atrio-ventricular (AV) dissociation. These tracings are from a 10-year-old who was mistakenly given for maintenance a double dose of digitalis preparations after mitral valve surgery. The combined toxic effects of digitalis are evident in **A** and **B** AIVR (rate, 64 beats/min) with ventricular bigeminy dissociated from the sinus rhythm (rate, 90 beats/min). There is AV block; the P waves in lead I are landing beyond the T waves. They should be conducted but are not. Digitalis was discontinued, and 4 days later, **C,** the rhythm reverted to sinus with first-degree AV block. Note the P-mitrale in lead I. *(From Marriott HJL, Conover M: Advanced concepts in arrhythmias, ed 2, St Louis, 1989, Mosby.)*

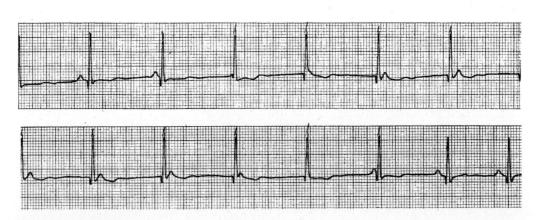

Fig. 17-5. Sinus bradycardia with a junctional escape rhythm. The sinus beats are not conducted (AV dissociation).

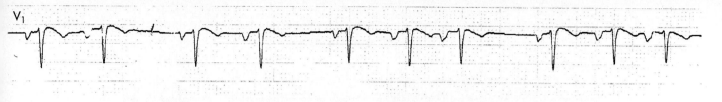

Fig. 17-6. Tracing of 3:2 and 4:3 sinoatrial (SA) Wenckebach that is due to digitalis intoxication. The first things one notices in this tracing are the group beating and the pauses caused by a missing P wave. When you "walk out" the PP intervals in the groups of three, you will see that the first PP interval of the group is longer than the second. The PP intervals shorten because the longest increment in SA conduction is between the first and second P wave of the group. In uncomplicated SA Wenckebach the PR intervals would be fixed; in this case they lengthen until the pause. *(Courtesy Linda Tune, RN, La Mesa, Calif.)*

discharges, which are never seen on the surface ECG; two of them are conducted to the atria, resulting in P waves. The groups of three reflect 4:3 SA conduction; there are four sinus discharges (not seen), and only three of them are conducted (three P waves). If this were a simple SA Wenckebach, the PR intervals would be fixed; rather, slight increments are seen in successive cycles. For example, in the sets of three (4:3 SA conduction) it is probable that had the fourth P wave occurred, it would have been nonconducted (AV Wenckebach).

ATRIOVENTRICULAR BLOCK

Digitalis prolongs the refractory period of AV nodal cells by vagal stimulation and by its direct effect on AV nodal cells. Often it is this precise effect that the clinician is seeking when attempting to slow the ventricular response to a rapid atrial rhythm (paroxsymal supraventricular tachycardia, atrial fibrillation, or atrial flutter). However, the AV node is influenced not only by vagal tone but also by sympathetic tone, which enhances AV conduction. Often the emergency setting of supraventricular tachycardia is associated with increased sympathetic tone, and digoxin alone is ineffective in slowing the ventricular response.[11] This is also true for the chronic administration of digitalis. In some patients during exercise the sympathetic nervous system may override the vagal effect of digitalis. Thus, to achieve control of the ventricular rate during daily activity, it is necessary for some patients to combine digitalis with another drug.

In therapeutic doses digitalis achieves its effect of AV block in part because some of the atrial impulses are conducted so slowly through the AV node that they fail to reach the ventricles and yet leave the AV node refractory to the next impulse (concealed conduction). In toxic doses, AV conduction can be compromised enough to cause symptomatic bradycardia or it may fail completely (third-degree AV block). Fig. 17-7 shows alarming prolongation of the PR interval during digitalis therapy—an early sign. The digitalis is discontinued until the PR normalizes, then the dosage is adjusted. Fig. 17-8 shows atrial fibrillation with high-grade AV block and a junctional escape pacemaker. A profound, life-threatening bradycardia caused

II

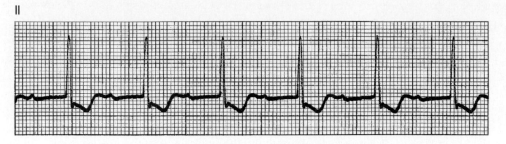

Fig. 17-7. Prolonged PR intervals, an early sign of digitalis intoxication.

V_1

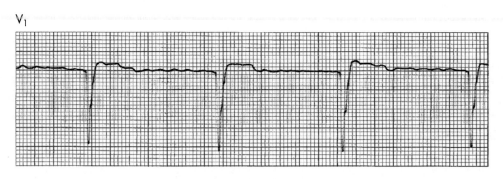

Fig. 17-8. Atrial fibrillation with profound AV block, a sign of digitalis intoxication.

by high-grade AV block in an acute digitalis overdose (suicide attempt) is shown in Fig. 17-9. Fig. 17-9, *A,* was recorded at admission. Fig. 17-9, *B,* shows conduction improvement with treatment.

ATRIAL TACHYCARDIA WITH BLOCK

Within 5 to 20 beats of the initiation of the tachycardias of digitalis intoxication a steady-state rate is usually established. This rate may vary slightly thereafter and increases along with the levels of digitalis.

In atrial tachycardia caused by triggered activity the focus is high in the right atrium, close to the sinus node, and there is usually AV block. The rhythm is exacerbated by hypokalemia, which often results from diuretics or loss through the gastrointestinal tract.[12]

ECG recognition

Atrial rate: 130 to 250 beats/min.
P waves: Similar in shape to sinus P waves (upright in leads II, III, and aV$_F$).
QRS complex: Narrow unless BBB is also present.
AV block: Usually present (2:1 or AV Wenckebach).

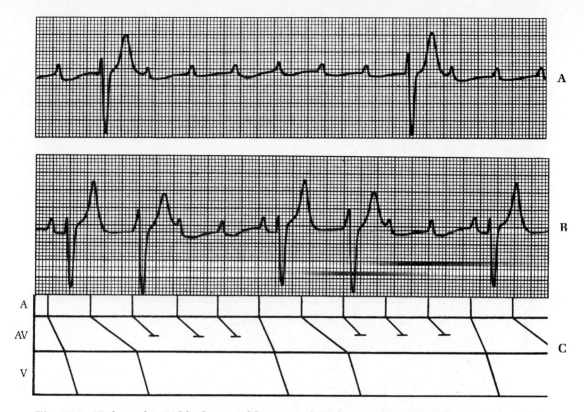

Fig. 17-9. High-grade AV block caused by acute digitalis overdose (suicide attempt). **A,** Recorded on hospital admission. **B,** Improved conduction after emergency treatment. The second beat in the pair is a conducted beat, as indicated in, **C,** the laddergram. The broad initial R wave of that beat is really a distortion by a P wave.

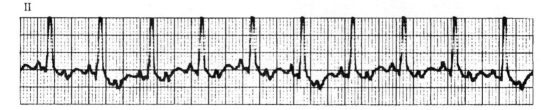

Fig. 17-10. Atrial tachycardia (200 beats/min) with 2:1 block. The signs of atrial tachycardia resulting from digitalis intoxication are upright P waves in the inferior leads and ventriculophasic PP intervals.

PP intervals: Often ventriculophasic, that is, the PP interval on either side of the R wave is shorter than the PP interval without an R wave. This is a vagal effect. When the aortic pressure influences the baroreceptors of the carotid body, the next atrial cycle (without an R wave) is longer.[13]

Best lead: II (the P′ wave is upright and similar in shape to the sinus P wave).

Fig. 17-10 shows atrial tachycardia with 2:1 block in a patient with digitalis intoxication. The atrial rate is 200 beats/min. The digitalis effect can be seen in the ST segment (the typical scooped-down appearance). Clues pointing to digitalis tox-

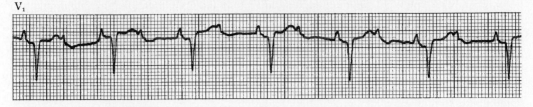

Fig. 17-11. Atrial tachycardia (130 beats/min) with 2:1 block. The marked ventriculophasic PP intervals are evident (see text).

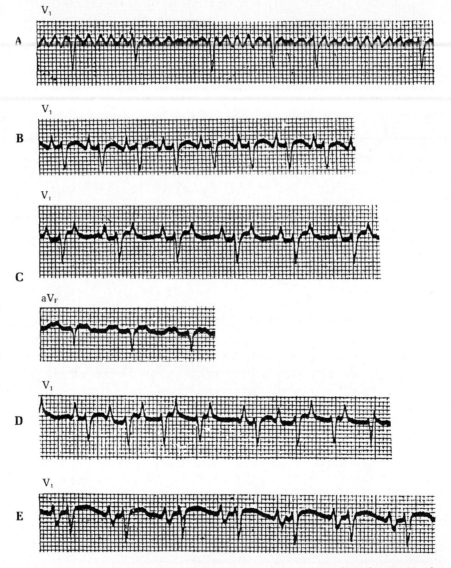

Fig. 17-12. A, Atrial fibrillation with AV block in a patient taking digitalis. **B,** Six days later. The rhythm converted to atrial tachycardia (160 beats/min) with 1:1 conduction. This sign of digitalis intoxication was not recognized, and more digitalis was given. **C,** Later the same day. Atrial tachycardia with 2:1 conduction. At this point the digitalis was discontinued. **D,** The next day. Conduction improved. Atrial tachycardia was still present with Wenckebach conduction. **E,** Normal sinus rhythm (4 days after the digitalis was discontinued).

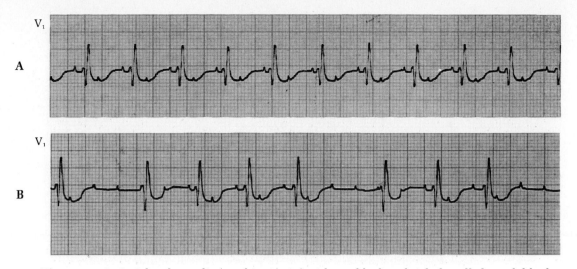

Fig. 17-10. A, Atrial tachycardia (220 beats/min) with 2:1 block and right bundle branch block (RBBB). **B,** Atrial tachycardia with a deterioration in AV conduction.

icity are (1) upright P′ waves in the inferior leads, indicating a focus high in the right atrium; (2) AV block; and (3) ventriculophasic PP intervals. (The difference between the PP interval with the R wave and the one without is about 0.02 sec, best seen in lead II.) The ventriculophasic PP intervals sometimes seen in atrial tachycardia resulting from digitalis intoxication may be so marked (Fig. 17-11) as to cause one to confuse it with bigeminal nonconducted premature atrial complexes (PACs).

When digitalis is discontinued because of atrial tachycardia and 2:1 block, often AV conduction improves before the rhythm converts to sinus. Such a sequence can be seen in a patient being treated for atrial fibrillation (Fig. 17-12) converted to atrial tachycardia and,when the digitalis was discontinued, to sinus rhythm.

In Fig. 17-13, *A,* the atrial rate is 220 beats/min in a patient with digitalis intoxication. (Note the digitalis effect in the ST segment.) There is no ventriculophasic effect in this case. (The PP intervals are all the same.) In Fig. 17-13, *B,* the block is more marked. Right bundle branch block (RBBB) is also present.

NONPAROXYSMAL JUNCTIONAL TACHYCARDIA

In clinical practice digitalis overdose has long been considered the most common cause of nonparoxysmal junctional tachycardia. Other causes are myocardial infarction, cardiac surgery, rheumatic fever, and hypokalemia. During nonparoxysmal junctional tachycardia, Wenckebach conduction from the junctional pacemaker can occur. The result on the ECG is group beating, which may be missed if there is also atrial fibrillation. It is important to recognize the first sign of digitalis intoxication in atrial fibrillation, that is, regularization of the rhythm or group beating; both are junctional rhythms, one without and one with exit block.

ECG recognition

P waves: May or may not be present.
QRS complex: Narrow unless BBB is also present.

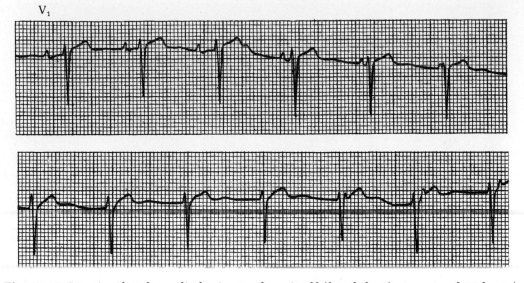

Fig. 17-14. Junctional tachycardia begins to show itself (fourth beat) at a rate of 74 beats/min. There is no retrograde conduction to the atria. The sinus rhythm continues to activate the atria, and the junctional focus activates the ventricles (AV dissociation).

Junctional rate: 70 to 140 beats/min; increases with exercise but rarely exceeds 140 beats/min. Carotid sinus massage has no effect, or there may be nodoventricular block.

Retrograde conduction: Conduction from the junctional focus to the atria is usually absent because of the AV block created by the digitalis; therefore AV dissociation is usually present.

Rhythm: Nonparoxysmal[15] (gradual onset)

Best lead: V_1 (In this lead junctional tachycardia can be differentiated from fascicular VT.)

Fig. 17-14 is a tracing of junctional tachycardia at a rate of 74 beats/min in a patient taking digitalis. Atrioventricular dissociation is present after the third complex.

Terminology

When the rate of the junctional rhythm is less than 100 beats/min, the term *accelerated idiojunctional rhythm* is often used. When the rate exceeds 100 beats/min, *junctional tachycardia* is used. This term is used in this book to refer to any accelerated junctional rhythm.

Junctional tachycardia during atrial fibrillation

Fig. 17-15 shows the development of junctional tachycardia in a patient with atrial fibrillation. Note the appropriately irregular ventricular response of atrial fibrillation (Fig. 17-15, *A*) that has developed into a regular rhythm (Fig. 17-15, *B*) at 80 beats/min. Although the atrial fibrillatory line is fine in these tracings, atrial fibrillation is easily recognized in Fig. 17-15, *A*, because of the expected irregular ventricular response. However, although the P waves are absent in Fig. 17-15, *B*, as they are in Fig. 17-15, *A*, the regularity of the junctional rhythm often causes the

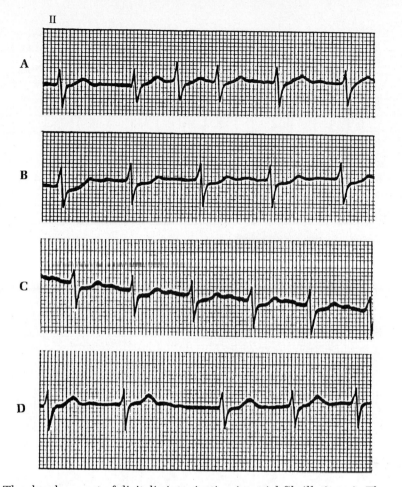

Fig. 17-15. The development of digitalis intoxication in atrial fibrillation. **A,** The ventricular response to atrial fibrillation is appropriately irregular. **B,** As the patient's condition became toxic, the rhythm began to regularize and was eventually regular at 80 beats/min, because of junctional tachycardia. **C,** The toxicity was not recognized until the rate approached 100 beats/min and the digitalis was discontinued. **D,** the rhythm is again irregular.

diagnosis of atrial fibrillation to be missed. This is a surprisingly consistent stumbling block. In Fig. 17-15, *C,* the rate is 100 beats/min; the digitalis was discontinued. In Fig. 17-15, *D,* the patient is no longer toxic, and the rhythm shows the appropriate irregularity of atrial fibrillation.

Even more of a stumbling block in atrial fibrillation is the recognition of junctional tachycardia when it is combined with Wenckebach exit block. In such a case the diagnostic ECG clue is *group beating,* usually in groups of two or three. Fig. 17-16 is a tracing of atrial fibrillation and junctional tachycardia with 4:3 Wenckebach exit block. Note the groups of three. In Fig. 17-17 junctional tachycardia of 98 beats/min suddenly drops a beat and lengthens the RR interval when 3:2 Wenckebach exit block develops, producing a bigeminal rhythm.

Hospitalized patients who have atrial fibrillation and are taking a digitalis glycoside should be monitored closely for the early signs of digitalis intoxication, that is, regularization of the rhythm and group beating. Patients who are not hospital-

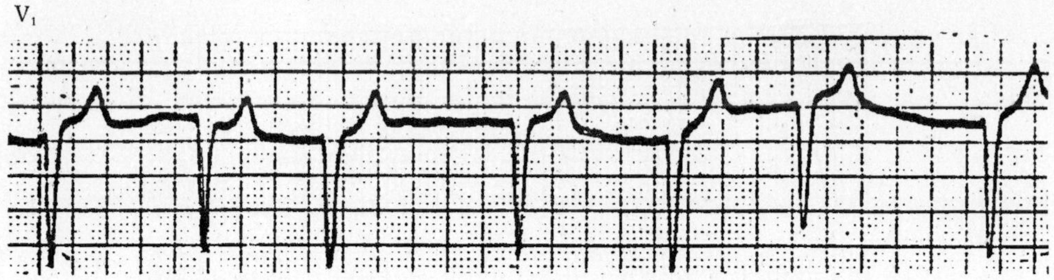

V₁

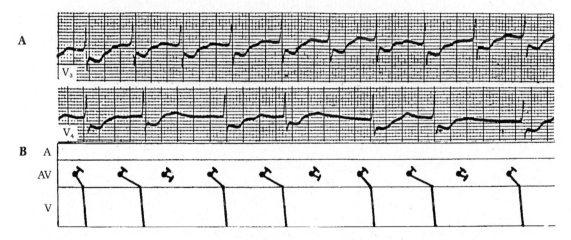

Fig. 17-16. Atrial fibrillation with junctional tachycardia and 4:3 Wenckebach exit block caused by excess digitalis. The group beating, shortening RR intervals, and pauses that are less than twice the shortest cycle are evident.

Fig. 17-17. A, Atrial fibrillation and junctional tachycardia. **B,** In the same patient the junctional tachycardia develops a 3:2 Wenckebach exit block. *(Courtesy Henry J.L. Marriott, MD.)*

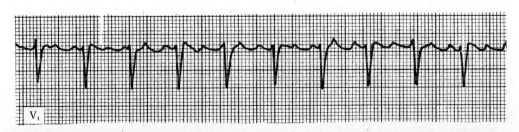

Fig. 17-18. Atrial flutter with junctional tachycardia. The regular ventricular rhythm (rate, 110 beats/min) is evident, yet the flutter waves have no fixed relationship to the QRS, a sign of AV dissociation.

ized should have regular 12-lead ECGs to evaluate for the same two eventualities. In both cases the digitalis is discontinued until a controlled ventricular response to atrial fibrillation is once again achieved, then the dosage is adjusted to avoid a recurrence.

Junctional tachycardia during atrial flutter. When atrial flutter is associated with junctional tachycardia, there is AV dissociation. This condition is recognized when the ventricular rhythm is regular, yet there is no fixed relationship between the flutter waves and the QRS. Fig. 17-18 was recorded in lead V$_1$. (The typical sawtooth pattern of atrial flutter is not present.) The P′ waves are positive peaks at regular intervals throughout the tracing. The ventricular rhythm is regular at 110 beats/min. Note that the flutter-QRS relationship varies, a sign of AV dissociation.

FASCICULAR VENTRICULAR TACHYCARDIA

Occasionally digitalis intoxication results in ventricular tachycardia. The focus is thought to be in one of the fascicles of the left bundle branch, resulting in an RBBB pattern and axis deviation; some cases have a left bundle branch block (LBBB) pattern indicating a right bundle branch focus. The mechanism of fascicular beats is explained and illustrated on p. 166. Other clinical settings in which fascicular VT has been reported are patients without heart disease[14] and those with herbal aconite poisoning.[15]

ECG recognition

Rate: 90 to 160 beats/min.
QRS complex: Usually incomplete RBBB pattern in V$_1$. The QRS duration is broad but less than 0.14 sec.
QRS axis: Right or left.
Best leads: V$_1$, I, and II (V$_1$ for the RBBB pattern and I and II for the axis deviation).

The RBBB pattern is caused by the origin of the impulse in the left bundle branch, so the right ventricle is the last to activate. However, because the impulse begins within the conduction system, the ventricular complex is not as wide as it is with other types of VT. Thus the pattern in V$_1$ is that of incomplete RBBB. In Fig. 17-19 note the digitalis effect in the sagging ST segment and the classic pattern of fascicular VT, RBBB pattern with a QRS of 0.12 sec. In the past this rhythm has commonly been mistaken for junctional tachycardia with RBBB aberration.

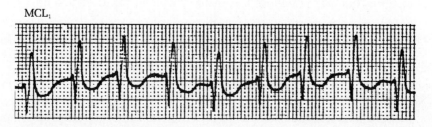

Fig. 17-19. Fascicular ventricular tachycardia (VT). The relatively narrow RBBB pattern (QRS, 0.12 sec), is typical of this condition. The sagging ST segment is an effect of digitalis. *(Courtesy Henry J.L. Marriott, MD.)*

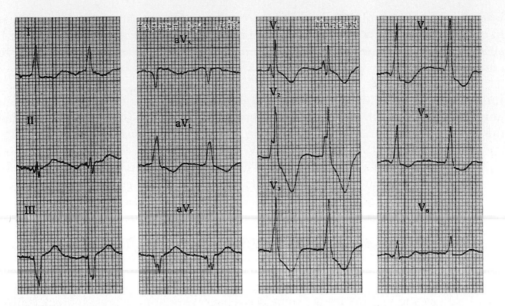

Fig. 17-20. Fascicular VT in a patient with congestive heart failure who was taking digitalis for chronic atrial fibrillation. Note the digitalis effect (scooped-down ST segment), the regular rhythm, the RBBB pattern in V_1, and left axis deviation, which indicate a posterior fascicular focus. *(Courtesy Kathy Brown, RN, Okanogan, Wash.)*

The axis deviation occurs because of the location of the ectopic focus in the fascicles. A focus located in the anterior (superior) fascicle has a right axis deviation, and a focus located in the posterior (inferior) fascicle has a left axis deviation.

Fig. 17-20 is a 12-lead ECG from a patient in congestive heart failure who was taking digitalis for chronic atrial fibrillation. Note the digitalis effect (scooped-down ST segment), the regular rhythm, RBBB pattern in V_1, and left axis deviation, which indicates a posterior fascicular focus.

BIFASCICULAR VENTRICULAR TACHYCARDIA

Bifascicular VT is sometimes called "bidirectional." The term implies that the QRS complexes during VT are changing direction in the frontal plane leads on a beat-to-beat basis. This life-threatening form of VT has long been recognized as an arrhythmia that most often occurs in digitalis intoxication, especially in older patients and in those with severe myocardial disease.[13] When seen in the setting of digitalis excess, this arrhythmia is a sign of advanced toxic effects and poor prognosis.[16]

ECG recognition

Rate: 90 to 160 beats/min[10]

QRS complex: Usually incomplete RBBB pattern in V_1. The QRS duration is 0.12 to 0.14 sec. The QRS alternates in height because of the alternating axis.

QRS axis: Right axis alternates with left, giving the bidirectional appearance seen in the limb leads; if only a precordial monitoring lead is available, the alternating axes may be missed.

Best leads: V_1, I, and II (V_1 for the RBBB pattern and I and II for the axis deviation).

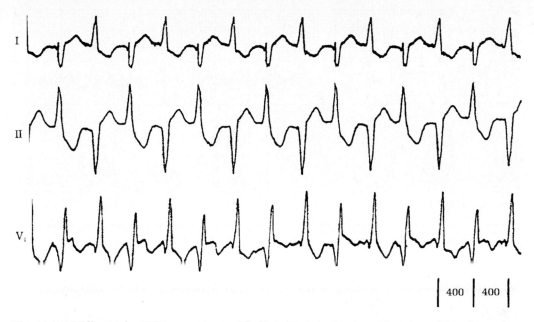

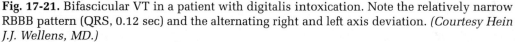

Fig. 17-21. Bifascicular VT in a patient with digitalis intoxication. Note the relatively narrow RBBB pattern (QRS, 0.12 sec) and the alternating right and left axis deviation. *(Courtesy Hein J.J. Wellens, MD.)*

Fig. 17-21 shows bifascicular VT in leads I, II, and V_1, in which all of the diagnostic features can be seen. Note the scooped-down ST segment (the digitalis effect). The pattern in V_1 is RBBB with a width of 0.12 sec. The alternating axis affects the shape of the QRS in V_1, causing the alternating heights. A normal axis has upright complexes in leads I and II. At no time in this tracing does that occur. When the complex in lead I is negative, lead II is positive (right axis deviation). When lead I is positive, lead II is negative (left axis deviation).

Mechanism. The focus alternates between the anterosuperior and posteroinferior fascicles, producing the typical pattern of RBBB and alternating axes (left to right).[17,18]

DOUBLE TACHYCARDIAS

The arrhythmias of digitalis toxicity have a tendency to double or triple in one patient. Often two tachycardias are combined or a tachycardia is associated with block, so the diagnosis is not immediately apparent. These pitfalls can be avoided if strict attention is paid to three steps. First, look at lead II and identify the atrial rhythm. Second, see if there is conduction. If there is, no further analysis is needed. If not, the third step is needed. Look at lead V_1 to evaluate the ventricular rhythm. Is it junctional or ventricular (fascicular)? Practice these steps in Figs. 17-22 and 17-23.

The ECG in Fig. 17-22 is from a patient with chronic obstructive pulmonary disease who was taking digoxin 0.25 mg/day.

1. What is the atrial rhythm? The P wave distorting the second ST segment

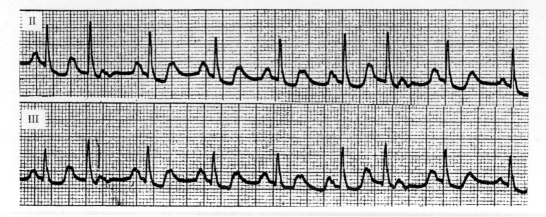

Fig. 17-22. Atrial tachycardia with 3:2 Wenckebach and 2:1 AV block. *(Courtesy William P. Nelson, MD.)*

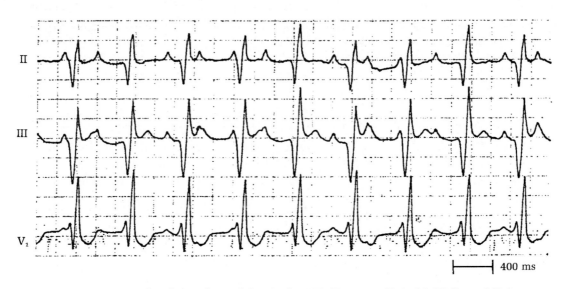

Fig. 17-23. Atrial tachycardia and fascicular VT. *(Courtesy Hein J.J. Wellens, MD.)*

gives a fix on the PP interval. The rest of the P waves can be found in T waves, in front of the R waves, and again in an ST segment. The atrial rate is 150 beats/min, and the P waves are upright in leads II and III, indicating atrial tachycardia as a result of digitalis intoxication.

2. Is there conduction? The irregular rhythm is your first clue to the presence of conduction. There is both 2:1 and Wenckebach 3:2 conduction.

Answer the same questions for Fig. 17-23.

1. What is the atrial rhythm? The P waves are upright in leads II and III at a rate of approximately 170 beats/min. This is atrial tachycardia.

2. Is there conduction? The regular ventricular rhythm without fixed PR intervals indicates that there is no conduction. Because of this, a third determination must be made.

3. Are the ventricular beats junctional or fascicular? Lead V_1 is the best lead to answer this question. The RBBB pattern (rSR′) in V_1 indicates that there is fascicular VT. This is a double tachycardia—atrial tachycardia and fascicular VT.

NONCARDIAC SIGNS OF DIGITALIS TOXICITY

The serum concentration of digitalis depends on many factors, including how much digitalis is bound to the membrane (where it cannot be measured). The ECG and the patient's symptoms are usually of more value in determining toxic effects.

Take a history that includes questions regarding neurologic symptoms such as headache, malaise, neuralgic pain, and pseudodementia (disorientation, memory lapses, hallucinations, nightmares, restlessness, insomnia, and listlessness).

Color vision

The patient should be queried regarding changes in the quality of color vision, especially red and green. Such symptoms are subtle and are not volunteered by the patient. Questions from the examiner regarding the patient's assessment of the present quality of color TV (especially the red and green colors), as compared with the past quality, may be revealing. One patient had recently purchased a new TV set in a frustrated search for better picture quality. Other visual symptoms include scotomas and flickering halos.

Gastrointestinal symptoms

The gastrointestinal symptoms of digitalis intoxication (anorexia, nausea, and vomiting) are mediated by chemoreceptors in the medulla rather than by a direct irritant effect of digitalis on the gastrointestinal tract.[2]

TREATMENT

Early recognition and intervention are important; when digitalis-induced arrhythmias are not recognized and digitalis is continued, the mortality rate is nearly 100%.[3] Those of us who care for patients taking digitalis are obliged to evaluate for the physical and ECG signs of the life-threatening condition of digitalis intoxication.

Management of early manifestations

For the early, more common manifestations of digitalis intoxication, such as occasional ectopic beats, marked prolongation of the PR interval, or a slow ventricular response in atrial fibrillation, the physician may judge a temporary withdrawal of the drug to be sufficient and may decide that the patient should have electrocardiographic monitoring. Once the patient's condition is stabilized, the dosage schedule is adjusted to prevent recurrence.[2]

Aggressive management of patients with serious arrhythmias or hemodynamic compromise[17]

1. Discontinue the digitalis.
2. Place the patient on bed rest. (Avoid sympathetic stimulation.)
3. Correct electrolyte abnormalities.
4. Active treatment of a rapid ventricular rhythm depends on the site of origin of the arrhythmia and its hemodynamic consequences.

5. If hemodynamic instability is present, emergency IV administration of Fab fragments of digoxin-specific antibodies is preferred. If digoxin antibodies are not available, phenytoin may be used, placement of a ventricular pacing lead.
6. Ventricular pacing is also indicated in cases of symptomatic bradycardia.

Fab fragments of cardiac glycoside-specific antibodies

High-affinity cardiac glycoside–specific antibodies are able to reverse the cellular effects of digoxin (i.e., inhibition of myocardial Na^+-K^+ ATPase pumps and monovalent cation active transport.[19]) Fab fragments are an improvement over the intact antibodies in the treatment of life-threatening digitalis intoxication. After IV infusion the smaller molecule of the Fab fragment has a greater rate and volume of distribution and reverses experimentally induced digoxin-induced arrhythmias more rapidly than does the intact antibody, and the response is relatively rapid, with cessation of fascicular VT within 1 hour.[2]

EMERGENCY APPROACH

The drug is, of course, discontinued, and the patient placed on bed rest (no sympathetic stimulation). Electrolyte abnormalities are corrected. When there is hemodynamic compromise, digitalis antibodies are considered or phenytoin is given. A ventricular pacing lead is inserted if phenytoin is used or if digitalis-induced bradycardia and hemodynamic deterioration are present.[10]

SUMMARY

Digitalis intoxication is diagnosed because of subjective and ECG symptoms; digoxin blood levels are used in conjunction with these findings. The ECG shows bradycardia (SA block and/or AV block); tachycardia (atrial, junctional, or fascicular); regularity in atrial fibrillation (junctional tachycardia or AV block with junctional escape); group beating in atrial fibrillation (junctional tachycardia with Wenckebach exit block); group beating in sinus rhythm (ventricular bigeminy, SA Wenckebach, or AV Wenckebach); *or* atrial flutter (with AV dissociation or high-degree AV block).

REFERENCES

1. Gadsby DC: The Na/K pump of cardiac myocytes. In Zipes DP, Jalife J, eds: *Cardiac electrophysiology from cell to bedside,* Philadelphia, 1990, WB Saunders.
2. Smith TW, Braunwald E, Kelly RA: The management of heart failure. In Braunwald E, ed: *Heart disease,* ed 4, Philadelphia, 1995, WB Saunders.
3. Dreifus LS, McKnight EH, Katz M et al: Digitalis intolerance, *Geriatrics* 18:494, 1963.
4. Powell AC, Horowitz JD, Hasin Y et al: Acute myocardial uptake of digoxin in humans: correlation with hemodynamic and electrocardiographic effects, *J Am Coll Cardiol* 15:1238, 1990.
5. Marcus FI: Use and toxicity of digitalis, *Heart Dis Stroke,* 1(No 1):27, 1992.
6. Rosen MR: Delayed afterdepolarizations induced by digitalis. In Rosen MR, Janse MJ, Wit AL, eds: *Cardiac electrophysiology,* Mount Kisco, NY, 1990, Futura.
7. Wit AL, Cranefield PF, Gadsby DC: Electrogenic sodium extrusion can stop triggered activity in the canine coronary sinus, *Circ Res* 49:1029, 1981.
8. Rosen MR: Cellular electrophysiology of digitalis toxicity, *J Am Coll Cardiol* 5:22A, 1985.
9. Vanagt EJ, Wellens HJJ: the electrocardiogram in digitalis intoxication. In Wellens HJJ, Kulbertus HE, editors: *What's new in electrocardiography,* The Hague, 1981, Martinus Nijhoff.
10. Wellens HJJ, Conover M: *The ECG in emergency decision making,* Philadelphia, 1992, WB Saunders.

11. Ewy GA: Urgent parenteral digoxin therapy: a requiem, *J Am Coll Cardiol* 15:1248, 1990.

12. Naccarelli GV, Shih HT, Jalal S: Clinical arrhythmias: mechanisms, clinical features, and management—supraventricular tachycardia. In: Zipes DP, Jalife J, eds: *Cellular electrophysiology from cell to bedside,* ed 2, Philadelphia, 1995, WB Saunders.

13. Zipes DP: Specific arrhythmias: diagnosis and treatment. In Braunwald E, ed: *Heart disease,* ed 4, Philadelphia, 1992, WB Saunders.

14. Martini B, Buja GF, Canciani B, Nava A: Bidirectional tachycardia: a sustained form, not related to digitalis intoxication, in an adult without apparent cardiac disease, *Jpn Heart J* 29:381, 1988.

15. Tsukada K, Akizuki S, Matsuoka Y et al: A case of aconitine poisoning accompanied by bidirectional ventricular tachycardia treated with lidocaine, *Kokyu To Junkan* 40:1003, 1992.

16. Grimm W, Marchlinski FE: Accelerated idioventricular rhythm, bidirectional ventricular tachcardia. In Zipes DP, Jalife J, eds: *Cellular electrophysiology from cell to bedside,* ed 2, Philadelphia, 1995, WB Saunders.

17. Wieland JM, Marchlinski FE: Electrocardiographic response of digoxin-toxic fascicular tachycardia to Fab fragments: implications for tachycardia mechanism, *PACE Pacing Clin Electrophysiol* 9:727, 1986.

18. Gorgels AP, Beekman HD, Brugada P et al: Extrastimulus-related shortening of the first post-pacing interval in digitalis-induced ventricular tachycardia: observations during programmed electrical stimulation in the conscious dog, *J Am Coll Cardiol* 1:840, 1983.

19. Hougen TJ, Lloyd BL, Smith TW: Effects of inotropic and arrhythmogenic digoxin doses and of digoxin-specific antibody on myocardial monovalent cation transport in the dog, *Circ Res* 44:23, 1979.

Atrioventricular Block

Pediatrics *261*
First-Degree Atrioventricular Block *261*
Second-Degree Atrioventricular
  Block *263*
Complete Atrioventricular Block
  (Third-Degree) *271*

Noninvasive Evaluation of the Site of
  Block *272*
Treatment *274*
Summary *274*

Atrioventricular (AV) block is the delayed conduction or nonconduction of an atrial impulse during a time when the AV junction is not physiologically refractory.[1] It is conventionally divided into three categories, first-, second-, and third-degree block.

> **first-degree AV block** Prolonged PR intervals.
> **second-degree AV block** Not all P waves are conducted; divided into types I and II. High-grade AV block is a type of second-degree AV block in which two or more consecutive P waves are not conducted.
> **third-degree AV block** Absence of AV conduction when the possibility to conduct is present.

Fig. 18-1 illustrates where in the conduction system these blocks are commonly located. Determination of the location and type of block has implications regarding immediate treatment and prognosis. The His bundle electrogram is, of course, the definitive means of determining whether the AV block is at the level of the bundle of His or the bundle branches, or both. However, there are four noninvasive interventions that give valuable information in this regard. They are summarized in Table 18-1 and discussed on p. 272.

Table 18-1. Noninvasive evaluation of atrioventricular block level

Intervention	Type I (nodal)	Type II (subnodal)
Atropine	Improves	Worsens
Exercise	Improves	Worsens
Catecholamines	Improves	Worsens
Carotid sinus massage	Worsens	Improves

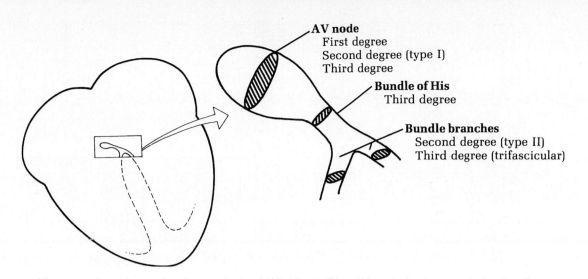

AV node
First degree
Second degree (type I)
Third degree

Bundle of His
Third degree

Bundle branches
Second degree (type II)
Third degree (trifascicular)

Fig. 18-1. Locations of atrioventricular (AV) block. The AV node is the usual site for first-degree AV block and type I second-degree block; the bundle branches are the usual site for type II second-degree block. Complete (third-degree) AV block may occur at any level but is most common in the bundle of His and the bundle branches.

PEDIATRICS

In children AV block is usually congenital and may occur alone or in association with another lesion. A common histologic finding is anatomic discontinuity between the atria and conduction system and between the AV node and the ventricles. Generally children are asymptomatic. Those in whom symptoms develop may require a pacemaker. The mortality rate is at its height in the neonatal period, is much lower during childhood and adolescence, and then increases slowly.[1]

FIRST-DEGREE ATRIOVENTRICULAR BLOCK
ECG recognition

PR interval: Longer than 0.20 sec; does not change from beat to beat (Fig. 18-2).
QRS complex: Normal in shape and duration unless there is another lesion lower in the conduction system. A narrow QRS usually indicates conduction delay within the AV node (prolonged atrial-His [AH] interval).
Atrioventricular conduction: All sinus beats are conducted to the ventricles.

Mechanism

The term "first-degree AV block" is a little misleading in that there is a prolongation of conduction rather than an actual block in conduction. Fig. 18-3 illustrates the parts of the heart involved in forming the PR interval (the atria, the AV node, and the His-Purkinje system). The impulse invades the AV node early in the formation of the P wave. Once this happens, the PR interval no longer depends on atrial conduction. Note also that the greatest part of the PR interval is due to the conduction time through the AV node, which is capable of lengthening that conduction

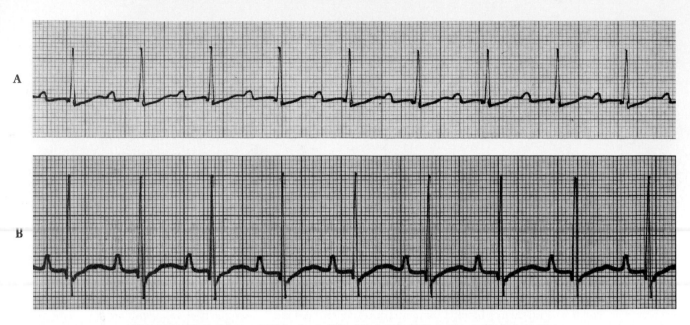

Fig. 18-2. First-degree AV block. **A,** The PR interval is 0.30 sec. **B,** It is 0.24 sec.

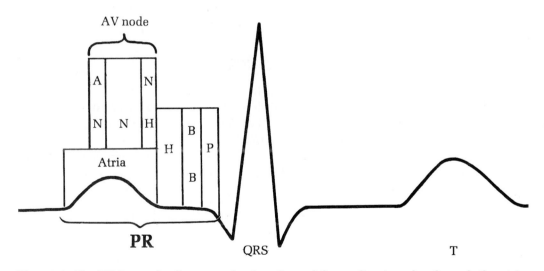

Fig. 18-3. The PR interval reflects conduction time of the cardiac impulse through the atria, AV node, His bundle *(H),* bundle branches *(B),* and Purkinje fibers *(P).* When the PR interval is long, it is usually the result of conduction delay in the AV node. *AN,* Atrionodal; *N,* node; *NH,* nodal-His.

time further in response to rapid rates or diseases. Conduction through the AV node can be likened to the stretch of a rubber band as opposed to the all-or-none behavior of the His-Purkinje system. A prolongation of the PR interval to 0.28 sec or more usually indicates AV nodal disease. However, the His bundle electrogram is the only definitive way to determine the level of block (AV node or His-Purkinje system) when the PR is prolonged.

Clinical implications

The clinical implications of a prolonged PR interval depend on the level of the lesion as determined by the His-ventricular (HV) interval of the His bundle electrogram. When the QRS duration is normal, a prolonged PR interval almost always reflects AV nodal delay. However, a PR that is not markedly prolonged may, in fact, be associated with disease in the His-Purkinje system, causing an alarmingly prolonged HV interval (greater than 100 ms).

Prolonged PR intervals occur in up to 13% of patients with acute myocardial infarction (MI) (usually inferior); 75% of these patients subsequently have type I AV block, and half of these then have high-grade or third-degree AV block with a dependable junctional escape pacemaker.[2] First-degree AV block is also seen in individuals with no history of cardiac disease and in healthy children.[1]

Physical signs

At bedside one may notice that in first-degree AV block the first heart sound diminishes in intensity with PR prolongation and that there is a long A to C wave interval in the jugular venous pulse.

Assessment of the jugular venous pulse

In examining the jugular pulse, the patient is positioned with the trunk at an angle of 15 to 45 degrees to the horizontal plane unless, of course, venous pressure is extremely high and the patient may need to sit upright. The right external jugular vein is the easiest to assess. Lighting should be oblique or tangential to the vein. Pulsation seen at the posterior border of the sternocleidomastoid muscle is a venous pulsation. (The arterial pulsation is at the anterior border.) Three separate pulsations can usually be identified in the venous pulse, as opposed to the artery, which has only one.

The A wave represents atrial contraction (when right atrial pressure rises); it is the most prominent. When the right atrium contracts against a closed tricuspid valve, "cannon A waves" can be seen.

The jugular C wave probably represents the onset of right ventricular systole; its origin is disputed.[3]

The jugular V wave begins during ventricular contraction and is the result of passive filling of the right atrium after the tricuspid valve closes.

Pediatrics

In children taking digitalis the PR interval may become prolonged; unlike in adults, such a development may represent digitalis intoxication. When the PR interval is prolonged in a child receiving digitalis, the physician decreases the amount of the drug being taken.[4]

Treatment

In adults the presence of first-degree AV block usually does not require therapy, whether digitalis is involved or not.

SECOND-DEGREE ATRIOVENTRICULAR BLOCK

Second-degree AV block is the nonconduction of some of the atrial impulses at a time when the AV junction is not physiologically refractory. The disease may be either in the AV node or within or below the bundle of His, each with different clinical implications, treatment, and prognosis. The QRS duration helps localize the level of block to above (narrow QRS) or below (broad QRS) the branching portion of the bundle of His. A prolonged PR interval with a broad QRS would point to a block in both the AV node and the bundle of His.

Second-degree AV block is usually divided into type I (AV Wenckebach or Mobitz type I) and type II (Mobitz type II). There is a third type, which is often moved back and forth between type I and type II; it is 2:1 AV block. It may have the pathologic features, treatment, and clinical implications of either type I or type II. In this book 2:1 AV block is given a separate classification.

Type I atrioventricular block (atrioventricular Wenckebach)

In classic AV Wenckebach the PR lengthens until finally one P wave is not conducted, which produces a pause. After the pause the sequence repeats itself.

ECG recognition

PR intervals: Become progressively longer until one P wave is not conducted and the sequence begins again.

QRS complexes: Narrow unless there is another lesion in the bundle branches. QRS complexes appear in groups because of the dropped beats.

RR intervals: Shorten if more than two P waves in a row are conducted. The shortening occurs because the second PR interval has the largest increment, causing the next R wave to be more delayed than the others in the group. The third PR interval of the group, although longer than the previous one, does not exhibit the same increment that the second in the series does.

In summary, the ECG signs of AV Wenckebach are as follows:

Group beating

Lengthening PR intervals

Pauses that are less than twice the shortest cycle

Shortening RR intervals (when three or more P waves are consecutively conducted)

The typical ECG of AV Wenckebach is illustrated in Fig. 18-4, and the ECG signs of the classic rhythm are listed. The tracing in Fig. 18-4 is 3:2 Wenckebach. That is, for every three P waves, only two are conducted. Fig. 18-5 illustrates 2:1 AV block and 3:2 Wenckebach in the same patient. Fig. 18-6 illustrates 4:3 Wenckebach.

Occasionally type I AV block is seen with a broad QRS (Fig. 18-6, *B*). This is usually the result of both AV nodal block and bundle branch block (BBB). In some instances there is BBB with Wenckebach-type conduction in the other bundle.

Mechanism. The disease in type I AV block is almost always in the AV node, rarely within the His bundle. The AV node normally has a slow-response action potential and slow conduction. Therefore any depressive influence, such as digitalis or ischemia, easily compounds the normal situation, causing the PR to lengthen until one P wave is not conducted; the sequence begins again, producing the group beating typical of Wenckebach periods.

Clinical implications. Type I AV block with a narrow QRS complex is more benign than type II and does not progress to a more advanced conduction problem. It is commonly associated with digitalis intoxication, acute inferior wall and right ventricular MI, acute myocarditis, or the period following open-heart surgery. In these

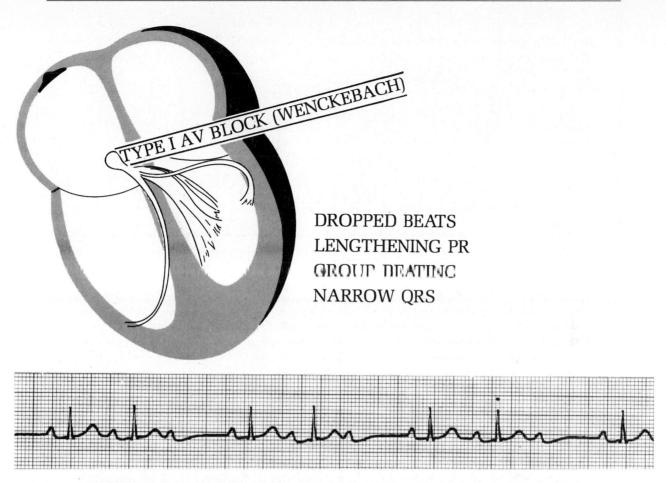

TYPE I AV BLOCK (WENCKEBACH)

DROPPED BEATS
LENGTHENING PR
GROUP BEATING
NARROW QRS

Fig. 18-4. Type I second-degree AV block is usually a function of the AV node and may be the result of inferior wall myocardial infarction.

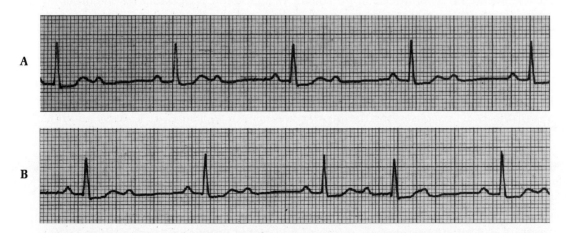

A

B

Fig. 18-5. In **A,** There is 2:1 block. The ECG signs of AV nodal disease are evident: PR intervals that are slightly prolonged (all identical) and a narrow QRS. **B,** Tracing from the same patient. There is 2:1 AV block at the beginning of the tracing and 3:2 AV Wenckebach at the center of the tracing. The lengthening PR interval (the fourth PR) and the nonconducted sinus P wave in the T of that beat are evident.

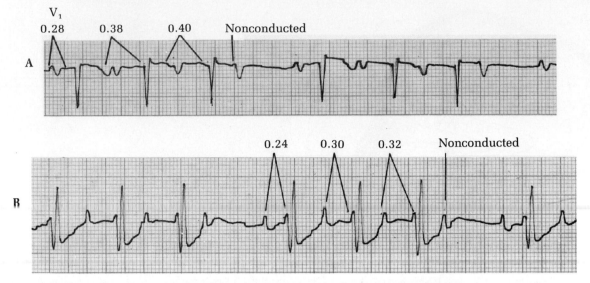

Fig. 18-6. Type I second-degree AV block (Wenckebach). **A** and **B,** The signs of typical Wenckebach periodicity: lengthening PR intervals and pauses that are twice the shortest cycle. **B,** Complicated by bundle branch block. There are two lesions, one at the AV node and the other in the bundle branches.

settings it is transient and requires only observation. If complete AV block develops because of inferior wall MI, the escape pacemaker is junctional and a pacemaker is rarely required. However, the development of the block in this setting identifies a high-risk patient with more extensive infarction. Such a patient can be identified at admission by the observation of ST-segment elevation in lead V_{4R} (p. 415), which also indicates a proximal right coronary artery occlusion and right ventricular MI.

Atrioventricular Wenckebach also occurs as a normal condition in trained athletes and may be related to their enhanced vagal tone. It is possible for the block to become more profound, resulting in syncope or presyncope. At this point it is necessary for the athlete to "decondition." In individuals without structural heart disease, chronic block at the level of the AV node is benign. When the block is associated with structural heart disease, the prognosis is linked to the heart disease.[1]

Physical signs. Second-degree AV block was actually first described without benefit of the ECG, by observing the jugular venous pulse. The *A*- to *C*-wave interval widens until an *A* wave is not followed by a *V* wave. There is a pause, and the sequence begins again. As the PR interval lengthens, the first heart sound diminishes in intensity.

Atrioventricular Wenckebach with junctional escape. The pause of the typical Wenckebach period is frequently interrupted with a junctional escape beat (Fig. 18-7) or, if digitalis is involved, with an accelerated junctional rhythm (Fig. 18-8).

In Fig. 18-7 the classic PR lengthening is evident, except that after the fourth P wave there is a junctional escape beat, which occurs at the same time as a sinus P wave and prevents that same P wave from being conducted.

The pauses in the tracing in Fig. 18-8 unmask an accelerated junctional focus.

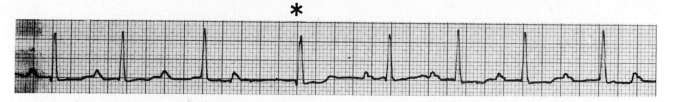

Fig. 18-7. Type I AV block with a junctional escape beat (*asterisk*). This is a common occurrence if the pause in the Wenckebach period is long enough. Junctional escape beats can confuse the diagnosis because they spoil the group beating pattern.

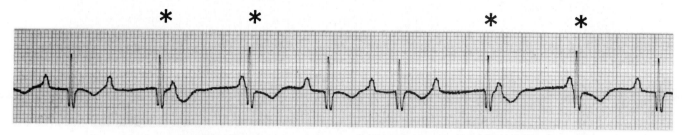

Fig. 18-8. Type I AV block with an underlying accelerated junctional rhythm (*asterisks*) resulting from digitalis intoxication. The accelerated focus in the AV junction is unmasked by the pauses. The clinical implications of this junctional rhythm are different from those of the normal junctional escape shown in Fig. 18-7.

The Wenckebach was the result of digitalis intoxication and so was the accelerated junctional rhythm. These Wenckebach periods might have had 3:2 conduction except for the interference from the junctional focus.

Atrioventricular Wenckebach and bigeminy. Fig. 18-9, *A,* illustrates a common Wenckebach conduction ratio, 3:2. This produces a bigeminal rhythm. The P waves are all sinus and right on time. The nonconducted P wave can be seen in the T waves before the pauses.

Fig. 18-9, *B,* is another bigeminal rhythm. The PR intervals are even lengthening. However, this bigeminal rhythm is caused by bigeminal premature atrial complexes (PACs). The second P wave of the group is premature and ectopic (− + instead of + − in shape).

Type II atrioventricular block

ECG recognition

PR intervals: The same from beat to beat and usually normal; some P waves are not conducted.

QRS complexes: Broad (0.12 sec or more).

The typical ECG of type II AV block is illustrated in Fig. 18-10. The clinical setting in this case was typical—acute anterior wall MI.

Mechanism. Type II AV block usually is within or below the bundle of His and is almost always associated with right bundle branch block (RBBB) and a long HV interval (greater than or equal to 950 ms).[2] The complete block of one bundle causes

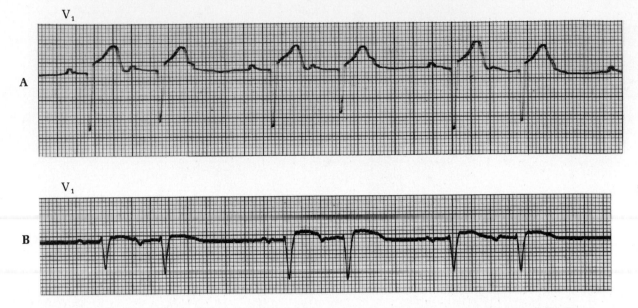

Fig. 18-9. Two bigeminal patterns with different causes. **A,** There is 3:2 AV Wenckebach. The P waves are on time, the PR lengthens, and there is a dropped beat. **B,** The second P of each group is a premature atrial complex (PAC), which looks like Wenckebach to the casual observer.

the ventricular complexes to be broad. Intermittent block of the other bundle causes dropped beats.

Clinical implications. Type II AV block is not as common as type I and is a more serious condition; disease is lower in the conduction system (at the level of the bundle branches). It often is later associated with Adams-Stokes syncope and deteriorates into complete AV block.[1] It is associated with anterior septal MI and chronic fibrotic disease of the conduction system. Its appearance in the setting of acute anteroseptal MI identifies a high-risk patient. Naccarelli et al.[4] called this particular form of heart block "treacherous and unpredictable." If the AV conduction deteriorates further, the complete heart block that results has a slow ventricular escape rhythm.

Physical signs. In type II AV block the diagnosis can be made as in type I, by observing the neck veins. There are intermittent *A* waves not followed by *V* waves. Because the PR intervals are fixed, the first heart sound maintains a constant intensity. The patient may have a sense of the heart skipping a beat.

Treatment. Most physicians insert a temporary pacemaker as soon as type II AV block is discovered. This is followed by insertion of a permanent pacemaker at a more convenient time. Such an approach has reduced the incidence of complete heart block, cardiac asystole, and sudden death in patients with type II second-degree AV block.[4]

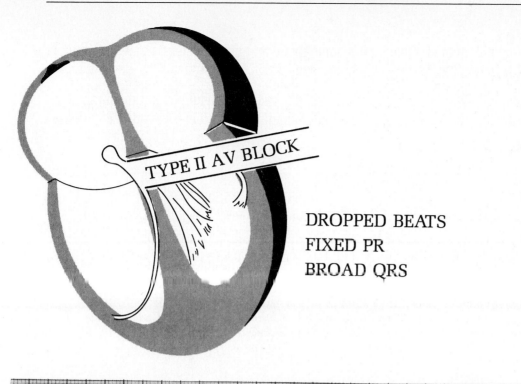

DROPPED BEATS
FIXED PR
BROAD QRS

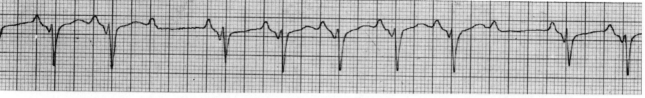

Fig. 18-10. In type II second-degree AV block the disease is in the bundle branches and is usually the result of anterior septal myocardial infarction.

Two-to-one atrioventricular block

ECG recognition

PR intervals: All the same; may be normal or prolonged. AV nodal disease is associated with a prolonged PR interval, whereas with subnodal disease the PR interval may be normal.

P waves: Sinus in origin.

AV conduction: There are two sinus P waves for every QRS.

QRS complex: May be narrow or broad. A narrow QRS is associated with AV nodal disease, and a broad QRS with disease in the bundle branches.

Compare Fig. 18-11, *A,* and Fig. 18-11, *B*. Both patients have 2:1 AV block, and both had acute MI, one of the inferior wall and right ventricle (Fig. 18-11, *A*) and the other of the anterior wall (Fig. 18-11, *B*). Both had profound bradycardia because of 2:1 AV block. The differences are in the clinical picture, the length of the PR interval, and the width of the QRS complexes. In the ECG with AV nodal disease there is a long PR interval and narrow QRS. In the ECG with disease in the bundle branches there is a normal PR and broad QRS.

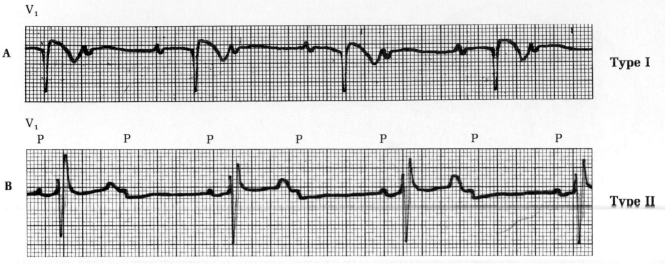

Fig. 18-11. Two-to-one AV block. **A,** Patient has inferior wall myocardial infarction with disease at the level of the AV node. The telltale long PR (0.20 sec) and narrow QRS are evident. **B,** Patient has anteroseptal myocardial infarction. The shorter PR interval and the broad QRS are evident.

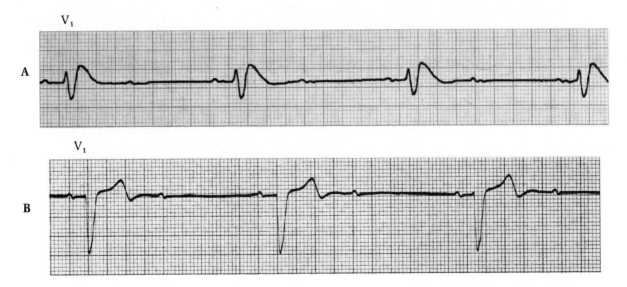

Fig. 18-12. **A** and **B,** signs of subnodal disease: 2:1 AV block with a broad QRS and a normal PR interval.

Two more tracings of type II AV block are shown in Fig. 18-12, *A* and *B*. These patients had acute anterior wall MI complicated by profound bradycardia (28 beats/min). When the anterior descending left coronary artery is involved, conduction problems are at the level of the bundle branches. In this case there is 2:1 block that is the result of involvement of the bundle branches. The diagnosis is made because of the clinical setting, normal PR interval, and the wide QRS.

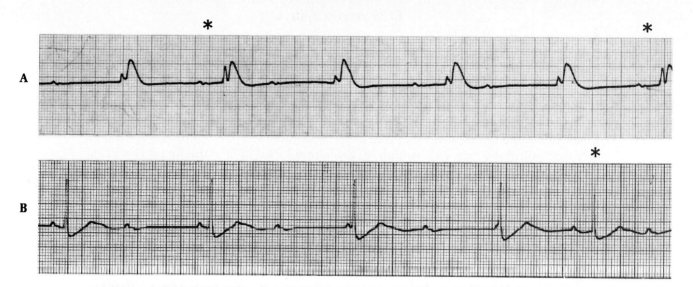

Fig. 18-13. High-grade second-degree AV block. **A,** There are only two sinus-conducted beats (*asterisks*), despite a sinus rate of 58 beats/min. **B,** Conduction occurs only at the (*asterisk*).

Mechanism. When the conduction ratio is 2:1, the disease may be nodal or subnodal, which may be determined by noninvasive interventions (discussed later in this chapter). Briefly, in AV nodal block, conduction improves with atropine, exercise, or catecholamines and worsens with carotid sinus massage. In subnodal block, conduction improves with carotid sinus massage and worsens with atropine, exercise, or catecholamines (Table 18-1).[2]

Clinical implications. The clinical implications depend on the level of block in the conduction system. Atrioventricular nodal disease is associated with acute inferior wall MI and, although the block may be complete, a pacemaker is usually not necessary. Subnodal disease is associated with acute anterior MI, and the patient may have syncope or hemodynamic deterioration. A temporary pacemaker may be indicated in a symptomatic patient with a broad QRS.

Physical signs. Two-to-one AV block may cause symptoms of bradycardia.

High-grade second-degree AV block

High-grade second-degree AV block is diagnosed when, at reasonable atrial rates of less than 135 beats/min, two or more consecutive atrial impulses fail to be conducted because of the block itself, not because of interference by an escaping subsidiary pacemaker.[3]

The tracing in Fig. 18-13, *A,* is from the same patient as that in Fig. 18-12, *A.* With a sinus rate of 58 beats/min, only two beats are conducted. In Fig. 18-13, *B,* conduction only takes place at the end of the tracing.

COMPLETE (THIRD-DEGREE) ATRIOVENTRICULAR BLOCK

Complete, or third-degree, AV block is diagnosed when no atrial impulses can be conducted to the ventricles. This is one form of AV dissociation.

ECG recognition

Atrial rhythm: Sinus or ectopic (atrial fibrillation or atrial flutter)

Ventricular rhythm: Independent (may be junctional or ventricular); usually regular, but may be irregular because of premature ventricular complexes (PVCs), a pacemaker shift, an escape pacemaker that has an irregular rhythm, or autonomic influences.

Ventricular rate: Depends on the level of block. Block proximal to the His bundle has an escape ventricular rate of 40 to 60 beats/min; acquired complete AV block has a ventricular rate of less than 40 beats/min.[1] The higher the focus is within the conduction system, the faster and the more dependable the ventricular rhythm is.

QRS duration: Depends on the level of block. A focus above the bifurcation of the His bundle produces a narrow QRS, as long as the bundle branches are conducting.

Pathology

Congenital third-degree AV block is usually located at the level of the AV node. In other cases the block may be located in the bundle of His or in the bilateral bundle branches (Fig. 18-14). The focus for the ventricles is usually located just below the block and may be above or below the His bundle bifurcation.

Clinical implications

In complete AV block the rate and dependability of the ventricular rhythm are related to the level of the lesion. An escape focus at the top of the bundle of His (nodal-His region) has a rate of about 55 beats/min, is relatively dependable, and often does not require insertion of a pacemaker. If the escape focus is at or below the branching portion of the bundle of His, however, the rate is slower and less dependable and the QRS is broad. Pacemaker insertion is often indicated.

Physical signs

Complete AV block may have all the symptoms of profound bradycardia, loss of atrial kick, and reduced cardiac output (presyncope, syncope, or angina).

Idiojunctional rhythm. Complete AV block with an idiojunctional rhythm is recognized because of narrow QRS complexes and AV dissociation. In Fig. 18-15 the P waves can be seen to occur regularly at a rate of 100 beats/min. They are totally independent of the ventricular rhythm (rate, 46 beats/min). The sinus node paces the atria, and the AV junction paces the ventricles. In congenital AV block the rate of the junction may be higher than 50 beats/min.

Idioventricular rhythm. Complete AV block with an idioventricular rhythm is recognized because of broad QRS complexes, AV dissociation, and a heart rate of less than 40 beats/min. In Fig. 18-16 the P waves are at a rate of 75 beats/min. They are regular and undisturbed by the ventricular rhythm of 36 beats/min.

NONINVASIVE EVALUATION OF THE SITE OF BLOCK

Since AV nodal block has a better prognosis and different treatment than subnodal block, it is important to determine the location of the block. The ECG supplies much information: a prolonged PR interval implicates the AV node, and a pro-

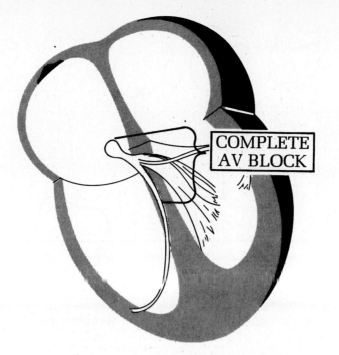

Fig. 18-14. Third-degree (complete) AV block may occur at the level of the AV node, the bundle of His, or the bundle branches.

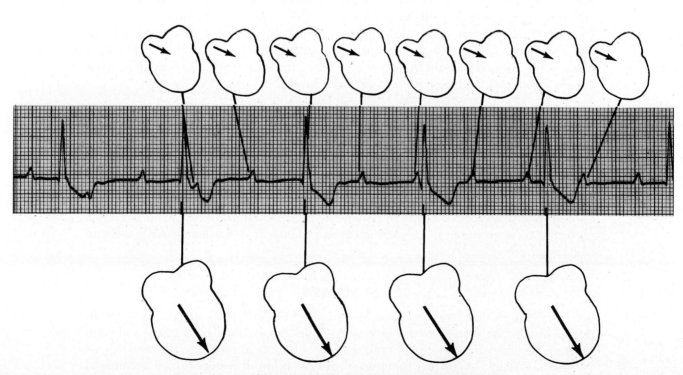

Fig. 18-15. Complete AV block with an idiojunctional rhythm.

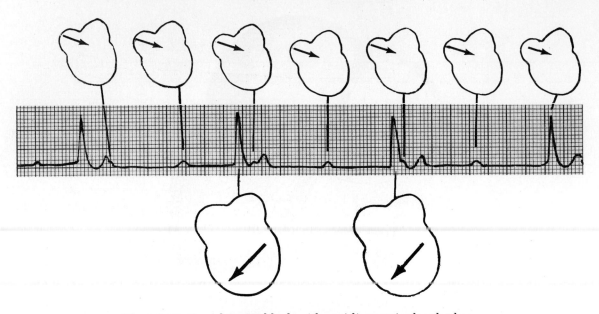

Fig. 18-16. Complete AV block with an idioventricular rhythm.

longed QRS duration implicates the bundle branches. Interventions that slow or improve AV conduction are also helpful. For example, if the sinus discharge and AV conduction are slowed with carotid sinus massage, the number of impulses reaching the bundle branches are fewer, so a block at that level should improve, whereas a block within the AV node would be compounded by such a maneuver. On the other hand, if the rate of the sinus node and the speed of AV conduction are increased with atropine, exercise, or catecholamines, impulses reach the bundle branches more frequently and would compound a block at that level, whereas a block at the AV node would be improved.[5] These three interventions tend to shorten the PR interval in both normal and diseased hearts.[4]

TREATMENT

In patients with symptomatic bradyarrhythmias, a temporary or permanent pacemaker is indicated. Appropriate drugs may be used until adequate pacing therapy can be initiated or if the block is likely to be temporary. For AV nodal disease, vagolytic agents such as atropine are used. Catecholamines such as isoproterenol may be used for AV block. In patients with acute MI, transcutaneous pacing is preferred to isoproterenol. In such cases isoproterenol is used only with extreme caution or not at all.[1]

SUMMARY

Atrioventricular block is conventionally divided into first-, second-, and third-degree block. The disease of first-degree AV block is commonly in the AV node and is recognized because the PR intervals are longer than 0.20 sec. Type I second-degree AV block (Wenckebach) is a function of the AV node. It is recognized because of group beating, lengthening PR intervals, shortening RR intervals, and dropped beats with pauses less than twice the shortest cycle. The QRS complex is narrow unless there is another problem in the bundle branches. In type II block the disease is in the bundle branches. It is recognized because of dropped beats, normal and fixed PR intervals, and broad QRS complexes.

In 2:1 AV block the disease may be either nodal or subnodal. This can be determined by His bundle electrogram, certain noninvasive techniques (atropine, exercise or catecholamines, and carotid sinus massage) and by the PR interval and QRS duration. In third-degree AV block the disease can be in the AV node, in the bundle of His, or in both bundle branches. The ECG shows AV dissociation and a slow idiojunctional or idioventricular rhythm.

REFERENCES

1. Zipes DP: Specific arrhythmias: diagnosis and treatment. In Braunwald E, ed: *Heart disease*, ed 4, Philadelphia, 1992, WB Saunders.
2. Lie KI, Durrer D: Acute and chronic aspects of conduction disturbances in acute myocardial infarction. In Befeler B, Lazzara R, Scherlag BJ, eds: *Selected topics in cardiac arrhythmias*, Mount Kisco, NY, 1980, Futura.
3. Willerson JT: Introduction: cardiac signs and symptoms. In Willerson JT, Cohn JN, eds: *Cardiovascular medicine*, New York, 1995, Churchill Livingstone.
4. Naccarelli GV, Willerson JT, Blomqvist CG: Recognition and physiologic treatment of cardiac arrhythmias and conduction disturbances. In Willerson JT, Cohn JN, eds: *Cardiovascular medicine*, New York, 1995, Churchill Livingstone.
5. Wellens HJJ, Conover M: *The ECG in emergency decision making*, Philadelphia, 1992, WB Saunders.

19

Potassium Derangements

Major Cellular Antiarrhythmic Functions   Hyperkalemia   *279*
  of Potassium   *276*   Summary   *283*
Hypokalemia   *276*

Potassium is excreted by the body in the urine, feces, and perspiration. Diuretics, vomiting, diaphoresis, and diarrhea can rapidly deplete the body of this vital ion (hypokalemia). Conversely, anuria can cause a potassium buildup (hyperkalemia). Both conditions may produce serious arrhythmias and even death. The potassium gradient across the membrane, along with the intracellular negativity generated by the sodium-potassium pump activity, determines conduction velocity and helps to confine pacing activity to the sinus node.

MAJOR CELLULAR ANTIARRHYTHMIC FUNCTIONS OF POTASSIUM

Potassium contributes to important antiarrhythmic functions as follows[1]:

1. Potassium prevents the action potential duration (and QT) from being too short (steady-state inward potassium ion [K^+] current).
2. Potassium accommodates rapid heart rates by shortening the QT interval (The delayed outward K^+ current fails to deactivate during electrical diastole in tachycardia.)
3. Potassium protects excitability in cases of hyperpolarization. (There is an increased influx of K^+ when the cell becomes too negative.)
4. Potassium slows the heart rate by increasing inward K^+ flux in response to parasympathetic stimulation. This inhibits postsynaptic potentials.

HYPOKALEMIA
ECG recognition

Progressive ST depression.
Progressive decrease in T-wave amplitude.
Advanced stage:
  Increase in U-wave amplitude. (The T and U waves fuse.)
  Increase in the amplitude and duration of the QRS interval.
  Increase in the amplitude and duration of the P wave.
  Slight prolongation of the PR interval.

Signs and symptoms

The following signs and symptoms of hypokalemia involve almost every system of the body:

Muscular: Weakness and atrophy.

Neurological: Tetany.

Cerebral: Irritability, lethargy, hallucinations, apathy, drowsiness, confusion, delirium, and coma. (The EEG is usually normal.)

Gastrointestinal: Nausea, vomiting, and ileus.

Carbohydrate metabolism: Impairment of glucose tolerance.

Renal: Symptoms result from the inability to concentrate urine (nocturia, polyuria, and polydipsia). Other renal manifestations of hypokalemia are related to the inability to maximally acidify urine because of stimulation of the production of massive amounts of renal ammonia by the hypokalemic kidney.

Treatment

The patient should, of course, have continuous monitoring with the ECG; repeatedly, potassium blood levels should be measured, and physical signs of hypokalemia (muscular weakness or paralysis) should be evaluated. Treatment consists of an increased dietary intake of or supplementation with potassium salts when possible.

Severe potassium deficiency. Intravenous (IV) potassium chloride is given (40- to 60-mEq/L concentrations at 20 mEq/hour, approximately 200 to 250 mEq/day).[4]

Prevention

The loss of potassium in patients taking diuretics can be minimized by using short-acting diuretics and by using the smallest effective dose.

HYPERKALEMIA
ECG recognition

The ECG changes resulting from hyperkalemia are shown in Figs. 19-3 to 19-7. If hyperkalemia is associated with sodium derangements, the duration of the QRS may be affected, hyponatremia prolonging and hypernatremia shortening it.

The ECG changes that occur as the degree of hyperkalemia progresses from mild to severe are listed next.

Mild hyperkalemia (less than 6.5 mEq/L)
1. Tall tented T wave (5.7 mEq/L), often symmetric with a narrow base; usually best seen in leads II, III, V_2, and V_4. The corrected QT (QTc) interval is not prolonged.[5]
2. Normal P wave and QRS complex.

Moderate hyperkalemia (6.5 to 8 mEq/L)
1. The QRS complex broadens. There is a wide S wave in the left precordial leads.
2. The QRS axis shifts superiorly (left axis deviation).
3. The ST segment deviates or disappears; that is, the terminal S wave becomes continuous with the tall tented T wave.
4. P wave amplitude and duration decrease (7 mEq/L).

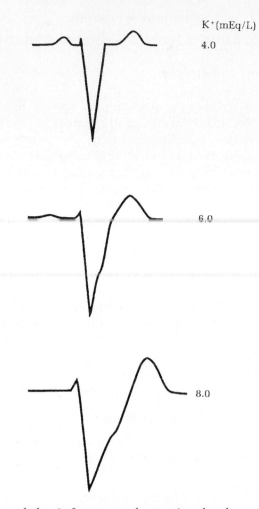

K⁺(mEq/L)

4.0

6.0

8.0

Fig. 19-3. Stages in hyperkalemia from normal potassium levels to plasma levels of 8 mEq/L. At 6 mEq/L the P wave flattens, the QRS broadens, and the ST segment disappears, with the S wave flowing into the tall tented T wave. At 8 mEq/L the P wave has disappeared and the QRS is even broader, with the S wave fusing with the T wave. *(From Wellens HJJ, Conover M: The ECG in emergency decision making, Philadelphia, 1991, WB Saunders.)*

K⁺ 6.8

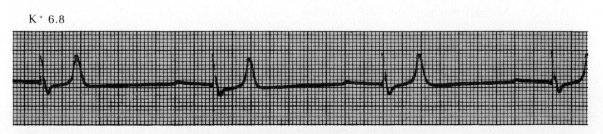

Fig. 19-4. Serum potassium level of 6.8 mEq/L.

K⁺ 7.3

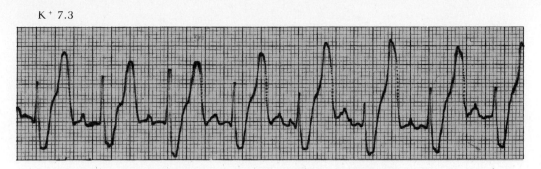

Fig. 19-5. Serum potassium level of 7.3 mEq/L.

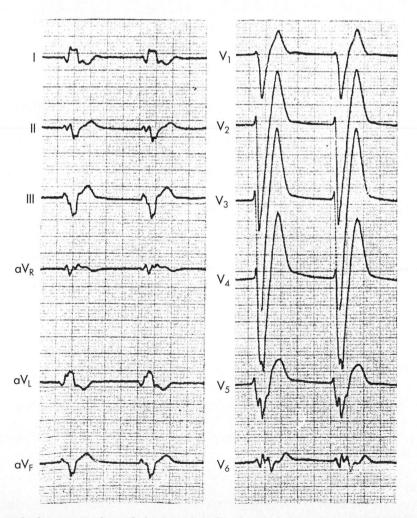

Fig. 19-6. Life-threatening hyperkalemia. Note the absence of P waves, broad QRS, left axis shift, lack of ST segment (in V_1 to V_5) and peaked T waves. *(Courtesy Hein JJ Wellers M.D.)*

II

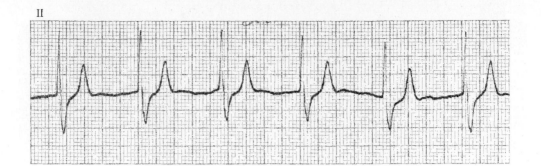

Fig. 19-7. Hyperkalemia. Serum potassium level of 8.3 mEq/L.

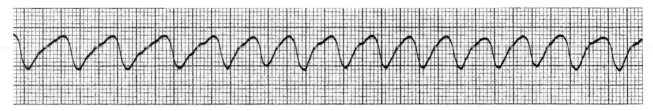

Fig. 19-8. The sine wave that occurs as a terminal event in hyperkalemia.

Fig. 19-4 is a tracing of moderate hyperkalemia. The QRS of 0.14 sec, the flattening of the P wave and long PR interval, and, of course, the tall tented T wave can be seen. The patient whose ECG tracing you see in Fig. 19-5 had a plasma potassium concentration of 7.3 mEq/L. In Fig. 19-5 the P wave has not yet flattened, but the distinctive merging of the ST segment with the tall tented T wave is apparent.

Severe hyperkalemia (greater than 8 mEq/L)
1. P wave duration increases, prolonging the PR interval.
2. P waves eventually disappear.
3. The QRS is broad and continuous with the T wave.
4. The QRS axis shifts.

There have been several reported cases of profound hyperkalemia without ECG manifestations.[6,7]

Fig. 19-6 is a 12-lead ECG from a patient with a potassium plasma concentration of 8.4 mEq/L. The absence of P waves, broad QRS, absence of ST segment, and left axis deviation are evident. Fig. 19-7 is a rhythm strip in lead II from a patient with a potassium plasma concentration of 8.3 mEq/L. Note the absent P waves, broad QRS, and tented T waves. In Fig. 19-8 an ECG that occurs before death is shown.

Treatment

Mild hyperkalemia. Identify and eliminate the cause, if possible. The usual cause of hyperkalemia is renal disease.

Moderate or severe hyperkalemia
1. Intravenous infusion of calcium gluconate, which immediately and briefly alters the effects of the excess potassium on the cellular membranes without lowering the plasma potassium concentration.

2. Intravenous infusion of glucose and sodium bicarbonate, which decrease the toxic effect of potassium by shifting potassium into the cells, even in patients who are not acidotic.
3. Administration of cation exchange resins.
4. In renal failure, hemodialysis or peritoneal dialysis.

Dosages

1. Calcium gluconate solution (10%), 10 to 30 ml IV infusion over 1 to 5 min with constant ECG monitoring).
2. Hypertonic glucose solution (10%), 200 ml to 500 ml in 30 min and 500 ml to 1000 ml over the next several hours.
3. Sodium bicarbonate (2 to 3 ampules) added to 1 liter 5% dextrose in 0.9% saline.

SUMMARY

Potassium is one of the most important ions in the body, serving in many antiarrhythmic roles at the cellular level, including control of action potential duration at different heart rates, protection of the excitability of the cell in cases of hyperpolarization, and serving as an important link in parasympathetic stimulation.

REFERENCES

1. Pennefather P, Cohen IS: Molecular mechanisms of cardiac K$^+$ channel regulation. In Zipes DP, Jalife J, eds: *Cardiac electrophysiology from cell to bedside,* Philadelphia, 1990, WB Saunders.
2. Aronson RS: Delayed afterdepolarizations and pathological states. In Rosen MR, Janse MJ, Wit AL, eds: *Cardiac electrophysiology,* Mount Kisco, NY, 1990, Futura.
3. Rosen MR: Cellular electrophysiology of digitalis toxicity, *J Am Coll Cardiol* 5:22A, 1985.
4. Wellens HJJ, Conover M: *The ECG in emergency decision making,* Philadelphia, 1992, WB Saunders.
5. Fisch C: Electrocardiography and vectorcardiography. In Braunwald E, ed: *Heart disease,* ed 4 Philadelphia, 1992, WB Saunders.
6. Szerlip HM, Weiss J, Singer J: Profound hyperkalemia without ECG manifestations, *Am J Kidney Dis* 7:461, 1986.
7. Hylander B: Survival of extreme hyperkalemia, *Acta Med Scand* 221:121, 1987.

20

Atrioventricular Dissociation

Causes   *284*
Physical Findings   *284*
Treatment   *285*
Sinus Bradycardia and Atrioventricular
   Dissociation   *285*
Nonparoxysmal Junctional Tachycardia
   With Atrioventricular
   Dissociation   *287*

Accelerated Idioventricular Rhythm With
   Atrioventricular Dissociation   *288*
Atrioventricular Block and
   Atrioventricular Dissociation   *289*
Summary   *291*

Atrioventricular (AV) dissociation is the independent beating of atria and ventricles. It is never a primary disorder but is always the result of a basic disturbance in impulse formation or conduction. Five main causes of AV dissociation are listed and a few examples are shown in this chapter.

CAUSES

1. Sinus bradycardia or sinus arrhythmia with a junctional escape rhythm. The activity of the escape pacemaker is not abnormal.
2. Acceleration of a latent pacemaker (nonparoxysmal junctional tachycardia, an accelerated idioventricular rhythm, or ventricular tachycardia). Such activity from latent pacemakers is pathologic.
3. Complete AV block.
4. Any combination of the first three causes listed.

PHYSICAL FINDINGS

1. Irregular cannon A waves in the jugular pulse.
2. Varying intensity of the first heart sound.
3. Beat-to-beat changes in systolic blood pressure.

   Any of the preceding clues indicates AV dissociation, although the absence of these clues does not rule out AV dissociation. For example, in atrial fibrillation with ventricular tachycardia (VT) there is AV dissociation without its usual physical or ECG signs. The physiologic aspects of the physical signs of AV dissociation have already been discussed on p. 284.

TREATMENT

Atrioventricular dissociation itself is not treated, since it is merely a symptom. The physician treats the underlying cause of the AV dissociation. For example, the treatment of VT with AV dissociation differs vastly from that of AV dissociation caused by complete AV block or sinus bradycardia and junctional tachycardia caused by digitalis intoxication.

SINUS BRADYCARDIA AND ATRIOVENTRICULAR DISSOCIATION
ECG recognition

The tracings in Fig. 20-1 are of AV dissociation caused by sinus bradycardia. In Fig. 20-1, *A*, the first four beats are junctional. (The sinus P wave is hidden within the QRS.) The P wave can be seen emerging from the third QRS as the sinus rate

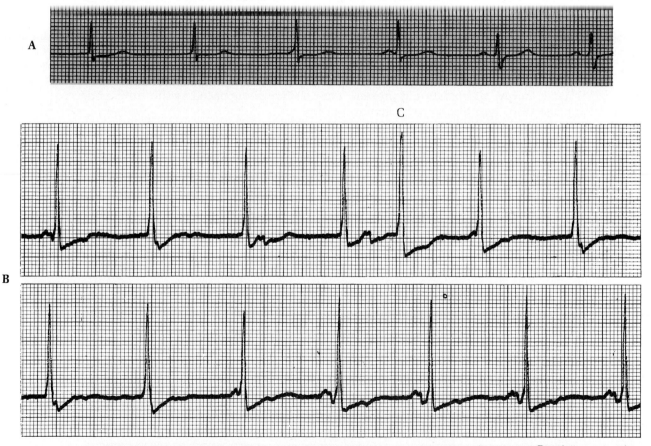

Continuous tracing

Fig. 20-1. Sinus bradycardia with atrioventricular (AV) dissociation. **A,** The sinus rate and that of the escape junctional focus are approximately the same. As a result, the junctional focus sometimes takes over. Note how the morphologic appearances of the junctional and sinus-conducted ventricular complexes differ. **B,** The sinus rate is 53 beats/min, and the junctional rate is 58 beats/min; AV dissociation results. There is capture *(C)* whenever the RP interval is long enough, in this case, 0.20 sec. There is acceleration of the junctional rate after the capture beat, a sign of triggered activity. This and the sinus bradycardia are signs of digitalis intoxication.

speeds up a little. By the fourth complex the sinus P wave is clearly visible in front of the QRS but is not conducted to the ventricles because the junctional focus escapes before the sinus P wave can be conducted into the bundle of His. By the fifth complex the sinus node has increased its rate enough to allow its impulse to be conducted to the ventricles (capture). In Fig. 20-1, *B,* the sinus rate is 53 beats/min and the junction is beating at 58 beats/min; there is one capture beat (Fig. 20-1, *C,*). Whenever the sinus P wave is far enough beyond the R (RP of 0.20 sec in this case), there is conduction. The capture beat resets the junctional rhythm.

The difference in morphologic appearance between the sinus-conducted beats and the junctional escape beats is evident in Fig. 20-1, *A.* Occasionally the junctional escape focus is a little offset within the nodal-His region. As a result, the wave front emanating from the ectopic focus is not precisely the same as it is for sinus-conducted beats. The resultant difference in morphologic appearance of the junctional escape complexes, when it exists, allows one to easily know at a glance when there is capture and when there is not.

Mechanism

When the sinus node slows to a rate below that of the AV junction, a junctional escape rhythm normally takes over as pacemaker of the ventricles. If the junctional focus does not have retrograde conduction to the atria, the term *idiojunctional* is used, and AV dissociation is present. The atria are being paced by the sinus node, and the ventricles by the AV junction.

Clinical implications

The clinical implications of AV dissociation resulting from bradycardia are those of the bradycardia and the loss of the atrial contribution to ventricular filling (the atrial kick). If the patient is tolerating this arrhythmia (has no symptoms related to hemodynamic impairment), no intervention is indicated.

V$_1$

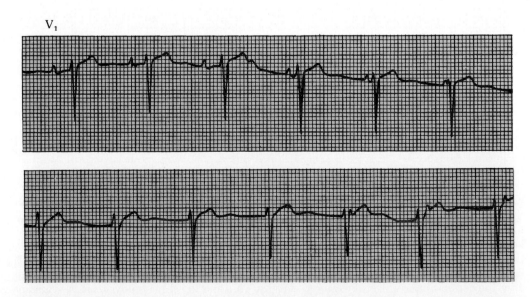

Fig. 20-2. Nonparoxysmal junctional tachycardia with AV dissociation (continuous strip).

NONPAROXYSMAL JUNCTIONAL TACYHYCARDIA WITH ATRIOVENTRICULAR DISSOCIATION
ECG recognition

Fig. 20-2 shows AV dissociation caused by nonparoxysmal junctional tachycardia. The first four beats are sinus conducted. By the fourth complex, although the sinus P wave is clearly visible in front of the QRS, it is not conducted to the ventricles because the junctional focus fires, causing the PR interval to shorten. The nonparoxysmal junctional tachycardia continues to overtake the sinus rhythm so that in the last three complexes the sinus P wave emerges behind the QRS.

Fig. 20-3 is another tracing of AV dissociation caused by nonparoxysmal junctional tachycardia. The junctional rate of 77 beats/min is unmasked in the presence of a sinus rate of 82 beats/min because of the pause following a premature atrial complex (PAC). Once the junctional rhythm gains control, there is a long period of isorhythmic AV dissociation during which both rates are almost identical. Aberrancy of junctional beats is evident in Fig. 20-3. Notice the marked difference in shape between the sinus-conducted beats and the junctional ones. Some of the junctional beats look broader than others because they are distorted by the isorhythmic sinus P waves.

Mechanism

When the AV junction accelerates to a rate greater than that of the sinus node, AV dissociation results. The sinus node paces the atria, and the junctional focus paces the ventricles. A common cause is digitalis intoxication.

Clinical implications

The clinical implications of AV dissociation caused by nonparoxysmal junctional tachycardia are those of the accelerated focus and the hemodynamic conse-

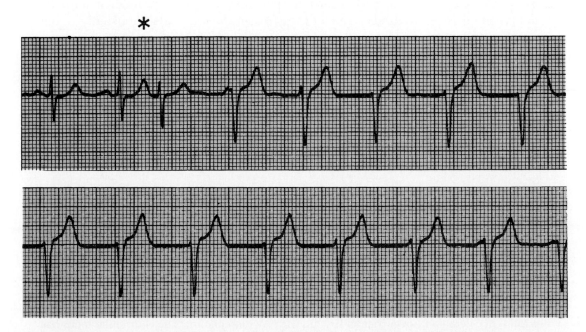

Fig. 20-3. A nonparoxysmal junctional tachycardia is unmasked by the pause following a premature atrial complex (PAC) (*asterisk*) (continuous strip).

quences of the loss of atrial kick. If digitalis intoxication is a factor, digitalis should be discontinued and the patient should be confined to bed (no sympathetic stimulation). Potassium levels should be checked and corrected. Another precipitating factor may be excessive catecholamines.

ACCELERATED IDIOVENTRICULAR RHYTHM WITH ATRIOVENTRICULAR DISSOCIATION
ECG recognition

Fig. 20-4 shows AV dissociation caused by an accelerated idioventricular rhythm. The fourth (and perhaps the third) and fifth beats are fusion beats (Fig. 20-4, *A*), as is the last beat in Fig. 20-4, *B*. The rhythm begins with a long coupling interval, a typical beginning for this reperfusion arrhythmia. The ECG typically shows the following:

1. Three or more successive ventricular ectopic beats
2. A rate of 50 to 120 beats/min
3. A long coupling interval to begin with
4. AV dissociation

Fig. 20-5 is an interesting tracing of atrial flutter with an accelerated idioventricular rhythm. In Fig. 20-5, *A*, there are three capture beats, the first of which is a fusion beat. In Fig. 20-5, *B*, the signs of AV dissociation during atrial flutter can be seen. The flutter-R relationship is changing with every ventricular beat. In atrial flutter with an intact AV conduction this relationship either is the same each time or alternates because of Wenckebach.

Mechanism

When a ventricular pacemaker accelerates to a rate greater than that of the sinus node, AV dissociation may result or there may be 1:1 retrograde conduction to the atria and therefore no AV dissociation. When the rate of a ventricular focus is greater than 40 beats/min, it is accelerated but does not become evident until its rate exceeds that of the sinus node. For this reason fusion beats are usually at the beginning and end of the run of ventricular beats.

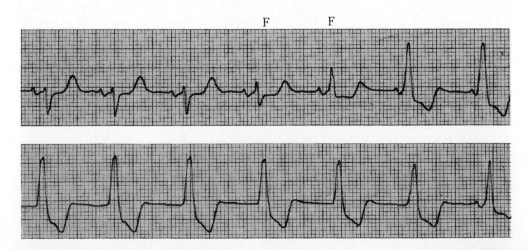

Fig. 20-4. Accelerated idioventricular rhythm with AV dissociation. The ventricular focus has a rate that is about the same as the sinus node and takes over with two (or three) fusion beats *(F).*

F

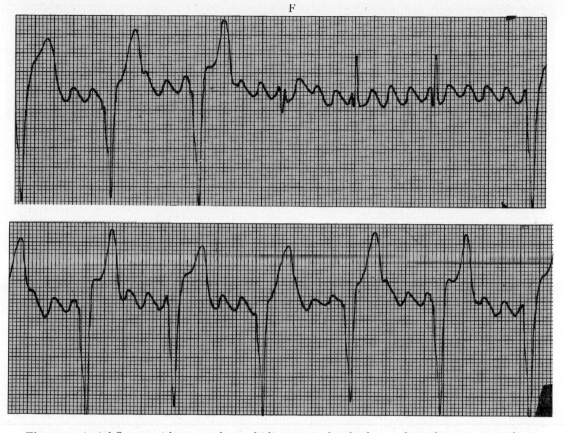

Fig. 20-5. Atrial flutter with an accelerated idioventricular rhythm and AV dissociation. There is one fusion beat *(F)*.

Clinical implications

Accelerated idioventricular rhythm with atrioventricular dissociation is often seen in the setting of acute myocardial infarction and is thought to be a reperfusion arrhythmia (spontaneous or following thrombolysis). No treatment is necessary unless associated with hemodynamic impairment.

Physical signs

When the ventricular rate is faster than the atrial rate, as seen in Fig. 20-4, the intensity of the first heart sound increases as the PR interval shortens, until finally there is a very loud sound ("bruit de canon") followed by a sudden softening in intensity. As the P waves "march through" the QRS, atrial and ventricular contractions coincide, causing a giant *A* wave in the jugular pulse.

ATRIOVENTRICULAR BLOCK AND ATRIOVENTRICULAR DISSOCIATION
ECG recognition

Complete AV block is recognized on the ECG because of total absence of conduction in the face of opportunities to conduct; that is, the rates of both pacemakers are not too fast. Fig. 20-6 is a tracing from a patient with complete AV block.

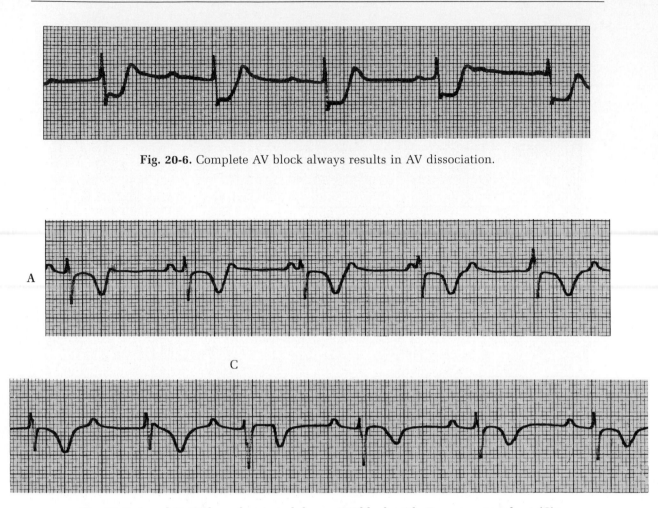

Fig. 20-6. Complete AV block always results in AV dissociation.

Fig. 20-7. A and **B,** High-grade, second-degree AV block with, **B,** one capture beat *(C).*

The atrial rate is 90 beats/min, and the ventricles are under the control of an idio-junctional focus at a rate of 50 beats/min. The first three P waves are far enough after the preceding T wave to have conducted, and yet they did not.

    Fig. 20-7, *A* and *B,* shows AV dissociation resulting from AV block. This time the block is not complete. Notice the conducted (capture) beat (Fig. 20-7, *B*). The atrial rate is 95 beats/min, and the junctional escape rate is 49 beats/min. When the RP interval is at least 0.68 sec, conduction takes place with a PR interval of 0.35 sec.

Mechanism

    Total AV block is included here for completeness. It is discussed more fully in Chapter 15. The term *complete AV block* or *third-degree AV block* implies the existence of a pathologic obstruction to conduction; the term *AV dissociation* does not. Atrioventricular dissociation means that the atria and the ventricles are under two different pacemakers. This could be due to any number of reasons, physiologic or pathologic. Thus, although complete AV block causes AV dissociation, AV dissociation is not necessarily complete AV block.

Clinical implications

The clinical implications of complete AV block depend on where the block is located. If it occurs early in the setting of inferior wall myocardial infarction, it is transient and is thought to be the result of increased parasympathetic tone or sudden ischemia that is relieved by the opening of the collateral circulation. This type of block responds to atropine or isoproterenol. Atrioventricular block that occurs late in the course of the myocardial infarction appears to be the result of metabolic alteration within the AV node caused by ischemia. A pacemaker may be indicated if there is hemodynamic impairment. In the setting of acute anterior wall myocardial infarction the clinical implications of complete AV block are ominous because the block is usually at the level of the bundle branches and requires a pacemaker.

SUMMARY

Atrioventricular dissociation is always the result of another condition such as sinus bradycardia, an accelerated lower pacemaker, or AV block. The clinical implications are evaluated according to the primary condition.

21

Fusion Complexes

Mechanisms   *292*   Atrial Fusion   *295*

ECG Recognition   *292*   Summary   *295*

Ventricular Fusion   *293*

In electrocardiography the term *fusion* is used to indicate that two vectors from two different foci have collided within the muscle mass of either the ventricle (ventricular fusion) or the atrium (atrial fusion).

MECHANISMS

When two opposing currents collide, they cancel each other out, causing a complex that is narrower or of lower amplitude than the ectopic beat alone. When the depolarization process is initiated from two different sites within the atria or the ventricles (Fig. 21-1), opposing cell masses have the same electrical potential. Therefore the mean vector can never at any moment in the process be very large, because it is the difference in potential within the muscle mass being activated that determines its strength. Of course, this difference in potential varies in accordance with how much muscle mass is captured by each opposing force.

Atrial fusion beats occur when an ectopic atrial focus and the sinus node discharge simultaneously or almost simultaneously (Fig. 21-1, *A*). Ventricular fusion beats occur when an ectopic ventricular focus discharges at the same time or almost the same time that normal conduction begins in the ventricles (Fig. 21-1, *B*).

ECG RECOGNITION

The principal ECG signs of fusion are as follows:
1. Complexes of low amplitude, caused by two vectors canceling each other out.
2. Complexes of shorter duration than that of the ectopic beats, seen both in atrial fusion beats and in ventricular fusion beats. The presence of two electrical forces causes the depolarization process to be completed more quickly.

The PR interval may be shorter or of the same duration as that of the underlying sinus rhythm, because fusion can take place as long as the sinus impulse is still traveling when the ectopic impulse discharges, or as long as the sinus impulse can enter the ventricles before the ectopic one is finished.

VENTRICULAR FUSION

In Fig. 21-2 an end-diastolic premature ventricular complex (PVC) is not early enough to completely capture the ventricles. The ectopic vector begins to activate the ventricles at almost the same time that the normal vector begins its course in the interventricular septum. The electrical forces thus cancel each other out, and a complex of lesser amplitude is produced. The duration of the depolarization process has been shortened from 0.12 to 0.05 sec. Notice also in Fig. 21-2 that the aberrant ventricular activity has caused an aberrant T wave.

Ventricular fusion beats are often seen at the beginning and end of an accelerated idioventricular rhythm. Because the rate of the idioventricular rhythm is often approximately the same as that of the sinus node, if the sinus node slows down only slightly the ventricular ectopic focus will discharge at the same time and the two forces will collide within the ventricle. Fig. 21-3 illustrates such a rhythm. The

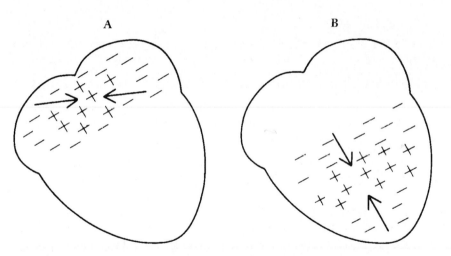

Fig. 21-1. A, Atrial fusion. **B,** Ventricular fusion.

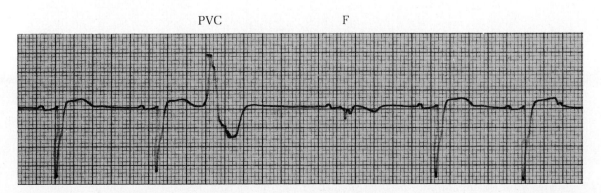

Fig. 21-2. Ventricular fusion *(F)*.

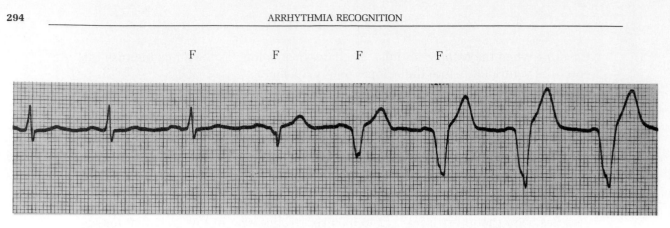

Fig. 21-3. An accelerated idioventricular rhythm. Note the changing shape of the fusion beats *(F)* as the ventricular ectopic focus dominates more completely with each beat.

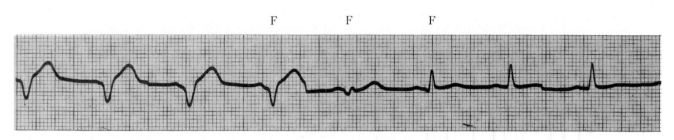

Fig. 21-4. An accelerated idioventricular rhythm. Note the three fusion beats *(F)* as the sinus-conducted impulse captures more and more of the ventricles until finally the ventricular ectopic focus is closed out altogether.

MCL₁

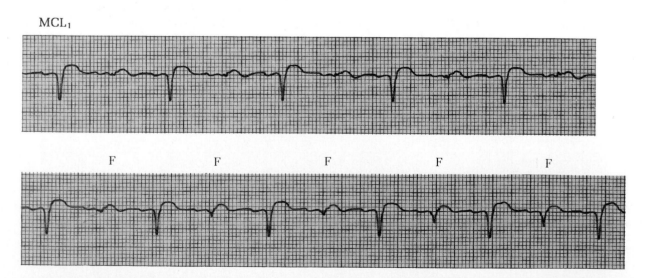

Fig. 21-5. Bigeminal end-diastolic premature ventricular complexes (PVCs) that are all fusion beats *(F)* (continuous strip).

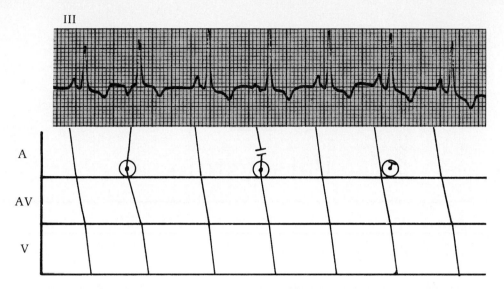

Fig. 21-6. Atrial fusion resulting from atrial parasystole. The fourth P wave is a fusion beat. The laddergram below the tracing depicts the mechanism. The atrial parasystolic focus is circled in the atrial (*A*) tier; note that the first atrial parasystolic force completely captures the atria, the second is a fusion beat, and the third is not manifested at all because of a perceding sinus beat and atrial refractoriness. In A tier the sinus conducted beats slant down and forward. Atrioventricular conduction is depicted in the AV tier. Ventricular conduction is normal, as shown in the V tier. *(From the Dr. Alan Lindsay Collection.)*

first two beats are probably totally sinus conducted. Notice the subtle difference in the shape of the third beat, a difference that you would not even notice were it not for what followed. The next three beats are also fusion beats. Note how the ectopic forces dominate more and more in each successive beat as the sinus-conducted impulse loses control of the ventricles. Fig. 21-4 (from another patient) illustrates the end of an accelerated idioventricular rhythm.

There probably is no other tracing as confusing to look at as that of a bigeminal end-diastolic PVC because such beats are usually fusion beats. Such a tracing is shown in Fig. 21-5. Some complexes are so isoelectric that only the T wave can be seen. If you "walk out" the P waves, you will find them to be right on time.

ATRIAL FUSION

Atrial fusion is shown in Fig. 21-6. In this case there is a parasystolic focus in the atria that happens to fire almost simultaneously with the sinus node, producing a fusion beat.

SUMMARY

Fusion beats, which can occur within the atria or the ventricles, are the result of the presence of two opposing currents within the same chamber. The two currents originate from two different places in the heart; usually one is normal and the other ectopic. The collision of forces results in an ECG complex that looks neither normal nor ectopic but is something in between, often narrower and of lesser amplitude than either the normal or the ectopic beat.

C H A P T E R
22
Parasystole

ECG in Parasystole   *296*   Mechanism   *298*
Modulated Parasystole   *297*   Clinical Implications   *300*

A parasystolic rhythm results from an ectopic focus surrounded by an area that protects it from being discharged by the depolarizations of the surrounding tissue. Such a focus can originate anywhere in the heart (atria, atrioventricular [AV] junction, ventricles), the most common location being ventricular. Two forms of parasystole have been described: "pure" and modulated.

Pure parasystole is sometimes called "traditional" or "classic." In the past, such a parasystolic focus was believed to be completely protected by an area of depressed excitability (entrance block) and uninfluenced by surrounding depolarizations. However, since the initial microelectrode studies of Jalife and Moe,[1] many investigators have shown that such an assumption cannot be made. According to Castellanos[1] group,[2,8] if impulses can exit across such a depressed zone, it is likely that the parasystolic focus is subject to some degree of modulation by electrotonic depolarizations arising in the surrounding tissue.

ECG IN PARASYSTOLE
No fixed coupling

Ventricular ectopic beats are often exactly coupled to the preceding complex. The parasystolic beat is usually not linked to a preceding beat; it is independent. An exeption is when the nonparasystolic rhythm modifies the parasystolic rate so that there is exact coupling (entrainment). That is, the parasystolic rate is changed so that it equals the nonparasystolic rate.[2]

Fusion beats

An occasional fusion beat is also a feature of parasystole, given a long enough tracing. If the parasystole is ventricular, the fusion beats result because the ectopic focus discharges just before or just as the sinus-conducted beat enters the ventricles. If the parasystole is atrial, fusion beats result because the ectopic focus discharges at the same time as or just before the sinus node. The fusion beats, obviously happenstance, are not necessary for making the diagnosis of parasystole.

Interectopic intervals

Some of the time the parasystolic focus may beat without being influenced in electrotonic fashion by the sinus (or dominant) rhythm. At such times the minimal time interval between interectopic beats is an exact multiple of longer time intervals. After what appears to be the minimal interval in a suspected tracing has been identified, the parasystolic rhythm can be "walked out." When the ventricles (or the atria in the case of atrial parasystole) are nonrefractory, an ectopic complex appears. Failure of the parasystolic impulse to appear when expected is called "exit block."

MODULATED PARASYSTOLE

A parasystolic focus is said to be modulated when its regular rhythm is disrupted by impulses arising in the surrounding tissues. In such a case, subthreshold electrotonic depolarizations are transmitted across the depressed barrier, prolonging or shortening the parasystolic cycle, depending on the amplitude of the electrotonic event and the relationship of the parasystolic and sinus beats to each other. If the sinus beat occurs early in phase 4 of the parasystolic rhythm, the next parasystolic beat is delayed. If the sinus beat occurs late in phase 4 of the parasystolic rhythm, the next parasystolic beat is early because it is captured by the invading impulse. The latter occurs because late in phase 4 the parasystolic focus is closer to threshold potential and a partial depolarization at this time across the zone of protection causes the parasystolic focus to fire prematurely.[2-6,10] In fact, a parasystolic focus can actually be entrained by the dominant pacemaker, causing fixed coupling of the parasystolic beat to the sinus beat.[3-5]

Fig. 22-1 is an example of classic ventricular parasystole. The ventricular ectopic beats have variable coupling intervals, there is a fusion complex (F), and the interectopic intervals are multiples of a common denominator. However, given a longer tracing, modulation of the rhythm would probably be demonstrated.

Fig. 22-2 shows atrial parasystole, which is less common and more difficult to diagnose than the ventricular variety. In the case shown in Fig. 22-2 a diagnosis is even more difficult because the parasystolic P waves are almost identical in shape to the sinus P waves. Recently a modulated parasystole originating in the sinoatrial (SA) node has been described.[1] The tracing in Fig. 22-2 is of atrial parasystole and may well be such a case. It fulfills the criteria given: (1) premature P waves having contour identical to sinus P waves, (2) variable coupling intervals, and (3) PP inter-

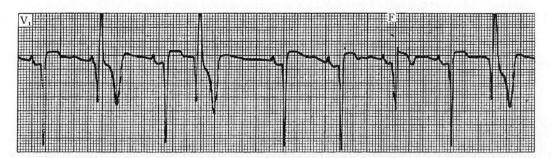

Fig. 22-1. Classic ventricular parasystole. The fusion beat *(F)* and the variable coupling intervals of the ectopic beats are evident. The interectopic intervals have a common denominator.

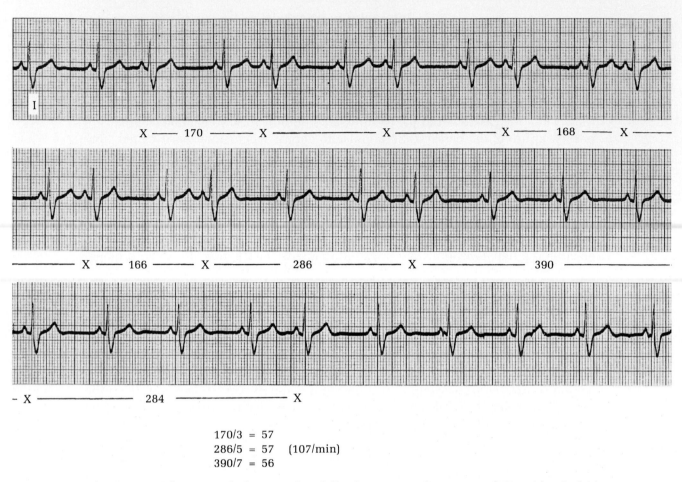

$$170/3 = 57$$
$$286/5 = 57 \quad (107/\text{min})$$
$$390/7 = 56$$

Fig. 22-2. Atrial parasystole (sinoatrial nodal). The parasystolic P waves *(X)* are identical in shape to the sinus P waves, there is no exact coupling, the interectopic intervals have a common denominator, and the parasystolic P wave resets the sinus node. *(Courtesy Dr. Alan Lindsay.)*

vals of the parasystolic-sinus pair not longer than the PP intervals of the sinus rhythm.

Modulated parasystole is shown in Fig. 22-3. The intrinsic cycle length of the ectopic parasystolic pacemaker is assumed to be 1300 ms. Modulation of the pacemaker was assessed only in bigeminal and trigeminal groupings.

MECHANISM

Parasystole is caused by a focus of altered automaticity or triggered activity.[2] This focus is surrounded by an area of protection, an abnormality that should not be confused with normal refractoriness. A variety of mechanisms have been postulated to explain the protected zone surrounding the ectopic focus. Although the ectopic focus is protected, it is not totally immune to the electrical activity going on around it and may change its rhythm because of what is called *electrotonic modulation*. When an impulse meets with the area of protection around the parasystolic focus, electrotonic potentials may be transmitted across the depressed tissue and

Expected firing of parasystolic pacemaker

Actual firing of parasystolic pacemaker

Presumed firing of parasystolic pacemaker

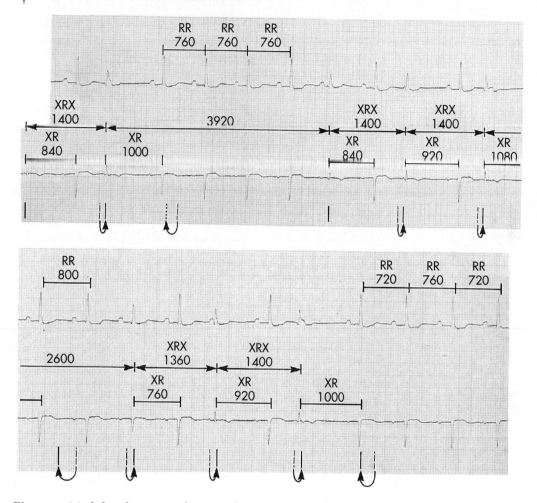

Fig. 22-3. Modulated parasystole. Note the presence of fusion beats and no fixed coupling of the ventricular ectopic beats, features typical of ventricular parasystole. The interectopic intervals, however, are not multiples because the rhythm of the parasystolic focus is influenced by subthreshold current being transmitted across the area of protection. Expected firing, actual firing, and presumed firing times of the parasystolic focus are identified. *RR*, R wave to R wave, that is, the interval between the two sinus conducted beats; *XRX*, interectopic intervals, "X" indicating the ectopic beats and "R" indicating the underlying rhythm; *XR*, the distance between a parasystolic beat and the next sinus conducted beat. *(Tracing courtesy Carol Fuller, RN, Portland, Ore. I am grateful to Charles Antzelevitch, PhD, [Gordon K. Moe Scholar]; Derge Sicouri, MD; and William Gans for their expert analysis of this figure.)*

may cause the ectopic focus to be delayed or accelerated. A beat that arrives early in diastole may cause the parasystolic discharge to be delayed. If the beat arrives late, the parasystolic discharge may be early.[1,6-9]

In addition to the preceding findings, experimental studies by Jalife and Moe[9] and others[1,3,10-13] showed that coupled beats can result from parasystolic rhythms and that the parasystolic focus could be modulated by a slight change in heart rate, ectopic pacemaker rate, level of block, and position of the parasystolic pacemaker relative to the block border.

CLINICAL IMPLICATIONS

Empirically the parasystolic rhythm is benign and is generally not treated. Although it would appear that the ventricular ectopic beats that are not precisely coupled to normal beats may easily fall on the T wave, in clinical practice this has not been the case. One report described ventricular fibrillation in a modulated parasystole with supernormal excitability.[14]

REFERENCES

1. Jalife J, Moe GK: Effects of electrotonic potentials on pacemaker activity of canine Purkinje fibers in relation to parasystole, *Circ Res* 39.801, 1970.
2. Castellanos A, Saoudi N, Moleiro F, Myerburg RJ: Parasystole. In Zipes DP, Jalife J, eds: *Cardiac electrophysiology from cell to bedside,* ed 2, Philadelphia, 1995, WB Saunders.
3. Antzelevitch C, Jalife J, Moe GK: Electrotonic modulation of pacemaker activity: further biological and mathematical observations on the behavior of modulated parasystole, *Circulation* 66:1225, 1982.
4. Jalife J, Antzelevitch C, Moe GK: The case for modulated parasystole, *PACE Pacing Clin Electrophysiol* 5:811, 1982.
5. Moe GK, Antzelevitch C, Jalife J: Premature contractions: reentrant or parasystolic? In Harrison DC, ed: *Cardiac arrhythmias,* Boston, 1981, GK Hall.
6. Wit AL: Cellular electrophysiologic mechanisms of cardiac arrhythmias, *Ann NY Acad Sci* 432:1, 1986.
7. Ferrier GR, Rosenthal JE: Automaticity and entrance block induced by focal depolarization of mammalian ventricular tissues, *Circ Res* 47:238, 1980.
8. Saoudi N, Letac B, Castellanos A: An electronic model for evaluating the dynamics of perfect pure parasystole in the human heart, *Amer J Cardiol* 75:730, 1995.
9. Jalife J, Moe GK: A biologic model of parasystole, *Am J Cardiol* 43:761, 1979.
10. Moe GK, Jalife J, Mueller WJ, Moe B: A mathematical model of parasystole and its application to clinical arrhythmias, *Circulation* 56:968, 1977.
11. Moe GK, Jalife J: An appraisal of "efficacy" in the treatment of ventricular premature beats, *Life Sci* 22:1189, 1978.
12. Rosenthal JE, Ferrier GR: Contribution of variable entrance and exit block in protected foci to arrhythmogenesis in isolated ventricular tissues, *Circulation* 67:1, 1983.
13. Antzelevitch C, Bernstein MJ, Feldman HN, Moe GK: Parasystole, reentry and tachycardia: a canine preparation of cardiac arrhythmias occurring across inexcitable segments of tissue, *Circulation* 68:1101, 1983.
14. Robles de Medina EO, Delmar M, Sicouri S, Jalife J: Modulated parasystole as a mechanism of ventricular ectopic activity leading to ventricular fibrillation, *Am J Cardiol* 63:1326, 1989.

PART III

ABNORMAL 12-LEAD ELECTROCARDIOGRAMS

23

Wolff-Parkinson-White and Other Preexcitation Syndromes

Classification of the Preexcitation
    Syndromes *303*
Wolff-Parkinson-White Syndrome *304*
ECG Recognition *306*
Degrees of Preexcitation *310*
Concealed Accessory Pathway *317*
Arrhythmias in Wolff-Parkinson-White
    Syndrome *318*
Circus Movement Tachycardia *318*
Orthodromic CMT (Rapidly Conducting
    Accessory Pathway) *318*
Emergency Response to PSVT *319*

Orthodromic CMT (Slowly Conducting
    Accessory Pathway) *323*
Antidromic CMT *325*
Atrial Fibrillation *328*
Radiofrequency Ablation *335*
Arrhythmias in Wolff-Parkinson-White
    Syndrome *318*
Nodoventricular and Fasciculoventricular
    Fibers *336*
Short PR Syndrome (Intranodal Bypass
    Tract) *340*
Summary *340*

Preexcitation exists when all or part of the ventricular muscle is activated by an atrial impulse earlier than would occur if activation had proceeded through a normal route or at a normal speed. Preexcitation syndromes are of interest because they often result in paroxysmal supraventricular tachycardia (PSVT) and atrial fibrillation, which, without intervention, may deteriorate into ventricular fibrillation (VF).

CLASSIFICATION OF THE PREEXCITATION SYNDROMES

There are several pathways by which the ventricles can be activated by a supraventricular beat earlier than anticipated. They are listed here with their new (and old) nomenclature:

1. *Accessory atrioventricular (AV) pathways* (Kent bundles) connect the atrium to the ventricle and result in Wolff-Parkinson-White (WPW) syndrome in its overt form. Accessory AV pathways are the most common type of preexcitation. Other AV connections mentioned are rare; they are not easily recognized on the surface ECG but require sophisticated intracardiac studies to be demonstrated.[1]

2. *Intranodal bypass tract* (James fiber) connects the atrium to the AV node and results in a short PR interval, a narrow QRS complex, and a tendency to PSVT (sometimes called *Lown-Ganong-Levine syndrome*).
3. *Nodoventricular, nodofascicular, or fasciculoventricular pathways* (Mahaim fibers) are connections from the AV node to the ventricle or into the bundle branch and from the His bundle or bundle branch to the ventricle.
4. *Atriofascicular bypass tract* (atrio-His fiber) connects the atrium to the His bundle.

WOLFF-PARKINSON-WHITE SYNDROME

Wolff-Parkinson-White (WPW) syndrome is a group of ECG findings (short PR, delta wave, and broad QRS) associated with the occurrence of tachycardias. When the ECG findings exist without the associated tachycardias, the term *WPW pattern* may be used.[2] As you will see, the accessory pathway and associated tachycardias can also be present without the ECG findings of the syndrome (latent or concealed accessory pathways).

Anatomic development

During early fetal development the heart is a single chamber; the atrial myocardium is continuous with the ventricular myocardium. The four chambers are formed with the invagination of the atrial and ventricular septa and the regression of muscle bands around the heart concomitantly with the formation of the annulus fibrosus (AV ring), which is normally a continuous sheet of fibrous tissue separating the atria from the ventricles. Accessory pathways are the result of faulty development of the AV ring, which may occur at almost any point around the annulus fibrosus as strands of normal myocardium bridge this insulating fibrous division between atria and ventricles.

Historical background

In 1930 Wolff et al.[2] described bundle branch block with a short PR interval in healthy young people prone to PSVT. This description was made without reference to AV bypass tracts. As early as 1893, however, Kent[3] had described in normal hearts AV connections that were located anteriorly, adjacent to the fibrous ring of the tricuspid valve. Before that, in 1876, Paladino also described AV connections.

In 1932 and 1933 Holzman and Scherf[3a] in Germany and Wolferth and Wood[3b] in the United States hypothesized that this AV connection, called *the bundle of Kent,* transmitted impulses from atria to ventricles and was responsible for the short PR interval and broad QRS complex of the WPW syndrome. By 1943 and 1944 Wood, Wolferth, and Geckeleler[4] and Ohnell[5] linked the ECG findings of short PR and broad QRS with postmortem histologic confirmation of the presence of accessory AV connections on the right and left sides of the heart. Fig. 23-1 illustrates such a connection.

Accessory pathway

An accessory pathway or an AV connection is an extra muscle bundle composed of working myocardial tissue[6] that forms a connection between atria and ventricles outside the conduction[7] system (thus the short PR and broad QRS) and may supply one arm of an AV reentry route (thus the tendency to develop PSVT).

The location of accessory pathways has historically been classified according

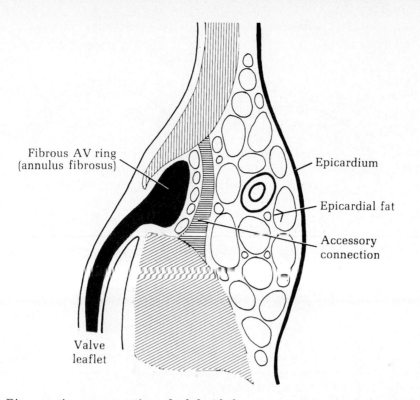

Fig. 23-1. Diagramatic representation of a left-sided accessory atrioventricular (AV) connection. The connection skirts through the epicardial fat, being outside the fibrous AV ring. (From Becker AE et al: Circulation 57:870, 1978.)

to quadrants: right anteroseptal, right free wall, posteroseptal, and left free wall. In the era of catheter ablation this classification is more refined (Fig. 23-2). The most common locations are the left free wall (50%) and posteroseptal (30%). Right free wall pathways occur in 13% of patients, and anteroseptal locations occur least frequently (7%).[1]

Surgical experience has demonstrated pathways located at any depth between the valve annuli and the epicardium. Experience with radiofrequency ablation suggests that the majority of left-sided pathways are subepicardial (juxtaannular), whereas right-sided pathways tend to be more variable in depth, some being closer to the epicardium and others midway between epicardium and endocardium.[8] The pathways may be single or multiple, active or inactive, and may possess the capability of conducting in both anterograde and retrograde fashion or only in retrograde fashion (concealed accessory pathway).[9] In approximately 60% to 70% of patients with an accessory pathway the diagnosis can be made by a knowledgeable examiner from the surface ECG when the patient is in sinus rhythm (overt WPW syndrome). The remainder of cases are concealed (30%) or latent. In such cases the diagnosis can be made by an alert and informed examiner from rhythm strips during the tachycardia.

Incidence

The estimated incidence of preexcitation from two large studies is 0.1% to 0.3% of the general population, with an annual incidence of new cases of 4:100,000 popu-

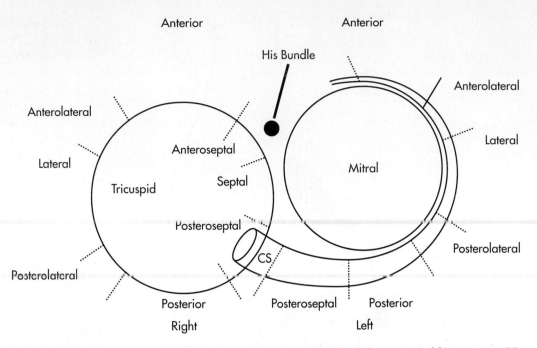

Fig. 23-2. Regional locations of accessory AV pathways in the left anterior oblique view. *CS,* Coronary sinus. *(From Naccarelli GV. In Willerson JT, Cohn JN, eds: Cardiovascular medicine, New York, 1995, Churchill Livingstone.)*

lation per year.[6,10] In one large study of 67,375 asymptomatic air force personnel, only 128 (0.19%) were found to have an overt WPW syndrome ECG pattern.[7] However, this condition is undoubtedly not noted in some individuals because of latent accessory pathways (minimal or no preexcitation), intermittent preexcitation, and concealed accessory pathways. Males are reportedly affected twice as often as females, and most patients do not become symptomatic until adolescence or adulthood.[11]

Genetics

In light of reports that family members of patients with WPW syndrome have a four times greater chance of having an accessory pathway than do people without a family history,[12] Wellens et al.[9] have suggested that the syndrome is inherited as an autosomal dominant trait.

ECG recognition (overt Wolff-Parkinson-White syndrome)

NOTE: It is important to remember that the classic ECG signs are not present in the concealed and latent conditions.

PR interval: Less than 0.12 sec.

QRS complex: A delta wave is present, which causes the QRS to be broader than 0.10 sec. A negative delta wave looks like a pathologic Q wave. Fig. 23-3 illustrates and explains the mechanisms of the short PR and delta wave.

T wave: Secondary T-wave changes may be present.

Associated arrhythmias: Paroxysmal supraventricular tachycardia (PSVT) and atrial fibrillation. The two most common types of PSVT are AV nodal reentry tachycardia (AVNRT) and circus movement tachycardia (CMT). AVNRT does not use an accessory pathway and is mentioned here because there is a

Table 23-1. Subjective symptoms during paroxysmal CMT (69 patients)

Symptom	No. of patients (%)
Palpitations	67 (97)
Dyspnea	40 (57)
Anginal pain	39 (56)
Perspiration	38 (55)
Fatigue	28 (41)
Anxiety	20 (30)
Dizziness	20 (30)
Polyuria	18 (26)

From Wellens HJJ et al. In Mandel WJ, ed: *Cardiac arrhythmias: their mechanisms, diagnosis and management,* Philadelphia, 1980, JB Lippincott.
CMT, Circus movement tachycardia.

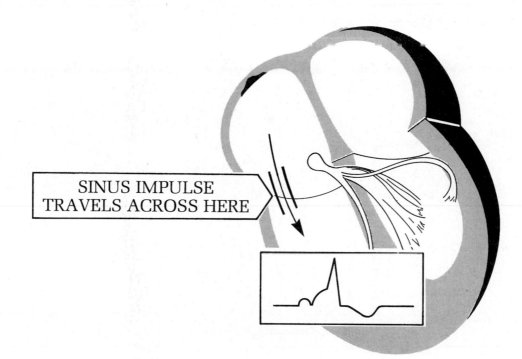

Fig. 23-3. In overt Wolff-Parkinson-White (WPW) syndrome the impulse initially arrives in the ventricles through an accessory pathway. Since this pathway conducts faster than the AV node, the PR interval is short. The delta wave (initial slurring of the QRS) is the result of initial ventricular activation outside the conduction system. There may also be secondary ST-T segment changes. The accessory pathway is a small fiber; it is diagramatically illustrated.

differential diagnosis between the two similar looking types of PSVT. Circus movement tachycardia uses the AV node for anterograde conduction and the accessory pathway for retrograde conduction. The differential diagnosis in PSVT is fully discussed in Chapter 11.

The patient's history is, of course, of great help in making the diagnosis. Many times, persons with an accessory pathway report being aware of frequent episodes of "palpitations" or, when queried, recall anginal pain and polyuria. These and other subjective symptoms during CMT are listed in Table 23-1.

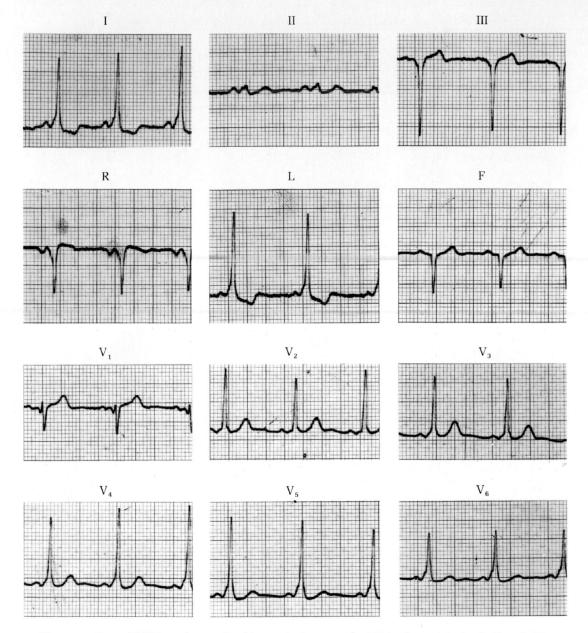

Fig. 23-4. Overt WPW syndrome. In this particular case the PR is shortest in leads II and aV$_L$ (0.08 sec). The delta wave is nicely seen in all leads except aV$_F$; in aV$_F$ the PR and QRS are normal because of isoelectric initial ventricular forces.

Table 23-2. Shortest normal PR intervals and longest normal QRS complexes according to age

Age	PR (sec)	QRS (sec)
0-6 mo	0.08	0.06
6 mo-3 yr	0.08	0.08
3-5 yr	0.10	0.08
5-16 yr	0.10	0.09
Older than 16 yr	0.12	0.10

Modified form Ferrer MI: *Electrocardiographic notebook,* ed 4, Mount Kisco, NY, 1973, Futura.

A 12-lead ECG of a patient with overt WPW syndrome is shown in Fig. 23-4. These ECG signs may be borderline or may not be seen in all leads because of an isoelectric delta wave (seen in Fig. 23-4 in lead aV$_F$) or factors influencing conduction time across the accessory pathway. Thus even in overt WPW syndrome, the diagnosis can be and often is missed. Often it is in the emergency department that the ECG during PSVT or a history of "palpitations" alerts one to the possibility of WPW syndrome. This may be the patient's only opportunity to receive the correct diagnosis and be referred for a cure (radiofrequency ablation of the accessory pathway).

PR interval

The short PR interval in overt WPW syndrome is the result of accelerated AV conduction across an accessory pathway. The sinus impulse enters the ventricle via a strand of cardiac muscle that does not involve the AV node or the His-Purkinje system. Because this strand of cardiac muscle has faster conduction than the AV node, the PR interval is short. The shortest normal PR intervals according to age are shown in Table 23-2.

Delta wave

Mechanism. The delta wave is the initial slurring of the QRS complex (a slow beginning) caused by the early arrival of the supraventricular impulse into the ventricle via the accessory pathway. When the sinus impulse arrives in the ventricle in this manner, it is outside the conduction system when it begins its journey (an "ectopic" beginning).

Polarity. The delta wave may be a positive or negative deflection (as illustrated in Fig. 23-5) or it may be isoelectric, as previously demonstrated in lead aV$_F$ of Fig. 23-4. Its polarity depends on the orientation of the preexcitation forces to the axis of the lead in question. An isoelectric delta wave is the result of the delta forces being perpendicular to the axis of a lead. If delta forces are flowing away from the positive electrode, the delta wave will be negative in that lead, producing an abnor-

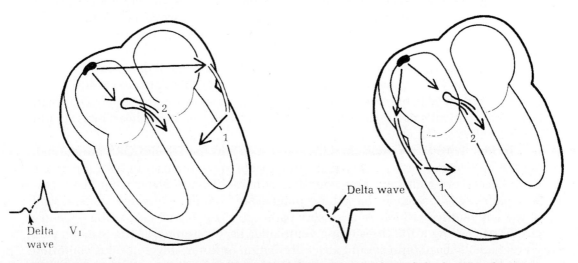

Fig. 23-5. Ventricular fusion caused by ventricular activation through both AV pathways—the accessory pathway and the AV node–His bundle.

mal Q wave (as seen in leads III and V_1 of Fig. 23-4). When this happens, the uninformed examiner may misdiagnose the condition as myocardial infarction (MI).

Size. The size of the delta wave depends on many factors but is ultimately the result of how far the preexcitation current is ahead of normal excitation in activating the ventricles.

Ventricular fusion. If the sinus impulse should happen to arrive in the ventricles simultaneously through both pathways (AV node/His bundle and accessory pathway), there would of course be no delta wave and the PR interval would be normal. However, because of the simultaneous activation of the ventricles from two sites, the QRS complex would be a fusion beat and the following abnormalities might exist:
- Abnormal Q waves
- Slurring of the ascending limb of the R wave
- Increased voltage of the QRS complex
- Axis shift

There would then be a differential diagnosis between WPW syndrome and MI, other interventricular conduction disturbances, and ventricular hypertrophy.[13]

Understanding the degrees of preexitation

An understanding of what can occur on the ECG when the ventricles are activated over two pathways is essential to successful recognition of WPW syndrome. It is not sufficient to simply learn the ECG signs of overt WPW syndrome; they are far to confining.

It is important to remember that when the ventricles are activated over two pathways, a fusion beat results. The characteristics of this fusion beat depend on the individual contributions of the two pathways. Fig. 23-6 illustrates different degrees of preexcitation, from maximal preexcitation to none, and how this affects the PR interval, the delta wave, and the shape of the QRS.

In Fig. 23-6, *A,* maximal preexcitation is present. Both ventricles are activated by the current passing through the accessory pathway. In such a situation the P wave may look like part of the QRS.

In Fig. 23-6, *B,* less than maximal preexcitation is present. The PR interval is still very short, with little or no PR segment. The excitation wave arrives in the ventricles first via the accessory pathway and then via the AV node, causing a fusion beat.

In Fig. 23-6, *C,* minimal preexcitation produces a very small delta wave, a longer PR interval, and a narrower QRS (another fusion beat). This appearance still qualifies as overt WPW syndrome because both measurements are abnormal. The small size of this patient's delta wave does not preclude life-threatening heart rates should atrial fibrillation develop.[1]

In Fig. 23-6, *D,* no preexcitation at all exists and the PR and QRS are normal, yet the patient has an accessory pathway capable of conduction in both directions (latent accessory pathway). This condition is more likely to occur when the accessory pathway is located at the farthest point away from the sinus node (lateral wall of the left ventricle). Such an accessory pathway is capable of supporting a reentry circuit or causing a life-threatening ventricular heart rate that at times may reach more than 300 beats/min should atrial fibrillation or flutter develop. This condition should not be confused with concealed WPW syndrome (discussed later), in which only retrograde conduction is possible in the accessory pathway.

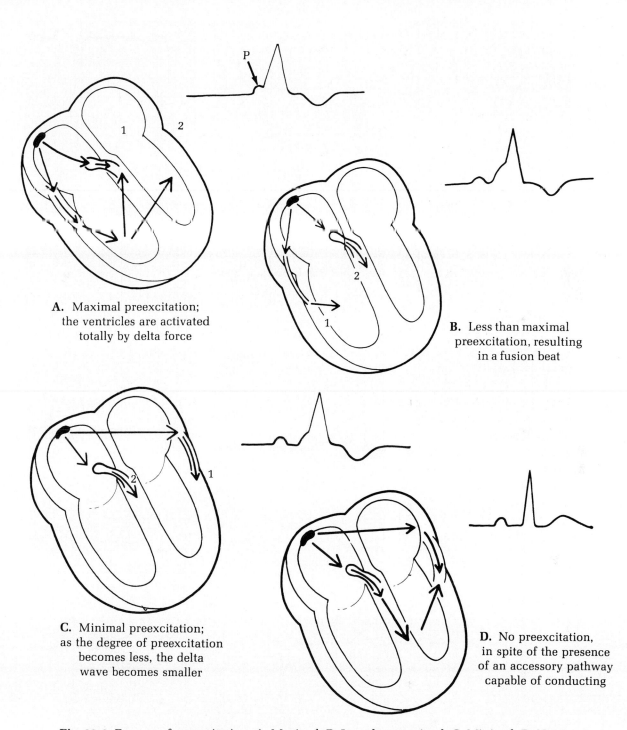

Fig. 23-6. Degrees of preexcitation. **A,** Maximal. **B,** Less than maximal. **C,** Minimal. **D,** None.

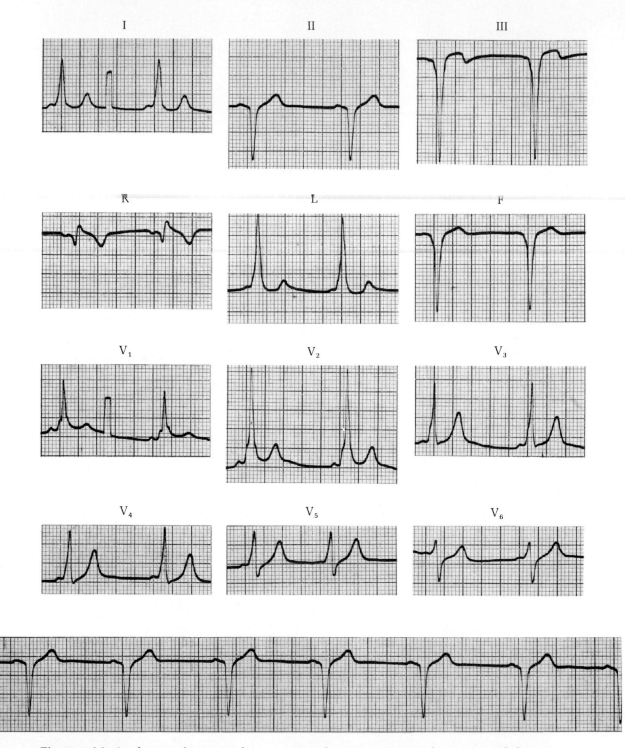

Fig. 23-7. Maximal or nearly maximal preexcitation from a posteroseptal or posterior left ventricular accessory pathway. The delta force actually interrupts the P wave in many leads. The QS waves in the inferior leads are the result of the orientation of the delta force toward the negative electrode of these leads.

Maximal preexcitation

The 12-lead ECG in Fig. 23-7 shows maximal preexcitation in a patient with a posteroseptal accessory pathway. In some leads the P wave is actually interrupted by the beginning of the delta wave, and the QRS is 0.16 sec in duration. Note the QS complexes in leads II, III, and aV_F, which along with the secondary changes in ST-T segment that often occur with preexcitation, may lead to misdiagnosis of inferior wall MI. The 12-lead ECG in Fig. 23-8 is another example of maximal or almost maximal preexcitation in a patient with a right lateral accessory pathway. Note that the delta wave is positive in leads I and II and in the precordial leads and negative in III, aV_R, and aV_F. A comparison of like leads in Figs. 23-7 and 23-8 of nearly

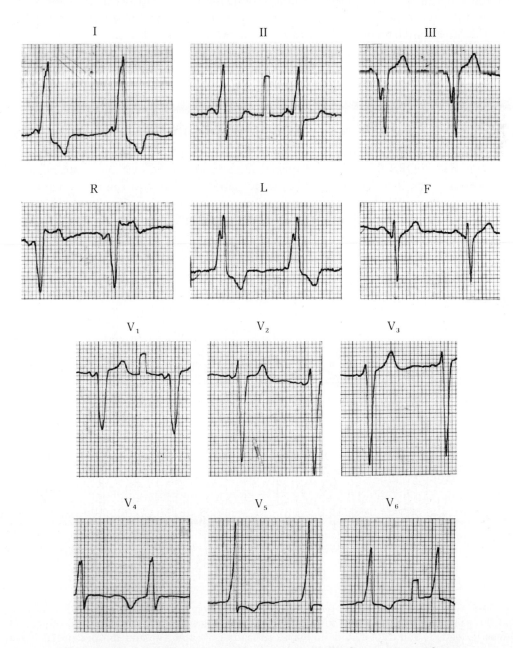

Fig. 23-8. Maximal preexcitation from an anteroseptal accessory pathway.

maximal preexcitation demonstrates how the location of the accessory pathway can produce QRS complexes that look completely different.

Less than maximal preexcitation: the fusion beat

In Fig. 23-9 the ventricular complex is a fusion beat, the result of initial activation over the accessory pathway (the delta waves) followed by activation via the AV node and His bundle.

In Fig. 23-10 one has to search all the leads for the short PR interval and the delta wave. Note that in leads II, III, aV_F, and V_1 the PR is 0.12 to 0.14 sec (quite normal), although the presence of abnormal Q waves (actually delta waves) in the inferior leads in this young patient makes one suspicious. However, in leads V_2 to V_6 the delta wave becomes a little more apparent, and the PR interval is 0.10 to 0.11 sec, just barely meeting the criteria for overt WPW syndrome.

Although the preceding diagnostic ECG signs do not jump out at you, the accessory pathway in the patient's heart supported life-threatening ventricular rates when atrial fibrillation developed. (The patient's ECG on admission is shown [see Fig. 23-21, A] and discussed later.)

The latent accessory pathway: no preexcitation

A latent accessory pathway is shown in Fig. 23-11, A. During sinus rhythm the PR interval and QRS duration are normal. Fig. 23-11, B, shows the potentially lethal results of atrial fibrillation in this same patient because of the existence of an accessory pathway that is capable of anterograde conduction. The mechanism of this life-threatening arrhythmia will be discussed shortly.

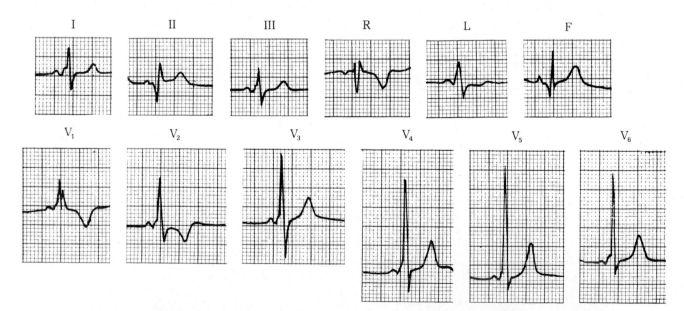

Fig. 23-9. Wolff-Parkinson-White syndrome, the result of a left lateral accessory pathway. Note that the ventricular complex is a fusion beat and that negative delta waves have produced Q waves in leads II and aV_F. The delta waves in leads I, III and aV_L and the precordial leads are nicely visualized.

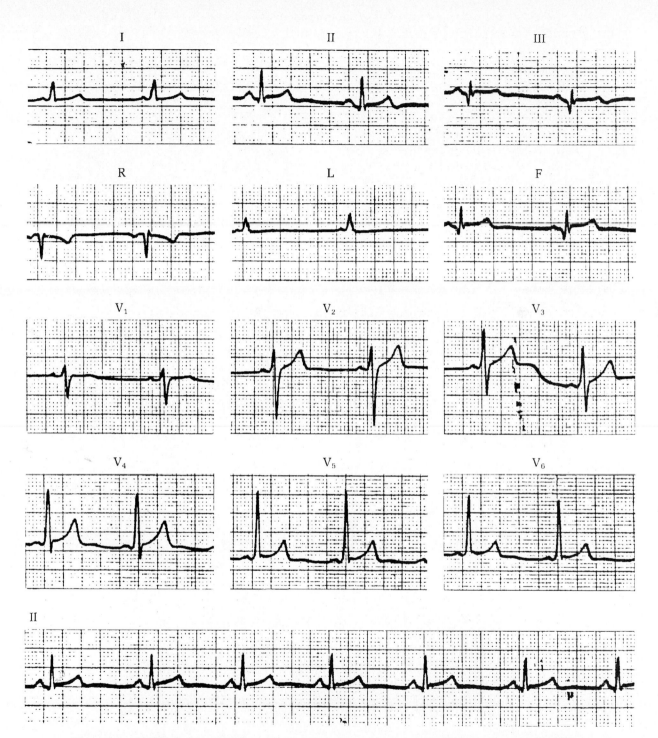

Fig. 23-10. Wolff-Parkinson-White syndrome with minimal preexcitation. The PR and QRS in leads II, III, aV$_F$, and V$_1$ are normal, although the abnormal Q waves in the inferior leads are probably delta waves. Delta waves are certainly evident in V$_2$ and V$_3$, where the PR is 0.11 sec, barely qualifying as an overt WPW syndrome. This tracing is from an 18-year-old man who was admitted with atrial fibrillation (see Fig. 23-20) and a heart rate of 250 to 300 beats/min caused by conduction over an accessory pathway. This is his postcardioversion tracing. *(Courtesy Kathleen Hester, RN, and Cathy Stark, RN, Concord, Calif.)*

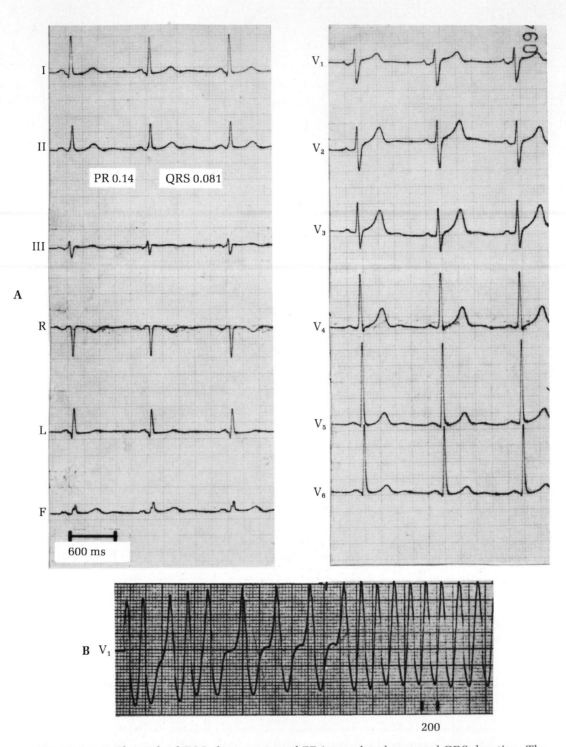

Fig. 23-11. A, The 12-lead ECG shows a normal PR interval and a normal QRS duration. The patient was admitted with an attack of atrial fibrillation **(B)** with a very high ventricular heart rate because of conduction from the atrium to the ventricles over an accessory pathway. (From Wellens HJJ et al. In Mandel WJ, ed: Cardiac arrhythmias, Philadelphia, 1980, JB Lippincott.)

T-wave changes

Because ventricular depolarization does not follow a normal sequence and is delayed, the repolarization process may also be out of sequence, causing secondary T-wave changes. The extent of these changes depends on the degree and the area of preexcitation.

Estimating the refractory period of the accessory pathway

Any degree of preexcitation is possible. However, it is not the size of the delta wave but the duration of the refractory period of the accessory pathway in the anterograde direction that identifies high-risk patients. This duration varies considerably among patients and is influenced by sympathetic tone.[14]

Wellens[15] has described three noninvasive ways of estimating the adequacy of the refractory period of the accessory pathway in the anterograde direction. The period is considered long enough to protect the patient from excessive ventricular rates should atrial fibrillation develop, as follows:

1. If preexcitation is intermittent.
2. If preexcitation disappears (not just lessens) with exercise (as a result of the catecholamines).[16] Wellens[1] exhorts care in this interpretation, since sympathetic stimulation during exercise speeds up AV nodal conduction and may diminish the area of preexcitation. Concurrent multiple ECG leads should be recorded with attention to the ECG after exercise. In cases of exercise-induced block in the accessory pathway, upon resumption of conduction through this pathway a sudden marked change in the ECG takes place.
3. If the PR and QRS normalize following intravenous (IV) administration of procainamide (10 mg/kg body weight over 5 min).[17]

NOTE: Before using procainamide for this purpose, one should become acquainted with the references, which indicate that hypertrophic cardiomyopathy should be ruled out by echocardiogram[18] and that because procainamide prolongs the refractory period of both the accessory pathway and the His-Purkinje system, it is given in a setting where complete heart block can be managed.[1]

Concealed accessory pathway

An accessory pathway is said to be "concealed" when it conducts only in a retrograde direction. Thus during sinus rhythm AV conduction proceeds normally, resulting in a normal PR interval and QRS duration (no preexcitation). Although conduction down a concealed accessory pathway is not possible, conduction up that pathway is. Thus the development of orthodromic circus movement tachycardia (CMT; AV reciprocating tachycardia) is possible. Should atrial fibrillation develop, patients with concealed accessory pathways are not at the same risk as those who have anterograde conduction in their accessory pathways. The concealed accessory pathway (no anterograde conduction) should not be confused with the latent accessory pathway, which is capable of anterograde conduction.

Incidence. In approximately 34% of patients with PSVT and no sign of preexcitation during sinus rhythm, electrophysiologic studies have demonstrated that there is a concealed accessory AV connection forming the retrograde limb of the reentry pathway.[19]

ECG diagnosis. Since the PR interval and QRS complex are normal during sinus rhythm, the diagnosis depends on the following:

1. Recording an adequate number of leads (at least I, II, III, V_1, and V_6) during the tachycardia and the same leads for comparison during sinus rhythm. The comparison helps locate the P' waves during the tachycardia.
2. Electrocardiographic observations made while the patient is having the PSVT, specifically, the location of the P' wave relative to the QRS (immediately following it), as discussed in Chapter 11.
3. Taking a good history.
4. Electrophysiologic studies.

ARRHYTHMIAS IN WOLFF-PARKINSON-WHITE SYNDROME

The most frequently occurring arrhythmias in patients with preexcitation are CMT and atrial fibrillation. In a series of 407 patients with WPW syndrome and cardiac arrhythmias, 265 had CMT, 76 had atrial fibrillation, and 66 had both.[19] Other arrhythmias are, of course, possible; any type of supraventricular tachycardia (SVT) results in rapid ventricular rates because of AV conduction via the accessory pathway.

The differential diagnosis in narrow and broad QRS tachycardias is discussed in detail in Chapters 11 and 14. The following is a discussion of the mechanisms, ECG recognition, and treatment of the common arrhythmias involving an accessory pathway, that is, the two forms of orthodromic CMT, antidromic CMT, and atrial fibrillation. Atrial flutter is of course also a possibility, but it is not as common.

Circus movement tachycardia

Circus movement tachycardia is a type of PSVT that is sustained by a reentry circuit using an accessory pathway and the AV node or using two accessory pathways. It may be orthodromic (narrow QRS) or antidromic (broad QRS). Two forms of orthodromic CMT are possible, the common form using a rapidly conducting accessory pathway and the relatively rare but persistent form using a slowly conducting accessory pathway.

Orthodromic circus movement tachycardia (using a rapidly conducting accessory pathway)

In symptomatic patients with WPW syndrome the most common arrhythmia is orthodromic CMT with a rapidly conducting accessory pathway. It is the mechanism in approximately 40% of all cases of symptomatic PSVT and is itself 15 times more common than antidromic CMT.[1]

ECG features
Rate: 150 to 250 beats/min.
QRS complex: Narrow (unless there is aberrant ventricular conduction).
Rhythm: Regular and paroxysmal.
P' waves: Located immediately following the QRS complex. The polarity of the P' wave depends on the atrial location of the accessory pathway, since atrial activation during CMT proceeds from the ventricle, through the atrial insertion to activate the atria. For example, with left-sided accessory pathways atrial activation is from left to right (toward the negative electrode of lead I); thus the P' wave is negative in lead I. With right-sided pathways it is positive in that lead.

Main diagnostic features

1. The P′ wave is separate from and follows the narrow QRS complex with a short RP interval.
2. QRS alternans (alternating heights of R peaks or depths of S nadirs) is frequently present and is helpful in the diagnosis when it persists after the first 3 to 5 sec.[19]

Locating the P′ wave during the tachycardia is necessary for the definitive diagnosis. Differentiating CMT from AV nodal reentry tachycardia and other forms of PSVT is an important diagnostic challenge because of the difference in long-term treatment. See Chapter 11 for a discussion of the differential diagnosis in PSVT.

Mechanism. The previously described (p. 137) common form of orthodromic CMT is supported by a reentry circuit using the AV node in an anterograde direction and a rapidly conducting accessory pathway in a retrograde direction. Study the illustration of this mechanism in Fig. 23-12, noting the initiation of the CMT by an early premature atrial complex (PAC) (Fig. 23-12, A), and then in Fig. 23-12, B, the sequence of the established circuit (atria, AV node, ventricles, accessory pathway, and over again). Note also the position of the P′ wave immediately following the QRS complex. In this common form of CMT the P′ wave is close to the preceding QRS because the accessory pathway conducts the ventricular impulse rapidly up to the atrium. This tachycardia is abruptly initiated by a critically timed PAC or premature ventricular complex (PVC), or when the sinus rhythm reaches a critical rate, such as during exercise or following the administration of a drug.[1]

Initiation with a PAC (Fig. 23-12)

Fig. 23-12, *A:* A PAC is blocked in the accessory pathway, passes down the AV node into the ventricles, and returns quickly to the atria via the accessory pathway.

Fig. 23-12 *B:* Establishing a reentry circuit (AV node, ventricles, accessory pathway, atria).

Fig. 23-23, *C:* Producing a typical narrow QRS tachycardia with a P′ wave immediately following the QRS complex.

Initiation with a PVC (Fig. 23-13)

1. A PVC has easy access to the accessory pathway.
2. The PVC is conducted in a retrograde direction up the accessory pathway to the atrium.
3. The impulse enters the AV node.
4. The impulse reenters the ventricles, establishing an orthodromic (narrow QRS) CMT.

Initiation with sinus tachycardia (Fig. 23-14)

1. During sinus tachycardia, such as would occur with exercise, a critical heart rate is reached in which conduction down the accessary pathway is blocked.
2. The impulse proceeds down the AV node to the ventricles.
3. The impulse then returns to the atria by the now nonrefractory accessory pathway, establishing a CMT.

Emergency response to paroxysmal supraventricular tachycardia

Record the tachycardia in 12 leads if possible. If this is not possible, at least 5 leads (I, II, III, V_1, and V_6) are important. If the tachycardia is terminated before adequate leads are recorded, a diagnosis cannot be made. Of course, a good clue to the supraventricular nature of the tachycardia is the observation of the "frog sign" in the neck veins (p. 151).

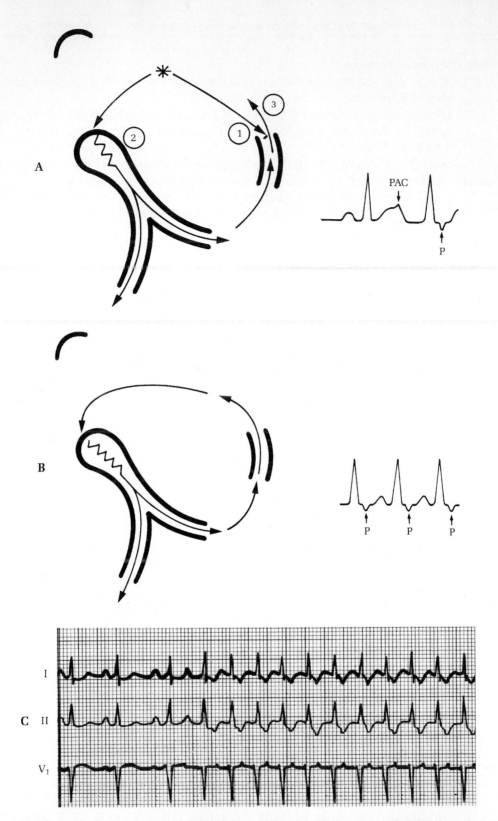

Fig. 23-12. A schematic representation of the mechanism of the onset of CMT. **A,** A premature atrial complex (PAC) is blocked in the accessory pathway *(1)*; the impulse passes down the AV node to activate the ventricles *(2)*; the impulse then returns to the atria in a retrograde direction across the accessory pathway *(3)*. **B,** A reentry circuit is established during which the ventricles and atria are activated in sequence. Note the location of the P' waves. **C,** The resulting ECG.

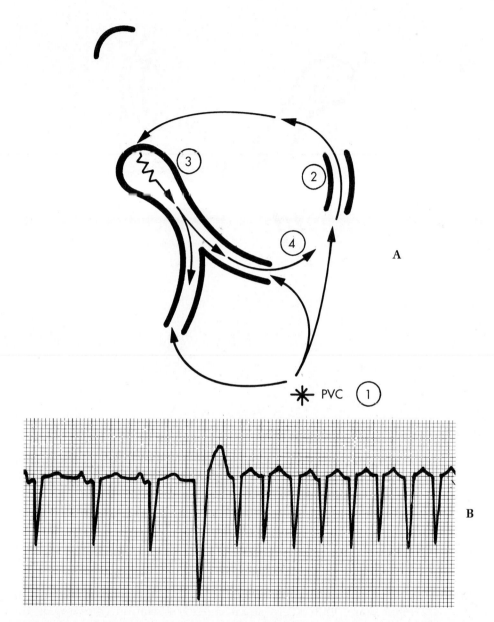

Fig. 23-13. A, A schematic representation of how a premature ventricular complex (PVC) can initiate orthodromic CMT. A PVC activates the ventricles *(1)*. It is also conducted in retrograde fashion up the accessory pathway *(2)* and returns to the ventricles via the AV node *(3)*, completing the circuit and beginning again *(4)*. **B,** The resulting ECG.

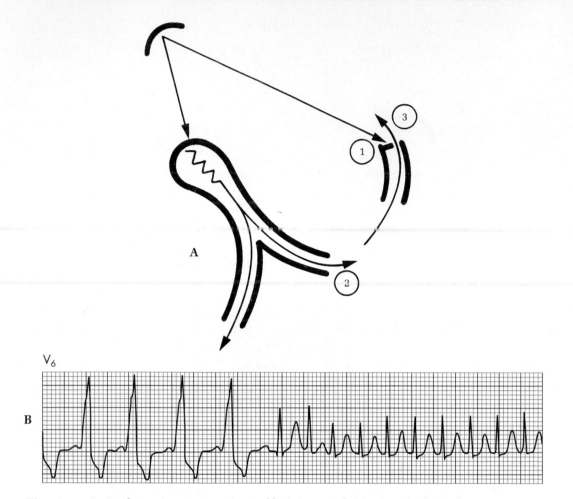

Fig. 23-14. **A,** A schematic representation of how a critical-rate sinus tachycardia can initiate orthodromic circus movement tachycardia (CMT). **B,** The resulting ECG. (**B** *courtesy Hein J.J. Wellens, MD, The Netherlands.*)

Treatment is aimed at interrupting the reentry circuit, first at the AV node and, if that fails, at the accessory pathway. Vagal maneuvers and calcium channel blockers block anterograde conduction through the AV node. Procainamide is the most effective of the drugs available to block accessory pathway conduction. The emergency approach to CMT proceeds as follows[1]:

1. Vagal maneuver. (Both carotid sinus massage (CSM) and gagging are strong vagal maneuvers. Others are squatting, leg elevation, blowing against a closed glottis, and cold water to the face.) This maneuver should be performed as soon as the tachycardia is recorded. The longer the wait, the more difficult it is to convert with a vagal maneuver because of the increasing dominance of the sympathetic nervous system.
2. Adenosine 6 mg IV, which may be increased to 12 mg and repeated at 1-min intervals, or the following.
3. Verapamil, 10 mg IV over 3 min; reduce to 5 mg if the patient is taking a beta blocker or is hypotensive. If unsuccessful, administer the following.
4. Procainamide, 10 mg/kg IV over 5 min.

5. To interrupt CMT, pacing or cardioversion are rarely required. However, if vagal maneuvers and drugs do not terminate the tachycardia or if the patient has hemodynamic instability at any time, electrical cardioversion is used.

After the resolution of the acute event the patient is referred to a center experienced in the treatment of the arrhythmias of WPW syndrome. A cure is available in the form of radiofrequency ablation.

Orthodromic circus movement tachycardia (using a slowly conducting accessory pathway)

Incessant or *permanent junctional tachycardia* and orthodromic CMT are terms given to a relatively rare and extremely debilitating type of PSVT.

ECG features
Rate: 130 to 200 beats/min.
QRS complex: Narrow.
Rhythm: Regular or paroxysmal.
P waves: Retrograde. The accessory pathway is located posterior-septally with the atrial insertion close to the coronary sinus ostium.[14] Thus the P′ waves are equiphasic or flat in leads I and V_1 and negative in leads II and III and leads V_2 through V_6.

Main diagnostic features
1. The persistence of the tachycardia.
2. The long RP interval (RP greater than PR).

The two types of orthodromic CMT are compared in Fig. 23-15. In Fig. 23-15, *A,* you will see that in CMT with a rapidly conducting accessory pathway the P′ wave closely follows the QRS; in Fig. 23-15, *B,* in CMT with a slowly conducting accessory pathway, the P′ wave is closer to the following QRS than it is to the preceding

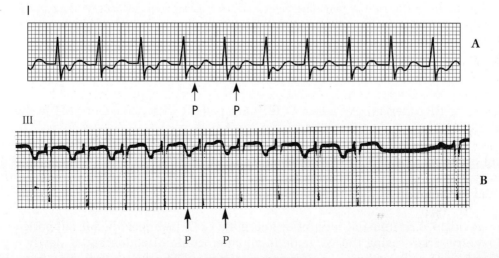

Fig. 23-15. The ECG in orthodromic CMT, **A,** with a rapidly conducting accessory pathway (short RP interval) and, **B,** with a slowly conducting accessory pathway (long RP interval). (*A courtesy Hein J.J. Wellens, MD, The Netherlands.*)

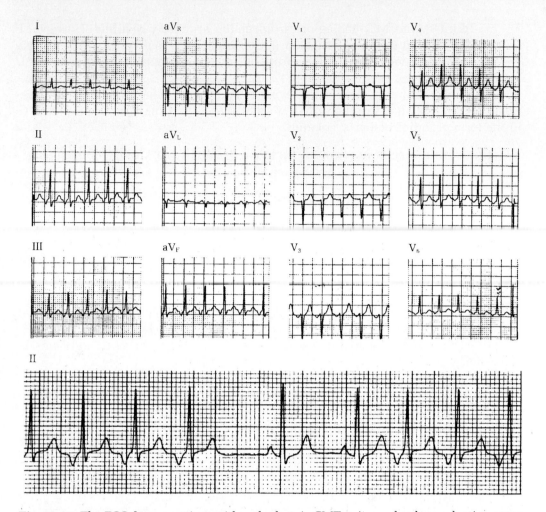

Fig. 23-16. The ECG from a patient with orthodromic CMT using a slowly conducting accessory pathway (the so-called incessant junctional tachycardia). In the lead II rhythm strip the tachycardia was transiently terminated by right-side carotid sinus massage (CSM). Termination without a retrograde P′ wave indicates that the vagal maneuver caused block in the accessory pathway (retrograde limb of the CMT) and illustrates its AV nodal–like properties. Note in that lead the spontaneous resumption of the tachycardia. *(From Yee R, Klein GJ, Sharma AD et al. In Zipes DP, Jalife J, eds: Cardiac electrophysiology, Philadelphia, 1990, WB Saunders.)*

one (long RP′ interval). A 12-lead ECG from a patient with persistent CMT is shown in Fig. 23-16.

    Patients may be unaware of the tachycardia, having lived with it as a prevailing condition. It is often not diagnosed until they seek medical attention because of symptoms of congestive heart failure resulting from their tachycardia-induced dilated cardiomyopathy.

Mechanism. The unusual form of orthodromic CMT just described is supported by a reentry circuit using the AV node in an anterograde direction and a slowly conducting accessory pathway in a retrograde direction. The slow conduction from the ventricle to the atria over the accessory pathway produces a long RP interval, so the retrograde P′ wave, along with the QRS that follows it, resembles a junctional beat (negative P′ in inferior leads immediately preceeding a QRS complex). The pathway in most cases is inserted into the ostium of the coronary sinus, although left-sided pathways with slow conduction have also been identified.[20] Because of a response similar to that of the AV node to drugs and vagal maneuvers, the slowly conducting accessory pathway is thought to have nodal-like tissue.

Treatment. Drugs are usually ineffective in treating the arrhythmia just described. Transvenous radiofrequency catheter ablation of the accessory pathway offers a complete cure and a dramatic cessation of the tachycardia. In many patients there is a dramatic improvement of ventricular function following the ablation of the accessory pathway.[21,22]

Antidromic circus movement tachycardia

Antidromic CMT is a reentry circuit using the accessory pathway in the anterograde direction (producing a broad QRS) and the AV node in the retrograde direction. Antidromic CMT commonly indicates multiple accessory pathways (at least 50% of the time).[23] Electrophysiologic studies are necessary to rule out ventricular tachycardia (VT). The ECGs from a patient with antidromic CMT caused by anterograde conduction down a left free wall accessory pathway are seen in Fig. 23-17.

ECG features
Rate: 150 to 250 beats/min.
QRS complex: Broad. As one would expect, the shape of the ventricular complexes exactly mimics those of VT, since the ventricles are being activated solely from the ventricular insertion of the accessory pathway.
Rhythm: Usually regular; however, it may be slightly irregular because retrograde conduction times vary through the fascicles of the left bundle branch to the atria. This fact may help to distinguish this type of broad QRS tachycardia from VT, which is regular 75% of the time, but may serve to confuse it with atrial fibrillation with conduction over an accessory pathway, which looks like VT but is irregular.
P waves: Although P′ waves are present following every QRS complex, they are usually not seen during this tachycardia because of the width of the QRS.

Main diagnostic feature. A broad QRS tachycardia with slow initial forces caused by excitation outside of the conduction system is the main diagnostic feature.

Mechanism. The mechanism of antidromic CMT is schematically illustrated in Fig. 23-18. Note that anterograde conduction proceeds down the accessory pathway and that initial forces are in the ventricular myocardium, where conduction is slower than it is in the conduction system. Initial penetration of the ventricle via an accessory pathway causes a relatively slow beginning to the broad QRS. Antidromic CMT begins as does orthodromic CMT, with a critically timed PAC, PVC, or a critical sinus rate, or because of a drug.

Emergency treatment. The treatment for antidromic and orthodromic CMT is the same as that of orthodromic CMT. The problem is that antidromic CMT is identical in morphologic appearance to that of VT.

Circus movement tachycardia with two accessory pathways

Circus movement tachycardia using two accessory pathways is another rare form of PSVT in which the QRS complexes are broad. Anterograde conduction is down one accessory pathway, and retrograde conduction is up another (Fig. 23-19),

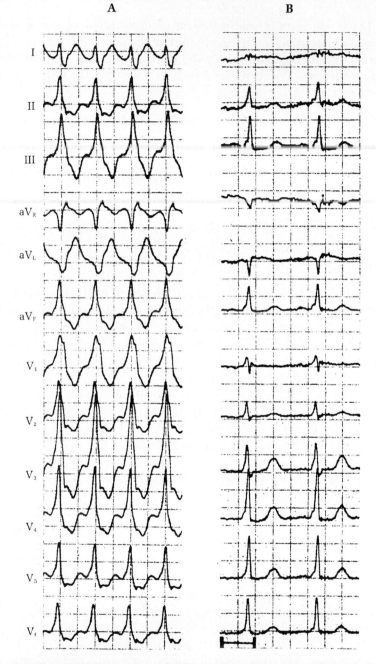

Fig. 23-17. A, Antidromic CMT. **B,** Sinus rhythm in the same patient shows a short PR interval and a delta wave caused by a left free wall accessory pathway. *(Courtesy Hein J.J. Wellens, MD, The Netherlands.)*

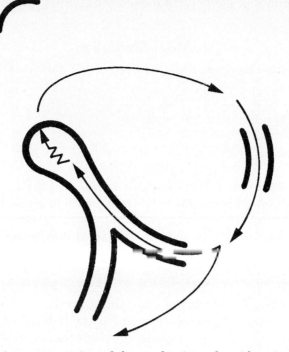

Fig. 23-18. A schematic representation of the mechanism of antidromic CMT. Anterograde conduction is down the accessory pathway, and initial ventricular forces are outside the conduction system, which explains the wide QRS with the relatively slow beginning.

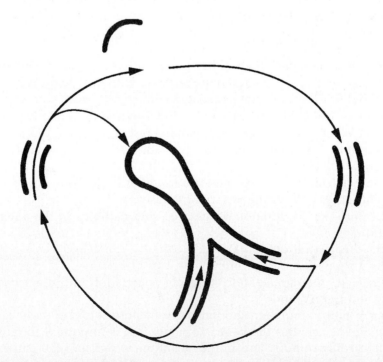

Fig. 23-19. A schematic representation of the mechanism of CMT using two accessory pathways. The resulting rhythm is identical to that of ventricular tachycardia (VT).

producing a rhythm that is identical to both VT and the previously described anti-dromic CMT.

Atrial fibrillation

Atrial fibrillation has been reported in 41 of 157 patients with WPW syndrome.

ECG features
Rate: Fast, usually more than 200 beats/min.
QRS complex: Broad.
Rhythm: Irregular.

Main diagnostic features. A fast, broad, irregular (FBI) rhythm is a diagnostic feature. If it were not for its irregularity, this broad QRS tachycardia (atrial fibrillation with conduction down an accessory pathway) would be identical to VT. Fig. 23-20 is a 12-lead ECG tracing from a patient with atrial fibrillation and AV conduction via an accessory pathway. A sinus rhythm strip in lead II is shown. Note the FBI features of this rhythm that are typical of atrial fibrillation and WPW syndrome. The sinus rhythm was recorded after cardioversion. Note the typical ECG features of WPW syndrome—short PR, broad QRS, and delta wave.

The emergency department tracings in Fig. 23-21 were taken during tachycardia and following conversion to sinus rhythm. Note that the typical features of atrial fibrillation with conduction over an accessory pathway (FBI) are evident. In the sinus rhythm (Fig. 23-21, *B*), however, the signs of preexcitation are subtle, so without the ECG during the tachycardia the diagnosis might be missed.

The tracings from an 18-year-old man in this potentially lethal case (Fig. 23-21) dramatically illustrate the importance of understanding the mechanism and ECG recognition of the arrhythmias of WPW syndrome, as well as the fact that an accessory pathway may be present without being detected during sinus rhythm on the 12-lead ECG.

Mechanism. The mechanism of atrial fibrillation with conduction over an accessory pathway is diagramatically illustrated in Fig. 23-22 with the typical ECG tracing.

When atrial fibrillation is not associated with an accessory pathway, the erratic electrical activity from the atria is slowed down by the AV node in its passage to the ventricles. When an accessory pathway is present, a very rapid ventricular response is possible. The mechanisms of the "FBI" features of atrial fibrillation in WPW syndrome follow.

Fast. The ventricular rate exceeds 200 beats/min. The following factors determine the ventricular rate during atrial fibrillation[1]:

1. Refractory period duration of the accessory pathway in the anterograde direction.
2. Refractory period of the AV node.
3. Refractory period of the ventricle.
4. Concealed anterograde and retrograde penetration into the accessory pathway and the AV node.[19]
5. Sympathetic stimulation shortens the refractory period of the accessory pathway and accelerates the ventricular rate.[24] It is important to terminate this tachycardia promptly and in the meantime to reassure the patient. There is a reflex sympathetic response to the fall in blood pressure that is associated with atrial fibrillation and the very rapid ventricular rate. Anxiety adds to this response.

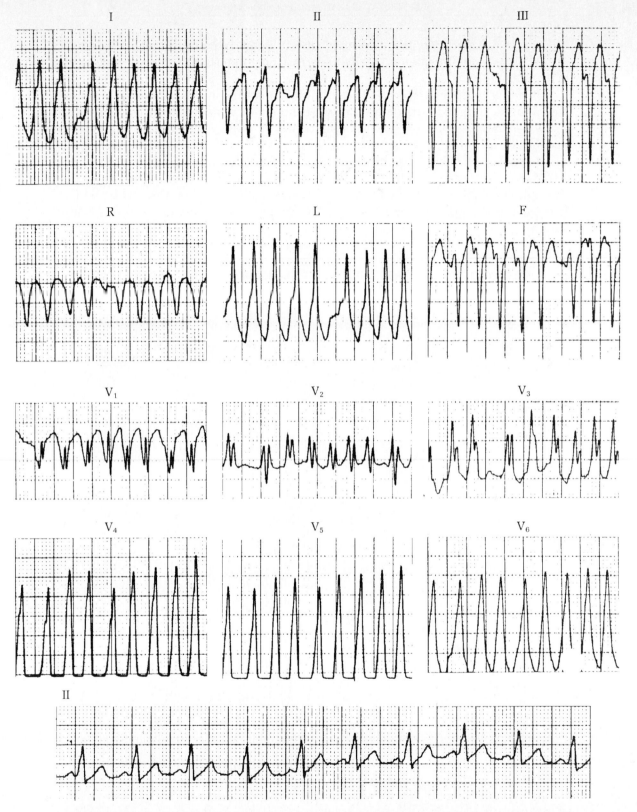

Fig. 23-20. A 12-lead ECG showing atrial fibrillation with conduction over an accessory pathway. Although the QRS has the shape of VT, the rhythm is irregular, typical of this mechanism. The lead II rhythm strip was taken after conversion to sinus rhythm. Note the short PR interval, delta wave, and broad QRS complex typical of overt WPW syndrome. *(Courtesy Ara Tilkian, MD, Van Nuys, Calif.)*

If the refractory period of the accessory pathway is short, the heart rate exceeds 300/min. This is a life-threatening arrhythmia that may deteriorate into ventricular fibrillation.

Broad. The QRS complex is broad (it looks just like a VT) because ventricular activation is initiated outside the normal conduction system. (Remember that this is not a reentry circuit and that it is the accessory pathway that must be blocked, not the AV node.)

Irregular. The rhythm is irregular because of rapid stimulation from the fibrillating atria, concealed conduction into the accessory pathway, and perhaps also because of changing refractoriness of the accessory pathway. This irregularity, which is typical, distinguishes atrial fibrillation with conduction over an accessory pathway from VT, which is usually regular.

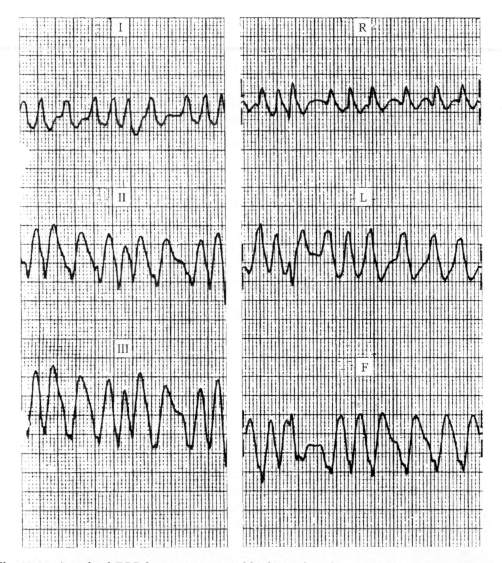

Fig. 23-21. A 12-lead ECG from an 18-year-old admitted to the emergency department. The signs of atrial fibrillation and WPW syndrome are evident. After conversion to sinus rhythm the signs of preexcitation are subtle and easy to miss. *(Courtesy Kathleen Hester, RN, and Cathy Stark, RN, Concord, Calif.)*

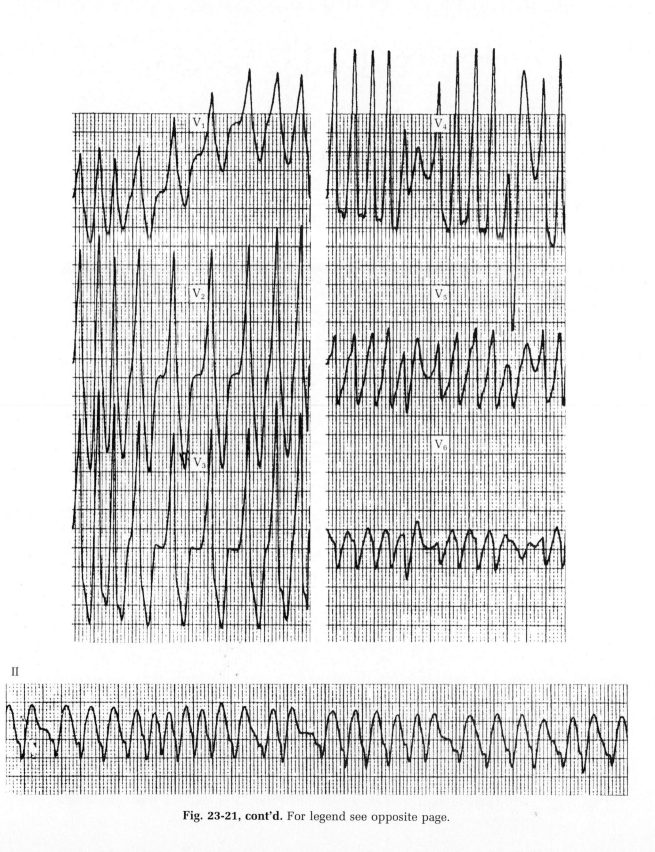

Fig. 23-21, cont'd. For legend see opposite page.

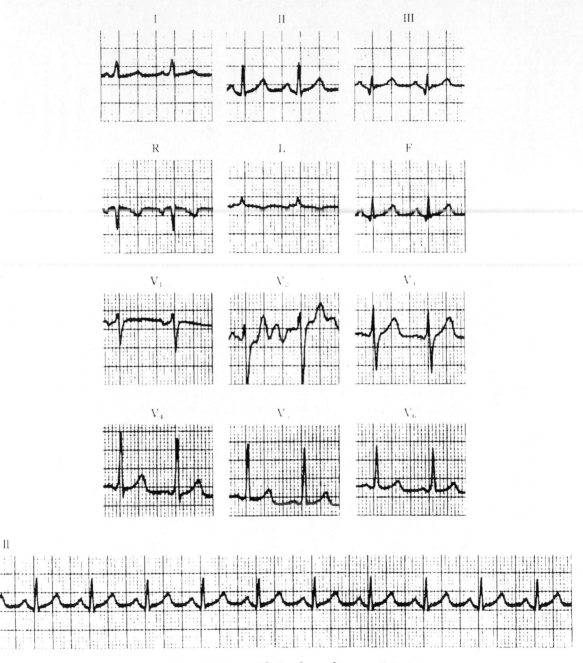

Fig. 23-21, cont'd. For legend see p. 330.

Emergency treatment. When a fast, broad, irregular rhythm presents itself in the emergency setting, one must do the following:

1. Obtain a 12-lead ECG during the tachycardia and one during sinus rhythm following conversion.
2. Administer procainamide 10 mg/kg body weight over 5 min. If procainamide does not slow down the rhythm and block the accessory pathway (complexes will become narrow as they pass down the AV node), the next step is as follows.

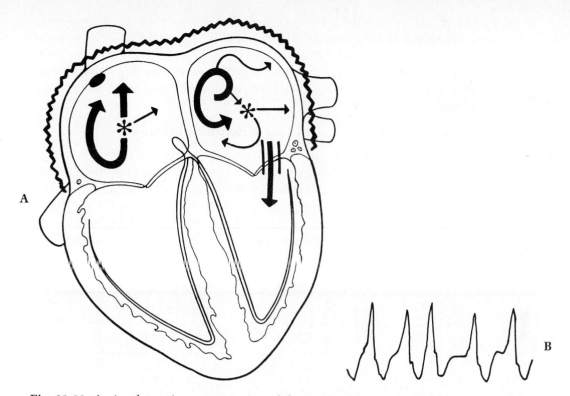

Fig. 23-22. A, A schematic representation of the mechanism of atrial fibrillation with conduction down an accessory pathway and, **B,** the resulting typical ECG tracing.

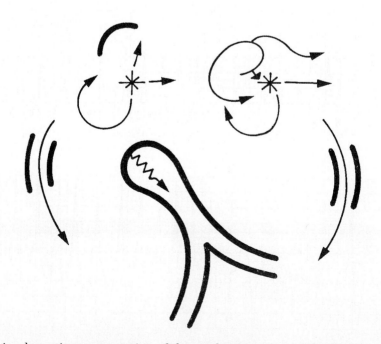

Fig. 23-23. A schematic representation of the mechanism of atrial fibrillation with conduction down a right-sided and left-sided accessory pathway.

3. Cardioversion, of course, is the first-line emergency treatment if there is severe circulatory impairment or if procainamide is ineffective. After conversion to a sinus rhythm the patient is referred to a center skilled in the treatment of patients with WPW syndrome. If procainamide did not work, this referral is in an emergency basis, because the patient cannot be protected from
recurrence.

Atrial fibrillation with two accessory pathways

As illustrated in Fig. 23-23, when atrial fibrillation occurs in a patient with two
accessory pathways, conduction into the ventricles has three pathways, the AV node
and the two accessory pathways. This results in an irregular rhythm and broad QRS
complexes of different shapes, depending on which pathway activates the ventricles
first. There would also be fusion beats. Fig. 23-24 illustrates the ECG during atrial
fibrillation in a patient with both right-sided and left-sided accessory pathways.

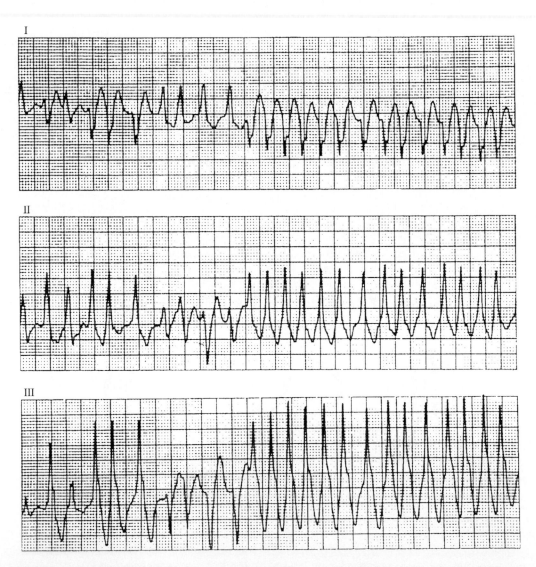

Fig. 23-24. Leads I, II, and III from a patient with atrial fibrillation and multiple accessory
pathways. *(From Yee R, Klein GJ, Sharma AD R et al. In Zipes DP, Jalife J, eds: Cardiac electrophysiology, Philadelphia, 1990, WB Saunders.)*

Locating the accessory pathway

The configuration and polarity of the P wave during orthodromic CMT help the examiner locate the atrial insertion site of the accessory pathway, whereas the axis of the delta wave during sinus rhythm helps locate the ventricular insertion site (Fig. 23-25). Because the atria are activated in a retrograde direction, this does not mean that the P′ wave will be always inverted in the inferior leads. For example, if the accessory pathway is left ventricular, the P′ wave is often negative in lead I. Its polarity in leads II and III depends on whether the left ventricular location is septal or posterior (negative) or left lateral (equiphasic or positive). If the accessory pathway is on the free wall of the right ventricle, the P′ waves are positive or biphasic in lead I and negative or biphasic in V_1 and may be positive in lead III and positive or equiphasic in lead II. Leads aV_R and aV_L are also helpful in locating the accessory pathway. If the P′ in aV_R is greater than the P′ in aV_L, there is a postero septal accessory pathway.

RADIOFREQUENCY ABLATION

The excitement over recent advances in the application of radiofrequency for the transvenous ablation of accessory pathways is well justified. This approach is a successful, less expensive, nonsurgical option for patients who suffer from and are threatened by the arrhythmias of WPW syndrome and AV nodal reentry tachycardia, among others. Jackman et al.[25] initially demonstrated in animals that radiofrequency current could be used to selectively destroy myocardial tissue in the anatomic location where some accessory pathways lie (underneath the mitral valve an-

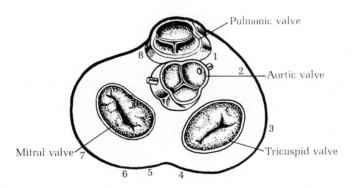

DELTA WAVE POLARITY

	I	II	III	(aV)	R	L	F	(V)	1	2	3	4	5	6
1	+	+	+	.	−		+	.			+	+	+	+
2	+	+	−	.	−	+	−	.		+	+	+	+	+
3	+		−	.	−	+		.		+	+	+	+	+
4	+	−	−	.	−	+	−	.		+	+	+	+	+
5	+	−	−	.	−	+	−	.	+	+	+	+	+	+
6	+	+		.	−		+	.	+	+	+	+	+	+
7	−		+	.	−	+		.	+	+	+	+	−	−
8	−	+	+	.	−	−	+	.	+	+	+	+	+	+

Fig. 23-25. Locating the accessory pathway by the delta wave polarity in the 12-lead ECG. *(Courtesy Hein J.J. Wellens, MD, The Netherlands.)*

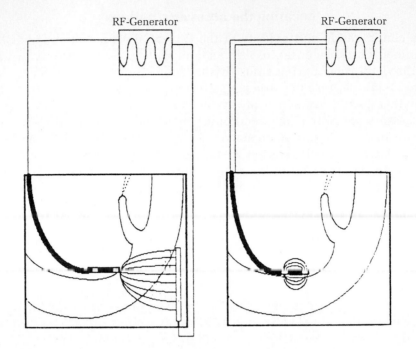

Fig. 23-26. Schematic diagram of radiofrequency (RF) circuit for unipolar *(left panel)* and bipolar *(right panel)* energy application. In a unipolar electrode configuration, high temperature and tissue necrosis occur at the "active" electrode because of high current density. No heating occurs at the "passive" electrode because it has a large surface that does not focus but disperses the current. In a bipolar electrode configuration two "active" electrodes are applied, resulting in a flow of current and heat development being focused between these electrodes. *(From Borggrefe Haverkamp W, M Hindricks G, et al. In Zipes DP, Jalife J, eds: Cardiac electrophysiology, Philadelphia, 1990, WB Saunders.)*

nulus at the AV junction between the atrium and ventricle). Soon after, this technique was used in clinical practice as a cure for patients with WPW syndrome.[26-28]

Radiofrequency ablation involves the use of unmodulated, high-frequency alternating current flow through tissue to cause heat, cell desiccation, and coagulation necrosis for the purpose of destroying troublesome areas and pathways in the heart. The closed electrical circuit required for cardiac ablation is achieved by a radiofrequency generator, connecting leads, and unipolar or bipolar electrodes. Unipolar and bipolar ablation are compared in Fig. 23-26.

NODOVENTRICULAR AND FASCICULOVENTRICULAR FIBERS

In 1941 Mahaim and Winston[29] described anomalous tracts between the lower AV node or bundle of His and the ventricles. The main anatomic types of Mahaim fibers are (1) nodoventricular fibers, which arise from the AV node itself and insert into the ventricle, and (2) fasciculoventricular fibers, which arise from the bundle of His or the bundle branches (Fig. 23-27).

ECG during sinus rhythm

The PR interval and QRS duration during sinus rhythm depend on the origin and insertion of the extra fiber, as well as its length and conduction time. Nodoven-

Mahaim fibers

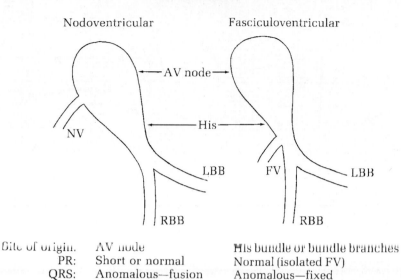

	Site of origin:	AV node	His bundle or bundle branches
	PR:	Short or normal	Normal (isolated FV)
	QRS:	Anomalous—fusion	Anomalous—fixed

Fig. 23-27. Diagramatic representation of the AV node and the two main varieties of Mahaim fibers. Nodoventricular (NV) fibers arise from the AV node itself, while fasciculoventricular (FV) fibers arise from the His bundle or the bundle branches. *LBB,* Left bundle branch; *RBB,* right bundle branch. *(From Gallagher JJ et al: Circulation 64:176, 1981.)*

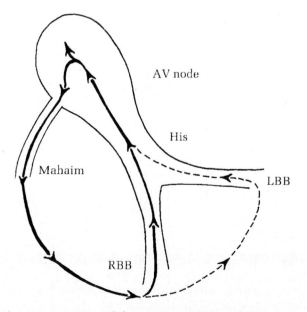

Fig. 23-28. Schematic representation of the reentry circuit underlying a reciprocating tachycardia. This reentry circuit uses a nodoventricular fiber. The nodoventricular fiber may insert into either the right ventricle or the RBB. The retrograde return circuit can conceivably be completed by either the RBB or the LBB. A portion of the reentry loop is confined to the AV node, and the atrium does not form a necessary link in the loop. *(From Gallagher JJ et al: Circulation 64:176, 1981.)*

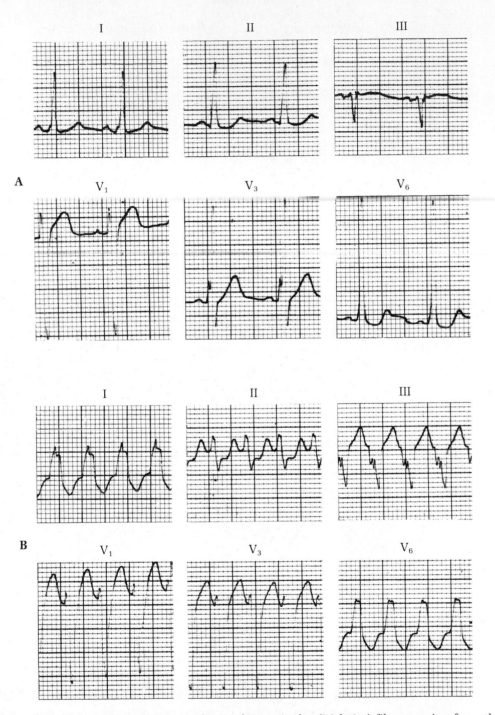

Fig. 23-29. Tracing from a patient with a nodoventricular (Mahaim) fiber running from the AV node to the posteroinferior part of the right ventricle. **A,** The ECG during sinus rhythm. **B,** The ECG during a supraventricular reentry mechanism. During tachycardia the ventricle is activated exclusively by way of the nodoventricular fiber (see Fig. 23-28). *(From Wellens HJJ et al. In Wellens HJJ, Kulbertus HE, eds: What's new in electrocardiography, The Hague, 1981, Martinus Nijhoff.)*

tricular fibers may be manifested by either a short or a normal PR interval. There may be a delta wave, and the QRS complex is often a fusion beat resulting from conduction over the extra fiber and over the normal pathway.

Paroxysmal supraventricular tachycardia resulting from nodoventricular fibers

When a supraventricular impulse is conducted in an anterograde direction down the extra fiber and not down the AV node, it may then return in a retrograde direction to the atria via the bundle branch(es), bundle of His, and AV node (Fig. 23-28). The resulting reciprocating SVT has a broad QRS complex because the ventricles are activated outside the conduction system. If the extra fiber inserts into the right ventricle, the QRS resembles left bundle branch block (Fig. 23-29). Thus there is usually an rS in lead V_1 and an RS in V_2 with left axis deviation.

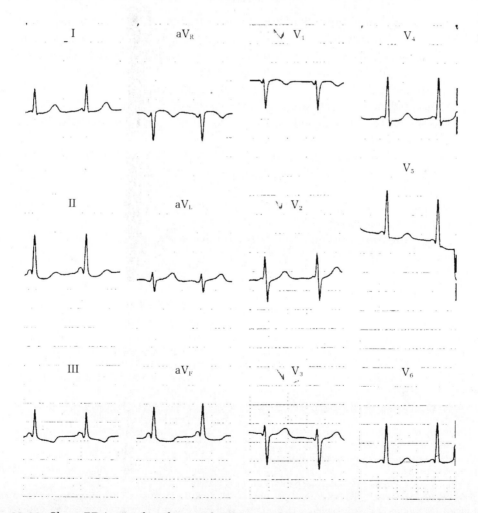

Fig. 23-30. Short PR interval and normal QRS complex of Lown-Ganong-Levine syndrome. (Courtesy Dixie Lee Hacker-Summers, Anchorage, Ala.)

SHORT PR SYNDROME (INTRANODAL BYPASS TRACT)

Although short PR intervals, normal QRS durations, and a tendency to SVTs were reported in 1938 by Clerc et al.[30] the syndrome is best known because of the emphasis given it by the work of Lown et al.,[31] who in 1952 reported that 11 patients with a short PR interval and a normal QRS complex had a much greater incidence of PSVT than did individuals with a normal PR interval. Thus the short PR syndrome is sometimes called the *Lown-Ganong-Levine syndrome.*

Note that (1) the syndrome is not said to exist simply because the PR is short. Supraventricular tachycardia (AV reciprocating tachycardia, atrial fibrillation, or atrial flutter) must also be documented and (2) a short PR interval may reflect error in measurement, a lower limit of normal, a child or an adolescent, increased heart rate, enhanced sympathetic activity, or ectopic atrial or junctional rhythms.

Fig. 23-30 is a 12-lead ECG tracing from an individual with Lown Ganong Levine syndrome. Note that the PR interval in this case is so short that there is no PR segment and that the QRS duration is normal.

SUMMARY

The most common type of preexcitation involves an AV accessory pathway, WPW syndrome. This syndrome consists of the ECG findings of short PR interval, delta wave, broad QRS complex, and the tendency to develop PSVT. The most common arrhythmias in such patients are orthodromic CMT (anterograde conduction over an accessory pathway and retrograde conduction over an accessory pathway) and atrial fibrillation, which results in very rapid rates.

Accessory pathways may exist in patients who do not manifest the ECG signs of preexcitation but who have the same tendencies to develop CMT and life-threatening atrial fibrillation. Patients with so-called concealed accessory pathways, although prone to PSVT, do not have excessively rapid heart rates with atrial fibrillation.

Because of the possibility of atrial fibrillation and deterioration into ventricular fibrillation and because there is a cure in the form of radiofrequency catheter ablation, identification and emergency treatment of symptomatic patients with accessory pathways are extremely important.

REFERENCES

1. Wellens HJJ: Pre-excitation. In Willerson JT, Cohn JN, eds: *Cardiovascular medicine,* New York, 1995, Churchill Livingstone.
2. Wolff L, Parkinson J, White P et al: Bundle-branch block with short P-R interval in healthy young people prone to paroxysmal tachycardia, *Am Heart J* 5:685, 1930.
3. Kent AFS: Researches on structure and function of mammalian heart, *J Physiol* 14:233, 1893
3a. Holzman M, Scherf D: Uber Elektrokardiogramme mit vorkurzten vorhol Kammer-Distanz und positiven P-Zacken, *z Klin Med* 121:404, 1932.
3b. Wolferth CC, Wood FC: The mechanism of production of short P-R intervals and prolonged QRS complexes in patients with presumably undamaged hearts. Hypothesis of an accessory pathway of auriculoventricular conduction (bundle of Kent), *Am Heart J* 8:297, 1933.
4. Wood FC, Wolferth CC, Geckeler GD: Histological demonstration of accessory muscular connections between auricle and ventricle in a case of short P-R interval and prolonged QRS complex, *Am Heart J* 25:454, 1943.
5. Ohnell RF: Preexcitation: a cardiac abnormality, *Acta Med Scand (Suppl)* 152:74, 1944.
6. Hiss RG, Lamb LE: Electrocardiographic findings in 122,043 individuals, *Circulation* 25: 947, 1962.
7. Smith RF: The Wolff-Parkinson-White syndrome as an aviation risk, *Circulation* 29:672, 1964.
8. Cox JL, Ferguson TB Jr: Surgery for the Wolff-Parkinson-White syndrome: the endocardial approach, *Semin Thorac Cardiovasc Surg* 1:34, 1989.

9. Wellens HJJ, Brugada P, Penn OC et al: Pre-excitation syndromes. In Zipes DP, Jalife J, eds: *Cardiac electrophysiology,* Philadelphia, 1990, WB Saunders.

10. Guize L, Soria R, Chaouat JC et al: Prévalence et évolution du syndrome de Wolff-Parkinson-White dans une population de 138048 subjets, *Ann Med Interne (Paris)* 136:474, 1985.

11. Yee R, Klein GJ, Guiraudon GM: The Wolff-Parkinson-White syndrome. In Zipes DP, Jalife J, eds: *Cardiac electrophysiology from cell to bedside,* ed 2, Philadelphia, 1995, WB Saunders.

12. Vidaillet HJ, Pressley JC, Henke E, et al: Familial occurrence of accessory atrioventricular pathways (pre-excitation syndrome), *N Engl J Med* 34:65, 1987.

13. Waller BF: Clinicopathological correlations of the human cardiac conduction system. In Zipes DP, Jalife J, eds: *Cardiac electrophysiology,* Philadelphia, 1990, WB Saunders.

14. Wellens HJJ, Bruguda P: Value of programmed stimulation of the heart in patients with Wolff-Parkinson-White syndrome. In Josephson ME, Wellens HJJ, eds: *Tachycardias: mechanisms, diagnosis, treatment,* Philadelphia, 1984, Lea & Febiger.

15. Wellens HJJ: Wolff-Parkinson-White syndrome. Part I, *Mod Concepts Cardiovasc Dis* 52:53, 1983.

16. Levy S, Bronstet JP, Clemency J: Syndrome de Wolff-Parkinson-White, *Arch Mal Coeur* 72:634, 1979.

17. Wellens HJJ, Braat SH, Brugada P et al: Use of procainamide in patients with the Wolff-Parkinson-White syndrome to disclose a short refractory period of the accessory pathway, *Am J Cardiol* 50:921, 1982.

18. Wellens HJJ Bär FW, Vanagt EJ: Death after ajmaline administration, *Am J Cardiol* 50:1087, 1982.

19. Josephson ME, Wellens HJJ: Differential diagnosis of supraventricular tachycardia, *Cardiol Clin* 8:411, 1990.

20. Okumura K et al: "Incessant" atrioventricular (AV) reciprocating tachycardia utilizing left lateral AV bypass pathway with a long retrograde conduction time, *PACE Pacing Clin Electrophysiol* 9:332, 1986.

21. O'Neill BJ, Klein GJ, Guiraudon GM et al: Results of operative therapy in the permanent form of functional reciprocating tachycardia, *Am J Cardiol* 63:1074, 1989.

22. Packer D et al: Tachycardia induced cardiomyopathy: a reversible form of left ventricular dysfunction, *Am J Cardiol* 57:563, 1986.

23. Wellens HJJ, Josephson ME: *Diagnosis of difficult arrhythmias,* Miami, 1987, Medtronic.

24. Wellens HJJ, Brugada P, Roy D et al: Effect of isoproterenol on the antegrade refractory period of the accessory pathway in patients with Wolff-Parkinson-White syndrome, *Am J Cardiol* 50:180, 1982.

25. Jackman WM, Kuck KH, Naccarelli GV et al: Radiofrequency current directed across the mitral valve annulus with a bipolar epicardial-endocardial catheter electrode configuration in dogs, *Circulation* 78:1288, 1988.

26. Jackman WM, Wang W, Friday KJ et al: Catheter ablation of accessory atrioventricular pathways (Wolff-Parkinson-White syndrome) by radiofrequency current, *N Engl J Med* 324:1605, 1991.

27. Calkins H, Souza J, El-Atassi R et al: Diagnosis and cure of the Wolff-Parkinson-White syndrome of paroxysmal supraventricular tachyardias during a single electrophysiologic test, *N Engl J Med* 324:1612, 1991.

28. Schlutr M, Geiger M, Siebels J et al: Catheter ablation using radiofrequency current to cure symptomatic patients with tachyarrhythmias related to an accessory atrioventricular pathway, *Circulation* 84:1644, 1991.

29. Mahaim I, Winston RM: Recherches d'anatomie comparee et de pathologie experimentale sur les connexions hautes du faisceau de His-Tawara, *Cardiologia* 5:189, 1941.

30. Clerc A, Levy R, Critesco C: A propos du raccourcissement permanent de l'espace P-R de l'éctrocardiogramme sans déformation du complexe ventriculaire, *Arch Mal Coeur* 31:569, 1938.

31. Lown B, Ganong WF, Levine SA: The syndrome of short P-R interval, normal QRS complex and paroxysmal rapid heart activation, *Circulation* 5:693, 1952.

24

Unstable Angina, Wellens Syndrome, and Left Main and Three-Vessel Coronary Artery Disease

Unstable Angina   *342*
Wellens Syndrome   *344*
Medical Treatment of Unstable
  Angina   *358*

Left Main and Three Vessel Disease   *360*
Summary   *360*

UNSTABLE ANGINA

U nstable angina is cardiac pain caused by severe transient myocardial ischemia resulting from severe coronary narrowing or coronary occlusion.

Incidence

Unstable angina has become the most frequent indication for admission to most coronary care units, being responsible for more than 570,000 hospitalizations annually in the United States. In more than 70,000 of those hospitalized with unstable angina, myocardial infarction (MI) develops, and some persons die suddenly. Of the patients admitted with acute MI, 30% to 60% have unstable angina before they reach the hospital.[1]

Type of pain

- Recent onset
- Sudden worsening of preexisting angina
- Occurs after a pain-free period
- Stuttering recurrence over days and weeks

Identifying characteristics

- Not "momentary" in duration
- Occurs at rest or is brought on by minimal exertion, commonly by walking or use of the arms
- Patient may describe "walking through" or "walking off" the pain
- During pain, blood pressure and heart rate are usually elevated, S_3 gallop is heard, and the patient resists lying down
- Relieved by sublingual nitroglycerin within a few (less than 5) minutes

Anginal pain

Anginal pain may radiate to the following:
- Any region above the waist
- Epigastric location (may confuse the diagnosis)
- Medial aspect of arms and the mandible (most characteristic location)
- Retrosternal area (highly specific)

NOTE: Localization of the pain to small areas is unusual.

Patients' common descriptions of anginal pain

- Tightness, heaviness, squeezing, choking, aching, burning, a weight, or numbness
- Duration: "Lasts about 2 minutes" (patients tend to overestimate)
- Builds up gradually, plateaus, and subsides gradually

Words and phrases patients use to describe angina pectoris[2] include the following*:

"A red hot poker"
"A shoe box in my chest"
"A toothache"
"Hot flame in the upper part of my mouth"
"An elephant on my chest"
"Jaw pain"
"Arthritis" (shoulder, elbow, or wrists)
"A bad feeling in the upper portion of my back"
"Tracheitis"
"A good feeling in my chest—-like I used to have in my side when I ran as a child"
"Sternal whisper"
"Dryness in my throat produced by effort or emotional stress"
"Smoke in my chest"
"Someone choking me from behind"

One patient in Hurst's study described severe, moderate, and mild discomfort as follows:

Severe discomfort: "A large fish hook stuck under my jaw" (hung up and suspended from a scaffold)
Moderate discomfort: "A small fish hook caught in my lower jaw"
Mild discomfort: "A needle and thread being pulled between two lower teeth"

Pain that is not anginal

- Occurs after, rather than during, exertion
- Caused by talking
- Caused by "lying on the left side"

*With thanks to J. Willis Hurst, MD.

- Occurs after, rather than during, coitus
- Precipitated exclusively by emotion
- Associated with palpitations, precordial tenderness, lightheadedness, or dysphagia
- "Sharp" (Anginal pain is not sticking or needlelike.)

Pathogenesis

Plaque fissure. During the pain of unstable angina there is increased thrombin generation. The most widely proposed mechanism for the increased thrombin formation that heralds the onset of the acute event is plaque fissure. The complicated events following plaque fissure are the following: exposure of endothelial collagen and its prothrombotic substrates to flowing blood, platelet aggregation, release of a vasospastic substance, coagulation, and thrombus formation.

A fibrous cap covers the atherosclerotic plaque. Thinning of this cap causes its delicate latticework of collagen to tear, usually at the junction of its attachment to normal intima, producing a fissure into the plaque. This tear constitutes an injury to the artery, which responds with the formation of a platelet-rich thrombus. The deeper the injury, the more layers of platelet deposition. For example, a mild injury such as endothelial denudation would result in a single layer of platelet deposition as long as the event was not accompanied by severe stenosis, which itself is a stimulus for enhanced platelet deposition. A deep injury, such as a tear into the internal elastic lamina of the artery or into the plaque fissure, results in platelet deposition within milliseconds; total occlusion may occur within minutes. The occluding lesion is typically complex with irregular, ragged borders (Fig. 24-1).[3]

Following the tearing event several things can happen to the thrombus, as illustrated in Fig. 24-2.

Fig. 24-2, A. The tear gets bigger until the lumen of the vessel occludes, resulting in acute MI and perhaps sudden death.

Fig. 24-2, B. It partially and perhaps critically obstructs the lumen, resulting in unstable angina with or without non–Q-wave MI and perhaps sudden death.

Fig. 24-2, C. It may be incorporated into the lesion and the fissure may heal over, resulting in no symptoms.

Fig. 24-2, D. It may become organized and may produce more symptoms.

Fig. 24-2, E. The thrombus may embolize.[4]

Transient intermittent lymphocyte activation. Doubts have arisen about the concept of plaque fissure being responsible for the events leading to unstable angina. The hypothesis is that the events precipitating unstable angina represent an acute, transient inflammatory state caused by lymphocyte activation that is intermittently triggered by unknown factors. Thus the string of events leading to the unstable pain is proposed to be exposure of lymphocytes to an inducer that triggers monocyte activation, increased thrombin generation, and thrombin formation.[5]

WELLENS SYNDROME

Wellens syndrome is a group of ECG signs that occur during the pain-free period in a patient with unstable angina, indicating critical stenosis high in the left anterior descending (LAD) coronary artery. The diagnosis is made because of specific T-wave changes in precordial leads on or shortly after hospital admission. Recognition of such a pattern and subsequent cardiac catheterization identify the need

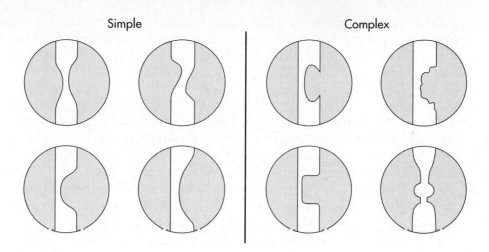

Simple   Complex

Schema of Discrete Lesions

Fig. 24-1. Schema of the most common coronary lesion geometries found at angiography (discrete simple vs. discrete complex lesions). *(From Ambrose JA, Israel DH: Am J Cardiol 68:78B, 1991.)*

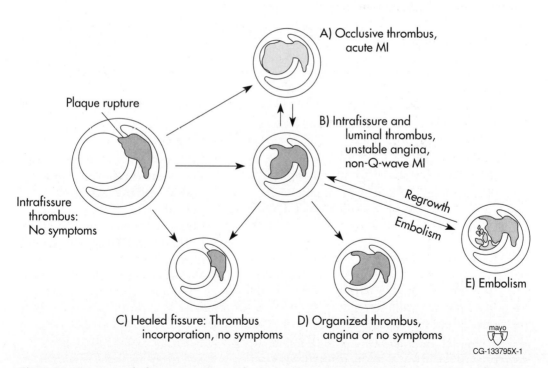

Plaque rupture

A) Occlusive thrombus, acute MI

B) Intrafissure and luminal thrombus, unstable angina, non-Q-wave MI

Intrafissure thrombus: No symptoms

Regrowth

Embolism

C) Healed fissure: Thrombus incorporation, no symptoms

D) Organized thrombus, angina or no symptoms

E) Embolism

CG-133795X-1

Fig. 24-2. Diagram of plaque rupture and arterial thrombus. Plaque rupture leads to the formation of a fissure. Flowing blood contacts intraarterial structures and forms an intrafissure thrombus. The thrombus may progress to a luminal thrombus causing, *A,* total occlusion, often associated with transmural or Q-wave myocardial infarction (MI). *B,* Incomplete occlusion resulting in unstable angina or non–Q-wave MI. *B to C,* The intraluminal thrombus may undergo endogenous lysis with healing of the fissure and no progression of disease or symptoms. *D,* The intraluminal thrombus may organize, leading to progression of disease with or without subsequent symptoms. *E,* A piece of thrombus may embolize distally. *(From Chesebro JH, Zoldhelyi P, Fuster V: Am J Cardiol 68:2B, 1991.)*

for bypass grafting or percutaneous transluminal coronary angioplasty (PTCA). Such intervention would prevent the development of extensive anterior wall MI. In view of the large area of the ventricle at risk, the recognition of this ECG pattern takes on critical importance.

Historical background

In 1981 and 1982 and again in 1985, 1986, and 1989 Wellens and others described in lectures[6,7] and publications[8-10] criteria by which critical stenosis high in the left anterior descending coronary artery could be diagnosed from specific ST-T segment changes on or shortly after admission to the hospital. The initial published study[8] involved 145 consecutive patients who were admitted because of unstable angina, of whom 26 had what is now recognized as Wellens syndrome, the classic pattern for critical proximal LAD coronary artery stenosis and imminent (mean period, 8.5 days) extensive anterior wall MI. Another study reported on 180 consecutive patients with unstable angina who had this distinctive, easily recognized ECG pattern.[10]

The term *Wellens syndrome* was first used by Ara G. Tilkian (Van Nuys, Calif.) and his cardiology group as an expedient way of communicating the need for urgency. Many patients all over the United States have benefited from this important study by the Wellens group and from Tilkian's encouragement to include Wellens's findings in three editions of this book.

ECG recognition

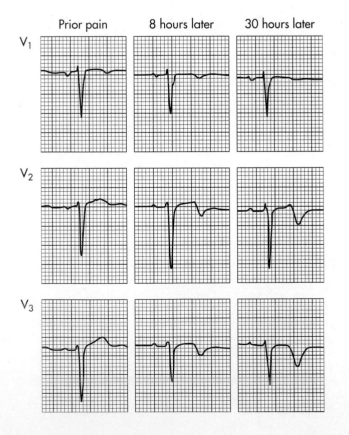

- **Prior angina**
- **Progressive, symmetric, deep T-wave inversion in leads V_2 and V_3 during pain-free periods**
- **Little or no enzyme elevation**
- **Little or no ST-segment elevation (≤ 1 mm)**
- **No loss of precordial R waves**

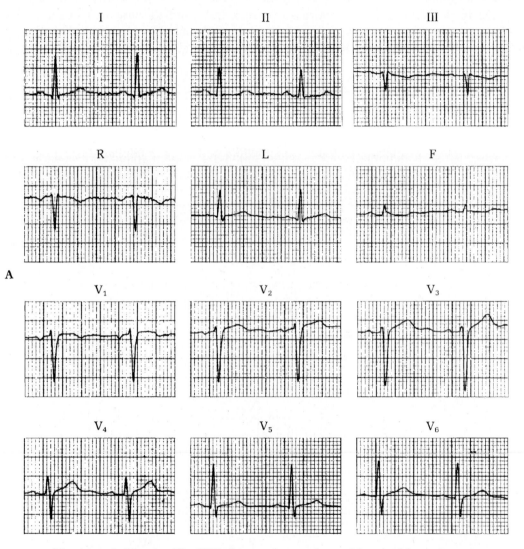

A

Fig. 24-3. A, Nonspecific ST-T changes in a patient with unstable angina.

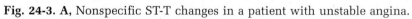

Continued.

The ST segment in leads V_2 and V_3 turns down into a negative T wave at an ST-T angle of 60 to 90 degrees. If the T wave is also inverted in V_1, this angle is wider. During chest pain these T-wave changes are replaced by positive T waves with either ST-segment elevation or depression. It is during this time that the coronary vessel is critically narrowed or occluding; the T-wave inversion of Wellens syndrome represents reperfusion.

Although leads V_2 and V_3 are the diagnostic leads for Wellens syndrome, the T-wave inversion is not necessarily limited to those leads. In a study involving 180 patients, the ST-T segment abnormalities seen in V_2 and V_3 were also found in lead V_1 in 121 patients, in lead V_4 in 136 patients, and sometimes in leads V_5 and V_6.[10]

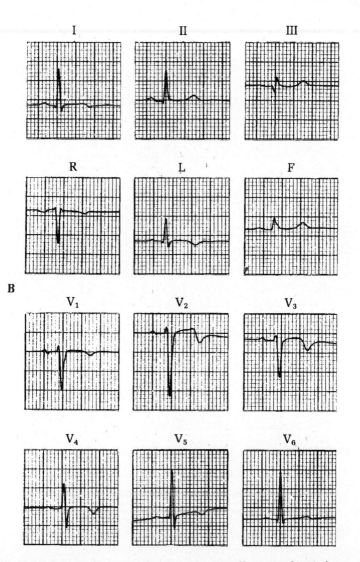

Fig. 24-3, cont'd. B, Eight hours later, definite signs of Wellens syndrome have appeared and the patient is pain free. Note in V_2 and V_3 the symmetric T-wave negativity and the takeoff of the negative T wave from the ST segment at an angle of about 80 degrees.

A series of 12-lead ECGs in Fig. 24-3 illustrate Wellens syndrome. The patient entered the emergency department because of pain at home. If the patient had been monitored on lead II or V_1 (as is common), this important sign would not have been noted and the patient would most likely have had a massive anterior wall MI. Fig. 24-4 is a drawing of the occlusion seen on arteriography in this patient. The location of the occlusion between the first and second septal branches is typical.

ECG during pain

Fig. 24-5 shows ECGs from a 69-year-old man with unstable angina who was admitted to the coronary care unit. His admission tracing (Fig. 24-5, *A*) showed Wellens syndrome. He was started on a regimen of heparin and nitroglycerin drips

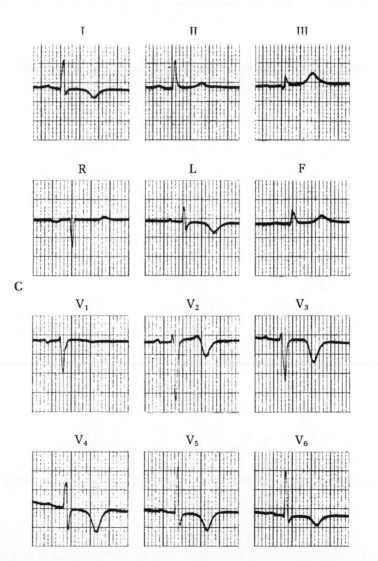

Fig. 24-3, cont'd. C, Ten hours later. This 12-lead ECG was taken just before cardiac catheterization. Note the deepening from the prior tracings of the symmetric T wave in leads V_2 to V_5. Lead II would have given no hint of these dramatic events. *(Courtesy Ara G. Tilkian, MD, Van Nuys, Calif.)*

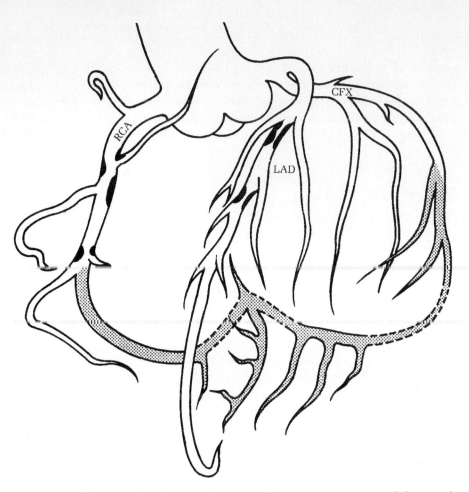

Fig. 24-4. Same patient as in Fig. 24-3. Drawing of the coronary arteries and their occlusions as seen with arteriography. The critical proximal left anterior descending (LAD) coronary artery stenosis is evident. *CFX,* Circumflex artery; *RCA,* right coronary artery.

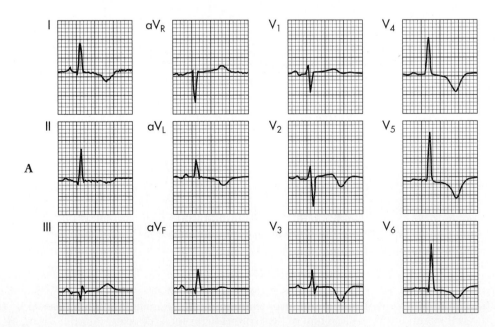

Fig. 24-5. For legend see opposite page.

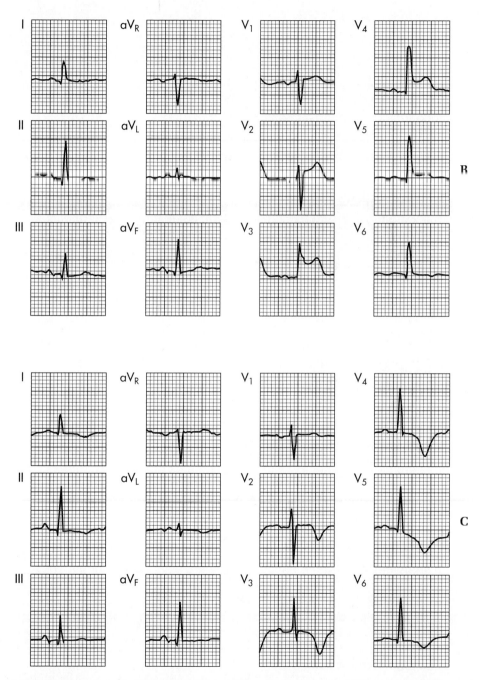

Fig. 24-5. A, Wellens syndrome on admission; the creatine kinase (CK) is 97, and the patient is without pain at the time. **B,** Eight hours later, during pain; the ST-segment elevation can be seen in V_2 to V_5. **C,** Ten hours after admission; the patient is without pain, and the T waves are deeper in the diagnostic leads V_2 and V_3. This diagnosis was made by Darlene Boomhower, RN, of La Mirada, Calif.

but continued to have unstable angina. Note that during pain (Fig. 24-5, *B*) there is ST-segment elevation as the coronary vessel critically narrows or occludes. The tracings in Fig. 24-5, *C*, were taken before coronary artery bypass surgery was performed. Note that the T waves in the precordial leads have deepened. His cardiac catheterization revealed 95% occlusion of the proximal LAD and 90% occlusion of the right

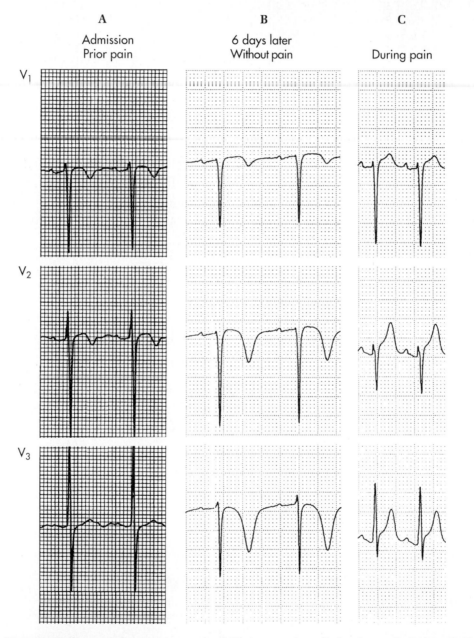

Fig. 24-6. A, Wellens syndrome seen on lead V_2 in a tracing obtained on admission. **B,** During pain the ST segments are elevated in V_1 to V_3. **C,** By the fifth hospital day all precordial T waves are inverted, deeply so in V_2 to V_4. The diagnosis of critical proximal LAD stenosis was made by Lyn Gilliam, RN, MN, CCRN, Columbia, S.C. Arteriography revealed 90% occlusion of the proximal LAD coronary artery.

coronary and circumflex arteries. He was discharged on his sixth hospital day without complications.

Fig. 24-6 is a series of ECGs from a 35-year-old woman who was complaining of "epigastric pain." During pain the ST segment is elevated, and following pain the signs of reperfusion (Wellens syndrome) are present. During the evolution of the dramatic changes taking place in leads V_2 and V_3, lead II remained the same and V_1 was not diagnostic, again emphasizing that patients with unstable angina must be monitored on lead V_2 or V_3. Cardiac catheterization revealed 90% occlusion of the proximal LAD. The patient had hypertension and a history of drug (cocaine) and alcohol abuse and was a heavy smoker.

Time frame for the development of the typical ECG findings

The typical ECG findings in Wellens syndrome (1) were present on admission or developed shortly thereafter in 60% of the 180 patients, (2) were present within 24 hours in the majority of the remainder of patients, or (3) were present within 2 to 5 days in a few patients. In the study by the Wellens group,[11] patients who had ECG signs at the time of admission had a longer duration of unstable angina and had a higher incidence of collateral vessels than did patients whose ECG signs developed later.

The 12-lead ECG in Fig. 24-7 was recorded on admission to the emergency department. The patient was a 51-year-old woman who was complaining of chest pain. The ECG changes of Wellens syndrome were present on admission; cardiac catheterization revealed 99% occlusion of the proximal LAD.

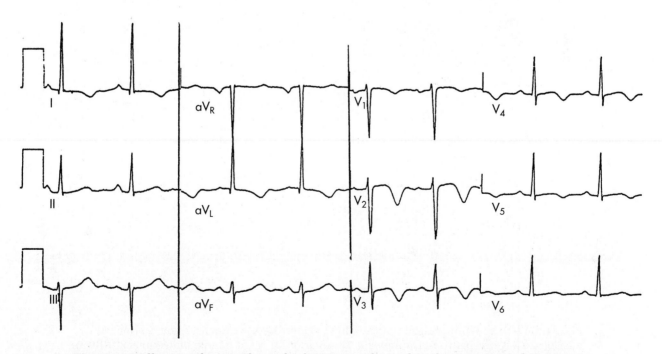

Fig. 24-7. Wellens syndrome. The 12 lead ECG was obtained in the emergency department, and the diagnosis made by Rebecca Fuller, RN, of Monterey, Calif. The patient was flown to San Jose, Calif. for cardiac catheterization. There was 99% occlusion of the proximal LAD.

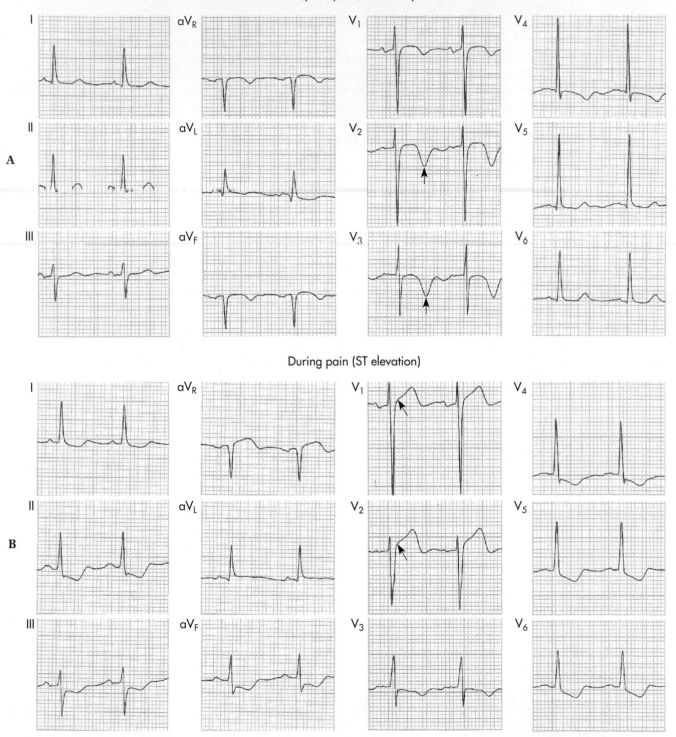

Fig. 24-8. Wellens syndrome with progression to anterior MI within a 12-hour period. **A,** Admission ECG (prior pain). **B,** During pain. **C,** Anterior MI, right bundle branch block (RBBB), and anterior hemiblock (LAH). The diagnosis of Wellens syndrome was made by Mary E. Thomas, RN, of South Whitley, Ind., but because of the patient's advanced age there was no cardiac catheterization.

12 hours later: Acute anterior wall MI, RBBB, LAH

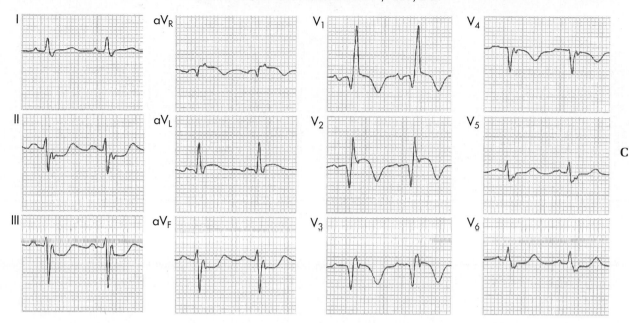

Fig. 24-8, cont'd. For legend see opposite page.

Fig. 24-8 shows a series of 12-lead ECGs taken during a 12-hour span without pain (Fig. 24-8, *A*), with pain (Fig. 24-8, *B*), and after having sustained anterior wall myocardial infarction, right bundle branch block, and anterior hemiblock (Fig. 24-8, *C*). This patient was not considered for intervention because of her advanced age (90 years).

Diagnostic monitoring leads

Often patients with unstable angina are admitted to telemetry units where nurses may not have the capability of monitoring on multiple leads. In such cases or in the intensive care unit or coronary care unit where this is also the situation the choice of monitoring leads becomes very important. It is not sufficient to simply admit the patient, monitor on lead V_1 or II, and await the next day's routine 12-lead ECG. Fig. 24-9 nicely illustrates the obvious development of Wellens syndrome in leads V_2 and V_3 while leads V_1 and II remain virtually unchanged.

If a unipolar V_2 or V_3 lead is not available for monitoring, the bipolar modified chest lead (MCL) MCL_2 or MCL_3 should be used. Fig. 24-10 demonstrates the use of MCL_3 to monitor a patient who was admitted with unstable angina. The 12-lead ECG obtained on admission showed no signs of an occluding coronary artery or reperfusion. The patient was monitored on MCL_3. When the T wave inverted, an emergency 12-lead ECG was ordered, the physician was called, and the patient was flown from Le Grande, Ore. to Portland. Cardiac catheterization revealed 95% occlusion of the proximal LAD.

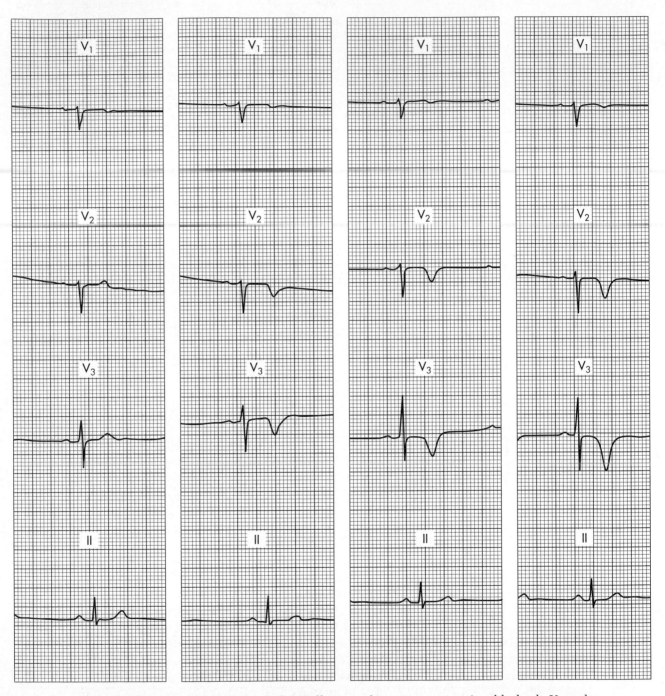

Fig. 24-9. The two diagnostic leads for Wellens syndrome are unquestionably leads V_2 and V_3. Classic picture of progressive, symmetric, deep inversion of the T wave in leads V_2 and V_3 in a patient with 97% occlusion of the proximal LAD. The T waves in leads V_1 and II do not change significantly.

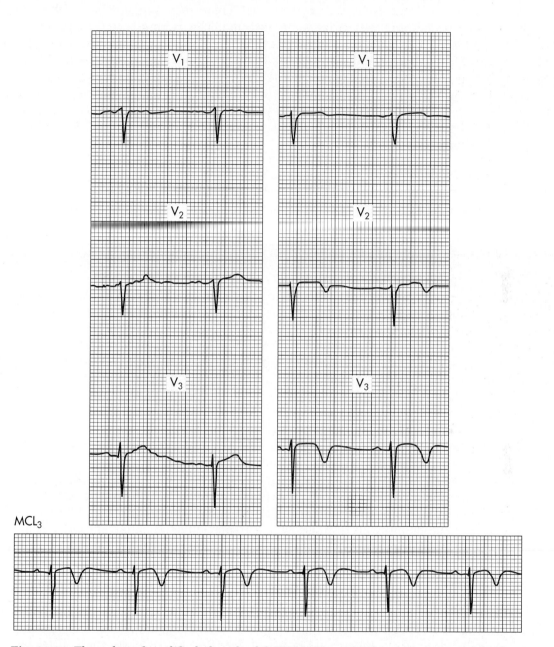

Fig. 24-10. The value of modified chest lead (MCL) MCL$_2$ or MCL$_3$ as a monitoring lead in patients with unstable angina. The patient was admitted with unstable angina. Five hours later the monitoring lead, MCL$_3$, showed Wellens syndrome and an emergency 12-lead ECG was obtained, confirming the diagnosis. Cardiac catheterization revealed 95% occlusion of the proximal LAD, total RCA occlusion, and 50% occlusion in both the left main and the CFX arteries. The diagnosis was made from the monitoring lead MCL$_3$ and the serial 12 lead ECGs by B.J. Brown, RN, and Norma Follett, RN, of Le Grande, Ore.

Emergency angiography

Because patients with Wellens syndrome without intervention may be imminently destined for massive anterior wall MI, emergency angiography to identify candidates for early revascularization is justified. The morbidity and mortality resulting from cardiac catheterization and revascularization surgery are less than those resulting from extensive anterior wall MI. In the past, in patients with the ECG findings that are now recognized as Wellens syndrome the condition has been diagnosed as either nontransmural or subendocardial ischemia (in the absence of enzyme changes) or subendocardial infarction of the anterior wall in the presence of slight enzyme elevation. However, patients with Wellens syndrome have not yet had the acute episode of MI.

MEDICAL TREATMENT OF UNSTABLE ANGINA

Treatment of unstable angina requires reduction of myocardial oxygen demand, coronary vasodilation (Beta-blockers, nitrates, calcium antagonists, bed rest), and rapid inhibition of intracoronary thrombus formation or extension.[18] Aspirin is an antiplatelet agent and heparin an anticoagulant; both are standard therapy for unstable angina. A study of 219 patients with unstable angina showed that a high dose of low molecular weight heparin during the acute phase was significantly better than aspirin alone or aspirin plus regular heparin.[19] However, neither heparin nor aspirin eliminate the risk of death, myocardial infarction, and recurrent ischemic pain. Heparin may be neutralized by activated platelets and inhibits only circulating thrombin, not clot-bound thrombin. Additionally, the risk of bleeding requires frequent adjustment of dosage and monitoring of anticoagulant effects.

Clinical tests suggest that direct thrombin inhibition (a new class of drugs) may be more effective in unstable angina than heparin. Hirulog is a synthetic, highly specific, direct inhibitor of free and clot-bound thrombin. This drug was designed after the model of hirudin, the natural thrombin inhibitor from the saliva of the medicinal leech *Hirudo medicinalis.* The antithrombotic action of hirudin in experimental animals was studied by Markwardt as early as 1982.[20] The encouraging results of the TIMI 7 trial[21] involving 410 patients with unstable angina agree with previous clinical experience with Hirulog.[22-25] When added to aspirin, Hirulog appears to be active and well tolerated with a stable activated partial thromboplastin time (aPTT) that does not require the dose adjustment needed for heparin.

Why not thrombolysis?

The concept of thrombolytics for patients with unstable angina is compelling because of its clearly beneficial effects in the early stages of MI for reducing mortality, limiting infarct size, and improving left ventricular function.[11,12] However, no beneficial clinical effects have been obtained by thrombolytic therapy for patients with unstable angina. In a double-blind, placebo-controlled, multicenter trial involving 159 patients with a typical history of unstable angina, no prior MI, and ECG signs of ischemia it was shown that although the angiographic picture improved with the thrombolytic therapy, there was an excess of bleeding complications and there was no clinical improvement.[13] This study confirmed the findings of others.[14,15]

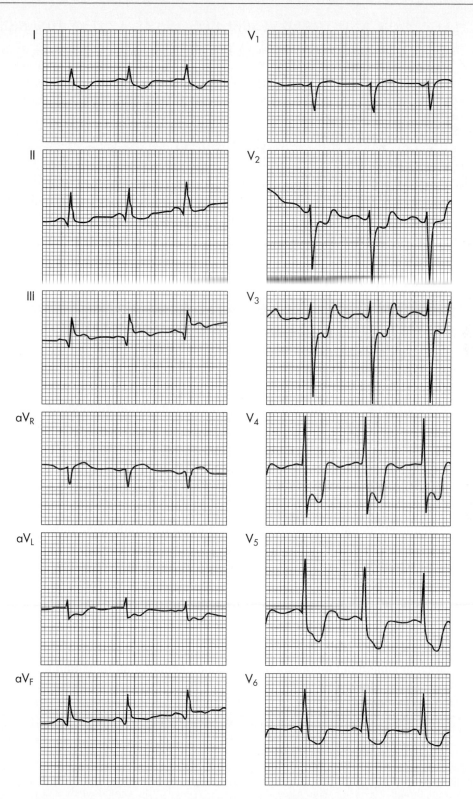

Fig. 24-11. The ECG pattern of left main stem disease. Note the llST segment elevation in leads V$_1$ and aV$_R$ and the ST segment depression in the remainder of the precordial leads and in leads I, II, and aV$_L$. The patient had an old inferior myocardial infarction. *(From Wellens HJJ, Conover M: The ECG in emergency decision making, Philadelphia, 1992, WB Saunders.)*

LEFT MAIN AND THREE-VESSEL CORONARY ARTERY DISEASE

Left main and three-vessel coronary artery disease can be diagnosed in patients with unstable angina from specific ST-T segment changes in the 12-lead ECG (Fig. 24-11). It is important to recognize this ECG pattern so that emergency cardiac catheterization can be performed and the myocardium revascularized before infarction occurs.

ECG recognition

- ST elevation in aV_R and V_1
- ST depression in eight or more leads

Record a 12-lead ECG during chest pain, since the tracing may be normal during a pain-free period. It is important to record the 12-lead ECG when the patient has pain. In a study involving 125 patients with left main coronary artery disease it was found that 25% have a normal ECG when they are without pain, even with as much as 91% to 99% occlusion of the left main coronary artery. In the same study the most frequently seen ECG pattern was ST depression in leads V_3 to V_5 and ST elevation in leads V_1 and aV_R. Lead V_4 showed ST depression in 67% of patients.[16,17]

SUMMARY

This chapter has discussed unstable angina and ECG patterns that are typical either of critical proximal LAD coronary artery stenosis (Wellens syndrome) or of left main or three-vessel coronary artery disease. Because revascularization procedures are now readily available, it is important to know how to recognize these ECG patterns so that emergency coronary arteriography can be performed to identify patients who are candidates for bypass graft or coronary angioplasty.

Wellens syndrome reflects reperfusion during unstable angina in the pain-free period and includes the ECG findings of progressive, symmetric T-wave inversion in leads V_2 and V_3 with no loss of precordial R wave and little or no enzyme elevation. Severe left main and three-vessel coronary artery disease is recognized because of ST elevation in two leads (V_1 and aV_R) and ST depression in eight other leads.

Although the ECG changes that are diagnostic of critical proximal LAD coronary artery stenosis are best recognized *outside* the episode of anginal pain, the abnormalities suggestive of severe left main or three-vessel coronary artery disease are most marked on the ECG recorded *during* an attack of chest pain.

REFERENCES

1. Wilcox I: Risk of adverse outcome in patients admitted to the coronary care unit with suspected unstable angina pectoris, *Am J Cardiol* 64:845, 1989.
2. Hurst JW, Logue RB: Angina pectoris: words patients use and overlooked precipitating events, *Heart Dis Stroke* 2:89, 1993.
3. Ambrose JA, Israel DH: Angiography in unstable angina, *Am J Cardiol* 68:78B, 1991.
4. Chesebro JH, Zoldhelyi P, Fuster V: Pathogenesis of thrombosis in unstable angina, *Am J Cardiol* 68:2B, 1991.
5. Neri Serneri GG, Abbate R, Gori AM et al: Transient intermittent lymphocyte activation is responsible for the instability of angina, *Circulation* 86:790, 1992.
6. Wellens HJJ: Characteristic electrocardiographic pattern indicating a critical stenosis high in left anterior descending coronary artery in patients admitted because of impending myocardial infarction. Presented at the symposium on new strategies in the management of ischemic heart disease, Scottsdale, Ariz. January 24-26, 1981.
7. Wellens HJJ: The electrocardiogram 80 years after Einthoven: The Bishop Lecture. Presented at the annual meeting of the American College of Cardiology, Anaheim, Calif., March 1985.

8. de Zwaan C, Bär RWHM, Wellens HJJ: Characteristic electrocardiographic pattern indicating a critical stenosis high in left anterior descending coronary artery in patients admitted because of impending myocardial infarction, *Am Heart J* 103:730, 1982.

9. Wellens HJJ: The electrocardiogram 80 years after Einthoven, *J Am Coll Cardiol* 7:484, 1986.

10. de Zwaan C, Bär FW, Janssen JHA et al: Angiographic and clinical characteristics of patients with unstable angina showing an ECG pattern indicating critical narrowing of the proximal LAD coronary artery, *Am Heart J* 117:657, 1989.

11. Gruppo Italiano per lo Studio della Streptochinasi nell'Infarto Miocardico (GISSI): Long-term effects of intravenous thrombolysis in acute myocardial infarction: final report of the GISSI study, *Lancet* 2:871, 1987.

12. ISIS-2 (Second International Study of Infarct Survival) Collaborative Group: Randomized trial of intravenous streptokinase, oral aspirin, both, or neither among 17,187 cases of suspected acute myocardial infarction: ISIS-2, *J Am Coll Cardiol* 12(suppl A):3A, 1988.

13. Bär FW, Verheugt FW, Col J et al: Thrombolysis in patients with unstable angina improves the angiographic but not the clinical outcome: results of UNASEM, a multicenter, randomized, placebo-controlled, clinical trial with anistreplase, *Circulation* 86:131, 1992.

14. Neri Serneri NGG, Gensini GF, Poggesi L et al: Effect of heparin, aspirin or alteplase in reduction of myocardial ischaemia in refractory unstable angina, *Lancet* 335:615, 1990.

15. Williams DO, Topol EJ, Califf RM: Intravenous recombinant tissue type plasminogen activator in patients with unstable angina pectoris: results of a placebo-controlled, randomized trial, *Circulation* 82:376, 1990.

16. Gorgels AP, Vos MA, Bär FW, Wellens HJ: An electrocardiographic pattern, characteristic for extensive myocardial ischemia, *Circulation* (suppl 2)78.1082, 1988.

17. Atie J, Brugada P, Smeetsdl JLRM et al: Electrocardiographic findings during and outside an episode of chest pain in patients with left main coronary artery disease, *Circulation* 80:0154, 1989.

18. Braunwald E, Jones RH, Mark DB, et al: Diagnosing and managing unstable angina, *Circulation* 90:613, 1994.

19. Gurfinkel EP, Manos EJ, Mejaíl RI, et al: Low molecular weight heparin versus regular heparin or aspirin in the treatment of unstable angina and silent ischemia, *J Am Coll Cardiol* 26:313, 1995.

20. Markwardt F, Hauptmann J, Nowak G, et al: Pharmacological studies on the antithrombotic action of hirudin in experimental animals, *Thromb Haemost* 47:226, 1982.

21. Fuchs J, Cannon CP, and the TIMI 7 Investigators: Hirulog in the treatment of unstable angina. Results of the thrombin inhibition in myocardial ischemia (TIMI) 7 trial, *Circulation* 92:727, 1995.

22. Sharma GVRK, Lapsey D, Vita JA: Usefulness and tolerability of Hirulog, a direct thrombin-inhibitor, in unstable angina pectoris, *Am J Cardiol* 72:1357, 1993.

23. Lidon R-M, Theroux P, Juneau M, et al: Initial experience with a direct antithrombin, Hirulog, in unstable angina: anticoagulant, antithrombotic, and clinical effects, *Circulation* 88:1495, 1993.

24. Cannon CP, Maraganore JM, Loscalzo J, et al: Anticoagulant effects of Hirulog, a novel thrombin inhibitor, in patients with coronary artery disease, *Am J Cardiol* 71:778, 1993.

25. Topol EJ, Bonan R, Jewitt D, et al: Use of a direct antithrombin, Hirulog, in place of heparin during coronary angioplasty, *Circulation* 87:1622, 1993.

25
Bundle Branch Block and Hemiblock

Structure of the Trifascicular Specialized
  Conduction System   *362*
Blood Supply to the Conduction
  System   *364*
Bundle Branch Block in Acute Myocardial
  Infarction   *364*
Chronic Bundle Branch Block   *365*
Pediatrics   *365*
Physical Findings   *365*
Comparison of lead V₁ in Right- and
  Left-sided Bundle Branch Block   *365*
Normal Ventricular Activation Time
  (Intrinsicoid Deflection)   *366*
T Wave Changes in Bundle Branch
  Block   *366*
Right Bundle Branch Block   *367*

Complete Versus Incomplete Right Bundle
  Branch Block   *371*
Left Bundle Branch Block   *372*
Alternating Right- and Left-sided Bundle
  Branch Block   *377*
Anterior Hemiblock   *377*
Posterior Hemiblock   *380*
Hemiblock with Right Bundle Branch
  Block (Bifascicular Block)   *381*
Differential Diagnosis in Anterior
  Hemiblock   *382*
Monitoring for Axis Shifts and for Right
  Bundle Branch Block   *383*
Trifascicular Block   *385*
Summary   *386*

One of the most distinctive examples of intraventricular conduction defect is the delay or obstruction of impulse conduction in one of the bundle branches. This chapter describes the anatomy, clinical implications, prognosis, mechanisms, and ECG patterns in bundle branch block (BBB) and hemiblock in acute myocardial infarction (MI) and in MI in its chronic form.

STRUCTURE OF THE TRIFASCICULAR SPECIALIZED CONDUCTION SYSTEM

Fig. 25-1 illustrates the specialized conduction system: right bundle branch (RBB) and left bundle branch (LBB) with its two main fascicles (anterior and pos-

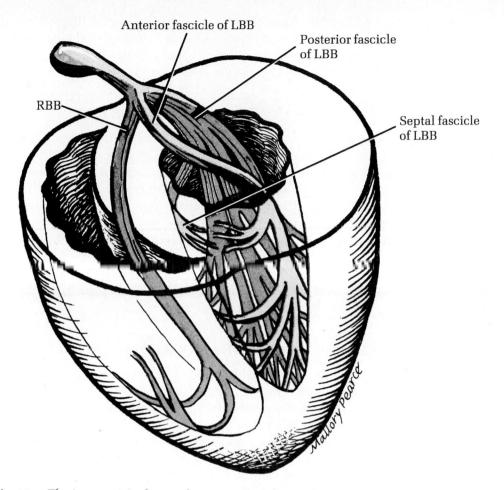

Fig. 25-1. The intraventricular conductive system shown through transparent walls. Note the anterior positions and similar constructions of the right bundle branch (RBB) and the anterior fascicle of the left bundle branch (LBB).

terior). A third division (septal) sends out connecting branches between the anterior and posterior fascicles. Note the broad, ribbonlike posterior fascicle and the long, thin anterior one that is similar in shape and position to the RBB. Three divisions of the LBB were described and illustrated by Tawara in 1906[1a] and then cast aside. Until the late 1960s, only two divisions, the right and left bundle branches, were described. From 1968 to 1973 Rosenbaum et al.[1-4] described the intraventricular conduction system as trifascicular (RBB and the two distinct divisions of the LBB) and coined the term "hemiblock" for the condition when conduction to half of the left ventricle is impaired. Rosenbaum's work gave clinicians a new insight into previously unexplained ECG phenomena and stimulated research into the electrical activation of the intraventricular conduction system. From this work evolved the terms *left anterior hemiblock, left posterior hemiblock, bifascicular block,* and *trifascicular block,* which have been widely used.

In 1972 Demoulin and Kulbertus[5] reminded us of the validity of Tawara's original 1906 model of the LBB as having three divisions instead of the two described by Rosenbaum. An LBB lesion is hardly ever confined solely to a distinct anterior or posterior division. Most of the time there is a network of septal fibers between the two main left branches that may be involved as well. However, the concept of two distinct divisions is useful in electrocardiography and clinical practice and continues to be employed to explain the axis shifts seen in acute MI.

BLOOD SUPPLY TO THE CONDUCTION SYSTEM

There are two main arterial systems supplying the conduction system. The left anterior descending (LAD) coronary artery supplies the anterior wall of the heart and the anterior two thirds of the septum. Its septal branch is the main blood supply to the proximal RBB and anterior division of the LBB and is vulnerable in anteroseptal MI. The posterior division of the left bundle branch has two blood supplies, the LAD and the right coronary artery (RCA). The posterior descending coronary artery is the RCA in 90% of individuals. It supplies the posterior third of the septum, and its atrioventricular (AV) nodal branch is the main blood supply to the AV node and bundle of His. Thus acquired right bundle branch block (RBBB) is more common in anterior wall MI and left bundle branch block (LBBB) in inferior wall MI.[6]

BUNDLE BRANCH BLOCK IN ACUTE MYOCARDIAL INFARCTION

When RBBB or hemiblock is acquired because of anterior wall MI, it signifies an occlusion in the proximal LAD coronary artery and extensive myocardial damage. In such cases there is a high chance of developing complete AV block, and despite the transient nature of the block and prophylactic pacing, the death rate is significantly higher than it would have been had this complication not occurred. Mortality is high, even if complete AV block does not develop.[7] Death results not from the AV block, but from pump failure. If pump failure does not cause death within the first few days, there is a 30% chance that death will come 1 to 3 weeks later in the form of sustained ventricular tachycardia or ventricular fibrillation. However, if the BBB existed before the infarction, the in-hospital mortality is lower. When inferior wall MI is associated with preexistent RBBB, hospital mortality is not affected.[6]

Determining on admission whether a BBB is new or preexisting is a challenge. One group[8] found that when BBB is present on admission in a patient with acute anterior wall MI, an age over 70 years and the classic triphasic rSR' pattern in lead V_1 (rather than a QR pattern) favors preexistent RBBB. These two patterns are compared later (see Fig. 25-4).

When LBBB is associated with acute MI, the significance is not as clear. LBBB itself is often associated with generalized left ventricular disease and is therefore a more ominous finding than is RBBB.[6]

Treatment

Because of the grave prognosis, aggressive treatment, as follows, is indicated when BBB complicates acute anterior wall MI[6]:

1. Thrombolytic therapy (intracoronary if intravenous [IV] therapy is not successful); if unsuccessful.
2. Emergency percutaneous transvenous coronary angioplasty is carried out.
3. A Swan-Ganz catheter is inserted to provide information about pump function.
4. Following reperfusion, if the BBB or fascicular block persists, temporary pro-

phylactic pacing is recommended. (The block is usually transient.) In this way, should complete heart block occur, there would be a smooth transition to a paced rhythm, avoiding the need for cardiopulmonary resuscitation.

5. Permanent pacing is reserved for persistent or recurrent high-degree AV block.

CHRONIC BUNDLE BRANCH BLOCK

Chronic BBB is rare in the young, but is a common finding in the elderly, becoming more common with age. Prognosis is related to the cardiac status. In patients with chronic BBB, widespread fibrosis is often present, especially if left fascicular block is also present. Diseases associated with BBB are coronary artery disease, hypertension, aortic valve disease, idiopathic degenerative diseases of the conduction system, and cardiomyopathy.

When LBBB is found on a routine ECG, it is usually associated with hypertensive ischemic, primary, or degenerative myocardial disease, which may be manifested on clinical examination, or it may not be associated with serious cardiac disease at all. The Framingham study[9] has concluded that when LBBB is newly acquired, the presence of underlying disease can be established by evaluating associated ECG findings such as QRS axis, P-wave morphologic appearance, polarity of the T wave in lead V_6, and tracings made before the LBBB.

PEDIATRICS

When found in conjunction with congenital cardiac abnormalities, BBB is usually not accompanied by heart disease and has an excellent prognosis. During surgery for congenital heart abnormalities the bundle branches (especially the right) are frequently damaged. Surgical repairs in which this finding is common are for ventricular septal defects, atrial septal defect, tetralogy of Fallot (50% to 100%), and complex intraventricular procedures such as the combination of ventricular septal defect, transposition of the great arteries, and pulmonary stenosis. Left axis deviation (left anterior hemiblock) is also present in up to 25% of surgical patients.[10]

PHYSICAL FINDINGS

In patients with complete RBBB, because of a delay in the pulmonic component of the second heart sound, persistent splitting is noted; that is, the two components (aortic second sound $[A_2]$ and pulmonic second sound $[P_2]$) are split on both inspiration and expiration but continue to exhibit normal respiratory changes. (The split is more marked during inspiration.) In patients with complete LBBB (or a right ventricular pacemaker), the right side of the ventricular septum is activated before the left, causing paradoxic (reversed) splitting of the second heart sound.[11,12] That is, the two components of the second heart sound separate during expiration and become single during inspiration.

COMPARISON OF RIGHT- AND LEFT-SIDED BUNDLE BRANCH BLOCK IN LEAD V_1

Bundle branch block causes the heart to be activated in a very lopsided manner—one ventricle after the other instead of both together. This characteristic is clearly reflected in lead V_1. Note in Fig. 25-2 that normally the deflection resulting

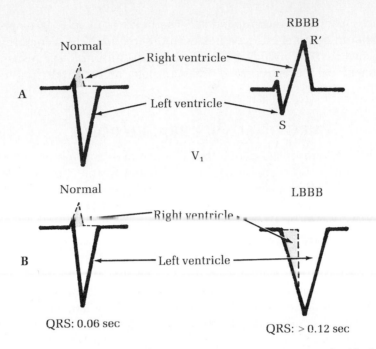

Fig. 25-2. The ventricular complex of **A,** RBB and, **B,** LBB is compared with the normal complex in lead V_1. The dotted lines indicate hidden events on the ECG. For example, right ventricular activation is normally effaced by left ventricular activation.

from activation of the right ventricle is buried in that from the left ventricle, resulting in a narrow rS complex in V_1. However, in RBBB the deflection representing right ventricular activation is delayed and becomes prominent, resulting in a broad terminal R′ wave and the typical rSR′ complex (Fig. 25-2, *A*). In LBBB, activation of both ventricles is also in sequence, but from right to left, resulting in a broad negative complex in V_1 (Fig. 25-2, *B*).

NORMAL VENTRICULAR ACTIVATION TIME (INTRINSICOID DEFLECTION)

The time from the beginning of ventricular activation (onset of the QRS complex) to that point at which the impulse arrives under a particular electrode is called the *ventricular activation time,* and the downward deflection that follows is the *intrinsicoid deflection.* Because V_1 is over the right ventricle and V_6 is over the left, we look to those two leads for the ventricular activation time for the right and the left ventricles, respectively.

Normally the impulse arrives over the thin-walled right ventricle early (0.02 sec); at that point the graph in V_1 begins its downstroke. Because the left ventricular wall is thicker than the right wall, it takes longer for the impulse to arrive under the V_6 electrode, and the graph peaks later. The onset of normal intrinsicoid deflections for the right and left ventricles are shown in Fig. 25-3.

T-WAVE CHANGES IN BUNDLE BRANCH BLOCK

Because depolarization is abnormal in BBB, so is repolarization. Thus the T wave is expected to be opposite in polarity to the terminal component of the QRS

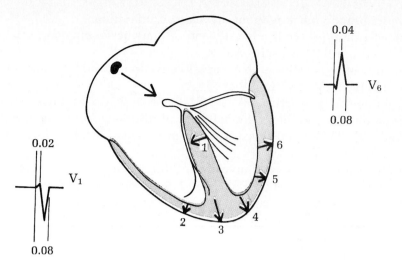

Fig. 25-3. Normal activation of the ventricles (arrows 1-6) as reflected in leads V_1 and V_6.

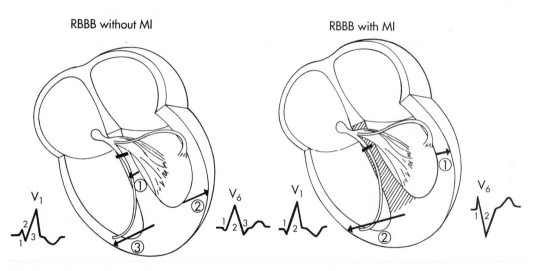

Fig. 25-4. Sequences in the activation of the ventricles in right bundle branch block (RBBB) without and with anteroseptal myocardial infarction (MI). In one, septal activation is intact; in the other it is not.

complex. This is known as a secondary change because it is a normal consequence of the BBB. If the direction of the T wave is the same as that of the terminal component of the QRS complex, myocardial disease is suspected.

RIGHT BUNDLE BRANCH BLOCK
Mechanism

Fig. 25-4 compares the mechanisms of ventricular activation in RBBB without and with acute anteroseptal MI. In both cases the two ventricles are activated one after the other instead of together, as they normally are.

Right bundle branch block without myocardial infarction
1. Septal activation proceeds normally and on time, producing an initial r wave in lead V_1 and a little q wave in lead V_6.
2. Septal activation is followed by normal activation of the left ventricle, producing an S wave in V_1 and an R wave in V_6.
3. The right ventricle is activated last and abnormally, the impulse gaining access transseptally. This produces the hallmark of RBBB—a late R wave in V_1 and an S wave in V_6. Thus the triphasic pattern in these two leads is formed.

Right bundle branch block with myocardial infarction
1. Septal activation does not take place because of necrotic and injured tissue. Initial forces are left ventricular, producing a Q wave in lead V_1.
2. Initial left ventricular forces are followed by late activation of the right ventricle, producing an R wave in V_1.

QRS complex in right bundle branch block with and without acute anteroseptal myocardial infarction

Duration: 0.12 sec or more.

Leads I, aV_L, and V_6: Terminal S wave.

Without acute anteroseptal myocardial infarction: Triphasic complex in V_1 (rSR′) and in V_6 (qRS).

With acute anteroseptal myocardial infarction: Biphasic complex in V_1 (QR); patterns in V_1 without and with MI are compared in Fig. 25-5.

    Fig. 25-6 is a 12-lead ECG of RBBB without MI. Note the triphasic patterns in V_1 and V_6 and the broad terminal S wave in leads I, aV_L, and V_6. Often the amplitude of the initial r wave is increased in RBBB in lead V_1 because normal septal activation involves a contribution from both sides of the septum with left-to-right activation dominating and a modest initial r wave is produced. When the RBB is blocked, activation of the septum is exclusively from left to right, producing a larger initial R wave. For the same reason the S wave is markedly reduced in lead V_1 in RBBB, even though this is the component reflecting the large left ventricular mean vector. The S wave reduction in lead V_1 occurs because the now stronger septal current opposes left ventricular activation. Thus some of the left ventricular forces are canceled out, producing a smaller S wave. Fig. 25-7 is a 12-lead ECG of RBBB with acute anteroseptal MI. Note the absence of the initial r wave in lead V_1; there is a Q wave instead. The patient also has left anterior hemiblock. Mortality is very high with such a pattern, which indicates a proximal LAD occlusion.

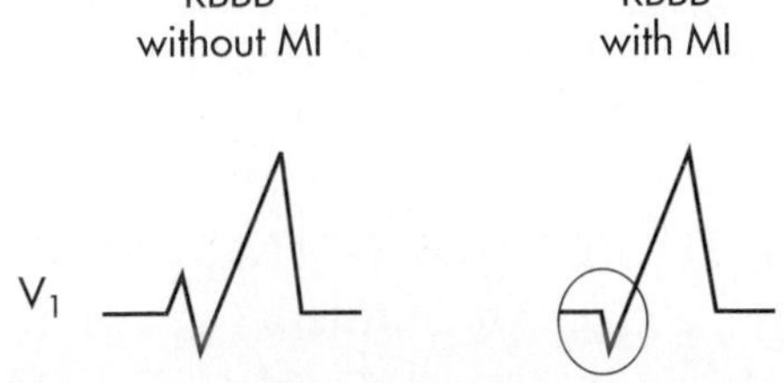

Fig. 25-5. Patterns of RBBB compared in lead V_1 (without and with anteroseptal MI).

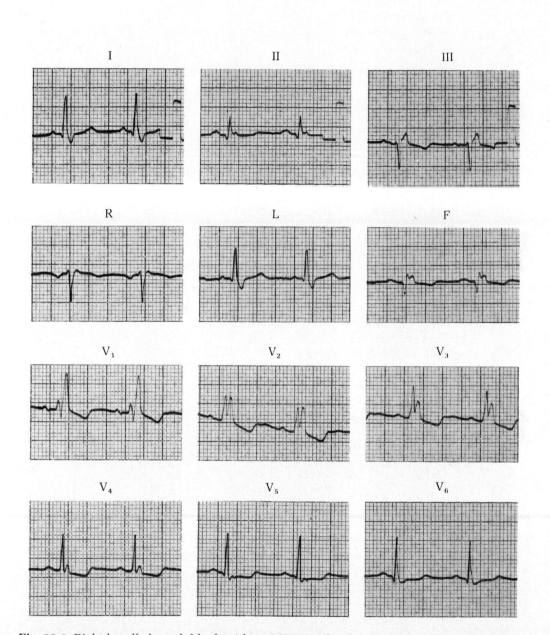

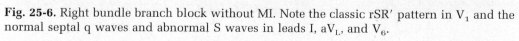

Fig. 25-6. Right bundle branch block without MI. Note the classic rSR′ pattern in V_1 and the normal septal q waves and abnormal S waves in leads I, aV_L, and V_6.

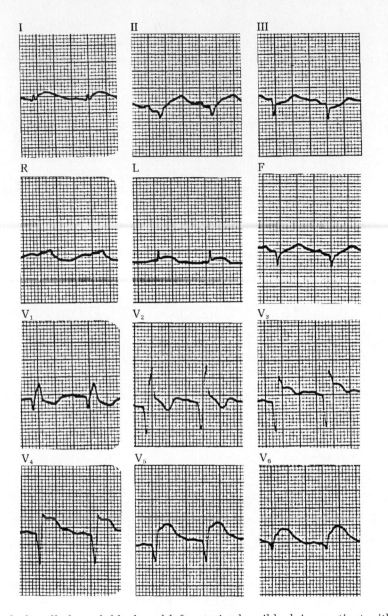

Fig. 25-7. Right bundle branch block and left anterior hemiblock in a patient with acute anteroseptal MI.

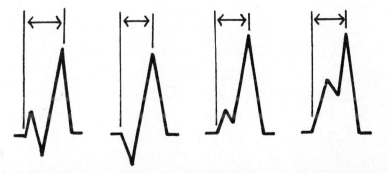

Fig. 25-8. Onset of intrinsicoid deflections and the ventricular activation time in different patterns of RBBB. The patterns have in common a ventricular activation time ≥0.07 sec.

Intrinsicoid deflection in right bundle branch block

The onset of the intrinsicoid deflection in lead V_1 occurs late (0.07 sec or more), the hallmark of uncomplicated or complicated RBBB. Fig. 25-8 shows that the different patterns seen in RBBB have one common denominator, the late R wave.

COMPLETE VERSUS INCOMPLETE RIGHT BUNDLE BRANCH BLOCK
Mechanism

The term "complete" in this context does not necessarily mean that there is no possibility for conduction to take place under any circumstances in the apparently blocked bundle. In fact, as you will see later in Fig. 25-16, there may be slow conduction in one bundle and rate-dependent block in the other (a very serious conduction problem). Such a situation would produce alternating right and left BBB.

ECG recognition

The ECG changes seen in incomplete RBBB include the following:
- QRS morphologic appearance like that of RBBB
- QRS duration of less than 0.12 sec

In Fig. 25-9 the QRS durations differ in complete and incomplete RBBB. The narrower QRS complexes follow pauses. There are two premature atrial contractions (one conducted [hidden in second T wave] and the other not conducted), producing pauses; after the pauses the QRS duration is only 0.10 sec, but the morphologic appearance is that of RBBB. After shorter cycles the duration of the QRS increases to 0.12 sec as the R' wave broadens.

In Fig. 25-10 are three examples of normal conduction following the compensatory pause afforded by a premature ventricular contraction. In these three patients normal conduction is possible if the bundle in question has a long enough rest, yet the QRS duration of the BBB complexes fulfills the criteria for "complete" RBBB.

Incomplete bundle branch block in athletes

The incidence of incomplete RBBB in all athletes is about 14% and is related to an increase in muscle mass of the right ventricular tip. Once athletic activity is discontinued, the RBBB pattern disappears. Affecting this percentage is the 10% epidemiologic incidence of incomplete RBBB in individuals who are 20 to 35 years of age.[13]

V_1

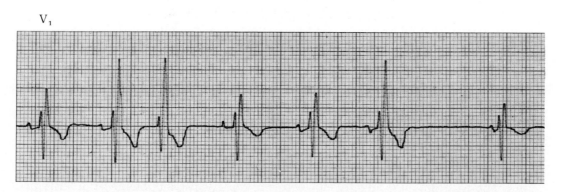

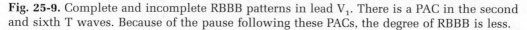

Fig. 25-9. Complete and incomplete RBBB patterns in lead V_1. There is a PAC in the second and sixth T waves. Because of the pause following these PACs, the degree of RBBB is less.

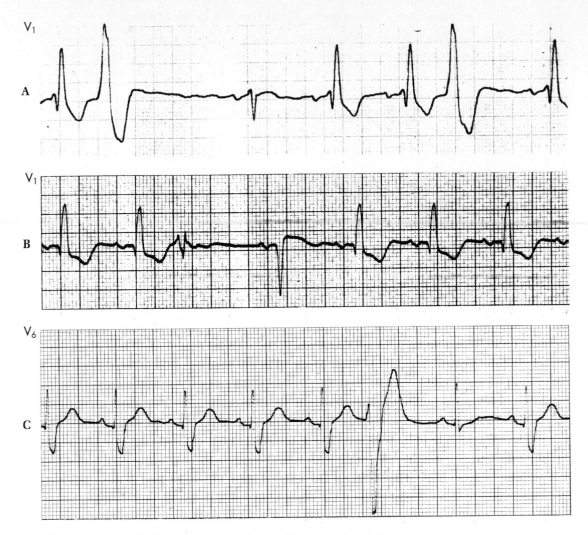

Fig. 25-10. **A** to **C,** Three examples of normal conduction following a compensatory pause.

LEFT BUNDLE BRANCH BLOCK
Mechanism

Fig. 25-11 compares the mechanisms of ventricular activation in LBBB without and with acute anteroseptal MI. In both cases the ventricles are activated from right to left.

Left bundle branch block without myocardial infarction. The right ventricle and the septum are activated simultaneously, followed immediately by left ventricular activation. Right ventricular activation is not seen. Thus the dominant current flow is away from lead V_1 (a negative deflection) and toward lead V_6 (a positive deflection). The ST segment is slightly elevated, and the T wave is opposite in polarity to that of the ventricular complex. Lead V_6 has no q wave and no S wave; it is totally positive.

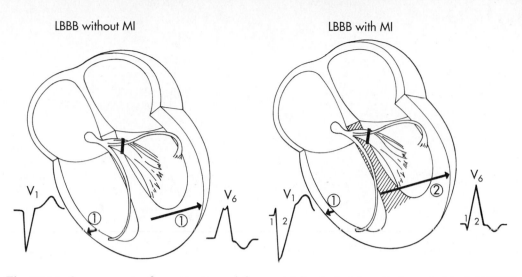

Fig. 25-11. Sequences in the activation of the ventricles in left bundle branch block (LBBB) without and with anteroseptal MI.

Left bundle branch block with myocardial infarction
1. Septal activation does not take place because of necrotic and injured tissue. Initial forces are right ventricular, producing a tall, thin R wave in lead V_1 and a Q wave in V_6.
2. The left ventricle is activated next, producing a deep S wave in lead V_1 and an R wave in V_6.

QRS complex in left bundle branch block with and without acute anteroseptal myocardial infarction

Duration: 0.12 sec or more, depending on the presence of associated ischemic heart disease or prior MI. The longer QRS duration in patients with LBBB and prior MI may be the result of prior damage of the distal specialized conduction system.[14]

Without acute anteroseptal MI: Lead V_1 has a QS or an rS pattern, and the downstroke of the S wave is swift and clean. Lead V_6 has an R wave that may be notched at the top (no q wave and no S wave).

With acute anteroseptal myocardial infarction: V_1 often has a tall, narrow r wave; V_5 or V_6 has a q wave. Patterns in V_1 and V_6 without and with MI are compared in Fig. 25-12.

The classic 12-lead patterns of LBBB without anteroseptal MI are shown in Figs. 25-13 and 25-14. The patients in Figs. 25-13 and 25-14 differ, however, in the seriousness of their condition and prognosis.

In Fig. 25-13 the frontal plane axis is in the left quadrant (left of 0 degrees) and the P wave reveals left atrial enlargement (P wave with a broad, negative trough in lead V_1 and notched in leads II and aV_F); these findings are associated with coronary disease, and congestive heart failure.[9]

In Fig. 25-14 the LBBB is associated with first degree AV block, an indication of a double lesion (AV node and left bundle branch). In about 30% of LBBB there is an initial small, narrow r wave in V_1 and V_2 (Fig. 25-14), probably the result of the early activation of the anterior papillary branch of the right bundle causing the thin anterior wall of the right ventricle to be activated first, and the initial forces to flow toward V_1, producing the initial, little r wave. In LBBB the two ven-

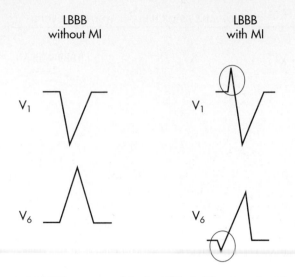

Fig. 25-12. Patterns of LBBB compared in lead V_1 (without and with anteroseptal MI).

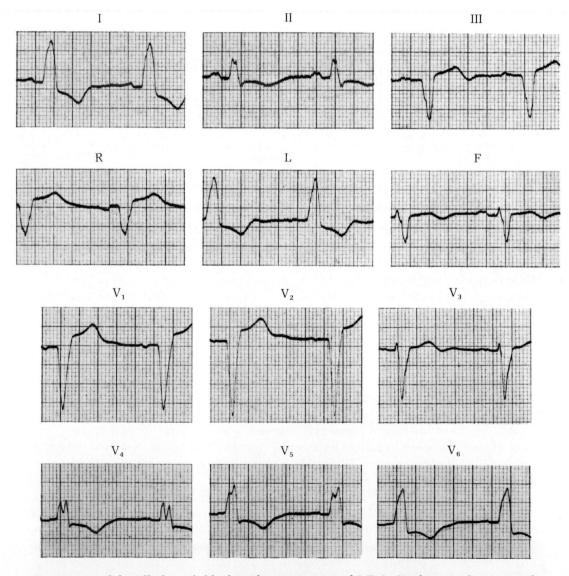

Fig. 25-13. Left bundle branch block without anteroseptal MI. In V_1 the complex is mainly negative, and in V_6, totally positive. There are other signs in this ECG that point to higher risk (see text).

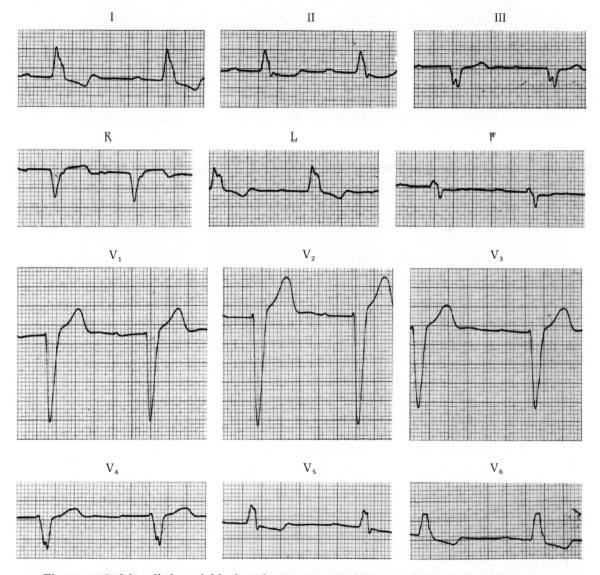

Fig. 25-14. Left bundle branch block without anteroseptal MI. Note the associated first-degree atrioventricular (AV) block, a sign of a double lesion (AV nodal and bundle branches).

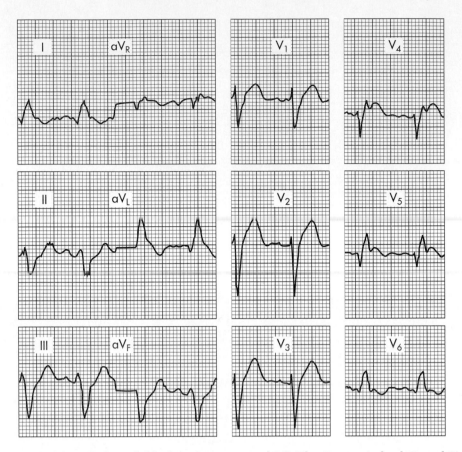

Fig. 25-15. Left bundle branch block and anteroseptal MI. The Q wave in lead V_5 and V_6 and the R wave in lead V_1 are evident. *(From Lyon LJ: Basic electrocardiography handbook, New York, 1977, Van Nostrand Reinhold.)*

tricles are activated one after the other, first the right ventricle and then the left, causing the main current to be leftward, away from V_1. This accounts for the broad, negative deflection in that lead and the broad positive one in V_6. An appreciation of the occasional occurrence of an rS pattern in lead V_1 with LBBB helps one to recognize this type of LBBB aberration on the rare occasions when it occurs.

Fig. 25-15 shows LBBB with anteroseptal MI. In the absence of septal activation, right ventricular activation can be seen and is reflected by the tall, skinny R wave in V_1 and the abnormal Q wave in V_5 and V_6.

ECG recognition of underlying cardiac disease in left bundle branch block

In the Framingham study[9] the associated ECG findings correlated with the prevalence of systemic hypertension, cardiomegaly, coronary heart disease, and congestive heart failure. The findings were as follows:

- A QRS axis of 0 degrees or to the left of 0 degrees (heart enlargement, coronary disease, and congestive heart failure).
- P-wave pattern of left atrial enlargement (hypertension and possible cardiac enlargement).

- Inverted T wave in lead V_6 in the first tracing after the development of LBBB. When the T wave was upright or biphasic in this lead in the Framingham study, the patients remained free of associated cardiovascular abnormalities.
- Abnormal ECG before onset of left bundle branch block.

In this study patients (1) without the axis shift, (2) without abnormal P morphologic appearance, and (3) without abnormal ECG before development of LBBB were six times more likely to remain free of all cardiovascular disease than were the 47 other patients who had one or more of these three ECG findings.

ALTERNATING RIGHT- AND LEFT-SIDED BUNDLE BRANCH BLOCK

Alternating RBBB and LBBB indicates disease in both bundles. Sometimes, only a one-sided BBB (which may be incomplete) is evident, and the block on the other side will not be seen until it is unmasked by an increase in the sinus rate. Such is the case in Fig. 25-16. At the onset of the tracing there is RBBB. When the cycle length shortens a little, the left bundle blocks as well (rate-related LBBB). However, because the block in the right bundle was incomplete (probably Wenckebach), the impulse now can proceed slowly down the right bundle (long PR interval with LBBB). The next sinus beat is blocked (the P wave hidden in the LBBB complexes), then conduction resumes down the LBB, and this cycle continues to produce a bigeminal pattern of LBBB with a long PR interval and RBBB with a short PR interval.

ANTERIOR HEMIBLOCK

There is no right-sided hemiblock. Therefore the shorter term "anterior hemiblock" is often used instead of "left anterior hemiblock." Another term in common usage is *anterior fascicular block.*

V₁

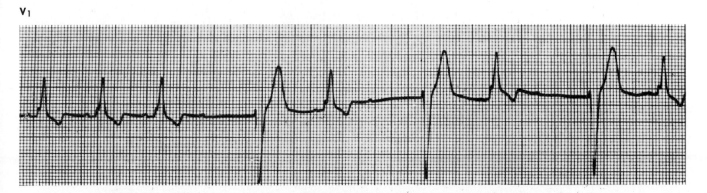

Fig. 25-16. Alternating LBBB and RBBB. In the first four beats there is RBBB. The left bundle is able to conduct as long as the rate is slow enough. When the rate speeds up, the left bundle blocks, unmasking the slow conduction through the right bundle branch (note the long PR interval with the LBBB beats). The next P wave blocks in both bundles, and the sequence begins again: (1) a short PR interval and conduction over the left bundle (RBBB), (2) block in the left bundle and slow conduction over the right bundle (LBBB with a long PR interval), and (3) block in both bundles. *(Courtesy Hein J. Wellens, M.D., Maastricht, The Netherlands.)*

Because the anterior fascicle of the conduction system is relatively thin and lies in the turbulent outflow tract, and because the anterior fascicle has only one blood supply, it is vulnerable to injury and block.

Mechanism

A block in the anterior fascicle is illustrated in Fig. 25-17; the block causes marked left axis deviation because the impulse activates the left ventricle through the posterior fascicle, spreading upward and to the left.

ECG recognition

ECG findings associated with anterior hemiblock include the following:
- **QRS axis:** Left; −40 degrees or greater.
- **QRS duration:** Normal (lengthens an average of 25 ms).
- **QRS morphologic appearance:** Small q waves in leads I and aV$_L$ (may be seen but are not necessary for the diagnosis[15] and are caused by the shift of initial forces [first 0.02 sec] inferiorly and to the right). There are small initial r waves in leads II and III.
- Fig. 25-18 is from a patient with acute anterolateral MI and anterior hemiblock. Note the marked left axis deviation, the normal QRS duration, the small q wave in leads I and aV$_L$, and the small r wave in the inferior leads.

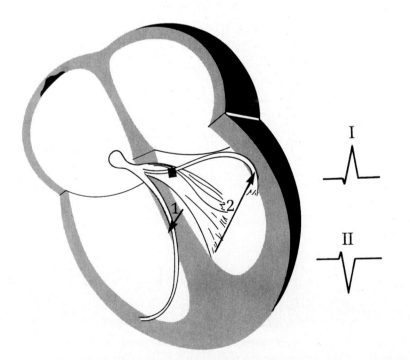

Fig. 25-17. The mechanism of the left axis deviation in anterior hemiblock. When the anterior fascicle is blocked, initial forces are septal (q wave in leads I and aV$_L$ and r wave in lead II). The left ventricle is then activated through the posteroinferior fascicle, causing left axis deviation.

Clinical implications

The anterior fascicle can receive its blood supply solely from the septal branch of the LAD coronary artery or may also be supplied by the AV nodal artery, a branch of the right coronary artery in 90% of individuals, which explains why, although left anterior hemiblock is considerably more common in acute anterior MI, it is also seen in the setting of inferior MI. Of all the conduction defects associated with acute MI, isolated left anterior hemiblock carries the lowest hospital mortality.

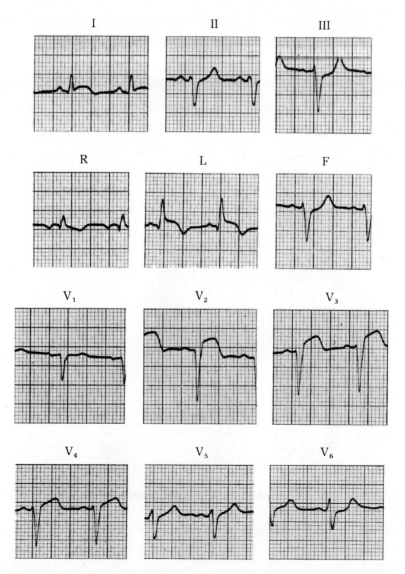

Fig. 25-18. Anterior hemiblock in a patient with acute anterior MI. The abnormal left axis deviation (greater than −30 degrees), the normal QRS duration, and the q waves in leads I and aV_L can be seen.

POSTERIOR HEMIBLOCK

The shorter term "posterior hemiblock" is often used instead of "left posterior hemiblock." Another term in common usage is *posterior fascicular block.*

The posterior division of the LBB, first division to branch from the bundle of His, is the conduction system for the posteroinferior wall of the left ventricle and the septum. It receives its blood supply from both the anterior descending left and the posterior descending right coronary arteries.

Mechanism

A block in the posterior fascicle is illustrated in Fig. 25-19. It causes marked right axis deviation because the impulse activates the left ventricle through the anterior fascicle, spreading downward and to the right and causing lead I to be mainly negative and leads II, III, and aV$_F$ to be mainly positive. The initial forces (first 0.02 sec) travel upward and leftward from the anterior papillary muscle. This is why there is a small initial r wave in leads I and aV$_L$ and a q wave in leads II, III, and aV$_F$.

ECG recognition

ECG findings associated with posterior hemiblock include the following:
- Right axis deviation of approximately +120 degrees
- q wave in leads II, III, and aV$_F$
- r wave in leads I and aV$_L$

When RBBB and right axis deviation are encountered, the diagnosis is always one of exclusion, distinguishing the acute from the chronic state and ruling out right

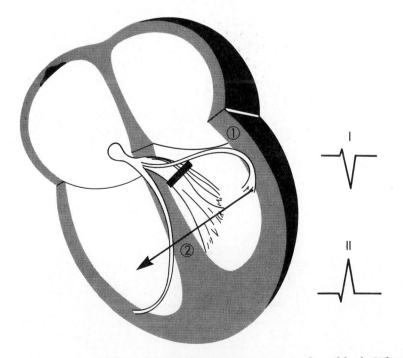

Fig. 25-19. The mechanism of the right axis deviation in posterior hemiblock. When the posterior fascicle is blocked, initial forces are the high, lateral left ventricular (r wave in leads I and aV$_L$ and q wave in lead II). The remainder of the left ventricle is then activated through the anterior fascicle, causing right axis deviation.

ventricular hypertrophy. Fig. 25-20 is from a patient with both posterior hemiblock and RBBB (bifascicular block). Note the right axis deviation, the q wave in the inferior leads, and the r wave in leads I and aV$_L$.

Clinical implications

Because of the width and the dual blood supply of the posterior fascicle, it is rarely completely compromised. If left posterior hemiblock does occur in the setting of acute MI (incidence 1.1%), it is almost always associated with RBBB and carries a poor prognosis (hospital mortality 71.3%).

HEMIBLOCK WITH RIGHT BUNDLE BRANCH BLOCK (BIFASCICULAR BLOCK)
Mechanism

In the setting of acute MI, anterior hemiblock is associated with RBBB more often than is posterior hemiblock because the right bundle and the anterior fascicle are similar in structure and share the same blood supply.

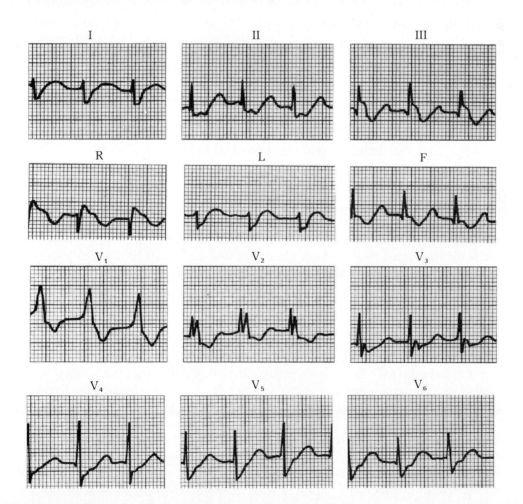

Fig. 25-20. Bifascicular block (RBBB plus posterior hemiblock) in a patient with evolving anterior wall MI. The abnormal right axis deviation and the small r wave in leads I and aV$_L$, as well as small q waves in the inferior leads, are evident.

ECG recognition

ECG findings associated with bifascicular block include the following:

- Pattern of RBBB with left axis deviation (RBBB plus left anterior hemiblock)
- Pattern of RBBB with right axis deviation (RBBB plus left posterior hemiblock) in the setting of acute MI and after having ruled out right ventricular hypertrophy.

    Fig. 25-20 shows bifascicular block involving the right bundle and the posterior division of the left bundle. Note the RBBB pattern with right axis deviation.

- It is possible for anterior hemiblock to obscure the ECG signs of RBBB, especially if the chest electrodes are placed too low. In such cases the R′ wave in lead V_1 and the telltale S waves in leads I and aV_L are abolished. You may be able to unmask the RBBB by placing the V_1 electrode one interspace above the conventional position or slightly to the right. This may reveal the classic terminal R′ wave of RBBB.[17]

Clinical Implications

In the setting of acute anteroseptal MI the incidence of bifascicular block comprising RBBB and left anterior hemiblock is 3.7%. Of these patients, 32% will have complete subnodal block and 48% will die before discharge. The incidence of bifascicular block comprising RBBB and left posterior hemiblock is only 1.1%, but the hospital mortality is high (71%). The percentage of those in whom complete subnodal block will develop is 47%.[14]

DIFFERENTIAL DIAGNOSIS IN ANTERIOR HEMIBLOCK
Inferior wall myocardial infarction

Inferior wall MI and anterior hemiblock may occur together, especially if some portion of the anterior wall is also involved or if the AV nodal artery supplies the proximal bundle branches. In some cases anterior hemiblock may obscure the signs of inferior wall infarction by abolishing the diagnostic Q waves in the inferior leads (II, III, and aV_F). The diagnosis of the combination of inferior MI and anterior hemiblock is also difficult because both abnormalities can result in left axis deviation. The degree of axis shift is helpful in the differential diagnosis because a large inferior infarction without anterior hemiblock can only produce a left axis shift of less than −30 degrees caused by loss of electrical forces from the inferior wall; however, if the axis is as far left as −60 degrees, hemiblock is almost certainly complicating the inferior wall MI.[3]

Marriott[18] gives us a helpful clue to the presence of anterior hemiblock: with or without inferior wall infarction, anterior hemiblock will produce a deep S wave in lead II, but never a terminal r wave. In lead aV_R there is commonly a terminal r or R wave with anterior hemiblock. Warner et al[15] have proposed the following criteria for the diagnosis of inferior MI and anterior hemiblock based on the relations between portions of the vectorcardiographic QRS loop in the frontal plane and the corresponding portions of the QRS complexes recorded by the limb leads: a terminal R wave in aV_R and aV_L with the peak of the R wave later in aV_R than in aV_L (requires simultaneous leads) and a Q wave present in lead II (can be of any magnitude).

In leads aV_R and aV_L measure the distance from the beginning of the QRS complex to the peak of the R wave. These leads must be simultaneous because the onset of the QRS may differ slightly from lead to lead as a result of isoelectric initial forces in one lead and not in the other.

Anterior wall myocardial infarction

Anterior wall infarction may also be masked by anterior hemiblock because of a small r wave in leads V_1 and V_2, which obscures the diagnostic QS wave. It may be that a low-lying V_1 electrode is recording an r wave because initial forces in anterior hemiblock are inferior and to the right. Moving the electrode up reveals the QS wave of anterior wall MI in the right chest leads.

MONITORING FOR AXIS SHIFTS AND FOR RIGHT BUNDLE BRANCH BLOCK

Leads I and II are best for detecting an axis shift. Fig. 25-21 illustrates that a left axis shift can be detected in lead II. Fig. 25-22 demonstrates that a right axis shift is seen best in lead I. Right bundle branch block is best detected in lead V_1. Fig. 25-23 illustrates that, especially in the presence of anterior hemiblock, when the QRS complex may broaden only slightly more, V_1 is the best lead for seeing

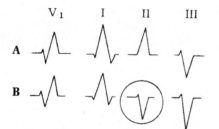

Fig. 25-21. A, Right bundle branch block without hemiblock. **B,** Right bundle branch block with left anterior hemiblock (LAH). The change is in lead II only.

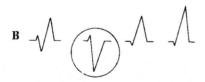

Fig. 25-22. A, Right bundle branch block without hemiblock. **B,** Right bundle branch block with left posterior hemiblock. The change is in lead I only.

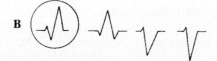

Fig. 25-23. A, Left anterior hemiblock without bundle branch block. **B,** Right bundle branch block with hemiblock. The change is best seen in lead V_1.

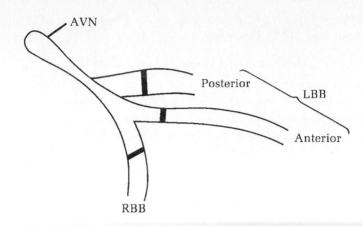

Fig. 25-24. Trifascicular block. *AVN, Atrioventricular node.*

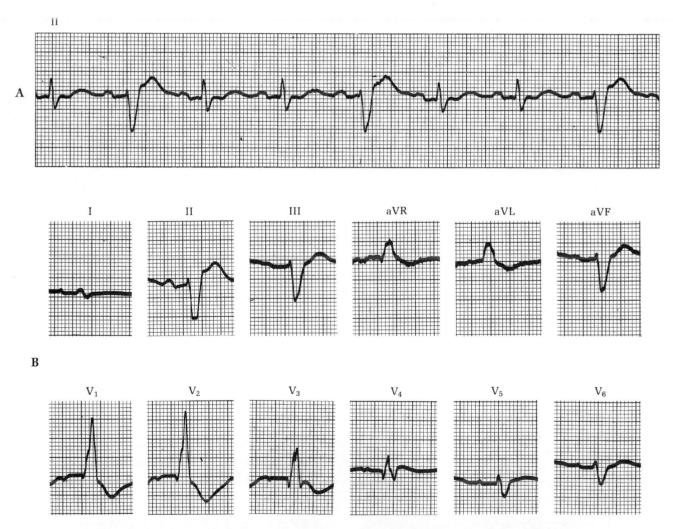

Fig. 25-25. A, Left axis deviation every third beat. Both the PR interval and the QRS complex are prolonged. **B,** Same patient, later. There is anterior wall MI and the intermittent LAH is now continuous. Right bundle branch block and a long PR interval (trifascicular block) are present.

RBBB because of the development of a broad terminal R′. It is also one of two leads that are helpful in differentiating aberrancy from ectopy, precisely because it reflects RBBB so well; V_6 is the other one.

TRIFASCICULAR BLOCK

Fig. 25-24 illustrates that the trifascicular block is located simultaneously in the three main fascicles of the intraventricular conduction system: the RBB and the anterior and posterior divisions of the LBB. If the block in all three of the fascicles is complete, the escape pacemaker is in the ventricles below the lesions. Thus the ventricular rate is that of a ventricular escape focus. If there is complete block in two fascicles and incomplete block in the third fascicle, AV conduction takes place, but usually with a prolonged PR interval. For example, RBBB, anterior hemiblock, and first-degree block may qualify as trifascicular if the first-degree block is in the posterior fascicle.

Fig. 25-25, *A*, was obtained in lead II from a patient with acute anterior wall MI. Lead II is the best lead for observing a shift of the axis to the left. In Fig. 25-25,

Table 25-1. Electrocardiographic recognition of bundle branch block and hemiblock

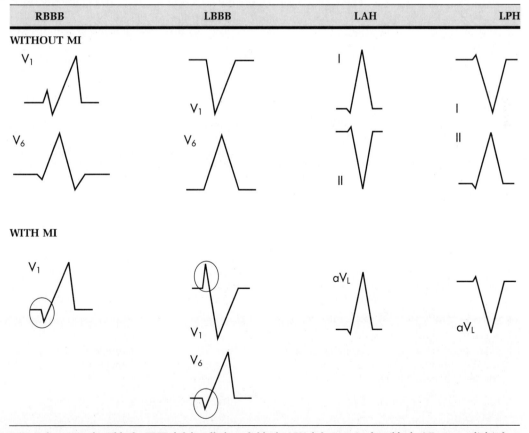

RBBB	LBBB	LAH	LPH

LAH, Left anterior hemiblock; *LBBB,* left bundle branch block; *LPH,* left posterior hemiblock; *MI,* myocardial infarction; *RBBB,* right bundle branch block.

A, there is abnormal left axis beyond −30 degrees every third beat; the QRS complex is broad, probably indicative of BBB; and the PR interval is long. Fig. 25-25, *B,* is from the same patient and shows trifascicular block as follows: (1) complete block of the right bundle (RBBB), (2) complete block of the anterior fascicle of the left bundle (left anterior hemiblock), and (3) a long PR interval, presumably the result of partial block of the posterior fascicle.

SUMMARY

The importance of recognizing BBB and hemiblock lies in the rapid identification of high-risk patients with acute MI. An appreciation for the mechanism of pathologic BBB adds to depth in the understanding of the 12-lead ECG and leads to a facility in recognizing functional BBB (RBBB or LBBB pattern) in the broad QRS tachycardia and in other critical clinical situations. Table 25-1 summarizes the ECG recognition of BBB and hemiblock and compares the patterns of LBBB and RBBB with and without anteroseptal MI and of anterior and posterior hemiblock.

REFERENCES

1a. Tawara S: *Das Reitzleitungssystem des Säugtierherzensm,* Jena, 1906, Gustav Fischer.

1. Rosenbaum MB: Types of right bundle branch block and their clinical significance, *J Electrocardiol* 2:197, 1969.

2. Rosenbaum MB, Elizari MV, Lazzari JO: Intraventricular trifascicular blocks: review of the literature and classification, *Am Heart J* 78:450, 1969.

3. Rosenbaum MB et al: Left anterior hemiblock obscuring the diagnosis of right bundle branch block, *Circulation* 48:298, 1973.

4. Rosenbaum MB, Elizari MV, Lazzari JO: *The hemiblocks,* Oldsmar, Fla, 1970, Tampa Tracings.

5. Demoulin JC, Kulbertus HE: Histopathological examination of the concept of left hemiblock, *Br Heart J* 34:807, 1972.

6. Wellens HJJ: Atrioventricular nodal and subnodal conduction disturbances. In Willerson JT, Cohn JN, eds: *Cardiovascular medicine,* New York, 1995, Churchill Livingstone.

7. Pasternak PC, Braunwald E, Sobel BE: Acute myocardial infarction. In Braunwald E, ed: *Heart disease,* ed 4, Philadelphia, 1992, WB Saunders.

8. Lie KI, Wellens HJJ, Schuilenburg RM: Bundle branch block and acute myocardial infarction. In Wellens HJJ, Lie KI, Janse MJ, eds: *The conduction system of the heart: structure, function and clinical implications,* The Hague, 1976. Martinus Nijhoff.

9. Schneider JF et al: Clinical-electrocardiographic correlates of newly acquired left bundle branch block: the Framingham study, *Am J Cardiol* 55:1332, 1985.

10. Perry JC, Garson A Jr: Arrhythmias following surgery for congenital heart disease. In Zipes DP, Jalife J, eds: *Cardiac electrophysiology from cell to bedside,* ed 2, Philadelphia, 1995, WB Saunders.

11. Perloff JK: Heart sounds and murmurs: physiological mechanisms. In Braunwald E, ed: *Heart disease,* ed 4, Philadelphia, 1992, WB Saunders.

12. Tilkian A, Conover M: *Understanding heart sounds and murmurs,* Philadelphia, 1994, WB Saunders.

13. Zehender M et al: ECG variants and cardiac arrhythmias in athletes: Clinical relevance and prognostic importance, *Am Heart J* 119:1378, 1990.

14. Hauer RNW et al: Long-term prognosis in patients with bundle branch block complicating acute anteroseptal infarction, *Am J Cardiol* 49:1581, 1982.

15. Warner RA et al: Electrocardiographic criteria for the diagnosis of combined inferior myocardial infarction and left anterior hemiblock, *Am J Cardiol* 51:718, 1983.

16. Davidson E et al: Atrial fibrillation: cause and time of onset, *Arch Intern Med* 149(2):457, 1989.

17. Sclarovsky S et al: Left anterior hemiblock obscuring the diagnosis of right bundle branch block in acute myocardial infarction. *Circulation* 60:26, 1979.

18. Marriott HJL: *Practical electrocardiography,* Baltimore, 1983, Williams & Wilkins.

C H A P T E R
26
Acute Myocardial Infarction

Pathophysiology of the Evolving
   Myocardial Infarction   *388*
Prognosis   *389*
Blood Supply to the Myocardium
   and Conduction System   *389*
ECG Signs of Myocardial Infarction   *391*
T Waves   *391*
ST Segment   *395*
Q Waves   *398*
Locating the Infarct   *400*
Anterior Wall Myocardial Infarction   *400*
Non-Q Wave Acute Myocardial
   Infarction   *407*
Inferior Myocardial Infarction   *409*
Right Ventricular Infarction   *415*
Peri-Infarction Block in Inferior
   Myocardial Infarction   *417*
Inferolateral Myocardial Infarction   *418*
Acute Posterior Wall Myocardial
   Infarction   *418*

Atrial Infarction   *420*
Emergency Approach to Acute Myocardial
   Infarction   *420*
Aggressive Therapy for High-Risk
   Patients   *421*
ECG Evaluation of Successful
   Reperfusion   *421*
Transporting Patients and Initiating
   Therapy   *422*
Eliminating Unnecessary Delays   *423*
Candidates for Thrombolysis   *424*
Contraindications to Thrombolytic
   Therapy   *424*
Effects of Prophylactic Antiarrhythmic
   Drug Therapy in Acute Myocardial
   Infarction   *425*
Differential Diagnoses   *426*
Summary   *426*

Each year approximately one and a half million individuals in the United States sustain a myocardial infarction (MI). One fourth of all deaths result from acute MI; 60% occur within the first hour.[1] Because of the availability of lifesaving and life-prolonging measures that preserve or reestablish coronary circulation, such as early thrombolysis, percutaneous transluminal coronary angioplasty (PTCA), and coronary bypass graft, the importance of the ECG in the early diagnosis and evaluation of the patient with chest pain and in the early recognition of reperfusion cannot be overemphasized. All emergency, prehospital, and critical care unit healthcare professionals should know how to do the following:

1. Use the ECG to identify patients with acute MI and the subgroups at high risk for MI.
2. Institute urgent thrombolytic therapy.
3. Recognize the ECG signs of successful and unsuccessful reperfusion.

PATHOPHYSIOLOGY OF THE EVOLVING MYOCARDIAL INFARCTION

The underlying pathophysiology of acute MI is the atherosclerotic plaque. This plaque may cause coronary arterial stenosis or may not be large enough to cause any obstruction to blood flow. Most atherosclerotic plaques are "inactive" in the sense that they do not become the site of thrombus formation and total occlusion, which causes acute MI. Most plaques are stable and progress slowly by buildup of lipid and macrophage complexes. Rapid plaque buildup is frequently caused by hemorrhage within a plaque—the unstable plaque—causing further compromise in the lumen of the coronary artery. These events generally do not cause acute MI but may present as accelerated or unstable angina. If the plaque is injured, ulcerates, or ruptures, it becomes a site for platelet aggregation, fibrin deposition, spasm, and thrombus formation. This active thrombus is the substrate and the anatomic and pathophysiologic basis of acute MI. If the active thrombus is only partially or intermittently occluding the coronary artery, the patient may present with acute coronary insufficiency of limited subendocardial MI or non–Q-wave MI. If the active

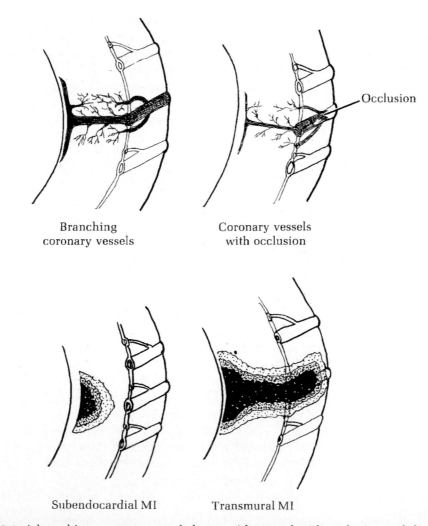

Fig. 26-1. A branching coronary vessel shown without and with occlusion and the resulting pathologic conditions.

thrombus totally occludes the vessel and stays occlusive, it usually causes the on-set of acute MI with acute ST-segment elevation and evolution into a Q-wave MI. The *initiating events* in acute MI are the plaque rupture and acute thrombus forma-tion at the site of the plaque.[2]

Following coronary occlusion, cellular changes in the myocardium begin im-mediately. If the ischemic condition is severe or prolonged, the area of ischemic tissue becomes more and more severely injured, cell functions cease, and irrevers-ible cell death ensues, producing a mass of necrotic tissue, which spreads from the central zone into a border zone. The resultant cellular pathophysiologic condition may produce life-threatening ventricular arrhythmias, especially in the first 15 to 30 min after coronary occlusion.[2]

Injured (ischemic) tissue is unable to contract (accounting for the systolic stretch during the acute stage of MI) but may be able to remain in a salvageable condition for some time and may return to normal function if flow is reestablished or collateral circulation develops and blood flow improves. However, if ischemia is severe and prolonged and blood flow is greatly impaired, cell death is inevitable. Fig. 26-1 demonstrates the pathologic process following a coronary occlusion and compares subendocardial and transmural infarctions. The surface ECG does not dis-tinguish between the two types of infarcts.

PROGNOSIS

The risk of dying during the first year after acute MI has been significantly re-duced over the last 20 years because of reperfusion procedures and the use of beta-blockers, aspirin, and angiotensin-converting enzyme (ACE) inhibitors.[3-5]

BLOOD SUPPLY TO THE MYOCARDIUM AND CONDUCTION SYSTEM

The coronary arteries and their major divisions are illustrated in Fig. 26-2. When the right coronary artery (RCA) provides the posterior descending branch, the term *dominant RCA* is used. When it is the left coronary artery (LCA) that does this, the term *dominant LCA* is used. Occlusion of the dominant RCA results in

Table 26-1. Features of atrioventricular conduction disturbances complicating acute myocardial infarction

Feature	Inferior MI	Anterior MI
Site of block	AV node	Bundle branches
Artery involved	RCA	LAD
Escape rhythm	Narrow QRS: heart rate, 40-60 beats/min; de-pendable	Wide QRS: heart rate, <40 beats/min; unde-pendable
Duration of block	Transient	Transient
Increase in hospital mor-tality (compared with same infarct location without block)	2½ times	4 times

From Wellens HJJ, Conover M: *The ECG in emergency decision making,* Philadelphia, 1991, WB Saunders.
AV, Atrioventricular; *LAD,* left anterior descending (coronary artery); *MI,* myocardial infarction; *RCA,* right coronary artery.

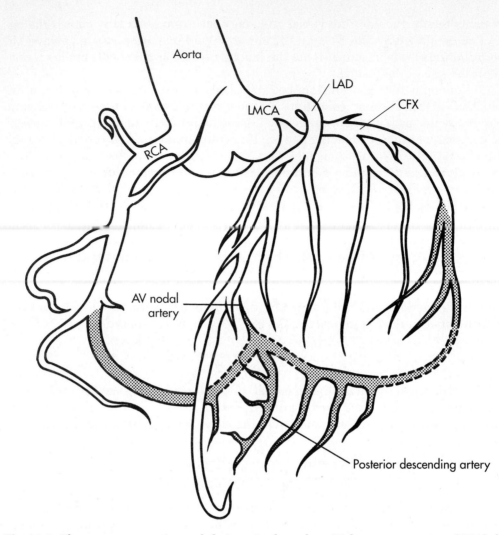

Fig. 26-2. The coronary arteries and their major branches. Right coronary artery (RCA), left main coronary artery (LMCA), left anterior descending (LAD) coronary artery, and circumflex (CFX) artery.

inferior MI. High-risk patients with inferior MI have proximal RCA occlusion in a dominant RCA, right ventricular MI, and atrioventricular (AV) block. Occlusion of the left anterior descending (LAD) coronary artery results in anterior MI. High-risk patients with LAD coronary artery occlusion have a proximal occlusion, right bundle branch block (RBBB), and/or hemiblock. Table 26-1 summarizes the features of AV conduction disturbances complicating acute MI.

Right coronary artery

In 90% of individuals the posterior descending branch of the RCA supplies the posterior third of the intraventricular septum and the posterior division of the left bundle branch (posterior fascicle). The RCA's *AV nodal branch* supplies the AV node and the proximal part of the bundle of His. Hence 20% of patients with acute inferior MI have high-degree AV nodal block.[6] Rarely the AV nodal artery may also supply the proximal bundle branches and, again rarely, the distal His bundle and the proximal bundle branches.[7,8] The RCA also supplies the right and left ventricles and, in some individuals, the posterolateral wall of the left ventricle.[9]

Left coronary artery

The LCA divides into the LAD branch and the circumflex artery. It is the LAD coronary artery that supplies the anterior and anterolateral walls of the heart and two thirds of the intraventricular septum. In most hearts, the first septal perforator from the LAD coronary artery provides the blood supply for the distal bundle of His and the proximal bundle branches.[8] In individuals with a dominant left coronary artery the posterior descending branch of the left bundle and the AV node are supplied by the distal branch of the circumflex coronary artery. The circumflex artery and its obtuse marginal branches supply the posterolateral wall of the left ventricle and, in some patients the inferior wall of the left ventricle.

ECG SIGNS OF MYOCARDIAL INFARCTION

The ECG signs of MI are T wave changes (ischemia), ST-segment displacement (injury), and abnormal Q waves (cellular death). Although oversimplified, this classification, first described in humans in 1920,[10] is useful in clinical practice.

After experimental coronary artery occlusion, almost immediately there are *T wave changes* (usually inversion) in the leads reflecting the involved surface and there is a loss of R-wave amplitude followed by an increase in amplitude; in clinical practice these initial changes are usually missed.

The preceding events are followed by a maximal *elevation of the ST segment.* As the pathologic condition progresses, the typically coved, elevated ST segment gradually evolves into inverted, symmetric T waves. *Abnormal Q waves* appear as early as 2 hours after the onset of chest pain in some patients and are usually fully developed within 9 hours.[9] This evolution of the ECG in patients with acute MI is dramatically altered with successful thrombolytic therapy (p. 422). Early signs include accelerated transient elevation of ST segment[11] followed by rapid reduction in ST segment elevation[12,13] and early T wave inversion.[14] See p.421 for ECG signs of reperfusion.

T WAVES

T waves reflect the repolarization of the myocardium. They are normally the same in polarity as the terminal QRS, asymmetric, and rounded. In MI, T-wave inversion is symmetric and pointed. As the infarction evolves, the elevated ST segments give way to inverted T waves. Such T waves are preceded by a typically

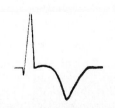

Fig. 26-3. The typical coved ST segment and inverted T wave of evolving myocardial infarction (MI).

coved, upward ST segment (Fig. 26-3). They may also reflect acute ischemia in the leads reflecting tissue near the injury. For example, a patient with acute anterior wall MI may have ST elevation in leads V_1 to V_4 and T-wave inversion in leads V_5 and V_6.

Normal T wave

The T wave is the result of the ventricular repolarization process. Although the process of depolarization proceeds from endocardium to epicardium, the process of repolarization proceeds in the opposite direction (epicardium to endocardium). This is thought to occur because the endocardium recovers more slowly than the epicardium as a result of the pressures of contraction and reduction in coronary blood flow. Thus T waves normally are inverted in lead aV_R and may be inverted or upright in V_1. They vary in leads V_0 and III, and they are normally positive in leads aV_L and aV_F but may be inverted if the QRS is less than 6 mm tall in those same leads.

Fig. 26-4 illustrates *current flow* (from negative to positive) during electrical systole and diastole. Depolarized tissue is negative, and repolarized tissue is positive. As illustrated in Fig. 26-4, although the processes of depolarization and repolarization are in opposite directions, the resultant current flow is in the same direction (endocardium to epicardium), producing a positive T wave.

Ischemic T wave

During *subendocardial* ischemia the sequence just described remains unchanged; that is, repolarization proceeds from epicardium to endocardium (positive T wave). In *subepicardial* ischemia, however, conduction is slowed in the epicardium, preventing it from initiating the repolarization process first. Instead the process begins in the endocardium, resulting in an inverted T wave. The mechanisms of normal and abnormal T waves are illustrated in Fig. 26-4. T-wave inversion of itself is by no means specific, since it may occur for many reasons.

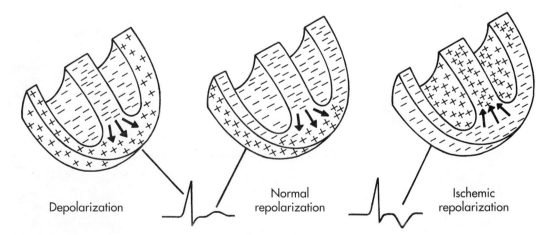

Fig. 26-4. Current flow during the processes of depolarization and repolarization; normal and ischemic repolarization are compared. The depolarization process proceeds from endocardium to epicardium, and the normal repolarization process proceeds in the opposite direction. Since current flows from negative to positive, the QRS complex and T wave are both positive. The ischemic repolarization process is opposite from normal, causing the T wave to be inverted.

T-wave inversions from causes other than myocardial infarction

Ischemia of unstable angina. In patients with unstable angina the progressive, deep, symmetric inversion of the T waves in leads V_2 and V_3 without loss of R waves in the precordial leads and with little or no enzyme elevation is not a sign of MI. These patients frequently have not yet had their infarction. Wall motion abnormalities may be observed on echocardiography in the absence of definite infarction—myocardial stunning. Such ECG signs may indicate critical proximal LAD coronary artery stenosis with possible brief periods of total occlusion and then spontaneous reperfusion (Wellens syndrome; see Chapter 24) and generally call for aggressive intervention, which may include emergency angiography and possible revascularization.

After periods of abnormal depolarization. When the ventricles are depolarized abnormally, as they are in ventricular tachycardia, Wolff-Parkinson-White (WPW) syndrome, and left bundle branch block (LBBB), the T wave may be inverted in the subsequent rhythms. For example, posttachycardia T-wave inversion may occur in the sinus rhythm following rapid pacing or ventricular tachycardia (VT).

In patients with WPW syndrome there is abnormal depolarization of the ventricles that is caused by the existence of an accessory pathway (Chapter 23), so the paroxysmal supraventricular tachycardia associated with this condition often has T-wave inversion in the leads that best reflect the delta wave during sinus rhythm, the delta wave representing a form of abnormal depolarization. These T wave changes can persist for days if the tachycardia was sustained for a long time.

In LBBB the ventricles are depolarized abnormally through the right bundle branch. Consequently, T-wave inversion may be seen in the sinus rhythm following the resolution of LBBB.

Normal variant. T-wave inversion may occur as a normal variant in young men, especially athletes, and in the right-side to midchest leads of children (the so-called juvenile T wave pattern), which may persist to adulthood.

Cerebrovascular accident. Deeply inverted, wide, blunted T waves may be the result of an acute cerebrovascular accident such as subarachnoid bleeding, major stroke, or trauma.

Acute pulmonary embolism. Precordial T-wave inversion is seen in some cases of acute pulmonary embolism after the first 24 hours.

Artifact. T-wave inversion may be an artifact produced either by the cardiac monitor (its filter), which should not be used to evaluate ST segments or T waves, or by sloppy application of electrode paste across the chest, in which case electrical potentials from the right chest may be transmitted to the left, causing T-wave inversions in midchest to left-side leads.

Hyperacute T waves

Marked T wave peaking may be present in the very early stages of acute MI, usually in association with ST elevation. The ECGs in Fig. 26-5, *A* and *B*, were taken 3 days apart. Note the tall, peaked T waves in leads V_1 to V_4 preceding the development of Q waves and elevated ST segments 3 days later.

In some patients with unstable angina, marked T wave peaking may be noted (hyperacute T waves) before the development of Wellens syndrome. Peaked T waves, like ST elevation, are indicative of acute occlusion. This occlusion could be the result of plaque rupture that is causing spasm, thrombus, platelets, or a combination of these. If the occlusion is total and unrelieved, it evolves into MI. If it is total but transient, there are varying degrees of ST-segment and T wave abnormalities and deep T-wave inversion. The approximate time frame for the occlusion and appearance of ECG changes is as follows:

<1 to 2 min: No ECG change.

5 to 30 min: ST-segment elevation and T-wave inversion.

Over an hour: Frequently there is infarction (ST elevation and perhaps Q waves).

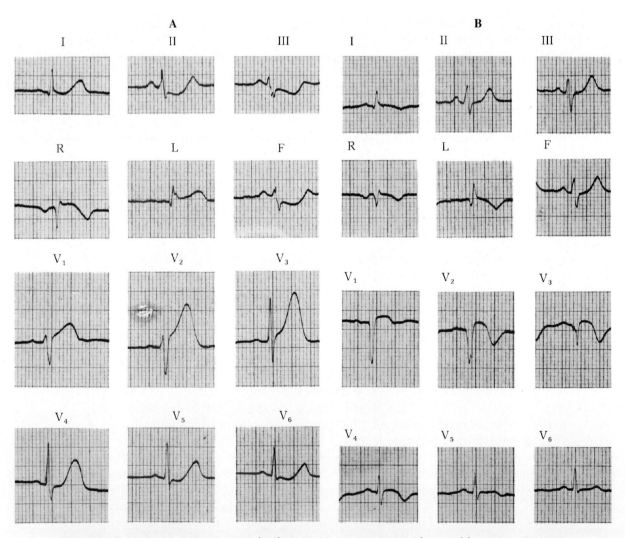

Fig. 26-5. A, Hyperacute T waves in leads V_1 to V_4 in a patient with unstable angina. **B,** Same patient 3 days later with acute anteroseptal MI.

ST SEGMENT
Acute injury

Prolonged (persistent) ST-segment elevation is a marker of acute ischemia and injury-infarction and is associated with elevated enzyme levels. Because of severe ischemia and lack of nutrients, the tissue immediately surrounding the center of the infarct is nonfunctional but may receive a blood supply from collateral circulation. This supply is sufficient to keep it alive but insufficient to maintain membrane integrity. The injured tissue has a different membrane potential from the healthy myocardium, and a current (current of injury) flows from the healthy tissue to the injured tissue during electrical systole (the ST segment) and in the opposite direction during electrical diastole (the TQ segment). Systolic and diastolic currents of injury are illustrated in Fig. 26-6.

Whenever there is a difference in electrical potential between myocardial cells, a current flows. Fig. 26-7, *A,* illustrates the ECG related to the action potential in the normal heart. Note that during the plateau of the action potential there is no difference in potential (where the dashed and the solid lines fuse). This lack of difference produces a normal isoelectric ST segment, and the normal sequence of repolarization results in a T wave that is the same in polarity as the QRS complex

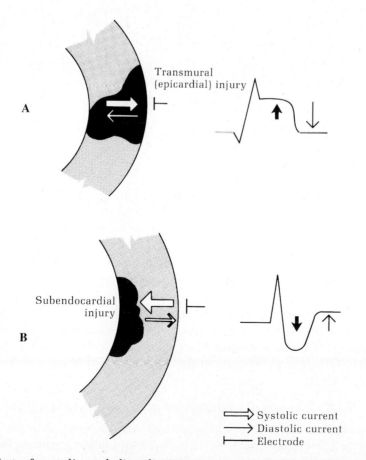

Fig. 26-6. Effect of systolic and diastolic injury currents on the ST segment because of **A,** epicardial injury and **B,** endocardial injury. *(Modified from Surawicz B et al: Am J Cardiol 41:943, 1978.)*

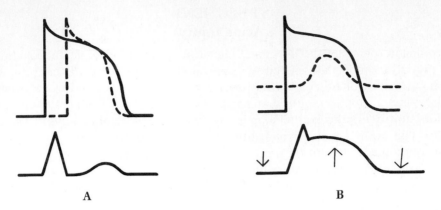

Fig. 26-7. Action potentials and the ECG from the normal heart **(A)** are compared with those from the ischemic and injured heart **(B)**.

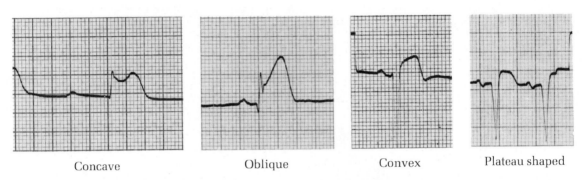

| Concave | Oblique | Convex | Plateau shaped |

Fig. 26-8. Different types of ST segment elevations in acute myocardial infarction.

(first cells to depolarize are the last to repolarize). In Fig. 26-7, *B,* the ischemic tissue has a membrane potential that is reduced to −60 mV and less. Note that in Fig. 26-7, *B,* the height of the action potential with the dashed line does not even reach the normal plateau. Thus a current flows throughout electrical systole and electrical diastole. The systolic current of injury displaces the ST segment upward, and the diastolic current of injury displaces the TQ segment downward. The result is an elevated ST segment. The greater the number of ischemic and injured cells present, the greater the displacement of the ST segment.

Fig. 26-8 illustrates the different types of ST elevation in acute MI—concave, convex, oblique, and plateau shaped. In most patients without thrombolytic therapy the ST segment falls rapidly within the first 12 hours, maintains a plateau, and then gradually normalizes.

ST-T changes not caused by myocardial infarction

Prinzmetal's angina. Prinzmetal's angina is caused by reversible severe coronary artery spasm and is characterized by an episode of chest pain associated with ST elevation that reverts to normal within a matter of minutes. In such cases, ST elevation indicates total occlusion and cessation of blood flow through the epicardial coronary artery. If the duration of the occlusion is short (usually minutes), the ST elevation resolves. This is the cause of the ECG pattern seen in Prinzmetal's angina. However, such a sequence is not necessarily associated with pain; it can be painless. There are two possibilities for the mechanism of the occlusion: (1) total spasm in an artery that is normal on angiography or (2) spasm superimposed on a fixed atherosclerotic obstruction, leading to 100% occlusion. If, on the other hand, the total occlusion is prolonged (20 to 40 min), the ST elevation does not resolve, enzyme levels rise, infarction develops, T waves become abnormal, and Q waves may develop.

Thus Prinzmetal's angina differs from a fixed infarction: Prinzmetal's angina is a temporary, reversible condition caused primarily by spasm and does not involve an acute thrombus, whereas in MI acute thrombus is primary, spasm may be contributing, and the occlusion is not self-limited.

Left main and three-vessel coronary artery disease. The more common type of unstable angina than Prinzmetal's angina is associated with diffuse depression of the ST segment, especially in leads V_3 and V_4, and ST elevation in leads aV_R and V_1. These ECG findings have frequently been shown to represent extensive myocardial ischemia and are commonly associated with left main or three-vessel coronary artery disease (Chapter 24). Urgent coronary arteriography and, frequently, revascularization are required.[15,16]

Acute pulmonary embolism. In acute pulmonary embolism ST elevation may be seen in the leads reflecting the dilated right side of the heart, V_1 and aV_R. When the ST elevation in V_1 is associated with an RBBB pattern and a positive T wave, it should raise the suspicion of acute pulmonary embolism.

Ventricular aneurysm. Ventricular aneurysm causes ST-segment elevation to persist after acute infarction caused by a current of injury generated from the myocardial cells bordering the aneurysm.

Pericarditis. ST elevation in pericarditis is often associated with pleuritic-type chest pain and is not accompanied by reciprocal ST changes. Frequently the ST-segment elevation is diffuse, involving multiple leads, and is accompanied by an increased sinus rate.

Artifact. ST-segment elevation may be caused by the low-frequency filter on the cardiac monitor or by poor electrode contact. Overdamping of the ECG stylus is another cause of ST elevation. It is recognized in the standardization artifact, which is slurred on its upstroke.

Nonspecific ST-T changes. *Nonspecific* describes ST-T changes that are outside the range of normal, including minor deviations of the ST segment, flattening of the T wave, and slight T wave inversions. Such changes should be monitored continuously in patients with unstable angina. Critical proximal LAD coronary artery stenosis is often initially manifested in these patients with a very slight negativity at the end of the T wave in leads V_1 to V_3.

ST-segment elevation in unstable angina. The ST segment elevates during pain in patients with unstable angina and critical proximal LAD coronary artery stenosis. When such patients are without pain, the ST segment may be only slightly elevated

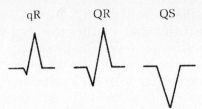

Fig. 26-9. Designation of the components of the QRS according to size and sequence. Lower case is used when the component is small.

or not at all elevated and there is deep, symmetric T wave inversion in leads V_2 and V_3 (Chapter 24). ST-segment elevation usually accompanies transient total occlusion of the vessel.

Q WAVES

A Q wave is a negative deflection that, when present, is the first component of the ventricular complex. An uppercase or a lowercase letter is used to indicate the size of the Q wave. Fig. 26-9 illustrates the differences between q and Q waves.

Normal q waves

Normal q waves reflect normal septal activation. They are narrow and small and are usually seen in leads I, aV_L, and V_6. They are less than 0.04 sec in duration and have less than 25% of the amplitude of the R wave. The dominant current in the intraventricular septum is from left to right. Thus the leads that record these initial forces have left-to-right lead axes with the positive electrode on the left side of the body, that is, leads I, aV_L, and V_6.

The axis of lead I is straight across the shoulders. Lead aV_L has an axis from the left shoulder to the center of the electrical field of the heart. Lead V_6 has an axis from a midaxillary position to the center of the electrical field of the heart. Fig. 26-10 illustrates the relationship of these three lead axes to normal septal forces. In leads I, aV_L, and V_6, septal forces move away from the positive electrode, producing a small q wave. In the electrically horizontal heart, normal septal q waves may also appear in leads V_4 and V_5, and in the electrically vertical heart, in leads II, III, and aV_F.

Pathologic Q wave

Abnormal Q waves are identified when there is an increase in duration and depth of normal Q waves or the appearance of "new" Q waves (not present in previous tracings). Thus changes in pattern may be just as significant as the size of the Q wave. Q waves are the classic diagnostic feature of myocardial necrosis. The possible processes for the appearance of pathologic Q waves on the 12-lead ECG are the following:

1. When electrically inactive tissue is present under the electrode, it records from the opposite wall of the heart (as if looking through a window).
2. When there is inactive tissue under the electrode, the wavefront must travel long distances around the inactive tissue. Abnormal Q waves reflect this delay. The larger and deeper the lesion, the larger the Q wave.[17]

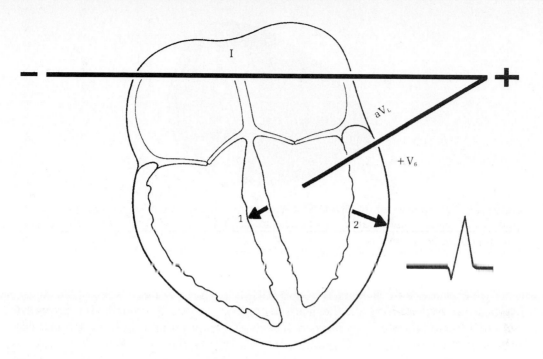

Fig. 26-10. Orientation of the initial QRS forces (septal) to the axes of leads I, aV_L, and V_6.

3. When there is conduction delay in the zone under the electrode, as in the early stages of acute MI, pathologic Q waves may appear. Thus, even with new pathologic Q waves, thrombolysis can still accomplish significant myocardial salvage, even after several hours of delay from the onset of pain.

Q waves from causes other than myocardial infarction

Normal variant. A QS complex may be normal in lead V_1 but rarely occurs in leads V_1 and V_2, simulating anteroseptal MI. A QS complex may also be a normal finding in leads III and aV_F. In the electrically vertical heart there may be a QS or Qr pattern in aV_L, simulating lateral wall infarction; the difference is that there are no other signs of MI, including ST-segment abnormalities, abnormal Q waves, or loss of R waves in the other lateral leads, I, V_5, and V_6.

Acute pulmonary embolism. Following acute pulmonary embolism (Chapter 24) a q wave often appears in leads V_1, III, and aV_F. In fact, because of this and because of the T wave changes that are sometimes seen in the precordial leads, such patients may be misdiagnosed as having acute inferior or anterior wall MI.

Infiltrative myocardial disease. In conditions such as amyloidosis, muscular dystrophy, and any other type of myocardial injury that causes a loss of electrical potentials and an inability to depolarize, abnormal Q waves may be seen.

Intraventricular conduction problems. Abnormal Q waves may be seen when intraventricular conduction is abnormal, such as in bundle branch block (BBB) and WPW syndrome.

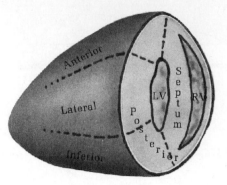

Fig. 26-11. The surfaces of the heart. Note that involvement of the anterior segment may extend to the septum (anteroseptal myocardial infarction) and the lateral wall (anterolateral). The inferior segment may extend to the posterior wall (inferoposterior), the lateral wall (inferolateral), or both (inferoposterolateral), and the right ventricle.

Ventricular hypertrophy. In the leads facing the ventricle opposite the hypertrophy, reciprocal Q waves may be seen. These may be prominent in hypertrophic cardiomyopathy.

LOCATING THE INFARCT

It is almost always possible to identify the location of an anterior, lateral, or inferior infarction. The key is an understanding of the surfaces of the heart and their reflecting leads. Apical locations are difficult, if not impossible, to determine on the surface ECG, and determining posterior locations has its own problems.

Echocardiography has proved invaluable in both the diagnosis and the localization of MI, especially when the clinical and ECG findings are not diagnostic or if complications of MI are suspected.

In Fig. 26-11 the cylinder of the left ventricle is portioned into anterior, septal, lateral, and inferior surfaces. The base of the heart is part of all of these surfaces. The anterior base of the left ventricle is the anterior septum. The inferior base is called "posterior." The leads reflecting these surfaces are discussed under their headings. The sensitivity of the ECG in localizing apical MI is very low. At times there are Q waves in precordial leads V_1 to V_4, and at other times, in the inferior leads. One source defines *apical* as Q waves present in leads II, III, and aVL and one or more of the leads V_1 to V_4.[18]

ANTERIOR WALL MYOCARDIAL INFARCTION
Reflecting leads

Anterior: V_3 and V_4
Anteroseptal: V_1 to V_4
Lateral: I, aV_L, and V_6
Anterolateral: I, aV_L, and V_3 to V_6
Extensive anterior: I, aV_L, and V_1 to V_6
High lateral: I and aV_L

Fig. 26-12 illustrates the proximity of the precordial leads to the anterior heart as follows:

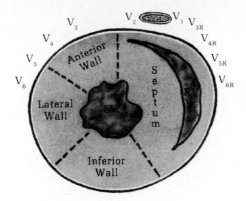

Fig. 26-12. Location of left and right precordial leads. Note the proximity of these leads to the surface of the ventricles. Leads V_2 and V_3 span the septum; leads V_2 to V_4 are over the anterior wall; and V_5 to V_6 are over the lateral wall. Lead V_{4R} is the best right-side precordial lead for detecting right ventricular MI.

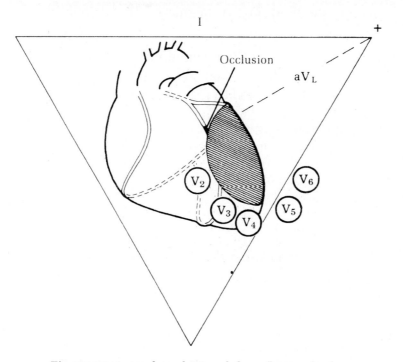

Fig. 26-13. Anterolateral MI and the reflecting leads.

- V_1 is over the anterior right ventricular surface.
- V_2 and V_3 span the septum.
- V_3 and V_4 are over the anterior wall of the left ventricle.
- V_5 and V_6 reflect the anterior and lateral walls of the heart, with leads I and aV_L reflecting the high lateral wall.

(Right-side chest leads V_{3R} to V_{6R} are also illustrated [Fig. 26-12]. As you will see, V_{4R} is useful in inferior wall MI in identifying high-risk patients and right ventricular MI.)

Fig. 26-13 is a diagram of muscle involved in an extensive anterolateral wall

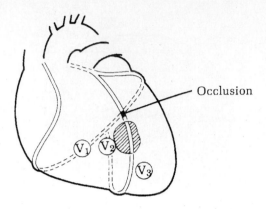

Fig. 26-14. Anteroseptal MI and the reflecting leads.

infarction and the relationship of the reflecting leads. Note that leads I and aV_L are close to the base of the heart. Fig. 26-14 shows a more circumspect anteroseptal infarction.

ECG recognition

1. ST-segment elevation in the precordial leads; leads I and aV_L may also be involved. The more leads involved and the higher the ST segment, the bigger the infarction.
2. Loss of R-wave progression (loss of anterior forces).
3. Symmetric T-wave inversion from an ST segment that is coved upward.

In Fig. 26-15 there are Q waves in leads V_1 to V_4 and ST elevation in leads V_1 to V_6 (anteroseptal and anterolateral). The Q waves in leads III and aV_F reveal an old inferior wall MI. The left-axis deviation points to left anterior hemiblock. In Fig. 26-16 the ECG signs of acute MI are seen in all of the superior leads (V_1 to V_6, I, and aV_L).

ECG identification of high-risk patients

High-risk patients with anterior wall MI are recognized on ECG in leads V_1, I, and II because of the development of RBBB or left anterior hemiblock, or both. Such findings are an independent marker of poor prognosis in patients with acute anterior MI. However, a study[19] involving 932 patients with Q-wave anterior MI showed that the absence of left ventricular (LV) failure identified a subgroup of patients with RBBB and low in-hospital (4%) and 1-year (5%) mortality. The authors found these patients to be comparable in mortality with patients who had neither LV failure nor RBBB. Chapter 25 discusses the ECG patterns of BBB.

Uncomplicated RBBB is recognized because of a broad QRS with an rSR' pattern in lead V_1. Right bundle branch block with MI is recognized because of a broad QRS with a QR pattern in lead V_1. Fig. 26-17, *A*, shows the serial tracings of a patient with acute anterolateral wall MI in whom left anterior hemiblock (Fig. 26-17, *B*) and RBBB (Fig. 26-17, *C*) subsequently develop. In Fig. 26-17, *C*, the typical rSR' pattern of uncomplicated RBBB is replaced by a QR pattern.

Fig. 26-18 shows anterior wall MI with RBBB without hemiblock. (Note the normal axis.) In Fig. 26-19 there are anterior wall MI (Q waves in leads V_1 and V_2), RBBB (late R wave in V_1), and left anterior hemiblock (extreme left-axis deviation).

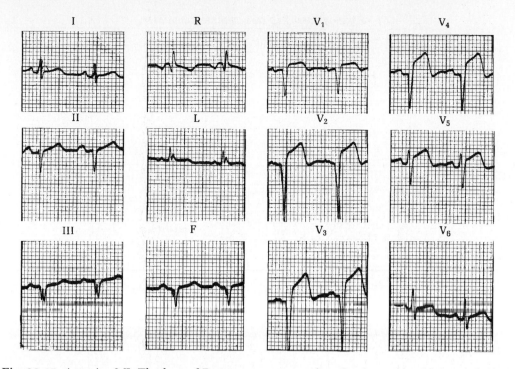

Fig. 26-15. Anterior MI. The loss of R-wave progression from lead V_1 to lead V_4 and the ST-segment elevation are evident. Limb leads show that anterior hemiblock has developed. (Note the negative complex in lead II.) Hemiblock and development of right bundle branch block (RBBB) identify high-risk patients.

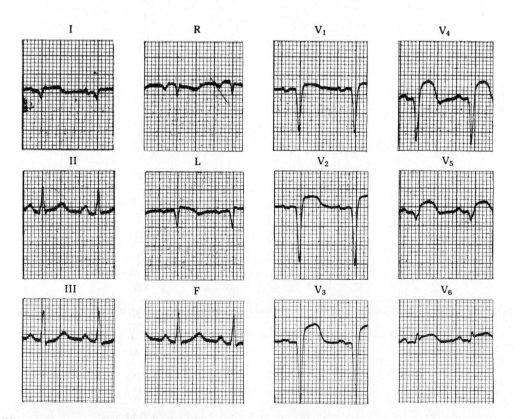

Fig. 26-16. Anterolateral MI. The loss of R-wave progression from lead V_1 to lead V_6 and the ST-segment elevation in those leads are evident.

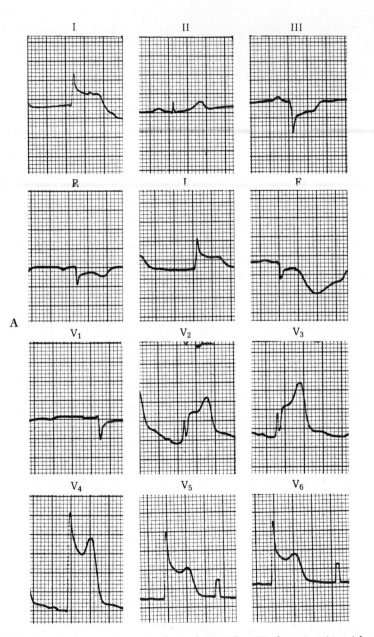

Fig. 26-17. A, ECG showing massive anterolateral MI. The ST elevation is evident in all the superior leads.

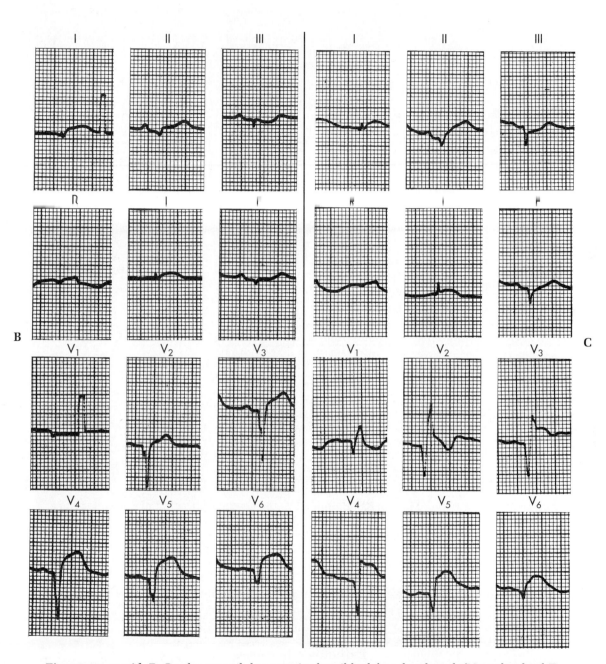

Fig. 26-17, cont'd. B, On the second day anterior hemiblock has developed. (Note that lead II has become negative.) **C,** By the third day RBBB has developed. *(Courtesy Peggy McKnight, RN, Las Vegas.)*

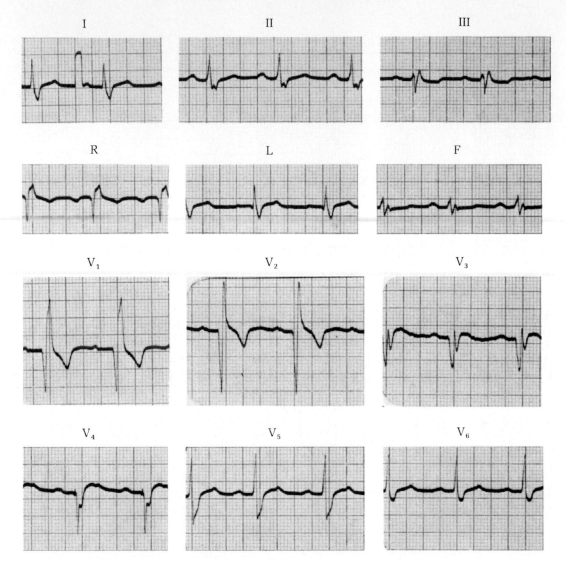

Fig. 26-18. Anteroseptal MI with RBBB. In lead V_1 the absence of the initial r wave is typical of uncomplicated RBBB. The appearance of RBBB identifies a high-risk patient. The QRS axis is normal; therefore hemiblock has not yet developed.

Immediately recognizing and reporting the development of BBB or hemiblock in patients with acute anterior wall MI is extremely important. Such a finding identifies a high-risk patient and is an indication for aggressive therapy.

Pathologic features

Anterior-wall MI frequently results from an occlusion of the proximal LAD coronary artery and may involve a combined lesion of the LAD coronary artery and RCA or left circumflex artery. The infarction may extend from the anterior wall into the septum (anteroseptal infarction) and to the left base, free wall, or apex; such infarctions are grouped under the term *anterolateral* or *extensive anterior wall MI*. The different pathologic features of Q-wave and non–Q-wave MI are discussed on p. 388.

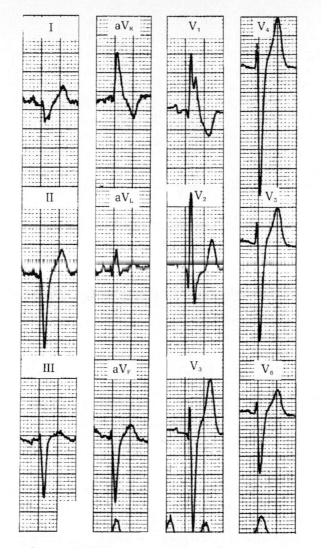

Fig. 26-19. Anteroseptal MI with RBBB and hemiblock. There is a Q wave in leads V_1 to V_3, along with a broad R wave. There is also left anterior hemiblock, as evidenced by the extreme left axis deviation. These ECG signs identify a high-risk patient.

Conduction abnormalities

In acute anterior wall MI the conduction problems that identify high-risk patients are BBB, hemiblock, and type II second-degree AV block.

NON–Q-WAVE ACUTE MYOCARDIAL INFARCTION

The diagnosis of non–Q-wave acute MI can be made only with characteristic elevations in levels of serum creatine kinase (CK) and creatine kinase–MB (CK_2). These patients may come to medical attention with transient (48 to 72 hours), nonspecific findings such as ST-segment depression or T wave abnormalities without the evolution of Q waves, or both. Although ST-segment depression has long been viewed as a sign of subendocardial ischemia, studies have shown that early ST-segment elevation occurs in both evolving Q-wave and non–Q-wave MI, being present in up to two thirds of cases of non–Q-wave infarction.[20,21] Furthermore, increased mortality has been observed in patients with MI who had ST-segment depression in *any* lead group, with or without ST-segment elevation in other ECG leads.[22]

Reflecting leads

- ST-segment depression in II, III, and aV_F: *Acute inferior non–Q-wave MI*
- ST-segment depression in I, aV_L, V_5, and V_6: *Acute lateral non–Q-wave MI*
- ST-segment depression in V_1 to V_4, as follows:

  Acute anterior non–Q-wave MI: If seen with evolving T-wave inversions and elevated enzymes

  Anterior wall ischemia: If seen with ST-segment elevation in the inferior leads and negative precordial T waves[21]

  Posterior wall ischemia[26]: If seen with ST-segment elevation in the inferior leads and positive precordial T waves[21]

ECG recognition

1. Symmetric, convex, downward ST-segment depression
2. ST-segment elevation in V_1 with ST depression in leads V_2 to V_4 that is not as marked as in acute posterior wall MI
3. Inverted or biphasic T wave with a terminally inverted segment in leads V_2 to V_3

   Fig. 26-20 shows non–Q-wave anterior MI; there is ST-segment depression in leads V_1 to V_6 and T-wave inversion in leads I, aV_L, and V_2 to V_6. Helpful in differentiating this type of MI from posterior MI are (1) the degree of enzyme level elevation (larger in acute posterior MI) and (2) the degree of ST-segment depression (more marked in acute posterior MI).[23]

   In contrast to Q-wave MI, in which there is a classic, evolving ECG pattern of ST elevation followed by development of Q waves in leads overlying the necrosis, there is not a specific ECG pattern in non–Q-wave MI; the diagnosis is based on the ECG and characteristic elevations of serum enzyme levels (CK and CK_2).

Pathologic features

The different pathologic features of Q-wave and non–Q-wave MI are discussed on p. 388.

Clinical significance

Non–Q-wave MI accounts for approximately 30% to 40% of acute MIs, a proportion that appears to be increasing. These patients have a smaller infarct size, better residual left ventricular function, and lower in-hospital mortality than do patients with Q-wave infarction.[24,25] Nonetheless, long-term survival is the same or less than that of patients with Q-wave infarction. Patients have a higher incidence of postinfarction angina and rate of recurrence than do patients with Q-wave infarction.[24] The factors related to mortality in the 1-year follow-up data for 515 patients surviving acute non–Q-wave MI were persistent ST-segment depression, a history of congestive heart failure, older age, and ST-segment elevation at discharge.[26] Patients with no ST-segment depression had approximately half the mortality of those with ST-segment depression.

The different clinical profiles of Q-wave and non–Q-wave MI have been attrib-

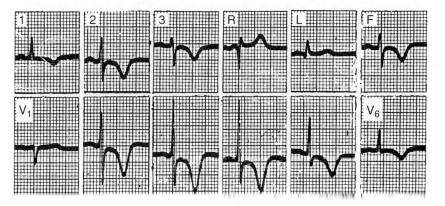

Fig. 26-20. Anterior non–Q-wave acute MI. The ST-segment depression in the precordial leads and the T-wave inversions in leads I, aV_L, and V_2 to V_6 are evident. *(From Boden WE, Kleiger RE, Gibson RS et al: Am J Cardiol 59:782, 1987.)*

uted to differing atheromatous plaque substrate. In the non–Q-wave variety the occlusion involves minimal nonulcerated luminal narrowing or severe stenosis, whereas in Q-wave MI there is moderate stenosis with an eccentric, ulcerated plaque.[27]

In the TIMI II study[27] involving 2634 patients, 29.1% had a non-Q-wave infart pattern and 70.9% a Q-wave infarct pattern within 24 hours of treatment with intravenous recombinant tissue-type plasminogen activator (rTPA). A greater percentage of non-Q-wave patients had normalization of the initial ST segment elevation during rTPA infusion; there were also more non-Q-wave patients with infarct-related artery patency and a predischarge resting left ventricular ejection fraction of 55%. In the Q-wave patients, new congestive heart failure during hospitalization, male sex, and anterior wall infarcts were more frequent than in the non-Q-wave group. After initial therapy (rTPA, heparin, and aspirin) for all patients, Q-wave and non-Q-wave patients were compared relative with their response to conservative treatment (coronary angiography and revascularization for recurrent spontaneous or exercise-induced myocardial ischema) and invasive treatment (coronary angiography, contrast left ventriculography, and PTCA). Early mortality and adverse clinical cardiac events were not significantly different in non-Q-wave and Q-wave MI.

INFERIOR MYOCARDIAL INFARCTION
Reflecting leads: II, III, and aV_F

Fig. 26-21 illustrates the proximity of leads II, III, and aV_F to the inferior wall of the heart. As a group, these leads are appropriately called *inferior leads.*

ECG recognition

ST-segment elevation, development of Q waves, and symmetric T-wave inversion in the inferior leads.

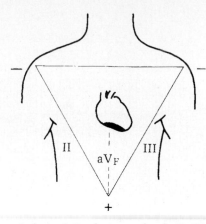

Fig. 26-21. Inferior MI relative to leads II, III, and aV_F.

Table 26-2. Major complications in acute inferior myocardial infarction (200 patients)

In-hospital outcome	No. of patients (%) TOTAL (%)	No. of patients in first 24 hours (%)
Death	7	13
Cardiogenic shock	16	10
Ventricular fibrillation	16	8
Sustained ventricular tachycardia	13	9
Complete atrioventricular block	8	3
Severe bradycardia	3	4
Required pacing	7	5
Myocardial rupture	3	2

High-risk patients

In one study involving 200 consecutive patients admitted with acute inferior MI, 20% died and 47% had major complications (Table 26-2).[28]

ECG identification of high-risk patients

1. ST-segment elevation in lead V_{4R} (proximal RCA occlusion and right ventricular [RV] infarction)
2. Complete AV block
3. Anterior precordial ST depression
4. Lateral ST elevation

NOTE: If the ECG changes are confined to leads II, III, and aV_F, the clinical problem is fairly benign, with a mortality of 4%.[29] High-risk patients may require more aggressive therapy when intravenous (IV) thrombolysis is not successful. Such therapy includes intracoronary thrombolysis and PTCA. The ST-segment elevation in V_{4R} usually disappears within 10 hours after the onset of pain; thus it is important to record this lead on admission.

Culprit coronary artery

In most cases of inferior MI it is the RCA that is involved. This artery supplies the AV node and the inferior wall of the heart in 90% of cases ("right dominance"). The circumflex artery performs this function in 10% of patients ("left dominance"). When the occlusion is in the RCA, it is the inferior posterior part of the ventricles that is infarcted.

Locating the occluded artery

The site of occlusion in inferior MI can be determined in two ways, one more specific than the other. They involve use of *lead V_{4R}* as one method, and use of *leads II* and *III* as the other. As you will see, ST-segment elevation in V_{4R} also identifies a patient with right ventricular infarction, and the patient is at high risk.

Lead V_{4R}. Patterns in this right chest lead can localize the occlusion[30] to the following:

Proximal RCA: ST-segment elevation greater than or equal to 1 mm; identifies a high-risk patient.

Distal RCA: No ST-segment elevation, but an ST segment with an upsloping shape.[30]

Circumflex artery: No ST-segment elevation and a downsloping ST-T segment. The preceding patterns are illustrated in Fig. 26-22. Before reading the legends, evaluate the 12-lead ECGs in Figs. 26-23 and 26-24 and identify the coronary artery involved. Further identify a proximal or distal occlusion.

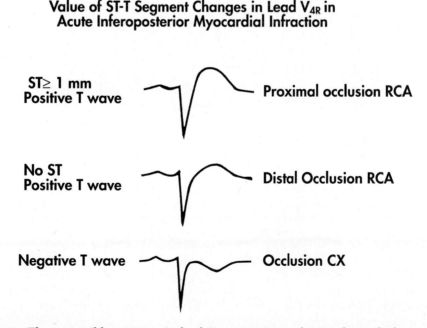

Value of ST-T Segment Changes in Lead V_{4R} in Acute Inferoposterior Myocardial Infraction

ST≥ 1 mm
Positive T wave — Proximal occlusion RCA

No ST
Positive T wave — Distal Occlusion RCA

Negative T wave — Occlusion CX

Fig. 26-22. Three possible patterns in lead V_{4R} in patients during the early hours of acute inferior MI. These patterns identify the location of the occlusion. *RCA,* Right coronary artery; *CX,* circumflex coronary artery. *(From Wellens HJJ, Conover M: The ECG in emergency decision making, Philadelphia, 1991, WB Saunders.)*

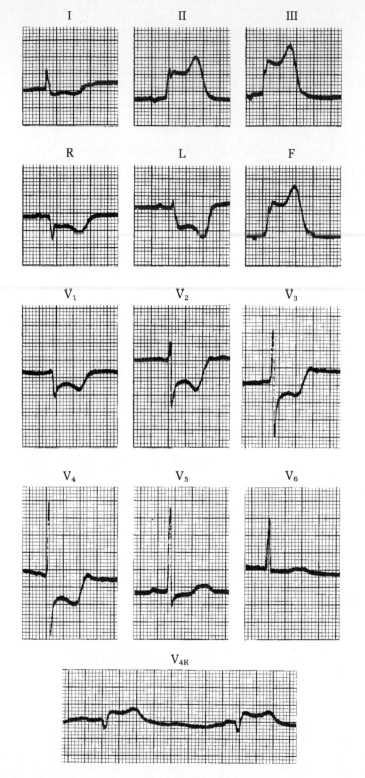

Fig. 26-23. Acute inferior and right ventricular MI. The ST-segment elevation is evident in leads II, III, aV$_F$, and V$_{4R}$. The ST-segment elevation in V$_{4R}$ identifies a patient with a proximal RCA occlusion and right ventricular MI who is at high risk for atrioventricular (AV) block. The RCA is also identified as the culprit lesion by comparing the ST-segment elevation in leads II and III; higher elevation in lead III than in lead II denotes RCA occlusion. *(Courtesy William P. Nelson, MD.)*

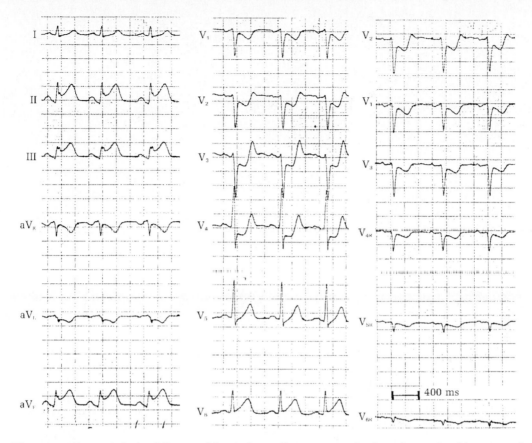

Fig. 26-24. Acute inferior MI caused by a circumflex artery occlusion, determined because of the negative T wave in lead V_{4R}. Also the ST segment is higher in lead II than in lead III, another sign of circumflex artery occlusion. *(From Wellens HJJ, Conover M: The ECG in emergency decision making, Philadelphia, 1991, WB Saunders.)*

Leads II and III. Comparison of the ST-segment elevation in leads II and III can also help differentiate between RCA occlusion and circumflex occlusion as follows:

 RCA occlusion: ST-segment elevation in lead III is greater than in lead II.

 Circumflex artery occlusion: ST-segment elevation in lead II is greater than in lead III.

In RCA occlusion the damage is to the inferior-posterior portion of the ventricles, placing the injury closer to the axis of lead III than to that of lead II. Because the injury current is between the axes of these leads, ST-segment elevation is dramatic.

In circumflex occlusion the damage is to the inferior lateral portion of the left ventricle, placing the injury closer to the axis of lead II than to that of lead III. In addition, the total ST-segment elevation in the inferior leads is smaller than that seen in RCA occlusion (given the same amount of infarcted tissue) because the injury current is between the axes of leads I and II (more remote from lead III).

The importance of recognizing circumflex occlusion is to alert the physician to its deceptively low ST segments. This knowledge would help in the decision to give or withhold thrombolytics in inferior MI with low ST-segment elevation.[31]

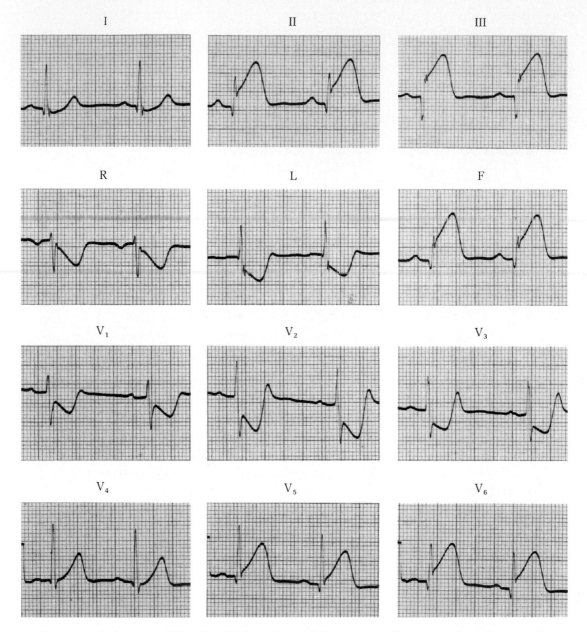

Fig. 26-25. Inferolateral MI. The ST elevation and Q waves can be seen in the inferior leads and in leads V_5 and V_6. The ST segment is higher in lead III than in II; this is a right coronary artery occlusion.

The preceding facts are illustrated in Figs. 26-23 and 26-24; in those cases lead V_{4R} is also available for confirmation. Before reading the legend in Fig. 26-25, determine which coronary artery is involved by comparing the ST-segment elevation in leads II and III.

Conduction abnormalities

Atrioventricular block occurs frequently in the setting of inferior MI and seems to indicate a larger infarct and increased mortality. Although with thrombolytic therapy the mortality rate of patients with AV block is somewhat lower than that of patients in the prethrombolytic era, the rate still remains relatively high. Mortality 1 year after discharge is increased in patients in whom AV block developed within 24 hours after thrombolytic therapy but not in those who had AV block before treatment.[32]

Conduction abnormalities at the AV nodal level can be expected in the form of second-degree AV block (usually type I) and complete AV block with a junctional escape pacemaker. Such conduction abnormalities occur in 20% of patients with acute inferior MI, are the result of proximal RCA occlusion, and identify a patient with RV infarction who is at higher risk had AV block not been present.[6,33] In such cases the in-hospital mortality rate is 23%, or 2½ times that of inferior wall infarction without AV block.[34] When third-degree heart block is present, the average mortality rate is 29%. The high mortality rates reflect a more proximal occlusion and more muscle damage. Other causes of AV block in acute inferior MI may be high vagal tone (Bezold-Jarisch reflex*), release of potassium and adenosine from inside the cells (both of which can cause heart block), and the presence of concomitant stenosis of the proximal LAD coronary artery, which would compromise the septal perforators and their rich network of collateral vessels that reach toward the AV nodal artery.

"Benign reciprocal changes" or worse prognosis?

Boden and Spodick[20] have explained that the difficulty in reconciling the term "benign reciprocal ECG changes" lies in the fact that the axes of the precordial leads are perpendicular to the axes of the limb leads. It is uncertain whether true electrical reciprocity can exist between lead axes that are perpendicular to each other. Therefore it is thought that reciprocal (electrically opposite) changes can occur only between leads in the same plane. For example, in the frontal plane leads, injury to the inferior wall typically results in ST-segment elevation in the inferior leads (II, III, and aV_F) and reciprocal ST-segment depression in the lateral wall leads (I and aV_L); furthermore, events occurring in the anterior and posterior walls are truly reciprocal or mirror images.

ST-segment depression in the precordial leads is an early finding in approximately half of patients with their first acute inferior MI (Figs. 26-23 to 26-25) and is thought by many investigators to indicate more extensive infarction and a worse prognosis than in patients without ST-segment depression, despite reperfusion therapy.[35] In one study precordial ST-segment depression in inferior MI was associated with a 1-year mortality rate that was six times that of patients without associated precordial ST-segment depression.[22]

RIGHT VENTRICULAR INFARCTION

Reflecting lead: Lead V_{4R}

ECG diagnosis

ST-segment elevation greater than or equal to 1 mm in lead V_{4R} (right precordial lead). In patients with acute inferior MI, ST-segment elevation of 1 mm or more in lead V_{4R} (Fig. 26-23) has a high sensitivity and specificity for detecting RV infarction,[36-39] pinpointing the site of occlusion in the proximal RCA and identify-

---

*When ischemia stimulates the afferent nerves adjacent to the AV node, increased vagal tone results. This produces sinus bradycardia, hypotension, and in some patients heart block.

ing patients at high risk for development of AV block. (In all patients with inferior wall MI the incidence of AV block is 11%.[40-42])

Recording lead V_{4R} in the coronary care unit

If lead V_{4R} is not routinely recorded on the 12-lead ECG at admission, it can be easily recorded on admission to the coronary care unit (CCU). Assuming that leads I, II, and III are in place (Einthoven's triangle), you now have the option to record any of the right- or left-side chest leads. Place the V recording electrode on the right side of the chest at the midclavicular line in the fifth intercostal space (same location on the right side of the chest as on the left precordium for the left-sided standard V_4 lead). For further discussion please review Chapter 1.

Pathophysiology

Right ventricular infarction occurs exclusively in patients with transmural infarction of the inferior-posterior wall with mandatory extension into the RV free wall.[29,43] Although the culprit lesion is usually the proximal RCA, a mid-RCA occlusion may also cause RV infarction; rarely is a dominant circumflex artery involved. Isolated RV infarction is seen in 3% to 5% of cases of MI (autopsy proven), usually associated with chronic lung disease and RV hypertrophy.[44]

Only 5% to 10% of patients with RV infarction have hemodynamic symptoms.[45] Should the patient come to medical attention in cardiogenic shock, the mortality rate is 35% and IV or intracoronary thrombolytic therapy has no impact. Hypotension and cardiogenic shock occur when the ischemia is enough to decrease the compliance and cause volume (pressure) overload in the right ventricle. Within a closed pericardial space this changes the curvature of the septum, which encroaches on LV function, decreasing LV preload and producing a hemodynamic situation consistent with LV tamponade. Because of this, patients with hemodynamic compromise caused by RV infarction may have elevated jugular venous pressure of 10 mm or more, a positive Kussmaul's venous sign (inspiratory increase in jugular venous distention), and clear lung fields. Hemodynamic monitoring is diagnostic, and findings are typical.

One common complication of RV infarction with inferior MI is the development of AV block. If the block is complete (third-degree AV block), the blood pressure falls precipitously and mortality is quite high. In such cases it is important to maintain AV synchrony because of the preload problem for the ventricles. If atrial fibrillation develops, DC cardioversion is attempted.[29]

Clinical implications: an overview

Right ventricular infarction is associated with serious hemodynamic consequences. This observation was made more than two decades ago by Cohn et al.[46] Since that time the following have been shown:

1. Right ventricular infarction is present in 19% to 51% of patients with acute inferior MI (postmortem studies).[47,48]
2. In most patients with RV infarction the condition does not manifest itself with its hemodynamic picture.[45,49]
3. The presence of RV infarction is a strong, independent prognostic parameter for life-threatening postinfarction tachyarrhythmias, AV block (45%), and poor short- and long-term outcome after inferior MI.[28,50-52]
4. Early diagnosis of RV infarction helps prevent mismanagement. In most patients the RV function improves rapidly and the response to reperfusion is

good; use of diuretics, nitroglycerin, and morphine is avoided because they decrease preload. However, in the 5% of patients who have hemodynamic compromise, knowledgeable medical treatment and informed hemodynamic monitoring help to avoid acute tamponade caused by RV volume overload squeezing the left ventricle. Early diagnosis allows anticipation of conduction problems and arrhythmias, which are aggressively treated; angioplasty improves the ischemic and hemodynamic condition. If cared for carefully, these patients improve in a few days as collateral flow increases and ischemia resolves.[29]

5. Lead V_{4R} (a right-side precordial lead) has a high sensitivity, specificity, and predictive accuracy in diagnosing RV infarction.[36-39,53,54]

Right ventricular infarction is common in inferior MI and carries with it a poor prognosis and increased incidence of life-threatening arrhythmias and AV block. In most patients this high-risk indicator is not recognized by physical signs. However, a recording of lead V_{4R} is a simple, promptly available means of establishing the presence of RV infarction. Such an ECG assessment should be routinely performed in all patients with acute inferior MI.[50]

PERI-INFARCTION BLOCK IN INFERIOR MYOCARDIAL INFARCTION

Peri-infarction block is the ECG manifestation of slowed conduction and delayed activation of fibers in association with or near the MI zone. It is possible that the ECG recognition of this condition may identify patients after MI who are at greater risk for sustained VT.[55]

History

It is necessary to explain the historical evolution of the term *peri-infarction block* because the meaning taken in the recent data is that of the original application in 1950, not that of later authors who equated it with hemiblock.

Peri-infarction block was described in 1950,[56] when it was recognized that although the electrodes close to and adjacent to the infarction could have a QRS duration of 0.11 sec or more, the electrodes in remote zones could have a normal QRS duration. The anatomic basis was demonstrated in the early studies by direct recordings from infarcted myocardium. When the electrode was over the center of the infarction, there was a QS pattern; when it was moved to the peri-infarction zone, there was a QR complex. Soon after these initial studies, peri-infarction block was equated with left anterior fascicular block.[57-61] Rosenbaum et al.[62] later correctly refuted this usage, but by this time the concept of peri-infarction block became one with hemiblock and slipped into oblivion. In 1985 an editorial by Scherlag et al.[63] suggested a link between the original concept of peri-infarction block and ventricular late potentials. The study by Flowers et al.[55] in 1990 demonstrated such a link.

Clinical significance

The data from the study by Flowers et al.[55] showed that patients who have had MI with the ECG pattern described for peri-infarction block may be at greater risk for sustained VT. There is apparently a link between the presence of the ECG pattern of peri-infarction block in inferior MI and ventricular late potentials, which are in turn linked to an increased risk for sustained VT and ventricular fibrillation

(VF).[64] This interesting and potentially useful information awaits further data and similar studies for anterior wall MI.

ECG recognition

Fig. 26-26 compares the 12-lead ECG from patients with and without peri-infarction block. Both patients have inferior wall MI with Q waves in leads II, III, and aV$_F$. However, the ECG without peri-infarction block has a narrow QRS complex in all leads, whereas the patient with peri-infarction block has a narrow QRS complex in all leads except II, III, and aV$_F$, which is caused by a distortion of the terminal forces.

Fig. 26-27 is a magnification of lead II in both patients. Note the broadening of the QRS complex in the peri-infarction block caused by a slurring of the downstroke of the R wave as compared to the swift downstroke of the R wave in the patient without peri-infarction block.

INFEROLATERAL MYOCARDIAL INFARCTION

Reflecting leads: Leads III, aV$_F$, V$_5$, V$_6$, I, and aV$_L$

ECG recognition

Leads II, III, and aV$_F$ (inferior wall)
Leads I, aV$_L$, V^5, and V$_6$ (lateral wall)
    ST segment elevation
    Q waves
    Inverted T waves
Fig. 26-25 shows an acute inferolateral MI.

ECG identification of high-risk patients

1. ST-segment elevation in lead V$_{4R}$ (proximal RCA occlusion and RV infarction)
2. Complete AV block
3. Anterior precordial ST-segment depression (posteroseptal involvement)

ACUTE POSTERIOR WALL MYOCARDIAL INFARCTION
Reflecting leads

Acute stage: Leads V$_3$ and V$_4$
Evolving stage: Lead V$_1$

ECG recognition

Acute stage: Horizontally depressed ST segments in leads V$_3$ and V$_4$.
Evolving stage: ST-segment depression resolves, and an R wave appears in lead V$_1$.

Because it is the endocardial surface of the posterior wall of the heart that faces the precordial leads (as opposed to the epicardial surface of the anterior wall), the ECG signs of acute posterior wall infarction are reversed (reciprocal changes). Therefore when evaluating for acute posterior wall MI, one looks especially in precordial leads for a depressed ST segment. In the acute stage the ST-segment is typically horizontally depressed, especially in leads V$_3$ to V$_4$. As the infarction evolves, the ST-segment depression gives way to an R wave in lead V$_1$. The R wave is, of course, a Q-wave infarction seen in reverse. Sometimes the ST-segment depression is downsloping.[23]

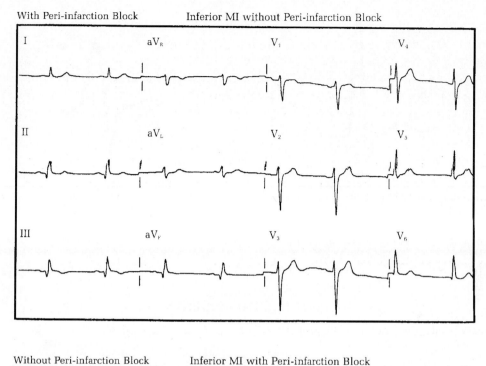

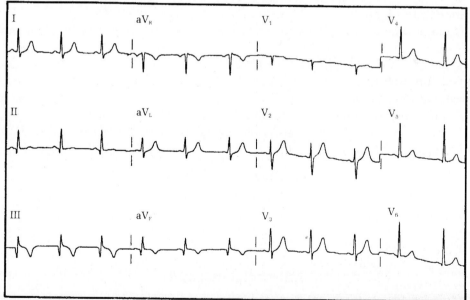

Fig. 26-26. Inferior MI with and without peri-infarction block. In the ECG without peri-infarction block, note the narrow QRS (duration, 0.09 sec) and the sharp descending limb of the R wave in leads II, III, and aV$_F$. In the ECG with peri-infarction block, note the broadened QRS (duration, 0.11 to 0.12 sec) and the distortion of the descending limb of the R wave in leads II, III, and aV$_F$. Also, in lead I the QRS complex is narrow. *(From Flowers NC, Horan LG, Wylds AC: Am J Cardiol 66:568, 1990.)*

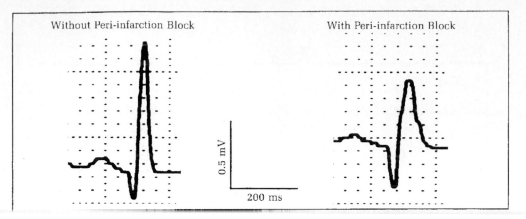

Fig. 26-27. An enlarged lead II complex from each electrocardiogram shown in Fig. 26-26. The contrast is evident between the sharpness of the descending limb of the R wave in the patient without peri-infarction block *(left)* and the slurred descent of the R wave in the patient with peri-infarction block *(right). (From Flowers NC et al: Am J Cardiol 66:568, 1990.)*

ATRIAL INFARCTION

Reflecting leads: Leads I, II, and III and leads V_1, V_2, V_5, and V_6

ECG recognition

One of the following is present:

PR-segment elevation is greater than 0.5 mm in leads V_5 and V_6 with PR-segment depression in leads V_1 and V_2.

PR-segment elevation is greater than 0.5 mm in lead I with PR-segment depression in leads II and III.

PR-segment depression is greater than 1.5 mm in precordial leads and greater than 1.2 mm in leads I, II, and III, combined with atrial arrhythmias.

P waves may also be abnormal in shape (W-shaped, M-shaped, notched, or irregular in configuration).

Clinical implications

Atrial infarction occurs in 7% to 17% of cases of MI (necropsy findings).[65] Because supraventricular arrhythmias often complicate atrial infarctions, its ECG recognition may influence the choice of therapy during the early stages of infarction.[66,67]

Differential diagnosis

Pericarditis, sympathetic stimulation, and atrial overloading that is due to left ventricular failure have been described as causes of PR-segment depression.[68]

EMERGENCY APPROACH TO ACUTE MYOCARDIAL INFARCTION

Early IV thrombolysis improves LV function and survival rates in patients with acute MI. In a study involving 41,021 patients with evolving MI it was found that a thrombolytic strategy consisting of accelerated tissue plasminogen activator (t-PA), that is, rapid IV administration of t-PA over a period of 1½ hours (two thirds of the dose is given in the first 30 min) along with IV heparin provides a survival benefit over previous thrombolytic regimens.[69,70] More important than the specific choice of the thrombolytic agent is its early administration.

Thrombolytic therapy can successfully be delivered in freestanding emergency departments, ambulatory health care centers, physicians' offices, ambulances, and patients' homes. Once treatment has begun, the patient's care should be managed in a facility from which the patient can be transferred to a tertiary care center should ischemia recur. Given the importance of early treatment, Braunwald[71] suggested that to obtain maximal benefit, paramedics, nurses, emergency medical technicians, and physicians' assistants should be trained in the recognition of candidates for thrombolysis and in the delivery of therapy.

AGGRESSIVE THERAPY FOR HIGH-RISK PATIENTS

The following is the emergency approach that is generally followed when dealing with high-risk patients with anterior wall MI (proximal LAD occlusion) or extensive inferior posterior MI (proximal RCA occlusion).

1. Prompt IV thrombolysis. If IV thrombolysis has not been successful, or if systemic thrombolytic treatment is contraindicated, the patient is taken to the cardiac catheterization laboratory where PTCA is performed. Intracoronary thrombolysis may also be used.

   In settings of acute high-risk MI, primary PTCA (angioplasty without thrombolysis) is being used with increasing frequency. Several studies have demonstrated its feasibility and benefits. Primary PTCA can achieve prompt reperfusion and help prevent the hemorrhagic risks of thrombolysis. This approach assumes the availability of a well-staffed, well-equipped cardiac catheterization laboratory and the ability to mobilize the team within 1 hour and achieve reperfusion within 2 hours.

2. In patients with hemodynamic instability or conduction abnormalities, a Swan-Ganz catheter with pacing electrodes is inserted during the catheterization procedure to gather information about pump function and permit emergency treatment.

3. If the patient survives the first few days, continuous ECG monitoring in a step-down unit is required because development of sustained VT or VF is possible 1 to 2 weeks after the onset of large anteroinferior wall infarction.

The follow-up care of the high-risk MI patient must be individualized, factoring in the degree of LV damage, differentiation of myocardial infarction versus myocardial stunning, absence of multivessel disease, and degree of reperfusion and flow established in the infarct vessel.

ECG EVALUATION OF SUCCESSFUL REPERFUSION

Thrombolysis is successful in achieving patency of the infarct vessel in 60% to 70% of patients.[72] Patients who do not respond to thrombolytic therapy are at high risk and may be candidates for emergency rescue angioplasty or coronary artery bypass surgery.[11,73] Therefore it is important to rapidly and noninvasively determine the presence of reperfusion. Typically there is an early peak of serum CK levels.[74]

The Wellens group[75] studied 61 patients who received thrombolytic therapy for acute MI in hopes of identifying clinical and ECG markers of reperfusion and avoiding emergency coronary angiography. Of the 44 patients who showed reperfusion on coronary angiography, 96% had relief of chest pain after 60 minutes. ECG signs of reperfusion were:

• Normalization of the ST segment (95%)
• Development of terminal T-wave inversion (64%)

- Accelerated idioventricular rhythm (42%)[74,76,77]
- A twofold increase in PVCs (74%)
- Transient increase in ST segment elevation and chest pain prior to ST normalization (69%)

ST-segment changes

Resolution of ST-segment elevation. Successful thrombolytic therapy is associated with rapid resolution of the ST-segment elevation.[78,79] Resolution of ST-segment elevation by 70% or more at 3 hours after the start of thrombolytic therapy has been shown to be a major predictor of favorable outcome.[80] Absence of ST-segment resolution of at least 30% at 3 hours after thrombolysis is highly specific (although not as sensitive) for lack of reperfusion.[13]

Schröder et al.[79] found that the extent of resolution of ST segment elevation conveys useful early information about prognosis after acute MI, as follows:

1. *Excellent survival rate.* Complete ST-segment resolution identifies such patients; however, there is a slightly higher probability of nonfatal reinfarction, suggesting that a predischarge stress test may identify patients who would benefit from early angiography and revascularization.
2. *Increasing risk of death risk over long term.* Partial ST-segment resolution after reperfusion for acute anterior MI identifies such patients, suggesting that they may benefit from vigorous adjunctive pharmacotherapy.
3. *Poor prognosis.* Lack of ST-segment resolution identifies patients who have a poor prognosis without reperfusion and who therefore may benefit from immediate coronary angiography and rescue PTCA or intracoronary thrombolysis.[79,81,82]

ST-segment elevation. Although early decrease in ST-segment elevation identifies the success of thrombolytic therapy for acute MI, frequently this decrease is preceded by a transient elevation above the level noted at the start of thrombolytic treatment.

Reperfusion arrhythmias

During MI the accelerated idioventricular rhythm (AIVR) has been shown to be a sign of reperfusion (spontaneous or as a result of thrombolytic therapy). Approximately half of the patients with reperfusion have an AIVR when the ECG is recorded continuously after thrombolytic therapy. This finding is of practical clinical importance in that it may help in the recognition of both spontaneous and thrombolytic-induced reperfusion in the absence of coronary angiography. For further discussion of the characteristics of the AIVR see p. 232.

Q waves and T-wave inversion

Successful reperfusion with thrombolytic therapy may accelerate the evolving ECG picture of infarction. Therefore rapid resolution of ST-segment elevation is followed by rapid development of pathologic Q wave and loss of R-wave amplitude. Matetzky et al.[83] found that early T-wave inversion after thrombolytic therapy (within 24 hours) predicts successful, effective reperfusion.

TRANSPORTING PATIENTS AND INITIATING THERAPY

When a patient comes to medical attention with the classic ECG signs of acute MI, prompt diagnosis and institution of treatment are critical. Speed is of the utmost importance, and the following are necessary[84]:

1. Well-trained emergency medical technicians with a physician-directed plan for quick effective response are needed. In some clinical trials thrombolytic therapy is being initiated in the field under the direction of a hospital-based physician. Evaluation of the patient in the field is carried out quickly with a specific protocol. In some communities thrombolytic therapy is instituted en route under the direction of the emergency department physician. The ECG may be transmitted via cellular telephone to an emergency department.

2. Patients must be taken to a nearby hospital equipped to manage patients with acute MI. Preferably the hospital should have facilities for cardiac catheterization, angioplasty, and cardiac surgery. If such facilities are not available, and if the patient's condition requires emergency intervention, the patient should be promptly transferred.

3. In the hospital emergency department the patient with suspected MI is rapidly assessed. Such suspicion is established by communication with the mobile unit before arrival so that an emergency department team is ready to respond when the patient arrives. Patients with chest pain or tightness, acute epigastric distress, or other symptoms of acute MI are placed on established protocol.

4. A "stat" 12-lead ECG with lead V_{4R} is obtained. Cardiac monitoring is continuous, vital signs are recorded frequently, and a physician sees the patient within the first few minutes of arrival. Delays of any kind should not be permitted in the admission and evaluation of this patient.

5. From the 13-lead ECG (12 standard leads plus lead V_{4R}), as well as the clinical assessment, high-risk patients are promptly identified. Echocardiography may be used selectively.

6. For patients with acute MI without contraindication to thrombolytic therapy, IV thrombolytic therapy is initiated by a trained emergency department physician and the staff, if this has not already been done en route. When systemic IV thrombolytic therapy is contraindicated or considered too hazardous, or when early large MI is suspected or the patient is in cardiogenic shock, emergency coronary arteriography may be performed with the aim of performing primary coronary angioplasty.

7. In rural areas where hospitals do not have special cardiac facilities or physicians trained in emergency cardiac care, a protocol should be established for telephone communication with nearby medical centers. Protocol for initiating thrombolytic therapy in patients from rural hospitals before transferring them to metropolitan centers has been shown to be safe and effective.

ELIMINATING UNNECESSARY DELAYS

The average time lapse from "911" call to IV thrombolysis is approximately 2.9 hours. In a study[85] involving eight U.S. cities the average time lapses were as follows:

From the "911" call to medic arrival	7.7 ± 9.0 min
Medic on-scene time	25.8 ± 8.9 min
Medic transport time	12.6 ± 6.6 min
From hospital admission to thrombolytic therapy	83.8 ± 55.0 min

Clearly the greatest delay is in the hospital, with one city (Salt Lake City) at 99.3 ± 44 min! The delays were in obtaining demographic data, recording the ECG, starting IV lines, obtaining a chest x-ray, obtaining laboratory samples, administering morphine sulfate and lidocaine, and awaiting cardiologist approval for thrombolytic therapy.

Following the study just mentioned the Cincinnati Heart Project successfully reduced delays by transferring the responsibility for initiation of thrombolytic therapy to the emergency physician. The authors[86] also found that the only change in the prehospital phase that reduced delay to thrombolysis was prehospital ECG transmission from the field. Current emphasis is on reducing delays by administering thrombolytic therapy in the field with the implementation of one of the following possible basic protocols:

1. A physician-operated mobile intensive care unit (ICU)
2. Prehospital physician evaluation followed by activation of the mobile ICU
3. Paramedic evaluation with cellular ECG transmission

The special taskforce[84,87] of the American College of Cardiology and the American Heart Association, from which most of these guidelines have been taken, advises that in the critical setting of acute MI there should be no unnecessary delays in initiating treatment, such as those consumed by "administrative procedures, for example, establishing insurance coverage" and "prolonged efforts to consult with the patient's private physician." Such delays "must not be allowed to occur" and are "inappropriate." Other causes for delay also occur. For example, patients with chest pain must wait their turn in busy emergency departments. Once admitted, there is another delay while a cardiologist is found to evaluate the need for thrombolysis, and such therapy may not be initiated until the patient is transferred to the CCU.[88] The sum of these delays reduces the potential benefit of thrombolysis. Evaluation of these delays by emergency department directors and hospital administrators is the first step in eliminating them. The goal is to start the IV thrombolytic treatment in the proper candidate within 30 min of arrival to the emergency care setting.

CANDIDATES FOR THROMBOLYSIS

There is general agreement that the patients who benefit most from thrombolysis are those with large infarctions who receive therapy early after the onset of pain. However, this does not necessarily rule out treatment for infarctions more than 6 hours after the onset of pain in patients who have ongoing clinical evidence of myocardial ischemia, nor is treatment contraindicated in elderly patients.[89] Although it is known that the risk of bleeding in older patients receiving thrombolytic therapy is higher than in younger ones, the benefits seem to outweigh the risks.[90] The Gusto Investigators[70] found that even at 24 hours, the mortality rate was reduced significantly (19%) with accelerated t-PA as compared with other regimens.

CONTRAINDICATIONS TO THROMBOLYTIC THERAPY
Absolute contraindications*

- Altered consciousness

*In such cases other reperfusion strategies are considered, such as PTCA or coronary artery bypass surgery.

- Active internal bleeding
- Suspected aortic dissection or pericarditis
- Recent head trauma
- Known spinal cord or cerebral arteriovenous malformation or tumor
- Known previous *hemorrhagic* cerebrovascular accident
- Intracranial or intraspinal surgery within 2 months
- Trauma or surgery within 2 weeks that could result in bleeding into a closed space
- Persistent blood pressure greater than 200/120 mm Hg
- Pregnancy
- Previous allergy to streptokinase product (but not a contraindication to use of other thrombolytic agents)

Relative major contraindications (individual evaluation of risk versus benefit)*

- Active peptic ulcer disease (recent)
- Gastrointestinal or genitourinary hemorrhage
- History of ischemic or embolic cerebrovascular accident
- Current use of oral anticoagulants
- Known bleeding disorder
- Major trauma or surgery within 2 weeks
- History of chronic uncontrolled hypertension (diastolic blood pressure greater than 100 mm Hg, treated or untreated)
- Subclavian or internal jugular venous cannulation or puncture of central noncompressible vessel
- Prolonged, traumatic cardiopulmonary resuscitation (CPR)
- Unwitnessed syncope or fall with potential central nervous system trauma

Relative minor contraindications

- Brief nontraumatic CPR
- Diabetic retinopathy
- Endocarditis

EFFECTS OF PROPHYLACTIC ANTIARRHYTHMIC DRUG THERAPY IN ACUTE MYOCARDIAL INFARCTION

The Cardiac Arrhythmia Suppression Trials (CAST I and CAST II) were initiated in June 1987 and showed increased mortality in patients receiving treatment with class IA (moricizine) and class IC (encainide and flecainide) antiarrhythmic drugs as compared with patients on a regimen of placebo.[91-93]

In 1993 Teo et al.[94] compiled data from 138 trials of more than 98,000 MI patients who were treated with antiarrhythmic agents and found that the routine use of any of the class I antiarrhythmic agents after MI is associated with a statistically significant increase in risk of death. In this study quinidine, in particular, showed a twofold increase in the odds of death, a finding consistent with other studies reporting threefold excess harm.[95] In fact, a harmful effect of quinidine in maintenance of sinus rhythm after cardioversion from chronic atrial fibrillation has also

---

*In instances when these contraindications have paramount importance, such as very recent trauma or surgery or active peptic ulcer disease with recent bleeding, they become absolute contraindications when weighed against a less than life-threatening and evolving acute MI.

been suggested.[96] Of particular interest was the lidocaine trial, which presumed that prophylactic use of lidocaine in acute MI may cause reductions in VF and VT but actually demonstrated *an increased risk of death* from asystole and bradycardia.[97]

The only class of agents that was conclusively shown to be beneficial was beta-blockers. In the preceding study[97] the limited data on amiodarone appeared to be promising and those on calcium channel blockers remained unpromising.

In the past, patients with acute MI were routinely given IV lidocaine prophylaxis for VT or VF. Post-MI arrhythmias were aggressively suppressed with antiarrhythmic drugs. The stunning results of the CAST study, as well as increased mortality noted with routine use of lidocaine in acute MI, have shown that such an approach may be harmful and have elicited a careful reevaluation of this problem.

DIFFERENTIAL DIAGNOSES
Acute pulmonary embolism

Acute massive pulmonary embolism (see Chapter 24) involving the main pulmonary arteries may simulate MI, especially since both conditions may present with chest pain, shortness of breath, and hypotension and may be associated with a fall in cardiac output, abnormal Q waves, ST-segment elevation, and T-wave changes. For example, right axis deviation with Q waves and T-wave changes in the inferior leads mimics inferior wall MI. Although the RBBB pattern and ST-segment elevation in lead V_1 leads one to suspect pulmonary embolism, especially if there is also a positive T wave in that lead, this pattern is also seen when RBBB is associated with acute anteroseptal infarction, acute pericarditis, and the "early repolarization" pattern, and it occurs in posterior wall MI. In acute pulmonary embolism the following differences help in the diagnosis, although none is truly specific:

1. The acute respiratory distress is more pronounced than would be expected in MI, unless the acute MI is accompanied by pulmonary edema.
2. The ECG, although abnormal, is not consistent with that usually seen in MI. For example, both inferior wall and anterior wall MI may be suggested in one 12-lead ECG; that is, Q waves may be seen in leads III and aV_F, but not in lead II, and these may be associated with changes in lead V_1.
3. The chest x-ray does not show pulmonary congestion, although there is severe dyspnea.
4. The diagnostic usefulness of the ECG is enhanced when combined with emergency echocardiography.

Wolff-Parkinson-White syndrome

Because the delta wave of Wolff-Parkinson-White syndrome (see Chapter 20) may be negative in some leads, it may look like an abnormal Q wave in some leads. It is possible that such a finding would lead the uninformed observer to mistake preexcitation syndrome for MI.

Pericarditis

The signs and symptoms of pericarditis can mimic those of acute MI: there may be chest pain, and there is ST-segment elevation. The diagnosis of pericarditis is based on (1) characteristic chest pain (sharp, pleuritic, and worse on inspiration), (2) no response to nitroglycerin, (3) pericardial rub, and (4) diffuse ECG changes that do not localize into right or left coronary artery distribution. The echocardiogram can be helpful in making the differential diagnosis because frequently there is pericardial effusion as a result of pericarditis.

Aortic dissection

The character of the pain differs slightly from that of acute MI, as follows: (1) Frequently there is posterior transmission, (2) there is no response to nitroglycerin, (3) the ECG may be normal or there may be ST-segment changes, especially if there is hypertension and hypertrophy, or (4) there may be ECG changes associated with pericarditis if the dissection involves the aortic root and there is pericardial hemorrhage. The diagnosis is made using chest x-ray films, computed tomographic scan, and, most important, echocardiography (especially transesophageal) and magnetic resonance imaging. Aortography is rarely needed for diagnosis.

Pancreatitis and cholecystitis

Pancreatitis and cholecystitis can present a clinical picture mimicking acute MI with chest pain. The differential diagnosis is made with abdominal ultrasound and determination of appropriate blood tests.

SUMMARY

The speedy diagnosis, identification of high-risk patients, and aggressive management of acute MI are extremely important in view of the potential benefits of early thrombolytic therapy or primary PTCA and the potential for myocardial salvage and reduction of mortality.

ST-segment elevation is the sign of acute myocardial occlusion and injury; the higher the elevation and the more leads involved, the more extensive the injury. If occlusion persists, the injury evolves into MI. The key to locating the infarct is understanding the coronary circulation, the surfaces of the heart, and their reflecting leads. Briefly, leads V_1 to V_4 reflect anterior wall MI; when this finding is combined with ST-segment elevation in leads I, aV_L, and V_5 to V_6, there is extensive anterolateral wall infarction. High-risk patients are recognized when RBBB or hemiblock appears. Leads II, III, and aV_F reflect inferior MI. High-risk patients are recognized when there is ST-segment elevation of 1 mm or more in lead V_{4R}. In selected patients emergency echocardiography is useful in the diagnosis, evaluation, and determination of possible complications in acute MI.

REFERENCES

1. American Heart Association: *1990 heart facts,* Dallas, 1990, The Association.
2. Fuster V: Mechanisms leading to myocardial infarction: insights from studies of vascular biology, *Circulation* 90:2126, 1994.
3. Hohnloser SH, Franck P, Klingenheben T et al: Open infarct artery, late potentials, and other prognostic factors in patients after acute myocardial infarction in the thrombolytic era: a prospective trial, *Circulation* 90:1747, 1994.
4. Pfeffer MA, Braunwald E, Moye LA et al: On behalf of the SAVE investigators: effect of captopril on mortality and morbidity in patients with left ventricular dysfunction after myocardial infarction, *N Engl J Med* 327:669, 1992.
5. The SOLVD Investigators: Effect of enalapril on survival in patients with reduced left ventricular ejection fractions and congestive heart failure, *N Engl J Med* 325:293, 1991.
6. Sugiura T, Iwasaka T, Takahashi N et al: Factors associated with late onset of advanced atrioventricular block in acute Q wave inferior infarction, *Am Heart J* 119:1008, 1990.
7. Frink RJ, James TN: Normal blood supply to the human His bundle and proximal bundle branches, *Circulation* 47:8, 1973.
8. Ross DL: Approach to the patient with bundle branch block. In Wellens HJJ, Kulbertus HE, eds: *What's new in electrocardiography,* The Hague, 1981, Martinus Nijhoff.
9. Schweitzer P: The electrocardiographic diagnosis of acute myocardial infarction in the thrombolytic era, *Am Heart J* 119:642, 1990.
10. Pardee HEB: An electrocardiographic sign of coronary artery obstruction, *Arch Intern Med* 26:244, 1920.
11. Shechter M, Rabinowitz B, Beker B et al: Additional ST segment elevation during the first hour of thrombolytic therapy: an electrocardiographic sign predicting a favorable clinical outcome, *J Am Coll Cardiol* 20:1460, 1992.
12. Barbash GI, Roth A, Hod H et al: Rapid reso-

lution of ST elevation and prediction of clinical outcome in patients undergoing thrombolysis with alteplase (recombinant tissue type plasminogen activator): results of the Israeli Study of Early Intervention in Myocardial Infarction, *Br Heart J* 69:241, 1990.

13. Clemmensen P, Ohman M, Sevilla DC et al: Changes in standard electrocardiographic ST-segment elevation predictive of successful reperfusion in acute myocardial infarction, *Am J Cardiol* 66:1407, 1990.

14. Matetzky S, Barbash G, Shahar A et al: The prognostic significance of early inversion of T waves after thrombolytic therapy for acute myocardial infarction, *Circulation* 84(suppl 2).63, 1991 (abstract).

15. Gorgels AP, Vos MA, Bär FW, Wellens HJJ: An electrocardiographic pattern characteristic for extensive myocardial ischemia, *Circulation* 70(suppl 2).1002, 1900.

16. Atie J, Brugada P, Smeets JLRM, et al: Clinical presentation and prognosis of left main coronary disease in the 1990s, *Eur Heart J* 12:495, 1991.

17. Mirvix DM et al: Electrocardiographic effects of experimental nontransmural myocardial infarction, *Circulation* 71:1206, 1985.

18. Fisch C: Electrocardiography and vectorcardiography. In Braunwald E, ed: *Heart disease, ed 4,* Philadelphia, 1992, WB Saunders.

19. Ricou F, Nicod P, Gilpin E et al: Influence of right bundle branch block on short- and long-term survival after acute anterior myocardial infarction, *J Am Coll Cardiol* 17:858, 1991.

20. Boden WE, Spodick DH: Diagnostic significance of precordial ST segment depression, *Am J Cardiol* 63:358, 1989.

21. Willich S, Stone PH, Muller JE et al: High-risk subgroups of patients with non-Q-wave myocardial infarction based on direction and severity of ST-segment deviation, *Am Heart J* 114:1110, 1987.

22. Krone RJ, Greenberg H, Dwyer EM et al: Long-term prognostic significance of ST segment depression during acute myocardial infarction, *J Am Coll Cardiol* 22:361, 1993.

23. Boden WE, Kleiger RE, Gibson RS et al: Electrocardiographic evolution of posterior acute myocardial infarction: importance of early precordial ST-segment depression, *Am J Cardiol* 59:782, 1987.

24. Kleiger RE: Frequency and significance of late evolution of Q waves in patients with initial non-Q-Wave acute myocardial infarction, *Am J Cardiol* 65:23, 1990.

25. Schechtman KB et al: Risk stratification of patients with non-Q-wave myocardial infarction: the critical role of ST segment depression, *Circulation* 80:1148, 1989.

26. Dacanay S, Kennedy, Uretz E et al: Morphological and quantitative angiographic analyses of progression of coronary stenoses: a comparison of Q-wave and non-Q-wave myocardial infarction, *Circulation* 90:1739, 1994.

27. Aguirre FV, Younis LT, Chaitman BR et al: Early and 1-year clinical outcome of patients' evolving non-Q-wave versus Q-wave myocardial infarction after thrombolysis. Results from the TIMI II study, *Circulation* 91:2541, 1995.

28. Zehender M, Kasper W, Kauder E et al: Right ventricular infarction as an independent predictor of prognosis after acute inferior myocardial infarction, *N Engl J Med* 328:981, 1993.

29. Bates ER: New perspectives on RV infarction and ischemia. Presented at the annual symposium of the Texas Heart Institute, Huston, Texas, September 24, 1992.

30. Braat SH, Gorgels APM, Bär FW, Wellens HJJ: Value of the ST-T segment in lead V4R in inferior wall acute myocardial infarction to predict the site of coronary arterial occlusion, *Am J Cardiol* 62:140, 1988.

31. Wellens HJJ Personal communication, November, 1994.

32. Berger PB, Ruocco NA, Ryan TJ et al: Incidence and prognostic implications of heart block complicating inferior myocardial infarction treated with thrombolytic therapy: results from TIMI II, *J Am Coll Cardiol* 20:533, 1992.

33. Tans AC, Lie KI, Durrer D: Clinical setting and prognostic significance of high degree atrioventricular block in acute inferior myocardial infarction: a study of 144 patients, *Am Heart J* 99:4, 1980.

34. Tans AC, Lie KI: AV nodal block in acute myocardial infarction. In Wellens HJJ, Lie KI, Janse MJ, eds: *The conduction system of the heart,* Leiden, 1976, Stenfert Kroese.

35. Bates ER, Clemmensen PM, Califf RM et al: Precordial ST segment depression predicts a worse prognosis in inferior infarction despite reperfusion therapy, *J Am Coll Cardiol* 16:1538, 1990.

36. Erhardt LR, Sjögren A, Wahlberg I: Single right-sided precordial lead in the diagnosis of right ventricular involvement in inferior myocardial infarction, *Am Heart J* 91:571, 1976.

37. Braat SH, Brugada P, de Zwaan C et al: Value of electrocardiogram in diagnosing right ventricular involvement in patients with an acute inferior wall myocardial infarction, *Br Heart J* 49:368, 1983.

38. Klein HO, Tordjman T, Ninio R et al: The early recognition of right ventricular infarction: diagnostic accuracy of the electrocardiographic V4R lead, *Circulation* 67:558, 1983.

39. Braat SH, Brugada P, den Dulk K et al: Value of lead V4R for recognition of the infarct coronary artery in acute inferior myocardial infarction, *Am J Cardiol* 53:1538, 1984.

40. Wilson BC, Cohn JN: Right ventricular infarction: clincial and pathophysiologic considerations, *Adv Intern Med* 33:295, 1988.

41. Dell'Italia LJ, O'Rourke RA: Pathophysiology and treatment of right ventricular myocardial infarction, *Curr Top Cardiol* 271-283, 1991.

42. Setaro JF, Cabin HS: Right ventricular infarction, *Cardiol Clin* 10:69, 1992.

43. Pasternak RC, Braunwald E, Sobel BE: Acute myocardial infarction. In Braunwald E, ed: *Heart disease,* Philadelphia, 1992, WB Saunders.

44. Kopelman HA, Forman MB, Wilson BH et al: Right ventricular myocardial infarction in patients with chronic lung disease: possible role of right ventricular hypertrophy, *J Am Coll Cardiol* 5:1302, 1985.

45. Lorell B, Leinbach RC, Pohost GM et al: Right ventricular infarction: clinical diagnosis and differentiation from cardiac tamponade and pericardial constriction, *Am J Cardiol* 43:465, 1979.

46. Cohn JN, Guiha NH, Broder MI, Limas CJ: Right ventricular infarction: clinical and hemodynamic features, *Am J Cardiol* 33:209, 1974.

47. Wartman WB, Hellerstein HK: The incidence of heart disease in 2,000 consecutive autopsies, *Ann Intern Med* 28:41, 1948.

48. Isner JM, Roberts WC: Right ventricular infarction complicating left ventricular infarction secondary to coronary artery disease: frequency, location, associated findings and significance from analysis of 236 necropsy patients with acute or healed myocardial infarction, *Am J Cardiol* 42:885, 1978.

49. Wellens HJJ: The electrocardiogram 80 years after Einthoven, *J Am Coll Cardiol* 7:484, 1986.

50. Zehender M, Kasper W, Schönthaler H, Olschewski M: In-hospital and long-term course after inferior myocardial infarction: prognostic impact of right ventricular infarction, *Circulation* 84(suppl 2):245, 1991.

51. Zehender M: Right ventricular infarction as an independent predictor of prognosis after acute inferior myocardial infarction, *N Eng J Med* 328:981, 1993.

52. Braat SH, de Zwaan C, Brugada P et al: Right ventricular involvement with acute inferior wall myocardial infarction identifies high risk of developing atrioventricular nodal conduction disturbances, *Am Heart J* 107:1183, 1984.

53. Braat SH, Brugada P, de Zwaan C et al: Value of lead V4R in acute inferior wall infarction to identify right ventricular involvement and risk of development of AV nodal block, *Am J Cardiol* 49:998, 1982 (abstract).

54. Croft CH, Nicod P, Corbett JR et al: Detection of acute right ventricular infarction by right precordial electrocardiography, *Am J Cardiol* 50:421, 1982.

55. Flowers NC, Horan LG, Wylds AC: Relation of peri-infarction block to ventricular late potentials in patients with inferior wall myocardial infarction, *Am J Cardiol* 66:568, 1990.

56. First SR, Bayley RH, Bedford DR: Peri-infarction block: electrocardiographic abnormality occasionally resembling bundle branch block and local ventricular block of other types, *Circulation* 2:31, 1950.

57. Grant RP, Murray RH: The QRS complex deformity of myocardial infarction in the human subject, *Am J Med* 17:587, 1954.

58. Grant LP: Left axis deviation: an electrocardiographic pathologic correlation, *Circulation* 14:233, 1956.

59. Grant RP, Dodge HT: Mechanisms of QRS complex prolongation in man: left ventricular conduction disturbances, *Am J Med* 20:834, 1956.

60. Davies H, Evans W: The significance of deep S waves in leads II and III, *Br Heart J* 22:551, 1960.

61. Bechwith JR: *Grant's clinical electrocardiography: the spatial vector approach,* New York, 1970, McGraw-Hill.

62. Rosenbaum MB, Elizari MV, Lazzari JO: The hemiblocks: new concepts of intraventricular conduction based on human anatomical, physiological and clinical studies, Oldsmar, Fla, 1970, Tampa Tracings.

63. Scherlag BJ et al: Peri-infarction (1950)–late potentials (1980): their relationship, significance and diagnostic implications, *Am J Cardiol* 55:839, 1985.

64. Simson MB: Signal-averaged electrocardiography: methods and clinical applications. In Braunwald E, ed: *Heart disease: a textbook of cardiovascular medicine,* ed 3, Philadelphia, 1989, WB Saunders.

65. Lowe TE, Wartment WB: Myocardial infarction, *Br Heart J* 6:115, 1944.

66. Neilsen FE, Andersen HH, Gram-Hansen P et al: The relationship between ECG signs of atrial infarction and the development of supraventricular arrhythmias in patients with acute myocardial infarction, *Am Heart J* 123:69, 1992.

67. Rechavia E, Strasberg B, Mager A et al: The incidence of atrial arrhythmias during inferior wall myocardial infarction with and without right ventricular involvement, *Am Heart J* 124:387, 1992.

68. Nagahama Y, Sugiura T, Takehana K et al: Clinical significance of PQ segment depression in acute Q wave anterior wall myocardial infarction, *J Am Coll Cardiol* 23:885, 1994.

69. International Society and Federation of Cardiology and World Health Organization Task Force on Myocardial Reperfusion: Reperfusion in acute myocardial infarction, *Circulation* 90:2091, 1994.

70. The Gusto Investigators: An international randomized trial comparing four thrombolytic strategies for acute myocardial infarction, *N Engl J Med* 329:673, 1993.

71. Braunwald E: Optimizing thrombolytic therapy of acute myocardial infarction, *Circulation* 82:1510, 1990.

72. Marder VO, Sherry S: Thrombolytic therapy: current status, *N Engl J Med* 318:1512, 1988.

73. Ellis SG, da Silva ER, Heyndrickx G et al: Randomized comparison of rescue angioplasty

with conservative management of patients with early failure of thrombolysis for acute anterior myocardial infarction, *Circulation* 90:2280, 1994.

74. Been M, de Bono DP, Muri AI et al: Coronary thrombolysis with intravenous unisoylated plasminogen-streptokinase complex GRL 26921, *Br Heart J* 53:253, 1985.

75. Doevendans PA, Gorgels AP, van der Zee R et al: Electrocardiographic diagnosis of reperfusion during thrombolytic therapy in acute myocardial infarction, *Am J Cardiol* 75:1206, 1995.

76. Gorgels APM, Vos MA, Letsch IS et al: Usefulness of the accelerated idioventricular rhythm as a marker for myocardial necrosis and reperfusion during thrombolytic therapy in acute myocardial infarction, *Am J Cardiol* 61:231, 1988.

77. Gressin V, Gorgels A, Louvard Y. Reconsidering arrhythmias as markers of reperfusion: combined arrhythmia and ST-Segment analysis during myocardial infarction, *J Electrocardiology* 26:262, 1993.

78. Goldberg S, Urban P, Greenspan A: Limitation of infarct size with thrombolytic agents: electrocardiographic indexes, *Circulation* 68(suppl 1):77, 1983.

79. Schröder R, Dissmann R, Brüggemann T et al: Extent of early ST segment elevation resolution: a simple but strong predictor of outcome in patients with acute myocardial infarction, *J Am Coll Cardiol* 24:384, 1994.

80. Dissmann R, Goerke M, von Ameln H et al: Prediction of early reperfusion and left ventricular damage by ST segment analysis during thrombolysis in acute myocardial infarction, *Z Kardiol* 82:271, 1993.

81. Califf RM, Topol EJ, Stack RS et al: Evaluation of combination thrombolytic therapy and timing of cardiac catheterization in acute myocardial infarction, *Circulation* 82:1543, 1991.

82. Gurbel PA, Davidson CJ, Ohmann EM et al: Selective infusion of thrombolytic therapy in the acute myocardial infarct–related coronary artery as an alternative to rescue percutaneous transluminal coronary angioplasty, *Am J Cardiol* 66:1021, 1990.

83. Matetzky S, Barabash GI, Shahar A et al: Early T wave inversion after thrombolytic therapy predicts better coronary perfusion: clinical and angiographic study, *J Am Coll Cardiol* 24:387, 1994.

84. ACC/AHA Task Force Report: Guidelines for the early management of patients with acute myocardial infarction: a report of the American College of Cardiology/American Heart Association Task Force on assessment of diagnostic and therapeutic cardiovascular procedures, *J Am Coll Cardiol* 16:249, 1990.

85. Kowalenko T, Kereiakes DJ, Gibler WB: Prehospital diagnosis and treatment of acute myocardial infarction: a critical review, *Am Heart J* 123:181, 1992.

86. Kereiakes DJ, Gibler B, Martin LH et al: Relative importance of emergency medical system transport and the prehospital electrocardiogram on reducing hospital time delay to therapy for acute myocardial infarction: a preliminary report from the Cincinnati Heart Project, *Am Heart J* 123:835, 1992.

87. ACC/AHA Task Force Report: Guidelines for the early management of patients with acute myocardial infarction: a report of the American College of Cardiology/American Heart Association Task Force on assessment of diagnostic and therapeutic cardiovascular procedures, *Circulation* 82:664, 1990.

88. Sharkey SW, Brunette DD, Ruiz E: An analysis of time delays preceding thrombolysis for acute myocardial infarction, *JAMA* 262:3171, 1989.

89. Kennedy JW: Expanding the use of thrombolytic therapy for acute myocardial infarction, *Ann Intern Med* 113:907, 1990.

90. Grines CL, DeMaria An: Optimal utilization of thrombolytic therapy for acute myocardial infarction: concepts and controversies, *J Am Coll Cardiol* 16:223, 1990.

91. The Cardiac Arrhythmia Suppression Trial (CAST) Investigators: Preliminary report: effect of encainide and flecainide on mortality in a randomized trial of arrhythmia suppression after myocardial infarction, *N Engl J Med* 321:406, 1989.

92. Echt DS, Liebson PR, Mitchell LB et al: Mortality and morbidity in patients receiving encainide, flecainide, or placebo: the Cardiac Arrhythmia Suppression Trial, *N Engl J Med* 324:781, 1991.

93. The Cardiac Arrhythmia Suppression Trial II Investigators: Effect of the antiarrhythmic agent moricizine on survival after myocardial infarction, *N Engl J Med* 327:227, 1992.

94. Teo KK, Yusuf S, Furberg CD: Effects of prophylactic antiarrhythmic drug therapy in acute myocardial infarction: an overview of results from randomized controlled trials, *JAMA* 270:1589, 1993.

95. Morganroth J, Goin JE: Quinidine-related mortality in the short-to-medium treatment of ventricular arrhythmias: a meta-analysis, *Circulation,* 84:1977, 1991.

96. Coplen SE, Antman EM, Berlin JA et al: Efficacy and safety of quinidine therapy for maintenance of sinus rhythm after cardioversion: a meta-analysis of randomized control trials, *Circulation* 82:1106, 1990.

97. MacMahon S, Collins, R, Peto R et al: Effects of prophylactic lidocaine in suspected acute myocardial infarction: an overview of results from the randomized controlled trials, *JAMA* 2:855, 1981.

27

Acute Pulmonary Embolism

Common Risk Factors   *431*

Pathophysiology   *432*

Signs and Symptoms   *432*

Physical Findings   *432*

Value of the ECG   *432*

Common ECG Findings in the Acute
   Phase   *433*

Value of the Echocardiogram   *434*

Other Available Tests   *436*

Differential Diagnosis   *436*

Treatment   *436*

Prevention   *437*

Summary   *437*

Acute pulmonary embolism is underdiagnosed in most clinical settings and is the most often missed diagnosis in cases of sudden death within the hospital. It accounts for approximately 300,000 hospitalizations and 50,000 deaths annually in the United States.[1] Weinberg[2] has described the following inscription on a tombstone in Bermuda:

> In memory of Richard Sutherland Dale
> Eldest son of Commodore Richard Dale
> of Philadelphia in the US of America
> and midshipman in the US Navy
> He departed this life at St. Georges, Bermuda
> on the 22nd day of Feb AD 1815
> age 20 years 1 mo 17 da
> He lost his right leg in an engagement between
> the US Frigate President and a squadron
> of his Brittanic Majesty's ship of war
> on the 15 da of Jan AD 1815
> His confinement caused severe complaint
> in his back which in a short time
> terminated his life

More than 180 years later, pulmonary embolism is all too often a cause of unexpected death.[2]

COMMON RISK FACTORS

Common histories in patients with pulmonary embolism are hypertension, diabetes mellitus, obesity, atrial fibrillation, and hyperlipidemia. Patients in an especially high-risk group are those undergoing orthopedic surgery or gynecologic surgery for cancer and immobilized medical patients. One study[3] found at autopsy pulmonary embolism in 27% of bedridden patients in a respiratory intensive care unit; half of the cases were not diagnosed before death. In the type of surgical patients just mentioned, pulmonary embolism may occur postoperatively as late as 1 month.

Other risk factors include the hypercoagulation state of occult cancer, use of oral contraceptives, the postpartum period, and especially the period after cesarean section.[4] Pulmonary embolism is the most common medical cause of maternal mortality associated with live births in the United States; the risk is much greater during the first 6 postpartum weeks than during the pregnancy itself.[5]

PATHOPHYSIOLOGY

In acute pulmonary embolism a central or peripheral pulmonary artery is suddenly obstructed. Significant obstruction results in the following pathophysiologic conditions:

- Acute pulmonary hypertension
- Right-side dilation
- Clockwise cardiac rotation
- Right ventricular failure
- Pulmonary infarction
- Marked ventilation-perfusion (V-Q) disturbance
- Acute lowering of the cardiac output

SIGNS AND SYMPTOMS

The most common signs and symptoms of acute pulmonary embolism are nonspecific: tachypnea, dyspnea, chest pain, and tachycardia (sinus).[4] One report[6] showed that pulmonary embolism should be considered in patients with syncope or near-syncope, even in the presence of an apparent arrhythmic cause, such as atrioventricular (AV) block. Other symptoms include hepatomegaly, palpable right ventricular impulse, increase in jugular venous *A* wave, increase in jugular venous distention, and palpable pulmonary artery pulsation.

PHYSICAL FINDINGS

Physical findings are related to acute right ventricular volume overload, right ventricular failure, and the increase in pulmonary artery pressure.[8] The following heart sounds may be heard:

- Tricuspid regurgitation
- Audible right ventricular fourth heart sound (S_4)
- Third heart sound (S_3)
- Narrow splitting of second heart sound (S_2) with an exaggerated pulmonic second sound (P_2)
- Pulmonary ejection murmur

VALUE OF THE ECG

Despite availability of lung scanning and pulmonary angiography, many emboli are found only on postmortem examination. A stunning estimation is that only *one of every three* cases of death-dealing pulmonary embolism is diagnosed while the patient is still alive.[4] Although the ECG signs of acute pulmonary embolism are not diagnostic, certain signs should raise a high degree of suspicion and elicit an order for an emergency sonogram for confirmation (elevated right ventricular end-diastolic diameter, tricuspid regurgitation, and elevated right ventricular systolic pressure). The Wellens group studied 49 consecutive patients who came to medical attention with acute symptoms and with subsequently proven pulmonary embolism.[9] The 12-lead ECG was reviewed in a blinded fashion to identify the ECG features of right ventricular overload. On the basis of the admission ECG alone a diagnosis of pulmonary embolism was suspected in 76% of patients. With the evaluation of serial tracings the diagnosis could be suspected in 82% of cases. Therefore it is imperative that emergency and critical care personnel be familiar with the ECG signs that warn of the possibility of acute pulmonary embolism and be prepared to institute emergency intervention. Speed is of the utmost importance. Serial 12-lead ECG tracings are necessary.

COMMON ECG FINDINGS IN THE ACUTE PHASE

The common ECG findings in the acute phase of pulmonary embolism are most likely the result of acute pulmonary hypertension with right atrial and ventricular dilation, hypoxia, and perhaps myocardial ischemia.[10] A diagnosis of pulmonary embolism is considered when three or more of the following ECG signs are present[9]:

- Complete or incomplete right bundle branch pattern, which may be associated with ST-segment elevation of more than 1 mm in lead V_1.
- S wave in leads I and aV_L (greater than 1.5 mm or an R:S ratio of less than 1).
- A shift in the transitional zone (p. 24) to lead V_5 or further left (clockwise rotation).
- Q waves in leads III and aV_F.
- Frontal plane QRS axis that is to the right of +90 degrees or indeterminate.
- Low-voltage (less than 5 mm) QRS complexes in the limb leads.
- T-wave inversion in leads III and aV_F or in leads V_1 to V_4 (a late sign).
- Arrhythmias (sinus tachycardia, atrial fibrillation, atrial flutter, premature atrial contractions (PACs) (right atrial), and premature ventricular contractions (PVCs) (right ventricular).
- Elevated ST segments in lead aV_R have also been described.[11]

In another study of 87 consecutive patients with minor to massive pulmonary embolism, the ECG changes most often noted (in 82% of patients) were those of acute right ventricular strain, such as complete or incomplete right bundle branch block (RBBB); S_1 (S wave in lead I), Q_3—T_3 pattern (Q wave and inverted T wave in lead III); inverted T waves in leads V_2 and V_3; and a shift in the frontal plane QRS axis to the right by 20 degrees or more.[8] In the preceding study no patient with vascular obstruction of two thirds or more had an ECG free of these signs. The RBBB and QRS axis shift correlated with the extent of embolization. These ECG signs are transient, and serial recordings are necessary.

Fig. 27-1 is a 12-lead ECG from a patient with acute pulmonary embolism. The sinus tachycardia and the emergence of an incomplete RBBB pattern (terminal r wave is beginning to appear) in lead V_1 can be seen. This reflects the abrupt stretching of the right bundle branch. There is also ST-segment elevation in leads V_1 and aV_R. There is clockwise rotation of the heart, another sign of acute pulmonary embolism. The transitional zone is between V_4 and V_5, whereas the normal location is

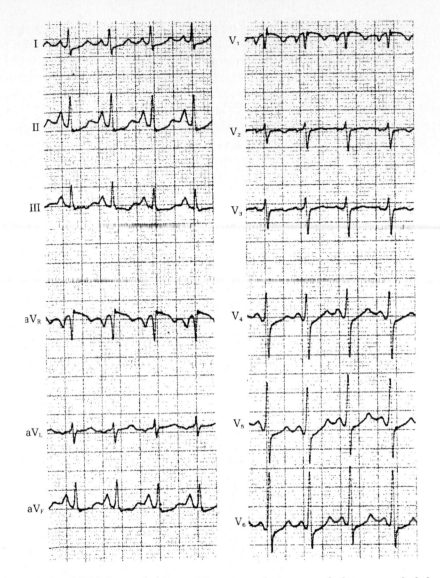

Fig. 27-1. A 12-lead ECG from a patient with acute pulmonary embolism recorded the day of the acute event. Note the sinus tachycardia, prominent P waves in leads II, III, and aV$_F$; S wave in lead I; incomplete right bundle branch block (V$_1$); and ST-segment elevation in leads V$_1$ and aV$_R$. *(From Brugada P, Gorgels AP, Wellens HJJ: In Wellens HJJ, Kulbertus HE, eds: What's new in electrocardiography, The Hague, 1981, Martinus Nijhoff.)*

V$_3$ to V$_4$. The tall P wave in lead II (P-pulmonale) is another reflection of the acute dilation of the right side of the heart.

Fig. 27-2, *A,* shows a normal preoperative ECG. Fig. 27-2, *B,* is from the same patient following acute pulmonary embolism. Note the development of sinus tachycardia, S$_1$ and Q$_3$ pattern, RBBB, and a shift in QRS axis from 0 to +30 degrees.

VALUE OF THE ECHOCARDIOGRAM

The echocardiogram visualizes the right side of the heart and central vessels, in particular, the pulmonary arteries, providing reliable information for the diagno-

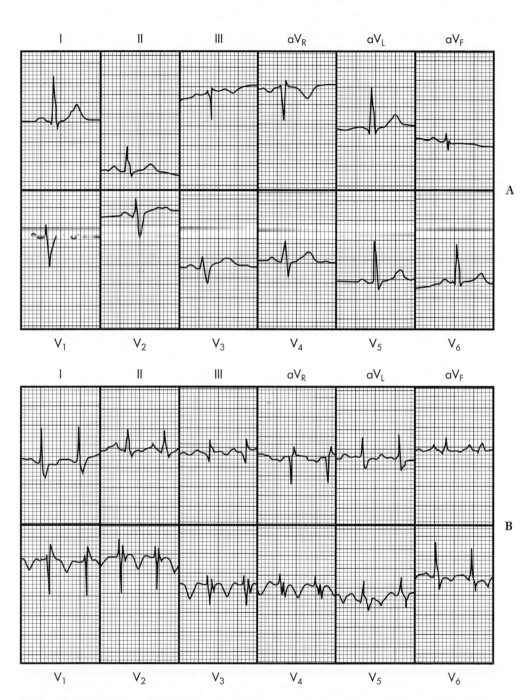

Fig. 27-2. Serial tracing. **A,** Before and, **B,** after acute pulmonary embolism. The following are evident: the acute development of sinus tachycardia, right bundle branch block, elevated ST segments in leads V_1 and aV_R, S_1 and Q_3 pattern, and a shift of the transitional zone from just before lead V_4 **(A)** to V_5 **(B).**

sis of pulmonary embolism. Echocardiographic diagnosis is primarily based on indirect signs such as right ventricular dilation and hypokinesis, bowing of the interventricular septum into the left ventricle, tricuspid regurgitation, and preserved left ventricular function.[12] Echocardiography also helps to exclude ventricular septal rupture, aortic dissection, and pericardial tamponade.[4]

OTHER AVAILABLE TESTS[4]

Chest x-ray helps to exclude lobar pneumonia, pneumothorax, and acute MI, although pulmonary embolism may exist along with these disorders.

Ventilation-perfusion lung scanning is a principal diagnostic test. The V-Q scan is most useful if it is clearly normal or demonstrates a high probability of pulmonary embolism. The diagnosis of pulmonary embolism, however, is not excluded if the scan is of intermediate or low probability when the clinical suspicion is strong. Such cases are usually followed by *selective pulmonary angiography.*

Ultrasonography of the leg veins is usually accurate in the diagnosis of proximal deep venous thrombosis when an outpatient is symptomatic.

Nonuseful tests

Room air arterial blood gas level or calculation of the *alveolar-arterial oxygen gradient* is not useful in excluding a diagnosis of pulmonary embolism and is not used as a screening test. *Ultrasonography of the leg veins* is inaccurate for asymptomatic inpatients, especially those with recent total hip or total knee replacement.

DIFFERENTIAL DIAGNOSIS

The ECG patterns in acute pulmonary embolism often resemble those of acute myocardial infarction (MI). For example, the abnormal Q waves, ST-segment elevation, and T-wave inversions that may occur in the inferior leads make one think of inferior wall MI, whereas the ST-segment elevation in lead V_1 and the RBBB may mimic anterior wall infarction. First of all, observing ECG signs of apparent MI in both inferior and anterior wall leads should alert the examiner to the possibility of acute pulmonary embolism. In addition, the dyspnea is usually much more pronounced in acute pulmonary embolism than in acute MI. Despite the severe dyspnea, a chest x-ray film does not show pulmonary congestion.

TREATMENT

1. Oxygen.
2. Analgesics.
3. Full-dose heparin. The major side effects of heparin are bleeding and thrombocytopenia (commonly heparin-induced platelet aggregation).[4]
4. Intravenous thrombolytic therapy is also used when there is hemodynamic instability, right ventricular dysfunction, a large pulmonary embolism, or extensive deep venous thrombosis. Contraindications include recent surgery or trauma.[4]
5. Emergency pulmonary thromboendarterectomy is rarely necessary but is lifesaving in patients with acute massive pulmonary embolism who do not respond to or who have absolute contraindications to thrombolytic therapy. This surgery is also considered a potential cure for patients with chronic pulmonary hyperten-

sion that is due to undiagnosed or inadequately treated prior pulmonary embolism.[13]

PREVENTION
Pharmacologic prophylaxis

Intensive preventive action is required for patients undergoing orthopedic or gynecologic cancer surgery and for immobilized medical patients. Goldhaber[4] suggested that moderate-dose warfarin be used for orthopedic patients and fixed low-dose heparin (5000 units three times a day) be used for gynecologic patients. In addition to pharmacologic prophylaxis, frequent change of body position and early mobilization, when possible, are important precautions.

Nonpharmacologic prophylaxis

Graduated compression stockings should be considered first-line prophylaxis in all hospitalized patients except those with peripheral arterial occlusive disease whose condition may be worsened by vascular compression. In patients at moderate to high risk the stockings may be used in combination with intermittent inflation of air-filled cuffs *(pneumatic compression boots)*. The compression stockings serve to oppose perioperative venodilation, and the compression boots prevent venous stasis in the legs and may stimulate endogenous fibrinolysis.[4]

Family history and young age

For patients with a family history of venous thrombosis or for young patients with venous thrombosis, Goldhaber[4] suggested that testing for a specific inherited hypercoagulable state may be justified. Such inherited states include deficiencies in antithrombin III, protein C, or protein S. The finding of acquired lupus erythematosis anticoagulant (which is typically associated with anticardiolipin antibodies) also may justify such testing.

SUMMARY

The common ECG findings in the acute phase of pulmonary embolism are the result of right ventricular failure and acute dilation of the right atria and right ventricle. Arrhythmias that occur in acute pulmonary embolism are sinus tachycardia, atrial fibrillation, atrial flutter, and right-sided PACs and PVCs. Electrocardiogram (ECG) changes reflecting the acutely dilated right side of the heart are RBBB, P pulmonale, right axis shifts of the P wave and QRS complex, elevated ST segments in leads V_1 and aV_R, clockwise rotation of the heart, and an S_1, Q_3, T_3 pattern. The preceding changes, which begin abruptly, require serial ECG tracings and are confirmed with Doppler echocardiography. Speed in diagnosing and treating acute pulmonary embolism is important because of the high mortality in untreated cases.

REFERENCES

1. Goldhaber SZ, Braunwald E: Pulmonary embolism. In Braunwald E, ed: *Heart disease,* ed 4, Philadelphia, 1992, WB Saunders.
2. Weinberg SL: President's page: pulmonary embolism—diagnosis on a tombstone, *J Am Coll Cardiol* 22:328, 1993.
3. Neuhaus A, Bentz RR, Weg JC: Pulmonary embolism in respiratory failure, *Chest* 73:460, 1978.
4. Goldhaber SZ: Recognition and management of pulmonary embolism, *Heart Dis Stroke 3:142, 1993.*
5. Morrison RB: Obstetrics. In Goldhaber SZ, ed: *Prevention of venous thromboembolism,* New York, 1993, Marcel Dekker.

6. Stollberger C et al: Syncope as a misinterpreted leading symptom of pulmonary embolism, *Dtsch Med Wochenschr* 111(12):443, 1986.

7. Akinboboye O, Brown EJ, Queirroz R et al: Recurrent pulmonary embolism with second-degree atrioventricular block and near syncope, *Am Heart J* 126:731, 1993.

8. Nielsen TT et al: Changing electrocardiographic findings in pulmonary embolism in relation to vascular obstruction, *Cardiology* 76(4):274, 1989.

9. Sreeram N, Cheriex EC, Smeets JLRM et al: Value of the 12-lead electrocardiogram at hospital admission in the diagnosis of pulmonary embolism, *Am J Cardiol* 73:298, 1994.

10. Fisch C: Electrocardiography and vectorcardiography. In Braunwald E, ed: *Heart disease,* ed 4, Philadelphia, 1992, WB Saunders.

11. Wellens HJJ, Conover M: *The ECG in emergency decision making,* Phildelphia, 1992, WB Saunders.

12. Come PC: Echocardiographic evaluation of pulmonary embolism and its response to therapeutic interventions, *Chest* 101(suppl): 153S, 1992.

13. Okubo S et al: Acute fatal pulmonary embolism: its prevention, diagnosis and treatment, *Respir Circ* 38(4):375, 1990.

C H A P T E R

28

Hypertrophy

Pathogenesis of Ventricular
  Hypertrophy   *439*
Diagnostic Tools   *439*
Left Ventricular Hypertrophy (LVH)   *440*
Right Ventricular Hypertrophy   *444*
Chronic Obstructive Lung Disease   *445*

Biventricular Hypertrophy   *446*
Normal P Wave   *447*
Left Atrial Abnormality   *447*
Right Atrial Abnormalities:
  P Pulmonale   *449*
Right Atrial Hypertrophy   *451*

PATHOGENESIS OF VENTRICULAR HYPERTROPHY

Increased metabolic demands or increased workload in the adult causes enlargement and structural alteration of myocardial cells and hyperplasia of nonmuscular cardiac components. Causes of cardiac hypertrophy are pressure and volume overload and neurohumoral factors. The two types of overload are compared with each other and with the normal heart in Fig. 28-1.

Pressure overload results when myocardial fibers generate increased systolic force or tension, as in aortic stenosis or systemic hypertension caused by another lesion. This results in *concentric hypertrophy* in which the ventricular wall thickens in relation to the ventricular cavity (Fig. 28-1).

Volume overload results when there is an increased end-diastolic wall stress, leading to *eccentric hypertrophy;* that is, the left ventricular wall thickness remains normal relative to the increase in the radius of the left ventricle (chamber dilation), as seen in Fig. 28-1. In this situation systolic pressure remains unchanged.

DIAGNOSTIC TOOLS

Echocardiography is superior to electrocardiography in the detection of mild hypertrophy and the monitoring of changes during progression or regression of chamber enlargement. Echocardiographic studies indicate that the ECG does not differentiate among concentric hypertrophy, eccentric hypertrophy, and dilation without hypertrophy, although the sensitivity of the ECG is greater in individuals with severe hypertrophy.[1] In addition, there is day-to-day variability of voltage measurements,[2,3] and young black individuals appear to have much higher voltages with normal ventricles than white individuals of the same age.[4,5] However, despite its

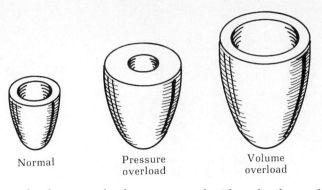

Normal   Pressure   Volume
overload   overload

Fig. 28-1. Pressure and volume overload are compared with each other and with the normal heart. *(Modified from Oparil S; J Am Coll Cardiol 5;57B, 1985.)*

limitations, the ECG remains a valuable tool for the detection of hypertensive target organ damage and is recommended as an essential test in the office evaluation of the hypertensive patient.[6,7]

LEFT VENTRICULAR HYPERTROPHY

Left ventricular hypertrophy (LVH) is causally related to high blood pressure.[8] Its presence in hypertensive patients points to hypertensive target organ damage. When there is ECG evidence of LVH, there is an associated increased risk for a number of cardiovascular diseases, including myocardial infarction, stroke, and congestive heart failure.[9] Left ventricular hypertrophy is also associated with an increased risk for arrhythmias and sudden death.[10] Moreover, risk has been shown to increase in step with increased QRS voltage or repolarization abnormalities to decline along with a decline in voltage or repolarization abnormalites, suggesting that regression of the ECG signs of LVH is associated with improved prognosis.[11] Antihypertensive treatment has been shown to decrease or reverse echocardiographic evidence of LVH in hypertensive patients.[12]

ECG recognition

- Increased QRS amplitude
- Late intrinsicoid deflection in lead V_6
- Widened QRS/T angle (left ventricular strain)
- Tendency toward left axis deviation

Increased QRS amplitude. QRS voltage (1) varies with age, being greater in the younger individual; (2) depends on the mean frontal plane QRS axis, being greater in the lead whose axis is parallel with the mean current flow; (3) is greater in individuals with a thin chest wall and is less in obese individuals, who may have LVH with normal QRS amplitude; (4) is less when there is lung disease; and (5) is greater in black children. Fig. 28-2 compares the normal QRS complex in leads V_1 and V_6 with that of LVH.

Intrinsicoid deflection. The intrinsicoid deflection is measured from the onset of the QRS complex to the peak of the R wave. It reflects the time required for peak

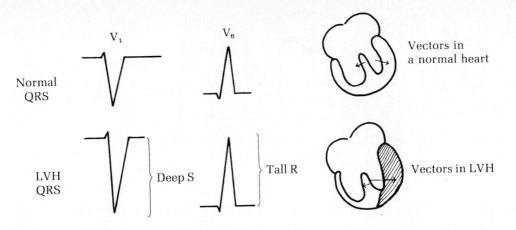

Fig. 28-2. The normal QRS complex in leads V_1 and V_6 compared with that of left ventricular hypertrophy (LVH).

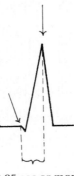

0.05 sec or more

Fig. 28-3. The intrinsicoid deflection in lead V_6 in LVH.

voltage to develop under a particular electrode. In lead V_6 the intrinsicoid deflection is delayed in LVH to 0.05 sec or more (Fig. 28-3), probably as a result of the extra time it takes to activate the hypertrophied ventricle. Although this delay in the intrinsicoid deflection is not specific, it occurs in 35% to 90% of cases.

Widened QRS/T angle. The *left ventricular strain* pattern denotes the pattern seen when the QRS/T angle widens because the ST segment and T wave are opposite in direction to that of the QRS. This pattern does not occur in uncomplicated hypertrophy but is associated with myocardial ischemia.

Left atrial involvement

Left atrial enlargement may be associated with LVH. The terminal P forces (left atrial) are best seen in lead V_1, where they produce a deep terminal trough on the ECG if the left atrium is enlarged (Fig. 28-4).

The 12-lead ECG in Fig. 28-5 represents LVH. Note the increased voltage of the QRS; the late intrinsicoid deflection in lead V_6; left axis deviation; the broad, deep negative component to the P wave in lead V_1; and the left ventricular strain pattern in leads I, aV_L, V_5, and V_6.

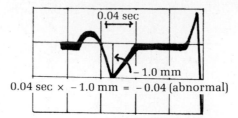

Fig. 28-4. The P wave in lead V_1 with left atrial enlargement.

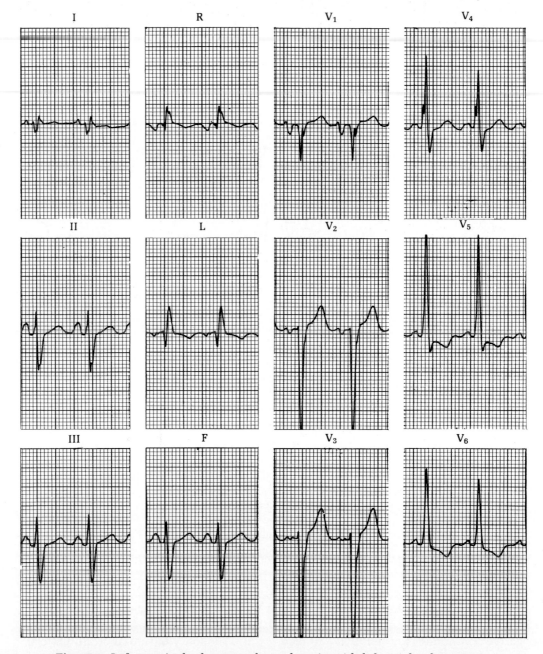

Fig. 28-5. Left ventricular hypertrophy and strain with left atrial enlargement.

Estes criteria and the use of Cornell voltage

The box below illustrates the Estes criteria for the diagnosis of LVH. The standard ECG is a poor screening test for the detection of LVH in individuals with essential hypertension. However, a study of 923 white untreated hypertensive individuals showed that a clinically relevant increase in the diagnostic accuracy of the ECG for detection of LVH can be achieved by a modification of the partition values of the Cornell voltage (S wave in V_3 plus the R wave in aV_L). A modified value of the Cornell voltage (greater than 2.4 mV in men and greater than 2.0 mV in women) had a sensitivity of 26% in men and 19% in women (overall, 22%); the specificity was 96% in men and 95% in women (overall, 95%).[13]

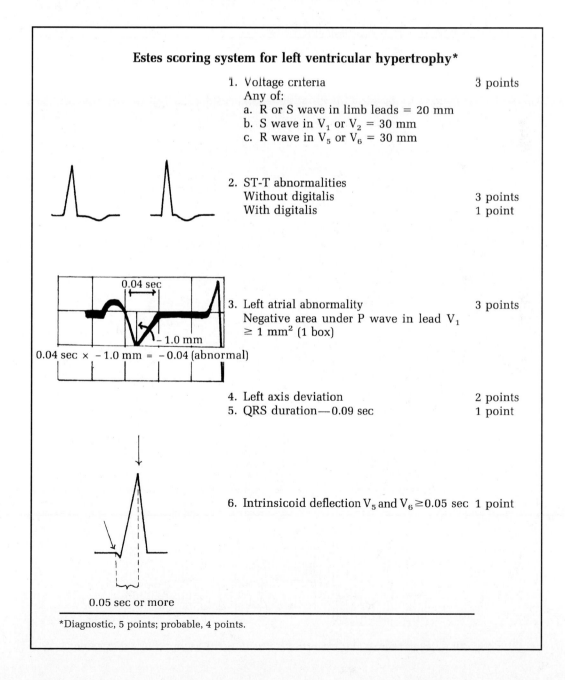

Estes scoring system for left ventricular hypertrophy*

1. Voltage criteria   3 points
   Any of:
   a. R or S wave in limb leads = 20 mm
   b. S wave in V_1 or V_2 = 30 mm
   c. R wave in V_5 or V_6 = 30 mm

2. ST-T abnormalities
   Without digitalis   3 points
   With digitalis   1 point

0.04 sec

−1.0 mm

0.04 sec × −1.0 mm = −0.04 (abnormal)

3. Left atrial abnormality   3 points
   Negative area under P wave in lead V_1
   ≥ 1 mm² (1 box)

4. Left axis deviation   2 points
5. QRS duration—0.09 sec   1 point

6. Intrinsicoid deflection V_5 and V_6 ≥ 0.05 sec 1 point

0.05 sec or more

*Diagnostic, 5 points; probable, 4 points.

RIGHT VENTRICULAR HYPERTROPHY

Right ventricular hypertrophy (RVH) is associated with conditions that cause the right ventricular mass to begin competing with the left ventricle, such as congenital pulmonary stenosis, tetralogy of Fallot, and primary pulmonary hypertension.

ECG recognition

- Right axis deviation in the frontal plane
- Tall R waves in the right precordial leads, which are sometimes preceded by Q waves, in which case there is frequently right atrial hypertrophy and tricuspid regurgitation (tall, peaked P waves in leads II, III, aV_F, and, occasionally, V_1, Fig. 28-6)
- Deep S waves in the left precordial leads

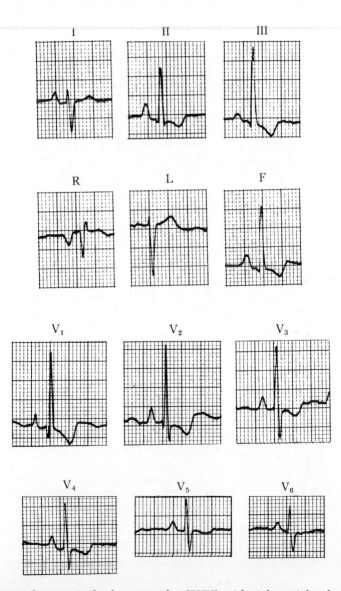

Fig. 28-6. Right ventricular hypertrophy (RVH) with right atrial enlargement.

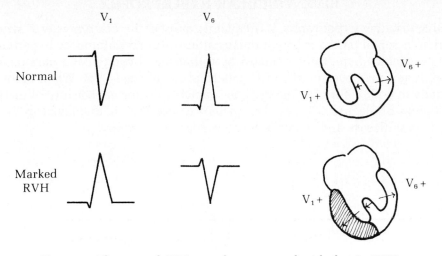

Fig. 28-7. The normal QRS complex compared with that in RVH.

- Slight increase in QRS duration
- Secondary ST-T abnormalities in the precordial and inferior leads (the T wave is opposite in polarity to the QRS).

NOTE: An incomplete right bundle branch block (RBBB) (rSR′ in V_1) pattern may signify RVH, dilation, or overload of the right ventricle, but it is most frequently the result of other factors. It is seen in mitral valve disease with pulmonary hypertension and atrial septal defect and disappears following corrective surgery.

Fig. 28-7 compares the patterns seen in leads V_1 and V_6 in the normal heart with those of marked RVH. The patterns present a mirror image of the patterns seen in LVH.

CHRONIC OBSTRUCTIVE LUNG DISEASE

In patients with chronic obstructive lung disease the lungs are overaerated and provide an insulating effect. This effect, along with the change in the spatial orientation of the heart, causes the ECG changes.

ECG recognition

- Peaked P waves in leads II, III, and aV_F (The amplitude increases with the severity of the disease.)
- Low R-wave amplitude (less than 0.5 mV in lead V_6 as the disease becomes more severe)
- Wide, slurred S waves in leads I, II, III, and V_4 to V_6 that are caused by the late QRS vector being oriented superiorly and to the right. (With more severe disease, the R:S ratio is equal to or less than 1 in lead V_6.)
- Right axis deviation and a dominant S wave in precordial leads (the most reliable signs of RVH in chronic lung disease)[2,6]
- Right axis deviation of the P wave

In emphysema the ECG voltage is low, the QRS axis is posterior and superior, and the P-wave axis is to the right of +60 degrees in the frontal plane. Right ventricular hypertrophy may also be present if there is an rSR′ pattern in right precordial leads, a slurred S wave in left precordial leads, and a prominent R wave in lead aV_R.

BIVENTRICULAR HYPERTROPHY

Biventricular hypertrophy is frequently present in *Eisenmenger's syndrome* (ventricular septal defect or patent ductus arteriosus and pulmonary hypertension). Right ventricular hypertrophy caused by pulmonary hypertension may be associated with and may obscure the ECG pattern of established LVH. When there is hypertrophy of both ventricles, the ECG may actually be normal because of the partial cancellation of electrical forces. The patient whose ECG is displayed in Fig. 28-8 had bilateral disease and probable biventricular hypertrophy.

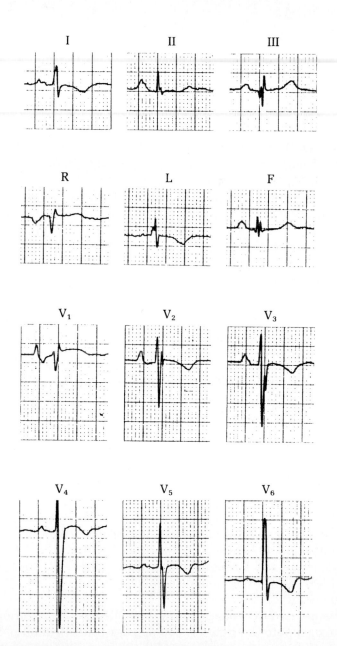

Fig. 28-8. A 12-lead ECG from a patient with hypertension. The notched, upright P wave in leads I, II, and V_4 to V_6 and the deep, broad terminal trough in lead V_1 are evident. *(Courtesy Ara G. Tilkian, MD, Van Nuys, Calif.)*

ECG recognition

- Right axis deviation in the limb leads
- Signs of LVH in the precordial leads
- A shift to the left of the transitional zone in the precordial leads (a less reliable sign)

NORMAL P WAVE

- Less than 3 mm high and less than 0.12 sec wide (Fig. 28-9, *A*)
- Upright in the left precordial leads and in leads I and II
- Usually diphasic in the right precordial leads
- P axis is about +60 degrees in the frontal plane
- Initial and terminal components corresponding to right (anterior) and left (posterior) atrial forces

LEFT ATRIAL ABNORMALITY

The pattern associated with left atrial enlargement reflects a conduction abnormality within the atria, not actual hypertrophy or dilation. The ECG pattern of left atrial abnormality is often present in hypertension and may transiently occur in pulmonary edema.

ECG recognition

- Prolonged P-wave duration
- Notched upright P wave in leads I, II, and V_4 to V_6
- A deep, broad terminal trough in lead V_1

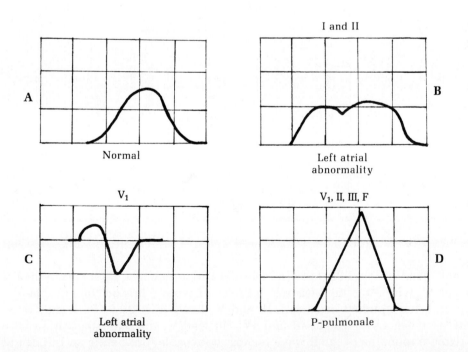

Fig. 28-9. A to **D,** The normal P wave compared with the P wave in left atrial abnormality and P pulmonale.

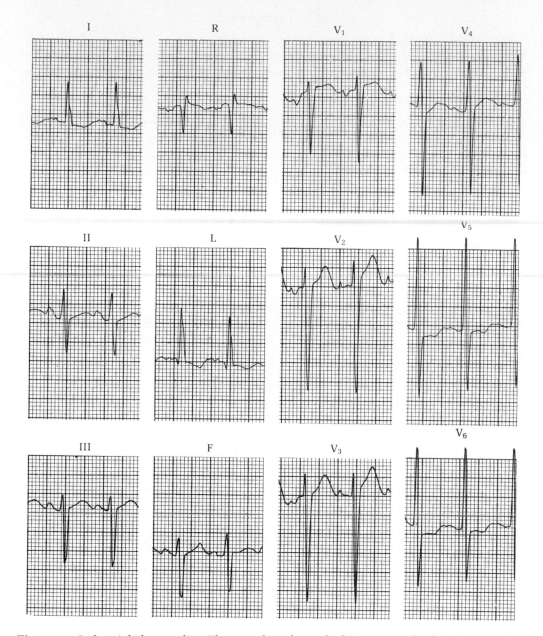

Fig. 28-10. Left atrial abnormality. There are broad, notched P waves in leads I, II, V_5 and V_6. The P wave in lead V_1 has a broad terminal trough. *(Courtesy Ara G. Tilkian, MD, Van Nuys, Calif.)*

Left atrial abnormality causes the initial and terminal components of the P wave to separate, widening the P wave to 0.12 sec or more. Thus on the ECG the P wave is upright and notched in leads I, II, and V_4 to V_6 (Fig. 28-9, *B*). It may be either positive or negative in leads III and aV_F. In lead V_1 the wide separation between the two components of the P wave is most noticeable, producing an initial upright component followed by an inverted component (Fig. 28-9, *C*). Left atrial abnormality is often accompanied by RVH.

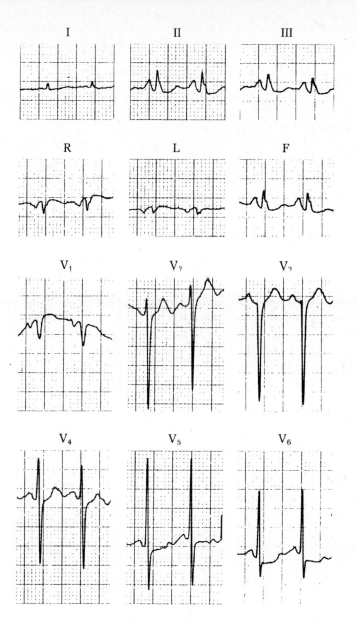

Fig. 28-11. P pulmonale. There are tall, peaked P waves in the inferior leads, and the P axis is rightward. *(Courtesy Ara G. Tilkian, MD, Van Nuys, Calif.)*

Fig. 28-10 is a 12-lead ECG from a patient with hypertension. The notched, upright P wave in leads I, II, and V_4 to V_6 and the deep, broad terminal trough in lead V_1 can be seen.

RIGHT ATRIAL ABNORMALITIES: P PULMONALE

The so-called P pulmonale pattern is probably the result of increased sympathetic stimulation (causing increased P amplitude) and low position of the diaphragm (causing the P axis to be rightward) associated with diffuse lung disease. The P pulmonale pattern aids in the evaluation of the severity of chronic obstructive lung disease (rightward P axis shift). The right axis deviation of the P wave is the best ECG change in evaluating the severity of chronic obstructive lung disease.

ECG recognition

- Tall, peaked P waves in leads II, III, and aV_F and sometimes in lead V_1 (Fig. 28-9, D)
- P axis to the right of +70 degrees

Fig. 28-11 is an ECG from a patient with chronic obstructive lung disease. Note the typical P pulmonale pattern.

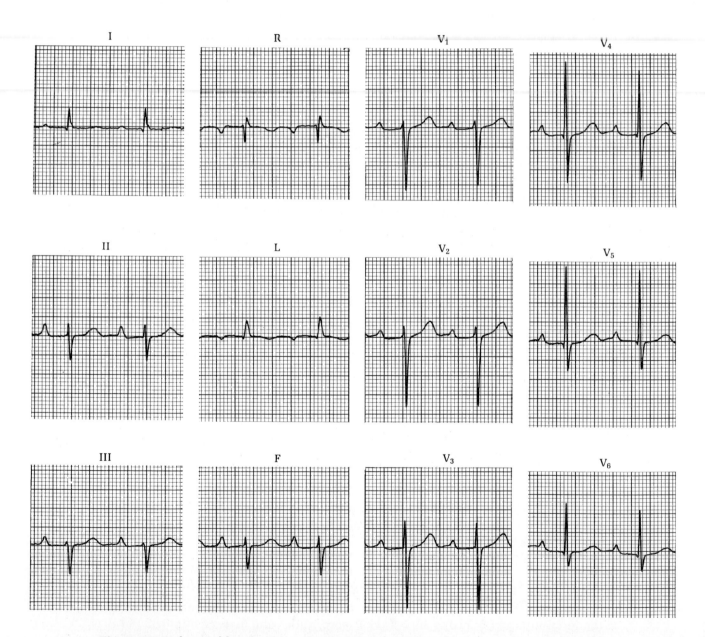

Fig. 28-12. Right atrial hypertrophy. There are tall, wide P waves in the inferior leads and in leads V_4 and V_5. *(Courtesy Ara G. Tilkian, MD, Van Nuys, Calif.)*

RIGHT ATRIAL HYPERTROPHY

In right atrial hypertrophy the major P vector is directed anteriorly. Right atrial hypertrophy results from congenital heart disease, tricuspid valve disease, and pulmonary hypertension.

ECG recognition

- Tall, wide P waves in the limb leads and right precordial leads
- Often associated with RVH

Fig. 28-12 is the ECG of a patient with right atrial hypertrophy caused by tricuspid valve disease (or pulmonary hypertension). The tall, wide P waves in the inferior leads and right precordial leads are evident.

REFERENCES

1. Norman JE Jr, Levy D, Campbell G, Dailey JJ: Improved detection of echocardiographic left ventricular hypertrophy using a new electrocardiographic algorithm, *J Am Coll Cardiol* 21:1680, 1993.
2. Farb A, Devereux RB, Kligfield P: Day-to-day variability of voltage measurements used in electrocardiographic criteria for left ventricular hypertrophy, *J Am Coll Cardiol* 15:618, 1990.
3. Van Den Joogen JP, Mol WH, Kowsoleea A et al: Reproducibility of electrocardiographic criteria for left ventricular hypertrophy in hypertensive patients in general practice, *Eur Heart J* 13:1606, 1992.
4. Xie X, Liu K, Stamlerdi GY: Ethnic differences in electrocardiographic left ventricular hypertrophy in young and middle-aged employed American men, *Am J Cardiol* 73:564, 1994.
5. Lee DK, Marantz PR, Devereux RB et al: Left ventricular hypertrophy in black and white hypertensives: standard electrocardiographic criteria overestimate racial differences in prevalence, *JAMA* 267:3294, 1992.
6. Frohlich ED, Apstein C, Chobanian AV et al: The heart in hypertension, *N Engl J Med* 327:998, 1992.
7. The fifth report of the Joint National Committee on Detection, Evaluation, and Treatment of High Blood Pressure, *Arch Intern Med* 153:154, 1993.
8. Levy D, Anderson KM, Savage DD et al: Echocardiographically detected left ventricular hypertrophy: prevalence and risk factors—the Framingham Heart Study, *Ann Intern Med* 108:7, 1988.
9. Sullivan JM, Vander Zwaag RV, el-Zeky F et al: Left ventricular hypertrophy: effect on survival, *J Am Coll Cardiol* 22:508, 1993.
10. Ghali JK, Kadakia S, Cooper RS, Liso YL: Impact of left ventricular hypertrophy on ventricular arrhythmias in the absence of coronary artery disease, *J Am Col Cardiol* 17:1277, 1991.
11. Levy D, Salomon M, D'Agostino RB et al: Prognostic implications of baseline electrocardiographic features and their serial changes in subjects with left ventricular hypertrophy, *Circulation* 90:1786, 1994.
12. Neaton JD, Grimm RH Jr, Prineas RJ et al: Treatment of Mild Hypertension Study: final results, *JAMA* 270:713, 1993.
13. Schillaci G, Verdecchia P, Borgioni C et al: Improved electrocardiographic diagnosis of left ventricular hypertrophy, *Am J Cardiol* 74:714, 1994.

29

Expert Bedside Monitoring

Digitalis Intoxication   *452*
Paroxysmal Supraventricular
  Tachycardia   *452*

Unstable Angina   *458*
Broad QRS Tachycardia   *458*
High Risk Myocardial Infarction   *462*

The ideal monitoring protocol would be to monitor in all 12 leads continuously. However, because in most hospitals in the United States this is not possible with the equipment that is available, this chapter will supply you with the minimal ECG lead requirements for monitoring patients in the acute settings of digitalis intoxication, premature supraventricular tachycardia (PSVT), broad QRS tachycardia, unstable angina, and acute myocardial infarction (MI). Table 29-1 is a summary of the diagnostic monitoring leads and the ECG patterns seen in them.

DIGITALIS INTOXICATION

Lead II

Use lead II initially to look for P waves that resemble sinus P waves during atrial tachycardia. In Fig. 29-1 the ectopic P waves in this atrial tachycardia closely resemble sinus P waves.

Lead V_1 or MCL_1

If no conduction or no P waves are present, you will need lead V_1 (or MCL_1) to determine whether the ventricular rhythm is junctional (rS pattern) or fascicular ventricular tachycardia (VT) (rSR' pattern). Chapter 17 discusses mechanism, ECG recognition, and treatment of digitalis intoxication. In cases of fascicular VT there will also be axis deviation (leads I and II). Atrial fibrillation with fascicular VT is shown in Fig. 29-2. The absence of P waves is noted in lead II, and the diagnosis of fascicular VT is made in V_1. Right axis deviation is noted in leads I and II.

Table 29-1. Diagnostic monitoring leads

Digitalis intoxication	PSVT	Unstable angina	VT	High-risk MI
II and/or V$_1$	I, II, III, V$_1$, and V$_6$	V$_2$ or V$_3$ s̄ pain	V$_1$, V$_2$, and V$_6$	Inferior, V$_{4R}$; anterior V$_1$, I, and II

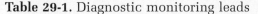

II: P in atrial tachycardia

CMT   AVNRT

Critical proximal LAD stenosis (Wellens syndrome)

V$_1$ positive complex

Inferior

V4R

If: No conduction or atrial fibrilltion

12-lead c̄ pain

Proximal RCA occlusion RV MI

R:S<1

ST ↑ V$_1$ and a V$_R$
St ↓ Eight other leads
Left main or three vessel coronary artery disease

V$_1$ negative complex
V$_1$ and V$_2$

V$_6$

Anterior
V$_1$ I II

or

Copyright 1992 by Mary H. Conover.
AVNRT, Atrioventricular nodal reentry tachycardia; *CMT,* circus movement tachycardia; *c̄,* with; *LAD,* left anterior descending (coronary artery); *MI,* myocardial infarction; *PSVT,* premature supraventricular tachycardia; *RCA,* right coronary artery; *RV,* right ventricular; *s̄,* without; *VT,* ventricular tachycardia.

PAROXYSMAL SUPRAVENTRICULAR TACHYCARDIA

Leads I, II, III, V$_1$, and V$_6$

During PSVT it is important at least to record leads I, II, III, V$_1$, and V$_6$. It is necessary to locate the P′ waves, which are not always visible in every lead; the leads in which they are visible are not the same for each patient. The finding of a pseudo-S wave in leads II and III or a pseudo-R wave in lead V$_1$ is diagnostic of atrioventricular (AV) nodal reentry tachycardia (Fig. 29-3). In lead I a negative P′ wave following the QRS is diagnostic of a left-sided accessory pathway (Fig. 29-4). These are the two most common mechanisms of PSVT (Chapter 11).

UNSTABLE ANGINA

Leads V$_2$ and V$_3$ without pain
A 12-lead ECG during pain

For patients with unstable angina, leads V$_2$ and V$_3$ are minimal requirements when the patient is without pain (Fig. 29-5) to assess for Wellens syndrome (Chapter 24), that is, critical proximal left anterior descending (LAD) coronary artery stenosis. During pain a 12-lead ECG is required to assess for left main or three vessel coronary artery disease (Fig. 29-6).

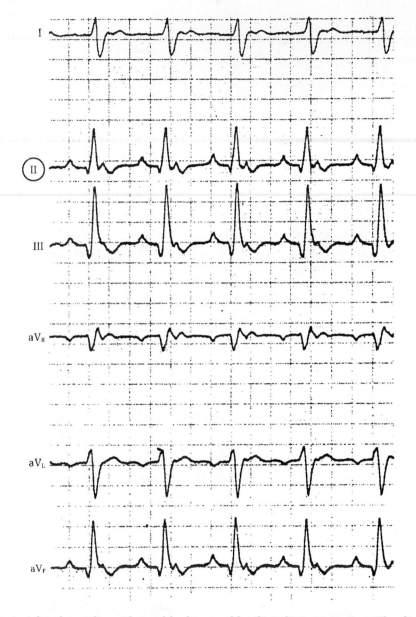

Fig. 29-1. Atrial tachycardia with 2:1 block caused by digitalis intoxication. The diagnosis is made in lead II because of the positive P wave, as well as the ventriculophasic PP intervals. The focus in this clinical setting is close to the sinus node, producing P′ waves that are positive in lead II and similar in appearance to sinus P waves. *(Courtesy Hein J.J. Wellens, MD, The Netherlands.)*

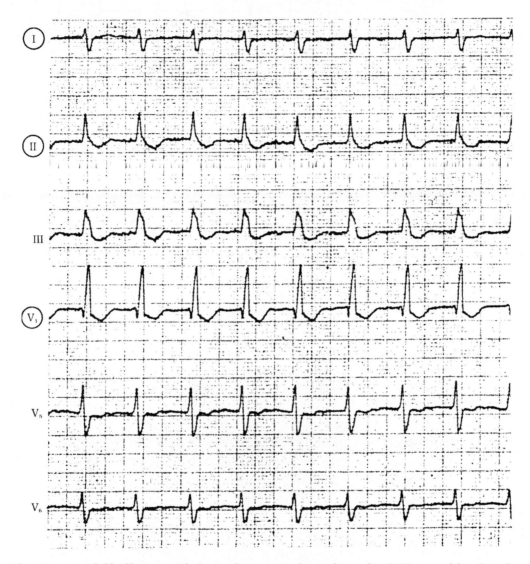

Fig. 29-2. Atrial fibrillation with fascicular ventricular tachycardia (VT) caused by digitalis intoxication. The diagnosis of atrial fibrillation is made in lead II (no P waves); absence of atrioventricular (AV) conduction is also noted in this lead (regular ventricular response). Lead V₁ shows a fascicular VT (rSR′ pattern). Leads I and II show right axis deviation, indicating a left anterior fascicular focus (see Chapter 17). *(Courtesy Hein J.J. Wellens, MD, The Netherlands.)*

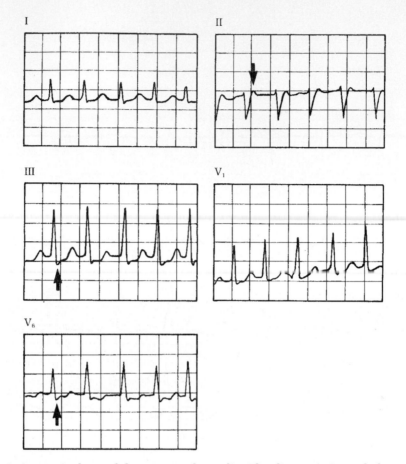

Fig. 29-3. Atrioventricular nodal reentry tachycardia. The diagnosis is made because the P′ wave is seen distorting the terminal QRS forces in leads V_1 (psuedo-r) and leads II, III, and V_6 (pseudo-S) *(arrows).*

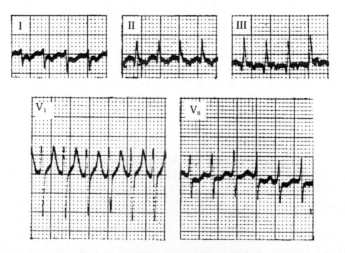

Fig. 29-4. Circus movement tachycardia. The diagnosis is made quickly because the P′ waves follow the QRS complexes and are separate from them. The P′ waves are clearly seen in the limb leads. In this case, a negative P′ wave in lead I is diagnostic of a left-sided accessory pathway. *(From Marriott HJL, Conover M: Advanced concepts in arrhythmias, ed 2, St Louis, 1989, Mosby.)*

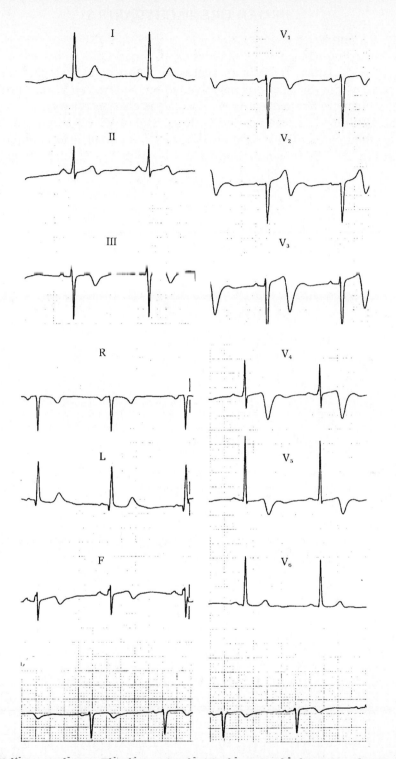

Fig. 29-5. Wellens syndrome. The diagnosis of critical proximal left anterior descending coronary artery stenosis is made because of the presence of unstable angina, along with the typical ST-T changes in leads V_2 and V_3, as described in Chapter 24 and noted here. When the patient is without pain, there is progressive deep, symmetric inversion of the T wave with little or no ST-segment elevation or elevation in creatine kinase level and there is no loss of precordial R waves. *(Courtesy Jerilyn Briten, RN, Nampa, Idaho.)*

BROAD QRS TACHYCARDIA

Leads V_1, V_2, and V_6

The recording of lead V_1 is mandatory in broad QRS tachycardia. If V_1 looks like VT, it is VT unless there is an accessory pathway. If V_1 looks like supraventricular tachycardia (SVT) and is negative, you must also see V_2 and probably V_6. If V_1 has the inconclusive pattern in V_1, lead V_6 is also necessary.

If the QRS in V_1 is positive and is diagnostic of VT (monophasic, biphasic, or taller left rabbit ear configuration) or SVT (rSR′), no other lead is required. For example, in Fig. 29-7 there is a monophasic R wave in V_1, which is diagnostic of VT.

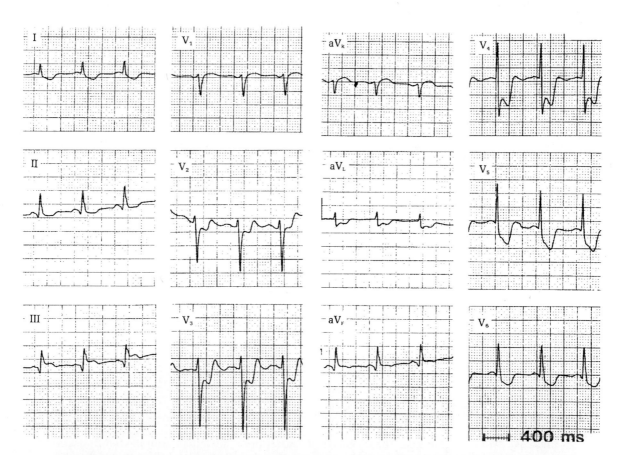

Fig. 29-6. Left main and three vessel coronary artery disease. The diagnosis is made because of the presence of unstable angina, the ST elevation in leads V_1 and aV_R, and the ST depression in at least eight other leads, as described in Chapter 24. *(Courtesy Hein J.J. Wellens, MD, The Netherlands.)*

If, however, one encounters a taller right rabbit ear configuration, lead V_6 is necessary for the diagnosis.

If the QRS in lead V_1 is negative and is diagnostic of VT (broad R, slurred S downstroke, or delayed S nadir), no other lead is necessary (Fig 29-8). If lead V_1 looks like SVT, one should also evaluate lead V_2 before deciding (Fig. 29-9).

Chapter 14 discusses aberration versus ectopy and will help to make you aware of the tachycardias that do not follow the rules. That is, the SVTs that look like VT use an accessory pathway to activate the ventricles. The VTs that look like SVT are fascicular VT, idiopathic VT, and bundle branch reentry VT.

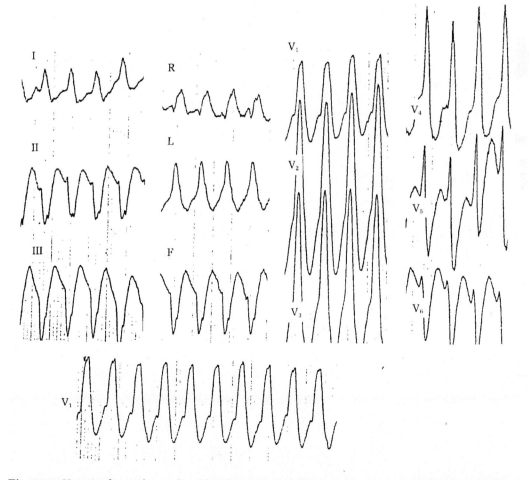

Fig. 29-7. Ventricular tachycardia. The diagnosis is made quickly because the QRS in lead V_1 is a monophasic R wave. Other clues are the deep S wave in V_6, QRS duration greater than 0.14 sec, left axis deviation, and signs of AV dissociation in lead I.

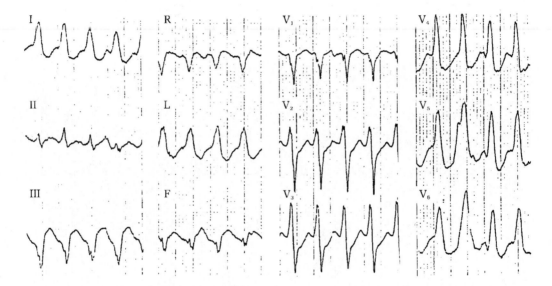

Fig. 29-8. Ventricular tachycardia. The diagnosis is made quickly because of the broad R wave, slurred S downstroke in lead V_1, the broad R wave in lead V_2, and the delayed S nadir in leads V_1 and V_2. Other clues are signs of AV dissociation in many leads, a fusion beat (lead II), and QRS duration greater than 0.14 sec. It was only necessary, however, to spot the slurred downstroke in lead V_1 to make the diagnosis.

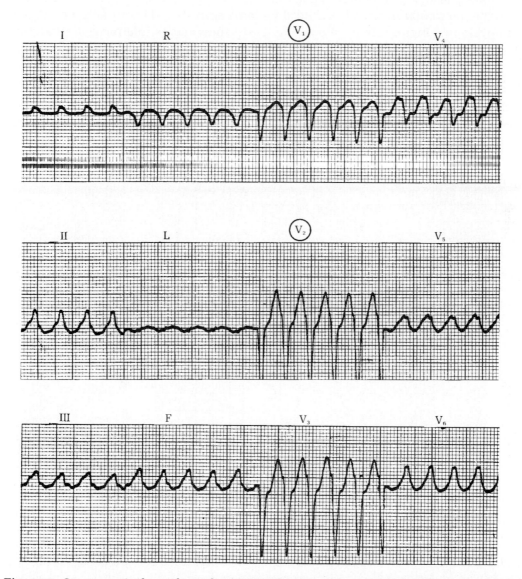

Fig. 29-9. Supraventricular tachycardia (SVT). The diagnosis is made because in leads V_1 and V_2 the S wave has a clean, swift downstroke. Both leads are necessary for this diagnosis because in some cases lead V_1 can look like SVT, but V_2 will confirm that the condition is VT.

HIGH-RISK MYOCARDIAL INFARCTION

Inferior MI high-risk assessment: Lead V_{4R}

Anterior MI high-risk assessment: Leads I, II, and V_1

The diagnosis of acute MI and the decisions regarding thrombolysis are made from the 12-lead ECG and lead V_{4R}. In monitoring patients with acute inferior wall infarction, lead V_{4R} is helpful in determining the coronary artery involved, absence of right ventricular infarction, the need for more aggressive therapy, and the chances of developing high-grade AV block. Fig. 29-10 shows acute inferior wall infarction in which involvement of the right ventricle, proximal right coronary artery occlu-

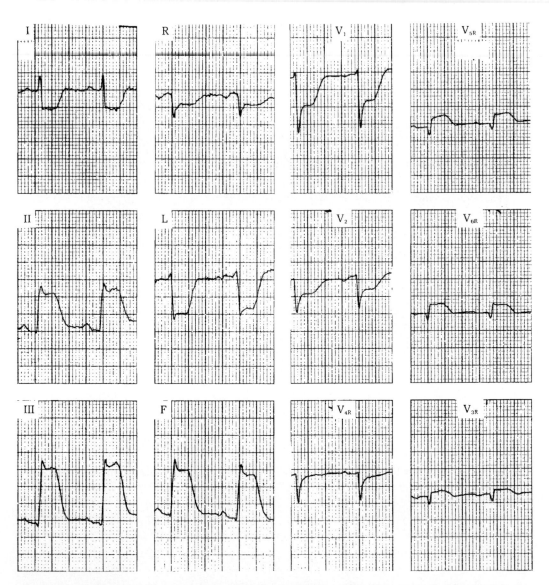

Fig. 29-10. Inferior wall and right ventricular infarction. The diagnosis of right ventricular infarction and high risk in a patient is made because of the elevated ST segment in lead V_{4R} (see Chapter 26).

sion, and risk of high-grade block were determined from the elevated ST segment in lead V_{4R} (Chapter 26). In monitoring patients with acute anterior wall infarction, leads V_1, I, and II are necessary to access the intraventricular conduction system. Bundle branch block can be diagnosed in lead V_1, and hemiblock in leads I and II (Fig. 29-11). It is important to recognize these conditions, since their appearance affects the prognosis and the approach to the patient.

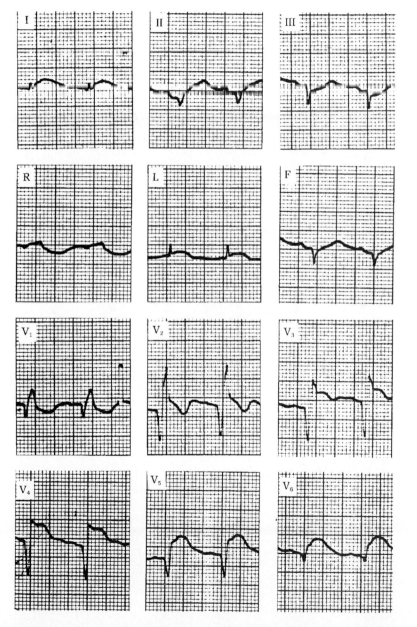

Fig. 29-11. Anterior wall myocardial infarction with right bundle branch block (V_1) and left anterior hemiblock (leads I and II) identify a high-risk patient. *(Courtesy Peg McKnight, RN, Las Vegas.)*

PART IV

SPECIAL DIAGNOSTIC AND THERAPEUTIC PROCEDURES

C H A P T E R
30

Signal-Averaged ECG and Fast Fourier Transform Analysis

EDWARD L. CONOVER

Problems in Analyzing Small ECG
  Signals   *467*
Signal Averaging   *468*
Time Domain Analysis of the
  Signal-Averaged ECG   *469*

Frequency Domain Analysis of the
  Signal-Averaged ECG   *470*
Other Analytical Methods   *475*
Summary   *476*

Patients surviving acute myocardial infarction (MI) may be at risk for development of life-threatening arrhythmias. In patients with a history of MI, certain low-level, high-frequency ECG signals have been observed and correlated with increased risk of developing spontaneous arrhythmias.[1-4] These distinctive signals, called *late potentials,* are high-frequency, low-amplitude events that occur late in and are continuous with the QRS complex. They apparently arise from delayed, disorganized activity in areas of the myocardium at the interface of fibrous scar tissue and normal tissue.[5-6] Because these late potentials are a very low-level phenomenon, special techniques and equipment have been developed to record them. Techniques such as the signal-averaged ECG (SAECG) are being used to evaluate late potentials and as a tool for other noninvasive studies, such as His bundle activity,[7] evaluation of the effect of surgical repair on congenital heart disease,[8] determination of left ventricular mass,[9] and effects of thrombolysis.[10-12]

PROBLEMS IN ANALYZING SMALL ECG SIGNALS

Although it is a demanding task to present the ECG of the electrical cardiac cycle in a noise-free manner, it is a much greater challenge to record and analyze microvolt-level ECG signals. The recording of the electrical cardiac cycle can be interfered with by noise from skeletal muscle movement, amplifier and instrumentation noise, power frequency and its harmonics, and tissue electrode interface. The small signals of late potentials are largely masked by larger, low-frequency signals (e.g., the ST segment) and noise.

Tissue-electrode artifacts can be minimized by lightly sanding the skin with fine sandpaper (no. 220), wiping with alcohol, and using silver–silver chloride electrodes. Shielding and twisting of input cables reduce power frequency noise, and investigations requiring extremely low noise levels enclose the patient and equipment in a Faraday cage. Muscle noise can be reduced by the use of muscle relaxants or spatial-averaging techniques.[13]

Further reduction of noise requires the use of sophisticated techniques that have been developed to separate the low-amplitude, high-frequency signals from the noise and low- frequency signals. These techniques are based on enhancing the characteristics of the signals that are desired while repressing the undesired ones.

SIGNAL AVERAGING

The objective of signal averaging is reduction of the noise that contaminates the ECG. Signal averaging can be accomplished by using either spatial averaging or ensemble averaging: both have unique advantages and disadvantages and are used according to the situation. Both techniques are based on the assumption that the noise is random, whereas the signal of interest is coherent and repetitive. Consequently, when several inputs representing the same event are added together, the coherent signal will be reinforced and the noise will cancel itself. The degree of noise reduction obtained is proportional to the square root of the number of inputs averaged. The key lies in obtaining multiple inputs representing the ECG and maintaining coherence. Spatial averaging averages multiple electrodes over a single complex; ensemble averaging uses a single vector electrode set over multiple complexes.

Spatial averaging

Spatial averaging uses from 4 to 16 electrodes to obtain the necessary multiple inputs.[14] These inputs are then averaged to provide the noise reduction. The noise reduction available from the use of spatial averaging is restricted by the practical limit on the number of electrodes that can be placed, the possibility that closely spaced electrodes will respond to a common noise source and not cancel effectively, and the theoretical limit of a two- to four-fold reduction in noise.

The advantage of spatial averaging is the ability to provide a signal-averaged ECG from a single beat, thereby allowing beat-to-beat analysis of transient events and complex arrhythmias.[13]

Ensemble averaging (signal averaging)

Ensemble averaging, as applied to cardiology, is commonly referred to as *signal averaging,* and this term will be used hereafter. Other terms for ensemble averaging are *temporal averaging* and *serial averaging.*

The multiple inputs necessary for signal averaging are gathered from standard orthogonal bipolar X, Y, and Z leads over a series of ECG cycles. Because the average can be taken over a large number of beats (typically 100 or more), the noise can theoretically be reduced by a factor of 10 or greater. The tacit assumptions underlying signal averaging are that the waveform is repetitive and can be captured without losing beat-to-beat synchronization.

Signal averaging is a computer-based process whereby each electrode lead input is amplified, its voltage measured or sampled at intervals of 1 ms or less, and each sample converted into a digital number with at least a 12-bit precision.[15] The ECG is thereby converted from an analog voltage waveform into a series of digital numbers that are, in essence, a computer-readable ECG of 100 or more QRS complexes. The digital QRS complexes are then aligned and averaged by a computer with a recognition template to reject ectopic or excessively noisy beats.

Fundamental to signal averaging is the establishment of a starting or fiducial point (usually a point on a fast-moving portion of the QRS) to use in aligning each of the series of QRS complexes. If the fiducial point is unstable (jitter) or the portion of the waveform of interest does not have a stable time relationship to the starting point, the waveform will be smoothed and high-frequency components lost.[16] To ensure that analysis uses valid data, the equipment often provides outputs to advise the user of the correlation coefficient and jitter. This signal-averaged data can be presented and analyzed in either the time domain or the frequency domain, or both.

TIME DOMAIN ANALYSIS OF THE SIGNAL-AVERAGED ECG

Time domain analysis, also referred to as high-pass filtering, presents the ECG as a function of time. After the individual lead signals have been signal-averaged, they are filtered and then combined to form the composite SAECG. Filtering removes the large, low-frequency components that would obscure the low-level, high-frequency late potentials. The following types of filters are commonly used in processing SAECG signals:

1. High-pass filters, which emphasize the high frequencies and minimize the low frequencies
2. Band-pass filters, which emphasize the midrange and high frequencies, minimizing both the low frequencies and the very high frequencies

Typically, the high-pass filters reject frequencies below 25 to 40 Hz, whereas the band-pass filters reject frequencies below 25 to 40 Hz and above 250 Hz.[13,15,17-20] The work of Vatterott, Bailey, and Hammill[17] and El-Sherif et al.[13] investigates the use of different filter frequency bounds. Generally a bidirectional four-pole Butterworth filter is used to minimize ringing and artifacts. After the X, Y, and Z leads have been signal-averaged and filtered, the vector magnitudes are combined $(X^2 + Y^2 + Z^2)^{1/2}$ to form the composite SAECG. Studies also have been made evaluating the filtered X, Y, and Z leads.[10,13]

Interpreting the time domain signal-averaged ECG

A typical filtered SAECG for a normal subject is shown in Fig. 30-1. Because very high gain is required to display the late potentials, the main portion of the complex exceeds the vertical range and is cut off or clipped. Investigation of late potentials centers around the magnitude and duration of the signals generated by the delayed depolarization of a portion of the myocardium. The areas of interest in the SAECG are the following:

1. Duration of the filtered QRS complex (QRSD), which is indicative of how long the completion of the QRS is delayed by late potentials.[15]
2. Amount of energy in the late potentials as given by the root mean square (RMS) voltage in the terminal 40 ms of the QRS complex (RMS40).[15]
3. Duration of the late potentials as indicated by the duration of the low-amplitude signals of less than 40 μV in the terminal QRS region (LAS40).[15,17]

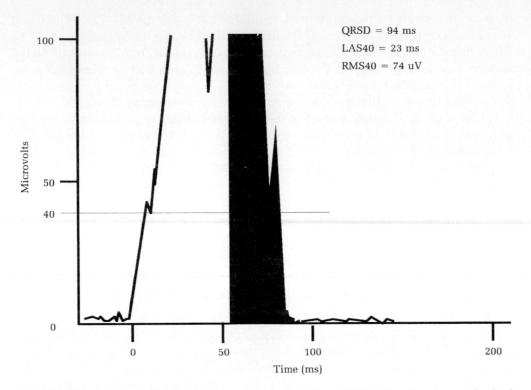

Fig. 30-1. Signal-averaged ECG depicting a normal subject. *QRSD,* The duration of the high-frequency QRS; *LAS40,* the duration of low-amplitude signals of less than 40 μV; *RMS40,* the root mean square voltage of the last 40 ms of the complex *(shaded area).*

The preceding values either can be read from the SAECG itself or can be derived by the computer system.

In Fig. 30-1 the time base starts at the onset of the filtered QRS, and the QRSD is 94 ms. The shaded portion defines the final 40 ms of the complex. RMS40 is computed from this portion of the complex. The duration of the low-amplitude signals (LAS40) is the interval from the intersection of the 40-μV line and falling edge of the QRS to the termination of the filtered QRS complex.

Defining a late potential and scoring an SAECG as normal or abnormal are highly dependent on technique. Although a consensus among investigators has yet to emerge, representative criteria for 40-Hz filtering are that late potentials exist when the filtered QRS complex is longer than 114 to 120 ms, when there is less than 20 μV RMS of signal in the terminal 40 ms of the filtered QRS, or when the terminal portion of the filtered QRS remains below 40 μV for longer than 38 ms.[1,6,15,21] Different criteria are used to enhance sensitivity or specificity, usually one at the expense of the other.[22] The criteria are altered if bundle branch block is present, and frequency domain analysis may be preferred.[23,24] Fig. 30-2 depicts an abnormal SAECG with late potentials present.

FREQUENCY DOMAIN ANALYSIS OF THE SIGNAL-AVERAGED ECG

Analysis of the SAECG using the frequency domain offers a different way of displaying the ECG, one in which it mathematically is broken into its component

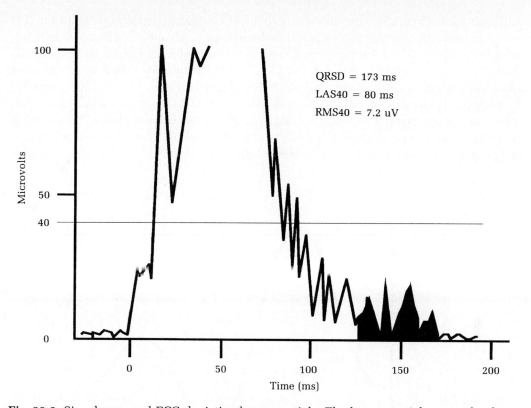

QRSD = 173 ms

LAS40 = 80 ms

RMS40 = 7.2 uV

Fig. 30-2. Signal-averaged ECG depicting late potentials. The late potentials cause the duration QRSD to be lengthened; a substantial portion of the increase is caused by the slowly decaying low-level signals in LAS40. The energy level in RMS40 is now composed of low-level signals and contains much less energy. *QRSD,* The duration of the high-frequency QRS; *LAS40,* the duration of low-amplitude signals less than 40 μV; *RMS40,* the root mean square voltage of the last 40 ms of the complex *(shaded area).*

frequencies, allowing the contributions of the individual frequencies to be examined.

Any continuous time domain waveform, for example, an idealized ECG, is composed of a series of sinusoidal components. This series consists of a fundamental frequency and a series of harmonics whose frequencies are integer multiples of the fundamental. The process usually used to accomplish the transformation from the time domain to the frequency domain is the fast Fourier transform (FFT). Frequency domain analysis plots the amplitude of the fundamental and its harmonics against frequency. The resulting display of information offers new insights into the SAECG.

In the same manner that a rainbow spreads the component color spectrum of sunlight across the sky, a frequency domain ECG spreads the constituent frequencies along the horizontal axis. Frequency domain plots are often referred to as *spectral plots* and are the spectrum of the time domain waveform. As would be expected, there is a certain mirror relationship between the time domain and the frequency domain.

Frequency domain

In the time domain ECG, events happening at different times are easy to discern. But events containing different frequencies occurring at the same time are very difficult to distinguish. The time domain SAECG attempts to compensate for this shortcoming through the use of filters, which tend to eliminate the undesired frequencies. These filters introduce artifacts that must be understood in reading the SAECG. In the frequency domain SAECG, events containing different frequencies occurring at the same time are easily discriminated; however, those of the same frequency but happening at different times pose a problem. Just as a filter is used in the time domain to reject signals occurring at unwanted frequencies, a "window" is used in the frequency domain to reject part of the waveform that occurs at unwanted times and select those occurring in the desired time slot. Fig. 30-3 depicts an arbi-

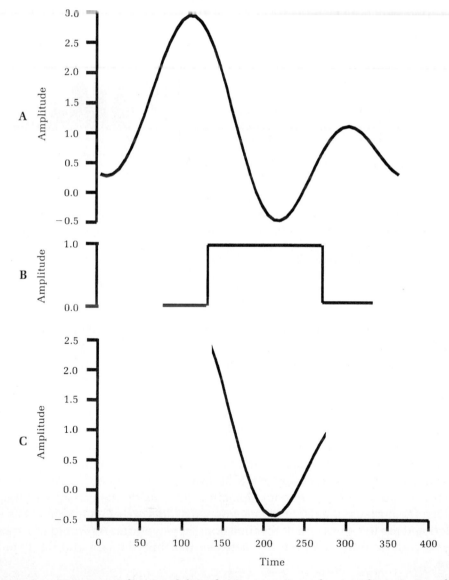

Fig. 30-3. A unity gain window used for selecting a section of a waveform **A,** An arbitrary waveform; **B,** a unity data window positioned to select a segment of the top waveform in **A. C,** The selected result. The window can be lengthened or shortened and moved horizontally to select the desired portion of the waveform.

trary waveform, a unity data window, and the portion of the waveform selected by the window. As the filter introduces some distortion in the time domain, so does the window in the frequency domain.

Methodology

Frequency analysis is performed using the signal-averaged inputs derived from Frank X, Y, and Z leads, although other corrected or uncorrected leads are used. Sampling rates of 1 kHz or greater are typically used. To eliminate filtering artifacts, the inputs are either unfiltered or filtered only to remove extremely low (less than 0.5 Hz) and extremely high (greater than 450 Hz) frequencies. Existing as an array of numbers in a computer, the ECG can be displayed, scaled, and manipulated. By positioning the cursor window over the desired part of the waveform, the

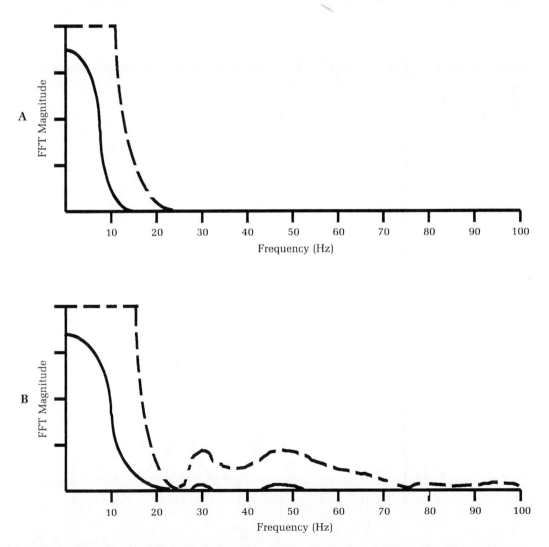

Fig. 30-4. Representative frequency domain tracings. **A,** A normal subject. **B,** The presence of high-frequency potentials is demonstrated. The dashed curve is a magnification ×10 of the solid curve. Evaluation of the fast Fourier transform *(FFT)* of an ECG is based on the areas or ratio of areas under the curve for different frequency ranges and the frequency and magnitude of peaks.

operator can make spectral plots of the entire QRS complex or any part of it. The terminal 40 ms of the QRS complex and the ST segment are of greatest interest. Once the window is positioned and its length set, either manually or under computer control, the computer calculates the FFT and displays the frequency domain tracing. Because the degree of late potential activity is indicated by the energy in the high-frequency components, the frequency domain tracing often shows the magnitude squared (power is proportional to the square of the voltage), giving the power spectrum. Fig. 30-4 shows a representative FFT tracing.

One of the basic assumptions made in using the FFT on a portion of any waveform is that the signal is continuous; that is, the start point and end point of the signal are at the same level. If this is not the case, false frequency responses will be produced in the FFT. To reduce these errors, window-shaping functions such as

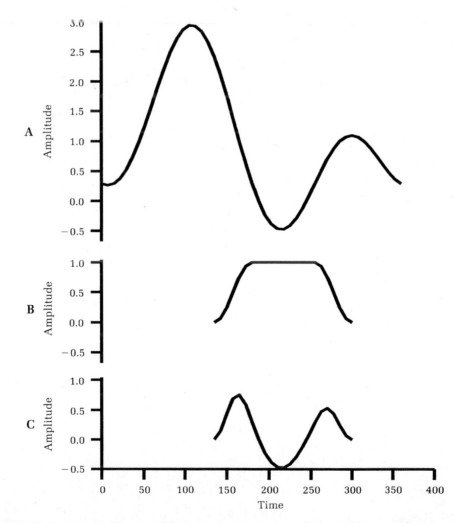

Fig. 30-5. A shaped window used for selecting a portion of a waveform. **A,** The same waveform as shown in Fig. 30-3. **B,** A shaped window. (The slope of the sides is exaggerated for illustration; each slope usually is only about 10% of the total window length.) **C,** The result of a sample-by-sample multiplication of the waveform **A** by the window. Portions of **A** that fall under the sloped sides are severely attenuated.

Blackman-Harris are used to smooth the data to zero at the boundaries and reduce the false side lobes. Fig. 30-5 depicts the use of a shaped window to reduce edge discontinuities.

Shaped windows can reduce the high frequencies in the ECG and, if the sloped edge of the window is positioned over the late potentials, severely attenuate them. The spectral resolution is related solely to the reciprocal of the length of the window. A window length of 100 ms provides a frequency resolution of 1/0.100 sec or 10 Hz. The fundamental will be 10 Hz, and the harmonics will be 20, 30, and 40 Hz and so forth. Longer windows provide greater resolution and vise-versa. But it must be kept in mind that short windows, in addition to having poorer resolution, attenuate more of the signal with the sloped sides of the window. Each point in the FFT algorithm accepts one point (a point being one sample) of the ECG complex. A commonly used FFT is one of 512 points, which accommodates up to a 512-ms window at a 1-kHz sample rate. However, the windows chosen are usually much shorter, and the remaining unfilled points are filled with zeros. The selection of the length and position of the window can have a great effect on the results of tests on the same data. In a patient with anterior wall MI and recurrent ventricular tachycardia (VT) Kelen et al.[25] have shown that a small change in the boundary of the analyzed segment, in the order of 10 ms, can result in changes in the area ratio of several hundred percent. Some researchers have conducted FFT analysis over the entire cardiac cycle.[26]

Interpreting the frequency domain signal-averaged ECG

The interpretation of the frequency domain SAECG is highly subject to technique. However, a common thread runs through the evaluation criteria, in that they evaluate the amount of high frequency energy present, usually by means of an area ratio. This is the ratio of area of the high-frequency portion of the spectrum divided by the total area of the spectrum. The definition of what the high-frequency spectrum comprises varies according to the individual researcher.[27] Pierce et al.[18] used the ratio of the area between 60 and 120 Hz to that of 0 to 120 Hz; while Cain et al.[28] relied on the ratio of the region of 20 to 50 Hz to the area of 10 to 50 Hz. The area ratio of the 40- to 120-Hz to the 0- to 120-Hz regions was used by Kinoshita et al.[29] In addition to the area ratios, some researchers also consider the frequency peaks.[28]

The Fourier transform analysis is a powerful tool, and the implications of its usefulness are still evolving. Research in the field is moving rapidly, but repeatable criteria for distinguishing risk are still emerging.[30] The use of the FFT requires that the researcher, and eventually the clinician, be aware of the limitations of this technique.

OTHER ANALYTIC METHODS

The analytic methods previously described have been combined in various configurations to improve screening accuracy. Among these methods are the following:

1. *Spectral temporal mapping* displays both time and frequency information in a three-dimensional plot. The plot is generated by dividing the ST segment into 20 to 30 segments. Each of the segments is of the same length (typically 80 ms) but starts a few milliseconds later than the previous segment. By stepping the window through each of these segments, the frequency components of each segment are computed using the FFT. The data are then

displayed as a three-dimensional surface map with amplitude on the vertical axis, frequency on the horizontal axis, and time on the Z axis.[31,32]

2. *Large electrode arrays.* Studies have been made using ensemble-averaging techniques on body map arrays of electrodes.[33-35] In these studies 28 to 87 body leads were used to gather ECG data. The data were then signal-averaged to reduce noise and evaluated. Tests in dogs have shown that the results of the body map array SAECG correlate more closely to the epicardial measurements than do the results of the standard three-lead SAECG.[34]

3. *Multivariate analysis.* Multivariate analysis statistically combines several factors that may affect the accuracy of determining risk factors. The factors combined are time domain SAECG, frequency domain SAECG, age, infarct location, number of diseased coronary vessels, left ventricular ejection fraction, infarct-related coronary artery patency, treatment received, delay between admission and SAECG recording, and delay between admission and coronary angiography.[32,36-38]

SUMMARY

Sophisticated techniques from the radar and communication disciplines such as signal averaging, digital filtering, and the FFT are being applied to the analysis of the ECG. These tools allow the researcher and diagnostician to examine portions of the ECG that were previously obscured by noise and artifacts. As the subject of the bulk of the clinical studies, the time domain signal-averaged ECG has emerged as an important tool in the evaluation of late potentials. Although the techniques and standards are still evolving, the time domain and frequency domain SAECGs alone or in combination with other tests and factors provide noninvasive tests to identify those MI patients at risk of sustained VT or sudden death.[39-41]

REFERENCES

1. Simson MB: Signal-averaged electrocardiography. In Zipes DP, Jalife J, eds: *Cardiac electrophysiology from cell to bedside,* ed 2, Philadelphia, 1995, WB Saunders.

2. Steinberg JS, Regan A, Sciacca RR et al: Predicting arrhythmic events after acute myocardial infarction using the signal-averaged electrocardiogram, *Am J Cardiol* 69:13, 1992.

3. Simson MB: Noninvasive identification of patients at risk for sudden cardiac death, *Circulation* 85(suppl 1):1, 1992.

4. Lindsay BD, Ambos HD, Schechtman KB et al: Noninvasive detection of patients with ischemic and nonischemic heart disease prone to ventricular fibrillation, *J Am Coll Cardiol* 16:1656, 1990.

5. Klein H, Karp RB, Kouchoukos NT et al: Intraoperative electrophysiologic mapping of the ventricles during sinus rhythm in patients with previous myocardial infarction: identification of the electrophysiologic substrate of ventricular arrhythmias, *Circulation* 66:847, 1982.

6. Simson MB, Untereker WJ, Spielman SR et al: The relationship between late potentials on the body surface and directly recorded fragmented electrograms in patients with ventricular tachycardia, *Am J Cardiol* 51:659, 1983.

7. Hombach V: The high-resolution electrocardiogram: clinical aspects. In El-Sherif N, Samet P, eds: *Cardiac pacing and electrophysiology,* ed 3, Philadelphia, 1991, WB Saunders.

8. Stelling JA, Danford DA, Kugler JD et al: Late potentials and inducible ventricular tachycardia in surgically repaired congenital heart disease, *Circulation* 82:1690, 1990.

9. Vacek JL, Wilson DB, Botteron GW et al: Techniques for the determination of left ventricular mass by signal-averaged electrocardiography, *Am Heart J* 120:958, 1990.

10. Leor MD, Hod H, Rotstein Z et al: Effects of thrombolysis on the 12-lead signal-averaged ECG in the early postinfarction period, *Am Heart J* 120:495, 1990.

11. Zimmermann M et al: Reduction in the frequency of ventricular late potentials after acute myocardial infarction by early thrombolytic therapy, *Am J Cardiol* 67:697, 1991.

12. Moreno FLL, Karagounis L, Marshall H et al: Thrombolysis-related early patency reduces ECG late potentials after acute myocardial infarction, *Am Heart J* 124:557, 1992.

13. El-Sherif N, Restivo M, Craelius W et al: The high-resolution electrocardiogram: technical and basic aspects. In El-Sherif N, Samet P, eds: *Cardiac pacing and electrophysiology*, ed 3, Philadelphia, 1991, WB Saunders.

14. Flowers NC, Shvartsman V, Kennelly BM et al: Surface recording of His-Purkinje activity on an every-beat basis without digital averaging, *Circulation* 63:948, 1981.

15. Breithardt G, Cain ME, El-Sherif N et al: Standards for analysis of ventricular late potentials using high-resolution or signal-averaged electrocardiography: a statement by a task force committee of the European Society of Cardiology, the American Heart Association, and the American College of Cardiology, *J Am Coll Cardiol* 17:999, 1991.

16. Ros HH, Koeleman ASM, Akker TJ: The technique of signal averaging and its practical application in the separation of atrial and His-Purkinje activity. In Hombach V, Hilger HH, eds: *Signal averaging technique in clinical cardiology*, New York, 1981, FK Schattauer Verlag.

17. Vatterott PF, Vailey KR, Hammill SC: Improving the predictive ability of the signal-averaged electrocardiogram with a linear logistic model incorporating clinical variables, *Circulation* 81:797, 1990.

18. Pierce DL, Easley AR, Windle JR, Engel TR: Fast Fourier transformation of the entire low amplitude late QRS potential to predict ventricular tachycardia, *J Am Coll Cardiol* 14:1731, 1989.

19. Nalos PC, Gang ES, Mandel WJ et al: Utility of the signal-averaged electrocardiogram in patients presenting with sustained ventricular tachycardia or fibrillation while on an antiarrhythmic drug, *Am Heart J* 115:108, 1988.

20. El-Sherif N, Ursell SN, Bekheit S et al: Prognostic significance of the signal-averaged ECG depends on the time of recording in the postinfarction period, *Am Heart J* 118:256, 1989.

21. Hood MA, Pogwizd SM, Peirick J, Cain ME: Contribution of myocardium responsible for ventricular tachycardia to abnormalities detected by analysis of signal-averaged ECGs, *Circulation* 86:1888, 1992.

22. Lander P, Barbari EJ, Rajagopalan CV: Critical analysis of the signal-averaged electrocardiogram, *Circulation* 87:105, 1993.

23. Buckingham TA, Lingle A, Greenwalt T et al: Power law analysis of the signal-averaged electrocardiogram for identification of patients with ventricular tachycardia: effect of bundle branch block, *Am Heart J* 124:1220, 1992.

24. Fontaine JM, Rao R, Henkin R: Study of the influence of left bundle branch block on the signal-averaged electrocardiogram: a qualitative and quantitative analysis, *Am Heart J* 121:494, 1991.

25. Kelen GJ, Henkin R, Fontaine JM et al: Effects of analyzed signal duration and phase on the results of fast Fourier transform analysis of the surface electrocardiogram in subjects with and without late potentials, *Am J Cardiol* 60:1282, 1987.

26. Cain ME, Ambos HD, Markham J et al: Diagnostic implications of spectral and temporal analysis of the entire cardiac cycle in patients with ventricular tachycardia, *Circulation* 83:1637, 1991.

27. Malik M, Kulakowski P, Poloniecki J et al: Frequency versus time domain analysis of signal-averaged electrocardiograms. I. Reproducibility of the results, *J Am Coll Cardiol* 20:127, 1992.

28. Cain ME, Lindsay BD, Arthur RM et al: Noninvasive detection of patients prone to life-threatening ventricular arrhythmias by frequency analysis of electrocardiographic signals. In Zipes DP, Jalife J, eds: *Cardiac electrophysiology*, Philadelphia, 1990, WB Saunders.

29. Kinoshita O, Kamakura S, Ohe T et al: Spectral analysis of signal-averaged electrocardiograms in patients with idiopathic ventricular tachycardia of left ventricular origin, *Circulation* 85:2054, 1992.

30. Engel TR, Pierce DL, Patil KD: Reproducibility of the signal-averaged electrocardiogram, *Am Heart J* 122:1652, 1991.

31. McClements BM, Adgey AAJ: Value of signal-averaged electrocardiography, radionuclide ventriculography, Holter monitoring and clinical variables for prediction of arrhythmic events in the survivors of acute myocardial infarction in the thrombolytic era, *J Am Coll Cariol* 21:1419, 1993.

32. Steinberg JS, Prystowsky E, Freedman RA: Use of the signal-averaged electrocardiogram for predicting inducible ventricular-tachycardia in patients with unexplained syncope: relation to clinical variables in a multivariate analysis, *J Am Coll Cardiol* 23:99, 1994.

33. Ho DSW, Denniss RA, Uther JB: Signal-averaged electrocardiogram: improved identification of patients with ventricular tachycardia using a 28-lead optimal array, *Circulation* 87:857, 1993.

34. Freedman RA, Fuller MS, Greenberg GM et al: Detection and localization of prolonged epicardial electrograms with 64-lead body surface signal-averaged electrocardiography, *Circulation* 84:871, 1991.

35. Shibata T, Kubota I, Ikeda K et al: Body surface mapping of high-frequency components in the terminal portion during QRS complex for the prediction of ventricular tachycardia in patients with previous myocardial infarction, *Circulation* 82:2084, 1990.

36. Shin HH, Sagar KB, Stepniakowski K et al: Increased prevalence of abnormal signal-averaged electrocardiograms in older patients who have hypertension with low diastolic blood pressure, *Am Heart J* 125:1698, 1993.

37. De Chillou C, Sadoul N, Briançon S, Aliot E: Factors determining the occurrence of late potentials on the signal-averaged electrocardiogram after a first myocardial infarction: a multivariate analysis, *J Am Coll Cardiol* 18:1638, 1991.

38. Nogami A, Iesaka Y, Akiyama J et al: Combined use of time and frequency domain variables in signal-averaged ECG as a predictor of inducible sustained monomorphic ventricular tachycardia in myocardial infarction, *Circulation* 86:780, 1992.

39. Elami A, Merin G, Flugelman MY: Usefulness of late potentials on the immediate postoperative signal-averaged electrocardiogram in pre-dicting ventricular tachyarrhythmias early after isolated coronary artery bypass grafting, *Am J Cardiol* 74:33, 1994.

40. Turitto G, Ahuja RK, Caref EB, El-Sherif N: Risk stratification for arrhythmic events in patients with nonischemic dilated cardiomyopathy and nonsustained ventricular tachycardia: role of programmed ventricular stimulation and the signal-averaged electrocardiogram, *J Am Coll Cardiol* 24:1523, 1994.

41. Guidera SA, Steinbert JS: The signal-averaged P wave duration: a rapid and noninvasive marker of risk of atrial fibrillation, *J Am Coll Cardiol* 21:1645, 1993.

C H A P T E R

31

Electrical Stimulation Therapies

JOHN R. BUYSMAN PhD

Organization of Arrhythmias with Respect
  to Electrical Therapies   *479*
Goals of Electrical Therapies   *479*
Electrical Therapies for Bradycardia   *480*
Electrical Therapies for Tachycardias

Resulting from Cellular
  Abnormalities   *481*
Electrical Therapies for Tachycardia
  Resulting from Reentrant Loops   *482*
Acknowledgment   *490*

All natural cardiac rhythms and arrhythmias result from ion currents within and between cardiac cells; thus the rhythms and arrhythmias can be altered, driven, or terminated by the application of electrical energy. A wide variety of electrical antiarrhythmic therapy devices have been developed to exploit these effects.

ORGANIZATION OF ARRHYTHMIAS WITH RESPECT TO ELECTRICAL THERAPIES

Table 31-1 organizes the known arrhythmogenic mechanisms (atrioventricular [AV] conduction failure, abnormal automaticity, triggered activity, and reentry) in a manner that facilitates visualizing how they are affected by artificial electrical stimulations. The normal electrical activity of the heart and arrhythmogenic mechanisms have already been discussed in Chapters 2 and 5.

GOALS OF ELECTRICAL THERAPIES

Since ventricular pumping is crucial for life, the most important therapeutic goal is to preserve, restore, or create useful ventricular rhythms. Atrial rhythms are

Table 31-1. Relationship of common arrhythmias to basic arrhythmic mechanisms

General problem	Specific problem	Typical problem location	Corresponding rhythm	Systemic result
AV conduction failure	Block	AV node, bundle of His, or Purkinje system	Heart block	Bradycardia
Abnormal cellular electrophysiology	Automaticity: too slow	Atria	Sinus bradycardia	Bradycardia
	Automaticity: too fast	Atria	Atrial tachycardia	Tachycardia
		AV node, junction	Junctional tachycardia	Tachycardia
		Ventricle	Ventricular tachycardia	Tachycardia
	Triggered activity	Atria	Atrial tachycardia	Tachycardia
		Ventricle	Ventricular tachycardia	Tachycardia
Reentry	Small-loop reentry in a single mass	Atria	Atrial tachycardia	Tachycardia
		AV junction	Junctional PSVT	Tachycardia
		Ventricle	Ventricular tachycardia	Tachycardia
	Large-loop reentry in a single mass	Atria	Atrial flutter	Tachycardia
		Ventricle	Ventricular flutter	Tachycardia
	Meandering or multiloop reentry in a single mass	Atria	Atrial fibrillation	Tachycardia
		Ventricle	Ventricular fibrillation	Tachycardia
	Atrioventricular loop	Atria and ventricle	AV reciprocation PSVT	Tachycardia

AV, Atrioventricular; *PSVT,* paroxysmal supraventricular tachycardia.

not usually critical to life if the ventricular rhythm is supported. However, useful atrial rhythms are highly important to cardiac performance factors affecting quality of life.

ELECTRICAL THERAPIES FOR BRADYCARDIA

The most common way to treat the bradyarrhythmias is to use artificial cardiac pacemakers. Artificial pacemakers apply tiny electrical shocks (stimuli) to the atria or ventricle, or both, at a desired rate and sequence, to cause them to contract at the rate and sequence. Each atrial stimulus produces a single atrial contraction, and each ventricular stimulus produces a single ventricular contraction.

The electrical stimuli are produced by an electronic device called a pulse generator and are conveyed to the heart via insulated wires called leads. At the cardiac end of each lead there is an exposed contact called the electrode, which touches the heart and conveys the stimulus into the cardiac cells nearby (Fig. 31-1). The electrical potential of the stimulus overwhelms the natural electrical potential of these cells, altering their membrane permeabilities, which in turn allows rapid influx of sodium, which produces depolarization. The depolarization then spreads by cell-to-cell conduction throughout the entire mass of cardiac tissue, causing the mass to contract.

New pacing methods are being continually developed for treating bradyarrhythmias, adding to an existing large volume of pacing methods for treating bradyarrhythmias. Because the combined volume of these methods is large, these methods are presented in Chapter 32.

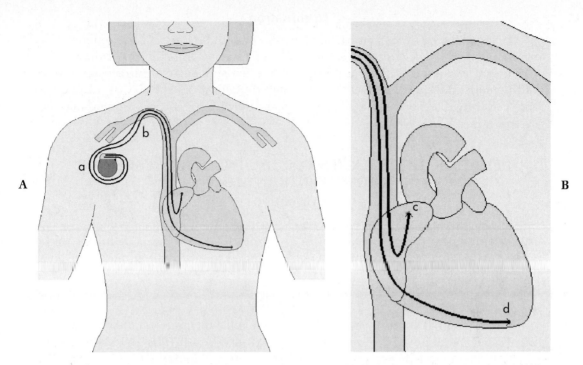

Fig. 31-1. Example showing use of a pacemaker to treat bradyarrhythmia. **A,** An implantable pulse generator *(a)* produces tiny electric pulses, which are conveyed to the heart by leads *(b).* Many systems employ two leads as shown here, one to pace the atria and another to pace the ventricle. **B,** At the tip of each lead (*c* and *d*) an electrode delivers the pulses to adjacent cardiac cells and depolarizes them. Depolarization then spreads by cell-to-cell conduction through the atrial and ventricular masses.

ELECTRICAL THERAPIES FOR TACHYCARDIAS RESULTING FROM CELLULAR ABNORMALITIES

Electrical therapies used for tachycardia of cellular origin are mainly electrical therapies of prevention, since electrical therapies for the termination of these tachycardias are crude and incidental.

Prevention

Some tachycardias are initiated by transient bradycardia. Pacing to prevent the bradycardia helps prevent the tachycardia.

Some drug therapies that control tachycardia may produce bradycardia, which renders the therapy impractical. Pacing can prevent the bradycardia, allowing the drug therapy to be used. Pacing, however, can mask signs of impending drug-induced ventricular proarrhythmia; thus caution is required in this application.

Excitable tissue that is mildly unstable can sometimes be stabilized by pacing the tissue at a cycle length less than its natural cycle length. This is known as *overdrive suppression.*

In many patients ablation of the offending cells can provide a lifelong cure and may be preferable to electrical stimulation therapies.

In rare cases of nontreatable atrial tachycardia and fast AV conduction, ablation of the AV node can block the conduction and ventricular pacing can be used to support the ventricular rate.

Termination

In emergencies of last resort, tachycardia of cellular origin can sometimes be terminated with high-energy electrical shocks from a defibrillator. Although the mechanism is not defibrillation, it appears that the shock can stun or upset the offending cells, altering their behavior for better or for worse. This use of massive force certainly lacks therapeutic eloquence and specificity, but it is sometimes successful.

ELECTRICAL THERAPIES FOR TACHYCARDIA RESULTING FROM REENTRANT LOOPS
Prevention

All the previously described preventive methods that calm excitable tissues can also be applied to prevent reentrant tachycardia. When the loop pathway can be located and is accessible, ablation may be preferred to electrical stimulation therapies.

Termination

For any loop to continue to propagate, there must be nonrefractory tissue available so that the depolarizing wavefront can advance into it. The key electrical termination therapies all work by artificially initiating depolarization of the tissue ahead of the advancing offending wavefront so that when the offending wavefront encounters the depolarized tissue, it will stop. After the tissues repolarize, it is hoped that a more normal depolarization pattern will spontaneously appear. To be successful, the artificially initiated depolarization must not initiate any new loops; otherwise the original offending loop will just be replaced by a new offending loop.

Historically, therapies developed along two approaches: the use of high-energy electrical shocks applied across the chest and the use of tiny, critically timed stimuli composed of pacing pulses that are applied directly to the heart.

High-energy shock therapies. The therapy of high-energy shocks was initially based on the concept that if all the cells in the heart could be depolarized simultaneously, there would be no nonrefractory tissue available to propagate the offending wavefront; hence the arrhythmia would terminate.

Since an artificially applied electrical potential can disturb the cell membranes of excitable cells, causing them to depolarize, a large electrical shock applied to the entire heart can depolarize the entire heart. Depolarization of the entire heart was initially accomplished by externally applying large electrodes onto the patient's chest and then delivering through them an enormous electrical shock from a bulky electrical apparatus. Although such devices could terminate all reentry tachycardia, they were mostly used to terminate fibrillation and so became known as defibrillators.

It later became apparent that it is not necessary to depolarize the entire heart; depolarizing just enough mass to prevent the wavefront from spreading is all that is needed. This concept is known as the *critical mass hypothesis.* Alternate hypotheses have been proposed—and some have merit—but the critical mass hypothesis is most commonly cited.

During a tachycardia, at any instant in time, part of the mass is depolarized (reverse-polarized and refractory) and part is nonrefractory (polarized). To terminate the tachycardia, it is necessary only to artificially depolarize the nonrefractory locations, since the rest is already depolarized. Of course, at any location the states of depolarization and nonrefractoriness are constantly varying, so this is not easy to do selectively. However, two distinctions can be made:

If the depolarization pattern is chaotic and has multiple loops, the locations of nonrefractory regions at any instant are unpredictable, so to ensure that all locations are reached, large shocks are required.

If the depolarization pattern is a well organized single-loop tachycardia, at any particular moment in each cycle a single location is nonrefractory while the rest of the mass is refractory. A smaller shock applied to a portion of the heart and synchronized to strike just at the moment when that portion is nonrefractory can depolarize that portion and prevent reentry into it and terminate the tachycardia. The concept of synchronizing a shock to the offending rhythm is called *cardioversion.**

In rare instances cardioversion may initiate new loops and cause fibrillation. Therefore cardioversion should be employed only by means of devices that also have high-energy shock capabilities so that if fibrillation should occur, a high-energy shock can be immediately delivered to terminate the fibrillation.

Automatic implantable cardioverter-defibrillator. In the 1970s the miniaturization of electronic components made possible an implantable device that monitored the ventricle and, when tachycardia was detected, automatically provided a high-energy shock to the heart. This device was known as the automatic implantable defibrillator, and a later version was known as the automatic implantable cardioverter-defibrillator (AICD). The device was typically implanted in the abdomen. Two small electrodes for sensing the electrical activity of the heart were attached to the ventricle to monitor the ventricular intervals. Two large patch electrodes were placed on the ventricles to deliver the high-energy shock (Fig. 31-2).

When a rapid tachycardia occurred, the depolarization wavefronts passed beneath the sensing electrodes at a high rate with short intervals. As each wave passed, it produced in the sensing electrodes a small electrical signal that was conducted by the leads to the electronic unit. The electronics analyzed the signals, and when the analysis indicated sustained tachycardia, the device delivered a high-energy shock. The shock was approximately 700 V and lasted for 5 to 8 ms.†

About 1990, transvenous leads with special high-voltage electrodes and sensing electrodes were developed. These are preferable to patch electrodes because the implant procedure for transvenous leads does not require thoracotomy.

Critically timed stimulation therapies (antitachycardia stimulation, also called antitachycardia pacing [ATP]). Antitachycardia stimulation therapy is based on the concept that in a single-loop tachycardia, any given location in the path becomes momentarily nonrefractory as the loop rotates. If during this brief moment the loca-

*The term *cardioversion* has had several definitions over many years, including (1) any method used to terminate a tachycardia; (2) any method using electrical shocks to terminate a tachycardia; (3) a method for terminating atrial flutter or fibrillation in which the shock is synchronized to occur during a ventricular depolarization (it is assumed that this method is less likely to trigger a ventricular arrhythmia); and (4) a method for synchronizing a shock to a regular tachycardia to terminate the tachycardia.

†High-energy shocks are customarily measured in Joules (J). External defibrillators deliver up to 360 J to the chest; about 10% to 20% of this amount reaches the heart. Automatic implantable cardioverter-defibrillators typically deliver directly to the heart 10 to 35 J for defibrillation and 0.1 to 10 J for cardioversion. All these shocks are painful, but fortunately they are very brief. By comparison, pacing stimuli are typically 0.000005 to 0.000025 J and are imperceptible.

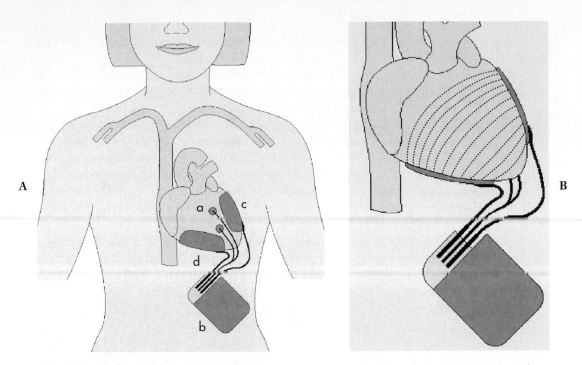

Fig. 31-2. Sketch of an automatic implantable cardioverter defibrillator (AICD). **A,** Cardiac signals are picked up by two small electrodes *(a)* and conveyed to the electronic device *(b),* where they are used to monitor the ventricular intervals. When fast tachycardia or fibrillation is detected, the device delivers a high-energy shock to two large, patchlike electrodes (*c* and *d*) placed on opposite sides of the heart. **B,** The manner in which the high-energy electrical field *(dotted lines)* between the patch electrodes stimulates a critical mass of the ventricles is shown.

Recently, the use of special transvenous leads for cardioversion and defibrillation has become more common than the use of patch electrodes; patches are now used only for special circumstances.

tion can be depolarized by a therapeutic action, the looping depolarization cannot enter it and the loop will terminate.

To apply this therapy, a pacing electrode is placed in or on the heart, and small electrical stimuli—essentially pacing pulses—are used to initiate depolarizations that can invade a small location in the path of the loop during the moment when that location is nonrefractory (Fig. 31-3). At least one invading depolarization must reach the loop simultaneously with the appearance of the nonrefractoriness. The timing is critical, since the invading depolarization must collide with the leading edge of the looping depolarization to terminate the loop, yet not start a new loop where the terminating loop is repolarizing.

Usually the stimulating electrode is some distance from the loop. Depolarizations spreading outward from the loop make this pacing site refractory much of the time, limiting the chances for therapeutic stimuli to start a depolarization. To overcome this limitation, a train of stimuli is applied at a fast rate, usually about 20% to 25% above the tachycardia rate, for several seconds. This is known as burst pacing. The first few paces may occur during refractoriness, but soon a pace occurs during nonrefractoriness and initiates a depolarization that spreads outward from the pacing site. This depolarization does not travel far toward the loop before it is blocked by a depolarization radiating from the loop; however, it also blocks the de-

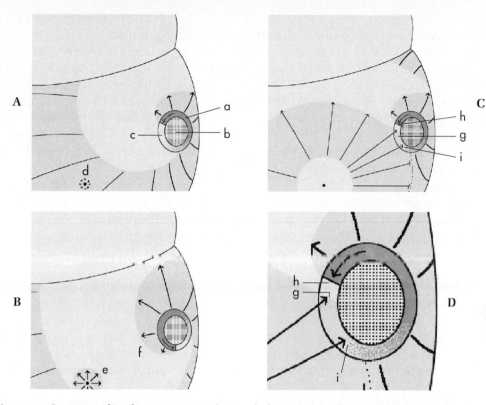

Fig. 31-3. Conceptualized termination of a single-loop reentry by antitachycardia pacing. **A,** Reentry loop *(a)* circles an anatomic obstacle *(b).* There is a region of repolarized tissue *(c)* that rotates as part of the loop. Stimuli are introduced through an electrode at a site *(d).* In this sketch the stimulus is unable to stimulate the tissue because the tissue is refractory *(medium shading).* **B,** Several cycles later a stimulus occurs when the tissue is nonrefractory *(light shading)* and initiates a new depolarization radiating outward *(e)* from the electrode site. This depolarization will collide with the depolarization *(f)* coming from the loop. This collision blocks the depolarization that is coming from the loop from reaching the pacing site and resetting the site; thus the pacing site will respond to the next pacing stimulus. Since the pacing rate is faster than the looping rate, this step will repeat again and again and the paced depolarizations will gain additional distance toward the loop with each succeeding cycle. **C,** Eventually, paced depolarizations reach the loop. After several more cycles the loop becomes nonrefractory at the location where the paced depolarization arrives (shown here and in enlargement, **D**), and the paced depolarization will enter the loop. **D,** The paced depolarization *(g)* will collide with the looping depolarization *(h)* and terminate the loop. It is hoped that the paced depolarization will react favorably with repolarizing tissue *(i)* of the loop so that another loop is not started in the same path.

polarization that is radiating from the loop from spreading to the pacing site and resetting the pacing site. After this event tissue around the electrode is driven by the pacing train, and each subsequent pace initiates a new paced depolarization. Since the rate of the paced depolarizations is faster than the rate of depolarizations from the loop, each successive paced depolarization travels a little farther toward the loop than the previous one, blocking the depolarizations from the loop. Eventually, paced depolarizations reach the loop, but they may not arrive coincident with the nonrefractoriness of the loop. However, since the depolarizations are reaching the loop at a rate slightly faster than the rotation rate of the loop, after several more cycles the nonrefractoriness of the loop will coincide with the arrival of a paced depolarization, invasion will occur, and the loop will terminate.

When the loop terminates, only the depolarizations from pacing remain. Since this rhythm is not looping, when the burst pacing stops, a natural, normal rhythm usually begins. Since the sinoatrial node may exhibit the phenomenon of overdrive suppression (either because of an atrial loop or via ventriculoatrial conduction if the loop is ventricular), a considerable pause may occur before the natural rhythm begins; to prevent this pause, it is customary after the burst to immediately pace at a moderate rate for a short time. This pacing allows the tissue to recover and lessens the chance that some other adverse arrhythmia will emerge.

Oftentimes depolarizations from the burst do not successfully enter the loop but instead only distort the loop. After the burst ends, the distorted loop may revert to the original form and the therapy then fails. More often, however, the distorted loop continues for several cycles and then spontaneously terminates, accomplishing the desired goal (see Tiered therapies and Figs. 31-5 and 31-6).

Sometimes the burst may initiate fibrillation. This is not uncommon in atrial applications, and atrial fibrillation of this cause usually spontaneously terminates in a few seconds to several minutes, accomplishing the desired goal. In ventricular applications initiation of fibrillation in the ventricle is infrequent; however, ventricular fibrillation virtually never terminates spontaneously and is fatal if not immediately terminated by other means. Thus burst pacing in the ventricle may be used only when high-energy shocks are available for ventricular defibrillation (see Tiered therapies and Fig. 31-7).

To improve the chance of termination, modern devices for burst pacing employ a variety of burst-pacing sequences. These devices monitor the natural heart intervals, analyze them, and then automatically select preprogramed burst sequences best suited to terminate the tachycardia. After each burst is applied the result is assessed. If the burst failed, another burst of the same or different design is tried. Some devices automatically select their first burst rate as a preprogramed percentage above the tachycardia rate, some select an increment or decrement rate, some set the number of paces in the burst or the duration of the burst, some modulate the intervals between the paces within the burst, and some adjust the time between successive bursts.

Antitachycardia pacing is quite successful for terminating single-loop tachycardia that has a regular pathway, but it is less satisfactory for multiloop or chaotic tachycardia. Ventricular fibrillation can almost never be terminated by antitachycardia pacing.

Antitachycardia pacemakers. In the 1960s a patient-activated implantable pacing stimulator for antitachycardia use was first available. This device was intended only for atrial applications, because atrial fibrillation, should it be induced, would not likely be life threatening. When the patient felt a tachycardia, he or she used a handheld transmitter to activate the burst pacing. In the 1970s automatic antitachycardia pacemakers were produced for atrial applications. These devices monitored the atria and, when a tachycardia was detected, produced atrial burst-pacing sequences. In the 1980s antitachycardia pacing sequences were added to certain conventional pacemakers, again for atrial applications. In addition, the standard pacemakers produced by some manufacturers for treating bradycardia can in the hospital setting be noninvasively linked to programers to perform complex antitachycardia pacing routines in either the atria or ventricles.

Tiered therapy

About 1990, implantable devices were developed in which a single device provided high-energy shocks, synchronized cardioversion, automated antitachycardia pacing, and conventional ventricular pacing, as needed. Devices with high-energy shock capabilities became generically known as implantable cardioverter-defibrillators or ICDs—a title that belies the important antitachycardia pacing and conventional pacing capabilities included in the newer devices (Fig. 31-4).

Implantable cardioverter-defibrillators that have a full range of automatic antitachycardia therapies, as well as conventional pacing for bradycardia, offer substantial advantages over any one therapy alone. For example, the conventional pacing can provide preventive benefits. Antitachycardia pacing can be used for single-loop reentrant tachycardia. High-energy shocks can be used for cardioversion, defibrillation, and termination of more resistant tachycardia. In addition, conventional pacing can prevent pauses following any tachycardia termination. Antitachycardia pacing and cardioversion can be employed in the ventricle, since, if ventricular fibrillation should occur, a high-energy shock can follow and terminate it. If ventricular flutter or fibrillation occurs for any reason, high-energy shocks can be immediately delivered with priority over other sequences (Figs. 31-5 to 31-9).

Serious natural arrhythmias such as fibrillation sometimes evolve naturally from simple arrhythmias. With multifunction devices the prevention of simple ar-

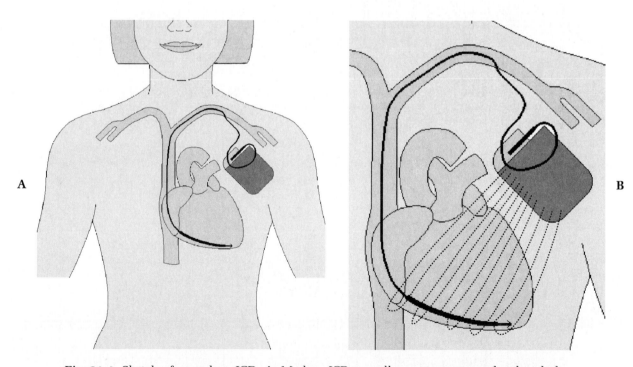

Fig. 31-4. Sketch of a modern ICD. **A,** Modern ICDs usually use transvenously placed electrodes. Two small electrodes at the tip of the lead provide pacing and sensing. The high-voltage shock is delivered between a flexible electrode (approximately 5 cm long) in the ventricle and the metal containment of the electronic device, which serves as the second electrode. **B,** The manner in which the high-energy electrical field *(dotted lines)* between the electrodes stimulates a critical mass of the ventricles.

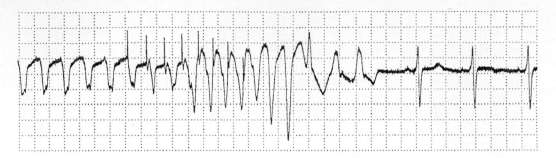

Fig. 31-5. Ventricular tachycardia terminated by antitachycardia pacing. A burst of eight pacing pulses was initially synchronized with the tachycardia and then decreased in interval with each successive pace. The paces modified the reentry path. Although modified reentry continued after the last pace, the new rhythm was not self-sustaining and terminated after several more cycles.

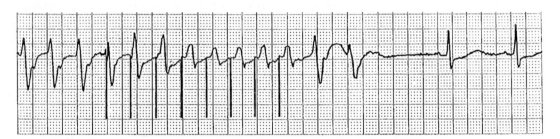

Fig. 31-6. Ventricular tachycardia terminated by antitachycardia pacing. A burst of eight paces modified the tachycardia; changes over the first five paces are evident. After the last pace the tachycardia seemed to reappear, but it was distorted too much to reestablish itself and so it terminated.

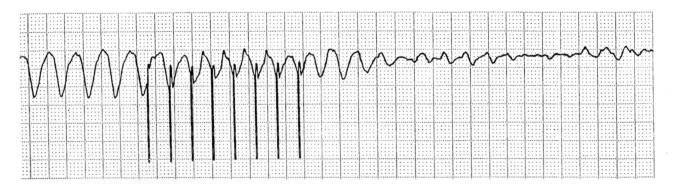

Fig. 31-7. Ventricular tachycardia accelerated by failed antitachycardia pacing. Laboratory demonstration showing a burst of eight paces, which modified the tachycardia into a reentry loop that converted to ventricular fibrillation. The importance of having backup ventricular defibrillation available whenever antitachycardia pacing is used in the ventricle is clear.

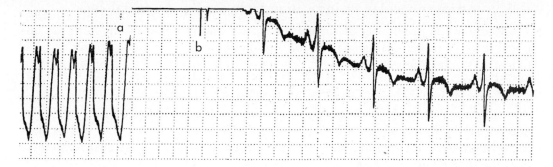

Fig. 31-8. Ventricular tachycardia terminated by cardioversion. A synchronized, low-energy shock of 0.2 J was applied to the ventricle *(a)* and terminated the tachycardia. This ICD also began backup pacing 1000 ms after the shock as can be partially seen off the upper edge of the paper *(b)*. Thereafter the native rate was faster than the pacing rate so sensing inhibited pacing.

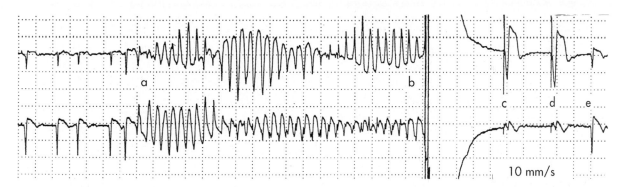

Fig. 31-9. Ventricular fibrillation terminated by high-energy shock. Tape-recorded episode of spontaneous ventricular fibrillation *(a)*. The ICD detected the rhythm and delivered a high-energy shock *(b)*, which terminated the ventricular fibrillation. When a natural rhythm did not return, backup pacing occurred *(c and d)* until a natural rhythm was sensed *(e)*.

rhythmias by pacing or their termination by antitachycardia stimulation helps prevent the emergence of serious arrhythmia, and in turn helps prevent the need for subsequent high-energy shocks. This benefit is highly significant in the ventricle, since avoiding ventricular fibrillation is always desirable. In addition, conventional pacing and antitachycardia pacing is painless, whereas high-energy shocks for cardioversion and defibrillation are very painful, although quick.

Generally the previously discussed devices are programed to respond to simple tachyarrhythmias in a stepwise manner, automatically trying the pacing termination routines first and then increasing in aggressiveness until success is achieved. This is known as *tiered electrical therapy.* Generally these devices are also programed to respond immediately to ventricular flutters and ventricular fibrillation by delivering an immediate high-energy shock, bypassing less aggressive tiers.

As of this writing, ICDs employing AV pacing have been designed but none have been released for sale by any manufacturer. Patients who need ICD therapies and dual-chamber pacing can have both an ICD and a dual-chamber pacemaker, provided these are arranged and programed to avoid adverse device interactions.

Atrioventricular reciprocation tachycardia: A special case

Many of the previously described preventive and termination methods are applicable to AV reciprocating tachycardia, but these methods are seldom used to treat this arrhythmia. Many patients with this arrhythmia now receive a permanent cure by ablation.

Conventional AV pacemakers can also be easily used to block AV reciprocation. If the AV interval is programed to a short value such as 70 ms, ventricular depolarization is forced to follow atrial depolarization so quickly that the ascending retrograde depolarization arrives at the atria while the atria are still refractory; thus the retrograde is blocked.

ACKNOWLEDGMENT

Thank you to Dr. Walter Olson of Medtronic, Inc., for sample ECGs.

C H A P T E R

32

Pacemaker Therapies for Bradycardias

JOHN R. BUYSMAN PhD

Pacing Concept *492*
Stimulation Concepts *492*
Sensing Concepts *494*
Pacemaker Timing *494*
Advanced Pacing *498*
Pacemakers that Provide a Responsive
   Heart Rate *498*
Applications of Advanced Pacing
   Concepts *499*

Retrograde (Ventriculoatrial)
   Conduction *505*
Tracking Limitations Caused by
   Atrioventricular Interval and
   Postventricular Atrial Refractory
   Period *508*
Special Features *513*
Maximizing Atrioventricular Synchrony
   with Ventricular Pacemakers *513*
Obtaining Assistance *514*

P acemakers—electronic devices that can repetitively stimulate depolarizations in cardiac muscle—are the principal therapy for treating bradyarrhythmias. In all bradycardias ventricular rate, at least, must be restored. Thus nearly all pacemaker systems are capable of *directly* pacing the ventricular muscle. In selected patients with *proven reliable conduction,* pacing need only be applied to the atrial muscle.

Atrial pacemakers function solely by stimulating the atria, *ventricular pacemakers* stimulate only the ventricles, and *atrioventricular (AV) pacemakers* can stimulate both the atria and the ventricles. The two former types are *single-chamber pacemakers,* and the latter type is a *dual-chamber pacemaker. Dual* refers to an atrial chamber *and* a ventricular chamber; it does not connote "left" or "right." The term *chamber* extends to include the whole atrial muscle or the whole ventricular muscle, as applicable.

Advanced pacemakers enhance the patient's *quality of life* by using the atria to restore the *AV synchronous sequence* of the heart and by producing a *varying* heart rate that is responsive to *dynamic* cardiac needs.

PACING CONCEPT

Electrical pulses can force cardiac cells to instantly depolarize. Thus to treat bradycardias, electronic pacemakers apply small electrical pulses *(stimuli)* to the atrial or ventricular muscle mass, or both, to trigger these muscle masses to depolarize at just the right moments to produce heartbeats at a desired heart rate and sequence. Each stimulus provokes a single depolarization within the muscle mass to which it is applied. The stimulus need only be applied to a small cluster of cells, since the depolarization there will spread throughout the muscle mass by cell-to-cell conduction.

The stimuli are produced by an electronic *pulse generator* and are delivered to the atrial or ventricular muscle mass, or both, through insulated wires called *leads.* At the cardiac end of each lead there is an exposed electrically conductive *electrode* that makes intimate contact with the cardiac tissue. The stimuli enter the cardiac tissue through this contact.

Stimulus artifacts on the ECG

When the electrical stimulus is delivered, it is usually recorded as a *stimulus artifact,* a "blip" on the ECG. Historically, with older model pacemakers the artifacts were large and obvious. Newer pacemakers now employ narrow pacing pulses, some with special recharge pulses. These are not displayed uniformly on digital ECG monitors and recorders, and some artifacts may be barely visible. Some monitors now employ a "pacemaker detect" feature that detects and replaces the real artifact with a standardized artifact mark.

STIMULATION CONCEPTS
Mechanisms of stimulation

When a pacing pulse appears at the electrode, an electrical field radiates from the electrode, penetrates the excitable cells, and triggers rapid depolarization of a few cells. This depolarization spreads by cell-to-cell conduction throughout the entire muscle mass, *capturing* the mass. Capture can be recognized as a depolarization observed immediately after the stimulus artifact (Fig. 32-1). The stimulus must be large enough to initiate rapid depolarization; that is, the stimulus must exceed a *threshold.*

Paced fusion and pseudofusion

If a native depolarization enters the ventricles about the same moment a ventricular pace is delivered, two depolarization patterns develop simultaneously, one from the native depolarization and the other from the pace-initiated depolarization,

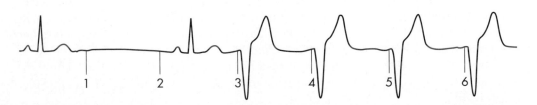

Fig. 32-1. Noncapture and capture (ventricular). Pacing stimuli *1* and *2* had insufficient strength to capture the ventricle. In the time between stimuli *2* and *3,* the pacing output was changed to a stronger setting. Stimuli *3* to *6* captured consistently.

and result in a *paced fusion* beat (Fig. 32-2). A premature ventricular contraction (PVC) and paced beat can also fuse. If a native depolarization has already passed the electrode by the time the stimulus is delivered, the stimulus will have no effect, since the tissue contacting the electrode is already depolarized. This occurrence is sometimes called *pseudofusion.* Similarly, a stimulus occurring during an ST segment will have no effect, since the ventricular tissue is refractory. Late in the T wave a stimulus may start another depolarization if the tissue at the electrode has already repolarized, but since parts of the ventricle are still refractory, an abnormal morphologic appearance on ECG results. An analogous process can occur in the atria.

Since pacing into refractory tissue serves no purpose, and since in rare cases pacing into relatively refractory tissue may be arrhythmogenic, nearly all pacemakers are designed with a feature that *senses* natural depolarization and then *inhibits* the delivery of a stimulus at this time.

Competitive pacing

The sensing feature can be turned off during certain standard pacemaker tests. With sensing turned off, the pacemaker is not inhibited by native beats. Pacing in the presence of native beats may result in *competitive pacing* with numerous fused beats (Fig. 32-3).

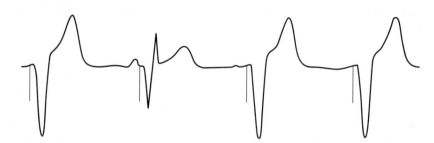

Fig. 32-2. Paced fusion (second complex). A pacing stimulus occurs immediately after the P wave and begins depolarizing the ventricles. The ECG complex begins showing the paced depolarization. Note the initial similarity to other paced depolarizations. Then normal conduction enters the Purkinje fibers, quickly completing depolarization of the ventricles and dominating the rest of the ECG complex. Repolarization is also affected, yielding a different T wave.

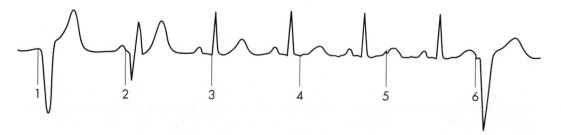

Fig. 32-3. Competitive pacing. When the sensing function is turned off, stimuli occur without regard to native depolarizations. Pace *1* results in a normal paced depolarization. Pace *2* is a fusion similar to that in Fig. 32-2. Pace *3* is fusion, but normal conduction is so far ahead that the complex appears normal; only a slight variation in the T wave is noticeable. Pace *4* and *5* fire into refractory muscle and hence do nothing. Pace *6* occurs after the muscle adjacent to the electrode has repolarized; thus it captures. However, the morphologic appearance shows that the depolarization pattern was shifted somewhat by remaining refractory muscle.

SENSING CONCEPTS

Pacemakers must coordinate pacing with the natural depolarizations occurring in the heart. For example, delivering stimuli to a refractory muscle is undesirable and must be avoided. Also, AV pacemakers coordinate ventricular pacing to follow natural atrial activity, so as to mimic natural AV synchrony.

To meet the preceding needs, pacemakers *sense* natural depolarizations and use the sensed information to control their timing functions.

Mechanisms of sensing

When depolarization occurs in cardiac muscle, ion movements during the initial depolarization process create a small voltage in the tissue. This voltage is carried by the lead into the pulse generator, where it is amplified and sent to various circuits to control the pacing functions.

Sensing involves only voltages close to the electrode; thus sensing is unrelated to the size of the surface complexes.

Undersensing and oversensing

Normal depolarizations are uniform; thus they are sensed uniformly beat after beat. Ectopic depolarizations vary; thus on rare occasions they may be unsensed by a normally operating pacemaker.

When a depolarization is not sensed, the pacemaker is said to be *undersensing*. When interference is sensed as if it were a depolarization, the pacemaker is said to be *oversensing*.

PACEMAKER TIMING

Pacemakers control the timing of their stimuli by continuously monitoring the *sequence* and *timing* between depolarizations occurring in the heart, both natural and paced, and by checking these against desired sequences and time-limit intervals electronically stored in the pulse generator. Whenever a natural depolarization fails to occur within an expected time, the pacemaker sends a stimulus to the delinquent muscle mass to produce a depolarization there.

Intercycle timing

A pacemaker uses an event from one cardiac cycle to set the time limit for the appearance of the next cycle. If the next cycle occurs naturally before the time limit expires, the existing time limit is canceled and reset for the next cycle. But if the next cycle fails to occur by the end of the time limit, the pacemaker instantly initiates a new cycle by pacing.

Cardiac cycles contain an atrial event and a ventricular event, or at least a ventricular event. An "event" is either a natural depolarization or a pace that initiates a depolarization. If the pacemaker uses the atrial event of one cycle to set the time limit for the appearance of the atrial event of the next cycle, the pacemaker employs A-A intercycle timing. If the pacemaker uses the ventricular event of one cycle to set the time limit for the atrial event of the next cycle, it employs V-A intercycle timing. Likewise, if the ventricular event sets the limit for the start of the next ventricular event, it is V-V cycle timing. Of course, a pacemaker that functions solely in the atria must use A-A timing, and a pacemaker that functions solely in the ventricle must use V-V timing. However, an AV pacemaker may use either A-A or V-A timing, and in varying circumstances it may alternate between them.

Historically some manufacturers reemployed the V-V timing circuits of their ventricular products to perform the V-A timing function in their AV products. Consequently the phrase "V-V timing" is often applied to AV pacemakers with V-A intercycle timing.

Atrioventricular timing schemes employ hierarchy; that is, certain events take precedence over others. For example, PVCs occurring between cycles cancel the present time limit and initiate a V-A intercycle time limit.

Timing mechanisms

The purpose of the pacemaker is to ensure an appropriate heart *rate,* but when analyzing pacemaker rhythms, it is easier to think in terms of time *intervals* expressed in milliseconds. The basic pacing rate in pulses per minute (equal to cycles per minute) can be converted to a basic interval by the following formula:

$$\text{Interval (ms/cycle)} = \frac{60,000 \text{ (ms/minute)}}{\text{Rate (cycles/minute)}}$$

Timing mechanisms are best understood by looking at the following examples.

Single chamber: A-A timing. A-A intercycle timing is illustrated by conventional atrial pacing in Fig. 32-4. The pacemaker is set such that the lowest rate to be permitted is 70 beats/min, which corresponds to 857 ms.

Single chamber: V-V timing. V-V intercycle timing is illustrated by ventricular pacing in a similar example in Fig. 32-5. A minimum rate of 60 beats/min is prescribed, corresponding to a 1000-ms time limit.

Atrioventricular pacing: the atrioventricular interval. Atrioventricular pacemakers have an additional time limit that ensures that each atrial beat is followed by a ventricular beat within a specified time interval, the *AV interval.* In nearly all applications each atrial event sets the time limit for the next ventricular depolarization, and if a ventricular depolarization does not occur before the end of the limit, the limit expires and a ventricular pace is immediately delivered.

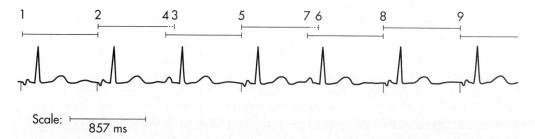

Fig. 32-4. A-A intercycle timing in a basic atrial pacemaker. The basic rate is programed to 70 pulses/min, corresponding to an A-A interval of 857 ms. A pace event at *1* sets a time limit that will expire 857 ms later, at *2.* When the time reaches *2,* the atria are paced and the time limit is reset for another 857 ms to expire, at *3.* Before the time reaches *3,* however, a native atrial depolarization occurs and is sensed at *4.* This event cancels the existing time limit and resets a new time limit for 857 ms to expire, at *5.* When the time reaches *5,* a pace occurs and the limit is reset again for *6.* At *7* a native depolarization is sensed and resets the time limit for *8,* and so forth.

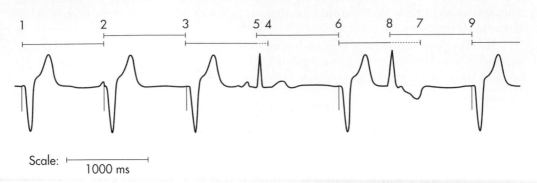

Fig. 32-5. Illustration of V-V intercycle timing in a basic ventricular pacemaker. The basic rate is programed to 60 pulses/min, corresponding to a V-V interval of 1000 ms. A pace at *1* sets a time limit to expire at *2*. When *2* is reached, a pace occurs, and the limit is reset to expire at *3*. At *3* a pace occurs, and the limit is reset to expire at *4*. However, a ventricular sense occurs at *5*, which resets the time limit to expire at *6*, where a pace occurs and resets the limit for *7*. However, at *8* a premature ventricular contraction is sensed, canceling the pace for *7* and resetting the limit to *9*.

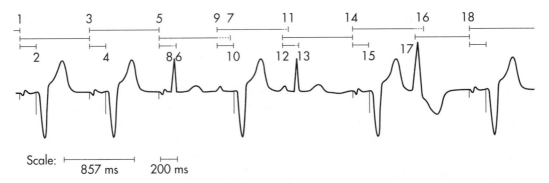

Fig. 32-6. A-A intercycle timing in a basic atrioventricular (AV) pacemaker capable of pacing and sensing both the atria and ventricles. The basic rate is programed to 70 pulses/min, and the AV interval to 200 ms, corresponding to an A-A interval of 857 ms and a special V-A interval of 657 ms following PVCs. The atrial pace at *1* sets a time limit of 200 ms ending at *2* for the appearance of a ventricular event, and a limit of 857 ms ending at *3* for the next atrial event. At *2* a ventricular pace is delivered. At *3* an atrial pace is delivered, and both time limits are reset for a ventricular event by *4* and an atrial event by *5*. At *4* a ventricular pace is delivered. At *5* an atrial pace is delivered, and both time limits are reset for a ventricular event by *6* and an atrial event by *7*. At *8* a ventricular event is sensed, which cancels the time limit for *6*. At *9* an atrial sense occurs and sets the time limit for a ventricular event by *10* and an atrial event by *11*. A ventricular pace occurs at *10*. An atrial sense occurs at *12*, which cancels the time limit for *11* and resets the time limits for a ventricular event by *13* and an atrial event by *14*. A natural ventricular depolarization occurs just before *13*, which cancels the limit for *13* but leaves the limit for an atrial event by *14*. An atrial pace occurs at *14*, setting a limit for a ventricular event at *15* and an atrial event at *16*. A ventricular pace occurs at *15*. The PVC occurring at *17* cancels the atrial event time limit for *16* and resets it 657 ms later, at *18*. At *18* an atrial pace is delivered.

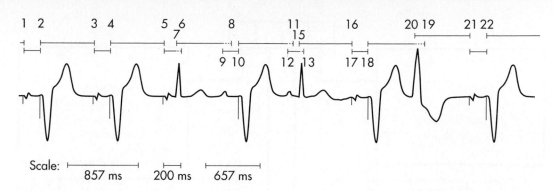

Fig. 32-7. Illustration of V-A intercycle timing in a basic AV pacemaker capable of pacing and sensing both the atria and ventricles. The basic rate is programed to 70 pulses/min and the AV interval to 200 ms, corresponding to an A-A interval of 857 ms and a V-A interval of 657 ms. The atrial pace at *1* sets a time limit of 200 ms, ending at *2* for the appearance of a ventricular event. At *2* a ventricular pace is delivered, and a time limit of 657 ms is set for the appearance of the next atrial event at *3.* At *3* an atrial pace is delivered, and the time limit for a ventricular event is set for *4.* At *4* a ventricular pace occurs, and the time limit for the next atrial event is immediately set to *5.* At *5* an atrial pace is delivered, and the time limit for a ventricular event is set for *6.* At *7* a ventricular sense occurs, canceling *6* and resetting for an atrial event by *8.* At *9* an atrial sense occurs and sets the time limit for a ventricular event by *10.* At *10* a ventricular pace occurs, and the time limit is set for an atrial event by *11.* An atrial sense occurs at *12,* which cancels *11,* and sets the time limit for a ventricular event by *13.* A ventricular depolarization occurs at *15* and sets the time limit for the next atrial event at *16,* and so forth. A PVC appears at *20,* canceling *19* and resetting the time limit for the next atrial event at *21.*

Dual chamber: A-A timing. Basic AV pacing with A-A intercycle timing is shown in Fig. 32-6. Each atrial event sets a time limit for the next atrial event. The minimum rate (the basic rate) is to be 70 beats/min (857 ms), and the maximum AV time limit is to be 200 ms. Remember, a PVC is a special event. It resets the atrial time limit to a value equal to the basic A-A cycle minus the atrioventricular time limit. (In the example in Fig. 32-6, 857 − 200 = 657 ms.)

Dual chamber: V-A timing. Basic AV pacing with V-A intercycle timing is shown in Fig. 32-7. Each ventricular event sets a time limit for the next atrial event. The basic rate is programmed to 70 beats/min (857 ms) and the maximum AV time limit is 200 ms. This means that the ventriculoatrial time limit is 657 ms.

Magnet mode

When a pacemaker is inhibited by natural depolarizations, there is no pacing to observe. Thus nearly all pacemakers contain a magnetic switch that, while activated by a magnet, produces *magnet mode operation,* allowing capture and some other functions to be assessed. In most brands this mode suspends sensing and produces constant pacing at a *magnet rate,* which may be the same as the basic rate or may be a special rate. To indicate the beginning of magnet mode, some pacemakers pace at an accelerated rate for about three cycles and then go to the magnet rate. In AV pacemakers the AV interval is typically shortened during the accelerated cycles. In patients who at present have AV conduction capability this shortening allows the ventricle to capture and to be observed before AV conduction occurs.

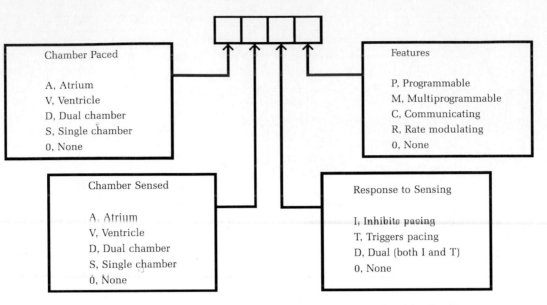

Chamber Paced

A, Atrium
V, Ventricle
D, Dual chamber
S, Single chamber
0, None

Features

P, Programmable
M, Multiprogrammable
C, Communicating
R, Rate modulating
0, None

Chamber Sensed

A, Atrium
V, Ventricle
D, Dual chamber
S, Single chamber
0, None

Response to Sensing

I, Inhibits pacing
T, Triggers pacing
D, Dual (both I and T)
0, None

Fig. 32-8. Four-letter code used to describe pacing modes (abridged).

ADVANCED PACING

Enhancing the quality of life in patients with paced heart rates centers on two important factors: *AV synchrony* and *a responsive heart rate.* Atrioventricular synchrony ensures that the normal mechanical cardiac sequence is maintained as much as possible, and it prevents certain arrhythmias precipitated by nonsynchrony. A responsive heart rate ensures that the patient's heart rate varies dynamically according to the patient's needs.

Most advanced pacemakers are of the AV type, although sole atrial pacing can provide AV synchrony in patients with intact conduction.

Pacemakers use a variety of timing schemes called *modes,* which are described by a five-letter code. The first four letters apply to pacing bradycardias and are shown in Fig. 32-8. The fifth letter is for antitachycardia pacing.

PACEMAKERS THAT PROVIDE A RESPONSIVE HEART RATE

Pacemakers that provide a responsive heart rate can automatically vary their pacing rate to match the needs of the patient. The mode of choice for a responsive rate depends on whether the atria are naturally responsive.

For patients with a naturally responsive atrial rate, a mode is used that *tracks* the natural atrial activity and synchronizes the ventricles to the atria.

For patients without a naturally responsive atrial rate a mode employing a *sensor* or another *measurement feature* is used, which monitors factors (other than atrial depolarizations) that reflect or correlate with cardiovascular needs. After processing, signals from the sensor determine what the desired rate should be, based on criteria programed into the pacemaker by a physician.

Sensor-controlled rate determination is revised cycle by cycle to match the patient's needs moment by moment. Pacing occurs at the sensor-determined rate unless superseded by sensing of a faster natural rate. In essence, the *processed sensor information modulates, or varies, the intercycle time limits* discussed previously. The sensor-determined rate is also called the *sensor-prescribed rate,* the *sensor-driven rate,* the *sensor-controlled rate,* or, most commonly, just the *sensor rate.*

Pacemakers that use sensors are referred to as *rate-modulating* or *adaptive-rate* or *rate-responsive* pacemakers. Atrial tracking pacemakers that have no sensors are by convention usually not referred to by these terms.

Sensors

Several physiologic parameters have been applied in clinical practice to control pacing rate. *Activity* is the most widely used. A sensor in the pacemaker monitors motion and vibration in the patient's body as a measure of the patient's activity. It then varies the pacing rate to match the activity. *Respiration, neurohumoral drive,* and *blood temperature* are also used. Future technologies may employ blood pH, contractility, oxygen saturation, or cardiac dimensions.

Rate prescriptions

All rate-modulating pacemakers and atrial tracking pacemakers have a lower rate limit and an upper rate limit. The pacemaker never paces slower than the lower rate limit or faster than the upper rate limit. Between these limits the rate is controlled by atrial tracking or the sensor, as conceptualized in Fig. 32-9, *A.* The lower rate limit is programable and is usually called the *programable lower rate limit* (PLRL), the *base rate,* or the *basic rate.*

In atrial pacemakers and ventricular pacemakers there is only one upper rate limit, which is programable and is usually called the *programable upper rate limit* (PURL). Of course, natural rates may exceed these limits, but the pacemaker will not.

In AV pacing there are additional factors that restrict the upper rate, and several upper rate restrictions may be present under varying circumstances. The terms applied to these upper rate limits, such as PURL, *maximal atrial tracking rate* (MATR), and *maximal sensor rate* (MSR), are not used identically by all manufacturers.

In rate-modulating pacemakers the sensor-controlled functions translate the sensor measurement into the sensor rate, which may be thought of as a dynamic or varying form of the lower rate limit (Fig. 32-9, *B*).

The *sensor threshold* is the level at which the parameter being monitored begins to take effect. Programing the threshold moves point "ST" left or right. The *rate response* controls the degree to which the rate is affected by the monitored parameter. Programing the rate response alters the slope of the response curve. At shallow rate-response curves the sensor rate may never reach the upper limit.

During atrial tracking of sinus rhythms the ventricular rate, of course, changes exactly as the atrial rate changes, as shown in Fig. 32-9, *C.* But during sensor control, some pacemakers employ *acceleration* and *deceleration* features, as depicted in Fig. 32-9, *D.* The acceleration and deceleration separately determine the quickness of the rate increase and decrease, respectively. Programing these features sets the slopes of the rate changes.

APPLICATIONS OF ADVANCED PACING CONCEPTS

The ECGs of advanced pacemakers are easy to interpret when understood in the context of how these pacemakers are applied; thus a brief review is presented here.

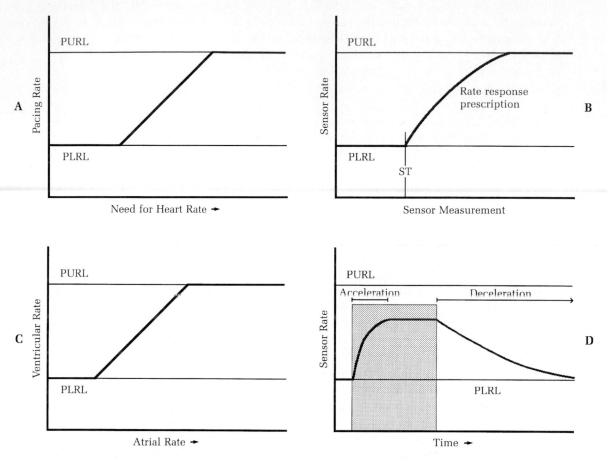

Fig. 32-9. Methods for determining the pacing rate. **A,** Concept of the rate-modulating pacemaker. The physiologic need for heart rate is translated to an appropriate pacing rate. When the need is minimal, the pacing rate is the programable lower rate limit (PLRL). At greater needs the pacing rates are faster and proportioned to the need. At even greater needs the pacing rate is held to acceptable limits by the programable upper rate limit (PURL). **B,** Sensor rate. A sensor measures a factor (other than atrial rate) that correlates with the physiologic need for heart rate. Sensor information is translated to a sensor rate by a rate-response prescription program. Whenever the sensor rate is between the rate limits and above the natural heart rate, pacing occurs at the sensor rate. **C,** Atrial tracking (dual-chamber pacemaker). In pacemakers with atrial tracking, which do not have a sensor, ventricular pacing tracks the atria. Thus the pacing rate varies between the rate limits according to the natural atrial rate. Sensor rates are often combined with and operate simultaneously with atrial tracking in rate-modulating dual-chamber pacemakers. In these applications, whenever the tracked atrial rate exceeds the sensor rate, ventricular pacing tracks the atrial rate. At other times the atria (and ventricles if necessary) are paced at the sensor rate. Thus the heart rate follows either the natural atrial rate or the sensor rate, whichever is higher. **D,** Acceleration and deceleration of sensor rate. Sensor rate during several minutes of exercise *(shaded area)* is shown. At the onset of the exercise the sensor quantitates the exercise, and the rate prescription program determines what the sensor rate should become. The sensor rate increases according to the programed acceleration, leveling at the desired rate. When the exercise ends, the sensor rate declines according to the programed deceleration. Any change in the intensity of the exercise would readjust the projected sensor rate.

Categorizing patients for pacing

PROVEN RELIABLE CONDUCTION with:

Atrial bradycardia

UNPROVEN CONDUCTION with one of the following:

Normal atrial rhythms
Intermittent atrial bradycardia/poor rate response to stress
Constant atrial bradycardia
Atrial fibrillation or flutter

An adequate ventricular rate is absolutely essential for life; thus every pacemaker system must, of course, meet this need. But for *quality of life,* each pacemaker must also ensure *AV synchrony* and a *responsive heart rate.* In this section the term *responsive heart rate* is used in a broad sense to include both atrial tracking and sensor-controlled, rate-modulating pacemakers.

Matching the pacemaker to the patient

From the viewpoint of pacing, all bradyarrhythmia patients can be placed into one of two groups, depending on the quality of their AV conduction. The smaller group includes only patients with *proven reliable conduction,* but who have atrial bradycardias. The larger group includes all patients who have *unsatisfactory or unproven conduction.* Unproven conduction is a critical distinction, since these patients must have pacemakers that can *directly* pace the ventricle.

The second group is further categorized according to the quality of the atrial rhythms. The atrial rhythms are assessed by looking at two factors: the natural rate at rest and the rate increase in response to stresses such as exercise and emotion (see the box above).

A method for selecting the best mode for each category is illustrated in Figures 32-10 through 32-15. Implicit in each case is that the mode must support life and, when possible, provide AV synchrony and a responsive heart rate.

Proven reliable conduction and atrial bradycardia (Fig. 32-10). To support life when there is proven reliable conduction, it is necessary only to pace in the atria. Atrioventricular synchrony occurs naturally as atrial activity conducts to the ventricle. Atrial sensing is used to inhibit pacing if there happens to be some natural atrial activity at times. To obtain a responsive heart rate, it is necessary to employ a sensor. This mode is atrial demand pacing with rate modulation, the *AAIR mode* in accordance with the code in Fig. 32-8.

The AAIR mode has not been widely accepted because of concerns that conduction disease may develop within a few years in some patients. Patients must be initially tested to validate conduction quality, and thorough, periodic follow-up tests are required to check for possible impending conduction problems.

ECGs for AAIR pacing are similar to those of atrial pacing as described earlier (Fig. 32-4), except that the A-A interval is controlled by the sensor. When increased rate is required, the rate-modulating function shortens this interval to produce the desired rate. The pacing rate will never be less than the PLRL or exceed the PURL.

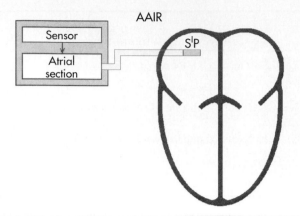

Fig. 32-10.* Application of a pacemaker to patients with proven reliable AV conduction but with atrial bradycardias. This is rate-modulated (sensor-driven) atrial demand pacing using the AAIR mode. There is no ventricular lead.

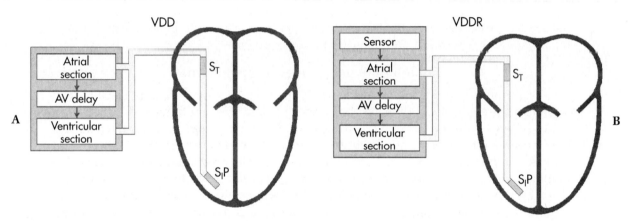

Fig. 32-11. A, Application of a pacemaker to patients with unreliable AV conduction but with normal atrial rhythm. This is atrial-synchronous ventricular-inhibited pacing, the VDD mode. Separate leads or a combined lead (shown here) can be used. **B,** Addition of a rate-modulating sensor provides a backup responsive heart rate if needed, the VDDR mode.

Unreliable conduction and good atrial rhythm. To ensure life when conduction is unproven, the pacemaker must be able to pace the ventricles, and it must sense to inhibit ventricular pacing if natural conduction appears before the AV interval time limit expires, or if ventricular ectopic depolarizations occur.

To provide AV synchrony and a responsive heart rate, the natural atrial rhythm can be tracked. The pacemaker should sense that rhythm and use it to trigger an AV interval, thereby synchronizing pacing of the ventricles shortly after each atrial contraction has finished, to mimic the natural AV timing of the heart.

The preceding functions are collectively described as the *VDD mode.* This mode is not widely used because all of its basic features are included in the more comprehensive DDD and DDDR modes (discussed later). The VDD mode is used only when a single transvenous lead is desired.

---

*Fig. 32-10 and similar illustrations represent the applications of a pacemaker to the heart. The large box represents the pacemaker, the light shaded lines represent the lead(s), and the dark shaded color on the lead(s) represents the location of the electrode(s). *S,* senses; *P,* paces; *I,* inhibits pace; *T,* triggers AV interval for tracking; *superscript,* applies to the atria; *subscript,* applies to the ventricles.

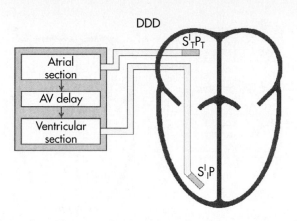

Fig. 32-12. The DDD mode. When two leads are used, it is common to also provide backup atrial pacing.

In a single lead application (Fig. 32-11, *A*), electrodes in the atria sense the atrial activity and initiate an AV delay in the generator, which in turn paces the ventricle if natural conduction is delayed or is blocked.

Atrial bradycardia may develop in some patients over time. To prevent ventricular bradycardia in this circumstance, backup ventricular pacing is provided at a lower rate limit, the PLRL. During backup pacing there is no AV synchrony, and in many patients retrograde conduction from the ventricle to the atria resets the atria and suppresses the resumption of atrial tracking. With a single lead, the atrial electrodes are not in close contact with the atrial wall; thus with movement, on rare occasions there may be a transient loss of atrial sensing. The ventricle will then be paced at the backup rate. Some pacemakers employ a sensor to provide a higher backup rate during activity *(VDDR mode)* (Fig. 32-11, *B*); at times, however, this feature can compete with the natural atrial rate and adversely disrupt AV synchrony.

When the atrial rate is close to the lower rate limit (or sensor rate), occasional rate cycles may decrease slightly below the limit. To salvage AV synchrony during these occasions, some VDD and VDDR pacemakers have a special feature in which an atrial sense that occurs immediately before the time limit for the ventricular pace will delay the ventricular pace to allow time for the atrial contraction to contribute to ventricular filling. This is known as "AV priority" or "sinus preference" timing. With this feature ECG reviewers may note tracked cycles that are longer than expected.

With a single lead, atrial pacing cannot be used because it requires a reliable electrode contact with the atrial wall. If a future need for atrial pacing is a possibility, separate atrial and ventricular leads are used with a pulse generator that has modes with the features of the VDD mode plus backup atrial pacing, for example, the DDD mode (Fig. 32-12).

If, in addition to atrial pacing, a future need for rate response is a possibility, a sensor is added, providing the DDDR mode discussed later (Fig. 32-13).

Some patients have occasional atrial tachycardias, and many have occasional PVCs that conduct in retrograde fashion into the atria. Pacemakers must be programed not to track these events. Simple programs that are used to manage these events also prevent desirable tracking of normally high atrial rates during exercise. To avoid this limitation, some newer pacemakers have complex timing algorithms, which are discussed later. In the subset of patients who have normally high atrial rates during exercise, it is most common to use pacemakers that can pace both the atria and ventricles with sensor-controlled rates (DDDR), since these pacemakers have the widest array of options for managing fast rates.

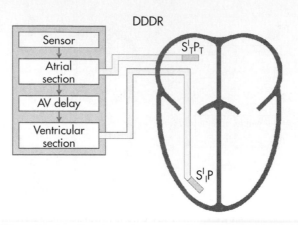

Fig. 32-13. The DDDR mode. Application of a pacemaker to patients with unreliable AV conduction and with intermittent atrial bradycardias.

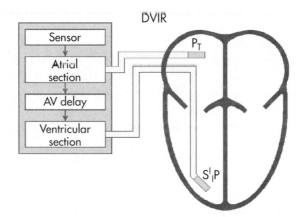

Fig. 32-14. The DVIR mode. Application of a pacemaker to patients with unreliable AV conduction and with constant atrial bradycardia.

Unreliable conduction and intermittent atrial bradycardia. To protect life, the ventricle must be paced when AV conduction is unreliable, and it must be sensed to inhibit ventricular pacing if there is conduction or ventricular ectopic activity. Since the atria do not always provide an adequate rate, a sensor should be used continuously to establish a varying rate that is appropriate for the patient's varying activity. Whenever the natural atrial rhythm is good (above the sensor rate), each atrial sense should inhibit pacing there and trigger an AV interval for pacing the ventricles. Whenever the natural atrial rate is inadequate (less than the sensor rate), the atria should be paced at the sensor rate and this should trigger an AV interval for pacing the ventricles. This is the *DDDR mode,* which is shown in Fig. 32-13.

Unreliable conduction and constant atrial bradycardia. Since AV conduction is unreliable, the ventricle must be paced and sensed. The atria must be paced, and this pacing must trigger an AV interval to synchronize the ventricular pace. Atrial sensing is not needed and is not used; not using atrial sensing prevents adversely tracking occasional atrial tachycardias and retrograde conductions that might occur. A sensor is used to provide a responsive heart rate. This is the *DVIR mode* (Fig. 32-14). If adequate natural atrial rates return, the pacemaker should be programmed to the DDDR mode.

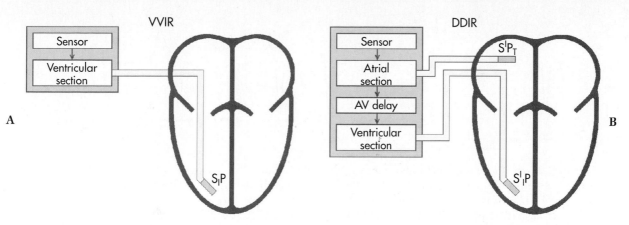

Fig. 32-15. A, The VVIR mode. Application of a pacemaker to patients with unreliable AV conduction and with atrial fibrillation. This is ventricular-inhibited rate-modulated ventricular pacing. **B,** If atrial fibrillation is intermittent, DDDR mode is preferred, but if tracking of the occurances of atrial fibrillation is a problem, a nontracking mode is used instead, such as the DVIR mode in Fig. 32-14 or the DDIR mode shown here. Newer pacemaker designs can automatically switch back and forth between DDDR and DDIR as needed.

Unreliable conduction and atrial fibrillation. To ensure life, the ventricle must be paced and sensed, as in previous cases. It is fruitless to pace or sense the atria while they are fibrillating. Atrioventricular synchrony cannot be obtained, but a sensor can be used to provide a responsive heart rate. This is *the VVIR mode* (Fig. 32-15, *A*).

The possibility of pharmacologic conversion of the atrial fibrillation should be reevaluated. With an implanted pacemaker present, drug therapy for treating the atrial fibrillation may be practical, since if drug-induced bradycardia happened to result it could be managed by the pacemaker. Particular caution must be used with proarrhythmic drugs, since pacing may obscure warning signs of impending fatal ventricular arrythmia. If atrial conversion is likely, DDDR pacing is preferable, especially with an automatic mode switching feature discussed later.

Conversion may not be maintained, and intermittent atrial tachyarrhythmias may occur. The pacemaker in DDDR mode may track these. If this is a problem and cannot be readily resolved through simple programing, a nontracking mode must be used, usually DVIR or DDIR. The DVIR mode does not sense in the atria and may pace into the atria during the arrhythmia. If the atrial arrhythmia is flutter, the pacing may occasionally terminate the flutter. However, if during sinus rhythm there are normal sinus rates above the sensor rate, competitive atrial pacing will occur. The DDIR mode senses in the atria to inhibit atrial pacing, but these senses do not initiate an AV interval. Instead the ventricular pace occurs at a time corresponding to the sensor rate (Fig. 32-15, *B*). In both modes atrial *paces* trigger AV intervals.

Some newer pacemakers operating in DDDR mode can detect atrial tachyarrhythmias and automatically switch to VVIR or DDIR modes for the duration of each arrhythmia. This feature is discussed later.

RETROGRADE (VENTRICULOATRIAL) CONDUCTION
Effects of retrograde conduction

In most normal hearts the conduction system can conduct backward. But what about in patients with poor forward conduction? In about a third of these patients the

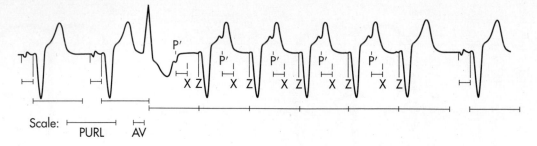

Fig. 32-16. Pacemaker-mediated tachycardia (PMT) caused by retrograde conductions. This pacemaker has a ventricular PURL, which functions by delaying any ventricular pace that would otherwise cause the pacemaker to exceed the upper rate limit. Following every ventricular event there is a limiting interval corresponding to the PURL. Any ventricular pace that would occur within this interval is delayed until the interval expires. Every ventricular event, including the PVC, resets the PURL interval. In the ECG the PVC conducts into the atria, producing a retrograde P wave at the first *P'* wave. This P wave is sensed and triggers an AV interval that expires at *X*. However, the ventricular pace is delayed until the PURL interval completes at *Z*. The pace resets the PURL interval again. The paced beat now sends a retrograde conduction to the atria. Since the preceding delay allowed the atria to repolarize, the atria accept the retrograde conduction and produce another retrograde P wave, and the cycle repeats. In the PMT shown, the retrograde mechanism fatigues and the PMT self-terminates.

conduction system can conduct backwards enough of the time to require consideration. A problem may occur in the atrial tracking modes if a ventricular beat conducts into the atria while the atria are not refractory, causing the atria to depolarize. This will be sensed through the atrial lead and trigger an AV interval to be followed by a ventricular pace. But the pace can be delayed by the upper rate limit function before it is delivered to the ventricles, and during this time the atria repolarize. When the delayed ventricular paced beat occurs, it initiates another retrograde conduction, which enters the atria, and the cycle repeats again and again (Fig. 32-16). This repetition creates a reentrant tachyrhythmia in which the pacemaker is the reentry mechanism. Tachycardias sustained by pacemakers are called *pacemaker-mediated tachycardias* (PMTs). Usually these repetitive retrograde conductions cause fatigue in the retrograde conduction path quickly, and the PMT self-terminates, although it can continue for hours. Most PMTs run at the upper rate limit of the pacemaker, but they can run at lower rates if the retrograde time or AV interval is long.

During normal operation the atria or the upper conduction system is still refractory at the time of ventricular depolarization; thus a retrograde conduction cannot enter the atria. However, an unsynchronized ventricular depolarization, such as a PVC, may occur when the atria are receptive, and a retrograde conduction may enter the atria.

A PVC is the most common cause of retrograde conduction, but there can also be retrograde conduction resulting from a paced ventricular beat that is out of synchrony. For example, the tracking of interference or a PAC invoking an upper rate limit for one cycle can result in a momentary loss of paced ventricular synchrony, allowing retrograde conduction to ascend.

Managing retrograde conduction (ventriculoatrial conduction)

Historically reviewers of pacemaker ECGs focused on the pacing rates, AV intervals, refractory periods, and modes as being constant. Now this has changed.

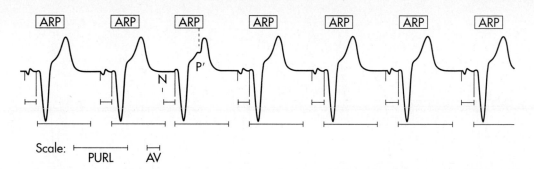

Fig. 32-17. Use of standard postventricular atrial refractory period (PVARP [ARP]) to ignore retrograde conductions following paced beats. Following the second complex, a momentary intense interference (noise [N]) caused a false atrial sense that inhibited the next atrial pace and triggered a subsequent ventricular pace, the third complex. Since the atria had not been paced and had not depolarized intrinsically, a retrograde conduction from the paced beat initiated a retrograde P wave, P'. The regular PVARP (ARP) covered this P' wave, preventing a PMT.

The newest pacemakers adjust their timing to *adapt* to the changing circumstances of the patient. Reviewers formerly evaluated whether the pacemaker was working correctly; now they must also determine whether it is adapting appropriately to meet the patient's needs.

Most of the special timing features relate to several methods used to manage ventriculoatrial conduction.

Postventricular atrial refractory periods. Refractory periods are special time intervals during which the principal response to sensed events are suspended. In most pacemakers atrial sensing is ignored during a period of time after each ventricular event; this period of time is known as the postventricular atrial refractory period (PVARP, or sometimes, just ARP).

Pacemaker-mediated tachycardias that are due to ventriculoatrial conduction cannot continue for more than one cycle without the sensing of atrial depolarizations caused by ventriculoatrial conduction from *ventricular-paced* beats. Retrograde conduction intervals for all paced beats in a given patient are consistent; thus a PVARP long enough to exceed the retrograde time causes the retrograde depolarization to be ignored. The PVARP also prevents certain unusual events from starting PMTs, as illustrated in Fig. 32-17.

Premature ventricular contractions often produce ventriculoatrial conduction with conduction times longer than the typical PVARP; thus they can readily initiate PMTs. Although such PMTs could be terminated quickly, some pacemakers also prevent them from starting in the first place. These pacemakers automatically extend the PVARP after each PVC, typically to 400 ms or more (Fig. 32-18). To detect PVCs, the pacemakers monitor the *sequence* of atrial and ventricular events. When a ventricular sense follows another ventricular event with no atrial event between the two, the sense is assumed to be a PVC.

Termination programs. In special situations, when the PVARP must be kept shorter than the ventriculoatrial conduction time, PMT termination programs may be used. These programs recognize a PMT and then initiate a special timing sequence to terminate it. Various methods are used. For example, one method monitors for atrial

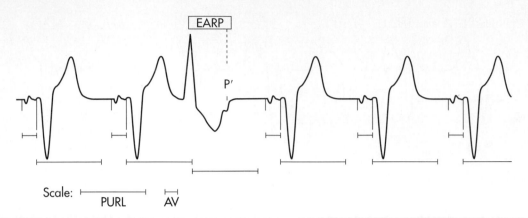

Fig. 32-18. Avoiding retrograde conductions from PVCs. The second ventricular event is followed by a sensed PVC, with no atrial event between. This sequence initiates an extended atrial refractory period *(EARP),* which causes the retrograde P wave to be ignored.

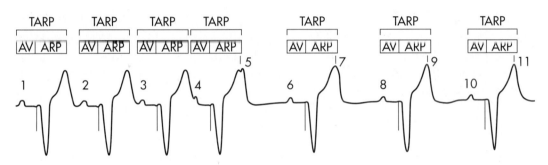

Fig. 32-19. Limitation of tracking rate caused by the total atrial refractory period (TARP). The trace illustrates a desirable, naturally increasing atrial tachycardia; the P waves are numbered. P waves *1* to *4* are tracked normally. As the length of the atrial cycle shortens, each new P wave becomes closer to the previous TARP. When the atrial cycle length becomes even shorter *(5),* the atrial sense occurs in the previous PVARP and is ignored and a cycle is skipped. The next P wave *(6)* is sensed, but the one that follows *(7)* is ignored. Likewise, *8* is sensed and *9* is ignored, and so forth. When the atrial cycle length becomes less than the TARP, every other P wave is sensed and 2:1 pacemaker block occurs.

senses occurring after the PVARP but within 400 ms after the ventricular pace. When eight such senses occur in a continuous manner, a PMT is assumed and a single, extended PVARP is applied to terminate it. Because tracking of high atrial rates during exercise can also be unintentionally detected as a PMT, termination sequences may occasionally be seen in ECGs during fast atrial tracking, generally appearing as skipped pace beats. To avoid excessive skipped beats, once a termination sequence is applied, it is not repeated for a minute or two.

TRACKING LIMITATIONS CAUSED BY ATRIOVENTRICULAR INTERVAL AND POSTVENTRICULAR ATRIAL REFRACTORY PERIOD

Although the PVARP limits tracking of retrograde conductions, it also limits tracking of normal, desirable sinus tachycardias during exercise.

Atrial sensing is refractory during the AV interval, as well as during the PVARP. Together, these two refractory periods form the *total atrial refractory period* (TARP).

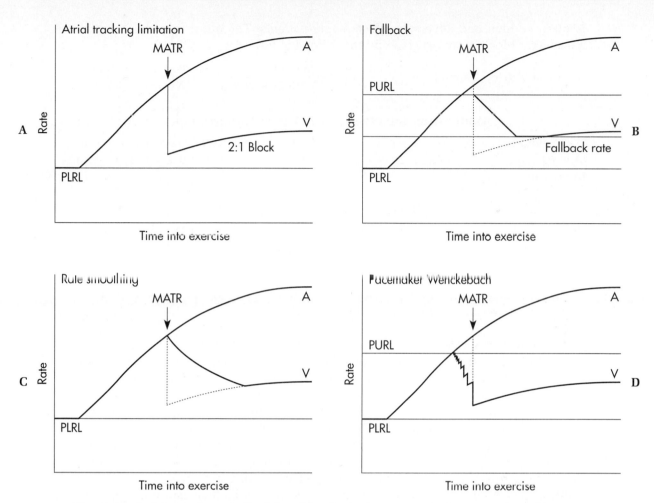

Fig. 32-20. A, Adverse impact of atrial tracking limitation on ventricular rate and synchrony in an exercising patient. The patient has complete heart block and a good atrial response. Before exercise the atria and ventricles are paced in synchrony at the PLRL. On exercise the atrial rate increases, and because of 1:1 tracking, the ventricular rate follows in synchrony. When the atrial rate surpasses the 2:1 block rate (maximal atrial tracking rate), the ventricular rate becomes half the atrial rate. The atrial rate continues to rise, but because of 2:1 tracking, the ventricular rate follows at half the atrial rate and there is ventricular synchrony with only every other atrial beat. Following exercise (not shown) 1:1 tracking resumes when the atrial rate declines below the 2:1 block rate. **B,** Fallback. After the atrial rate reaches an upper rate limit and after an onset delay to avoid responding to premature atrial contractions (PACs), the rate declines gradually, in contrast to the sudden drop shown in **A. C,** Rate smoothing during upper rate limitation. As the atrial rate increases above the upper limit, tracking is curtailed. However, the ventricular rate of each cycle is permitted to decrease only by a programed percentage of the rate of the previous cycle, producing a gradual reduction in rate. **D,** Ventricular upper rate limit. When the atrial rate exceeds the PURL, Wenckebach-like pacing occurs. As the atrial rate increases, the ratio of block increases, eventually reaching 2:1 pacemaker block. The *average rate* (shown) decreases because of increasing dropped beats, declining to half the atrial rate when half the beats are dropped, thereby producing a gradual, stepped reduction in rate.

When sensing a fast atrial rate, if the P-wave to P-wave cycle length is less than the TARP, a P wave that starts a TARP will be tracked but the next one will be ignored, since it occurs before the end of the TARP. Then the next one will be tracked, and the following one ignored. Thus every other P wave is tracked, and the ventricular rate is half the atrial rate, analogous to 2:1 AV block, as sketched in Fig. 32-19. The result of 2:1 pacemaker block is graphed in Fig. 32-20, *A.* The ventricular rate drop is often sudden and adversely affects some patients. The atrial rate above which pacemaker block occurs is given by the following formula:

$$\text{Block rate (cycles/min)} = \frac{60,000 \text{ (ms/minute)}}{\text{AV (ms/cycle) + PVARP (ms/cycle)}} = \frac{60,000 \text{ (ms/minute)}}{\text{TARP (ms/cycle)}}$$

Moderating the effects of 2:1 pacemaker block

Several methods were developed to make the change to half rate occur gradually. Although these methods have been superseded by better methods, they remain in common use.

Fallback. The pacemaker recognizes when the atrial rate is exceeding upper rate limits and then lowers the ventricular rate steadily to a predetermined rate. Tracking resumes when the atrial rate eventually comes down (Fig. 32-20, *B*).

Rate smoothing. The pacemaker does not allow the rate to change by more than a given percentage of the rate of the previous "R-R" cycle. Tracking resumes when the atrial rate becomes low enough (Fig. 32-20, *C*).

Ventricular upper rate limit. The pacemaker does not allow any ventricular cycle length to be less than an interval corresponding to the programed ventricular upper rate limit. When the atrial rate exceeds the upper rate limit, each ventricular pace is delayed until the limit interval finishes. Thus the atrial beats advance, but ventricular paces are held to the upper rate limit. This stretches the AV intervals. When the atria advance into a PVARP of a previously delayed pace, the atrial sense is ignored and a "skipped beat" occurs. A normal AV interval resumes after each skipped beat, but the AV interval lengthens with subsequent cycles until another skip occurs, producing a Wenckebach-like effect, as sketched in Fig. 32-21. As a result of programing the ventricular upper rate limit to be less than the 2:1 block rate, Wenckebach will precede 2:1 pacemaker block, causing a *stepped* reduction in rate to the 2:1 rate (Fig. 32-20, *D*).

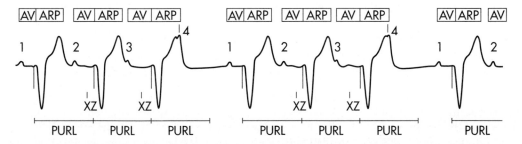

Fig. 32-21. Ventricular upper rate limit, most commonly called the PURL. In this case the atrial rate is slightly faster than the PURL. The first P wave *(1)* is tracked normally. The second and third P waves *(2 and 3)* are tracked, but the PURL delays their ventricular paces from *X* to *Z* in each case. The fourth P wave *(4)* occurs just before the end of the PVARP *(ARP)* and is ignored. On the next P wave the sequence repeats. In each sequence the first AV interval is in normal synchrony, the next few are lengthened, and the last is dropped: a Wenckebach-like rhythm. The ventricular rate within the sequence is at the PURL, but because of dropped beats, the average rate is less than the PURL.

Maintaining desirable heart rates during exercise

Fast heart rates are normal and desired during exercise. New methods have been developed to maintain tracking over a wider range and to provide sensor-driven rates with AV synchrony.

Rate adaptive sense-initiated AV intervals (RA-SAV). As can be seen in the block-rate formula, shortening the AV interval allows faster rates to be tracked. Some newer pacemakers automatically monitor the natural atrial rate and shorten their AV interval accordingly. In some pacemakers the AV interval changes abruptly when the atrial rate crosses certain limits. In the newest designs, the AV interval changes gradually according to the rate.

If 2:1 block is encountered, and the pacemaker has a sensor-driven rate, the pacing rate does not drop below the sensor rate.

In the newest designs, the pace-initiated AV interval (PAV) is shortened as well so that transitions between pacing and tracking are smooth. In patients with different intraatrial conduction times for paced compared with sensed events, to compensate, the PAV can be programed differently from the sense-initiated AV interval (SAV).

ECGs, especially at high rates, may show a variety of AV intervals. The controlling features are programable and specific to particular brands. During pacemaker evaluations, ECGs should always be recorded by the pacemaker's programer, because the programer records the pacemaker's internal timing markers along with the ECG, which greatly simplifies analysis.

Sensor varied postventricular atrial refractory period. Shortening the PVARP also allows faster rates to be tracked. In some patients it appears that the VA conduction time shortens during exercise, and the PVARP may be shortened accordingly. In some pacemakers the PVARP can be programed to shorten according to the sensor rate.

Sensor-driven rate-modulated atrioventricular pacing. Sensor-driven rate pacing is often used to provide AV pacing above the 2:1 pacemaker block rate. If the sensor rate is above the atrial rate, AV pacing occurs uniformly at the sensor rate. If the sensor rate is a little below the atrial rate, the sensor fills in the skipped beats (Fig. 32-22).

Managing pacing during occasional atrial tachycardias

Occasional atrial tachycardias must not be allowed to trigger pacing of the ventricles at a high rate. To prevent this type of triggering, tracking modes have special features.

Programable upper rate limit. The PURL feature limits the maximum rate at which the pacemaker can pace the ventricles.

Total atrial refractory period. Once one atrial event initiates a TARP, no other atrial event can be sensed until the TARP has ended. Thus no two atrial events can be sensed at a cycle length less than the TARP. The maximum atrial rate that can be fully tracked is the MATR defined earlier. The PVARP portion of the TARP may also be used to manage ventriculoatrial conduction, which usually determines the minimum PVARP.

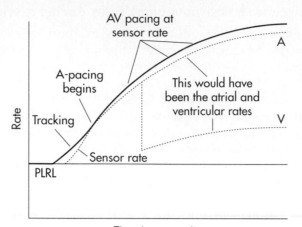

Fig. 32-22. Sensor-driven rate-modulated pacing to achieve rates above the 2:1 pacemaker block rate (maximal atrial tracking rate). Without this feature, the device in the patient shown in Fig. 32-20, **A** would have tracked until the atrial rate reached the maximal atrial tracking rate and then would have paced the ventricles at half the atrial rate. With a sensor programed to provide a rate slightly faster than the natural atrial rate, the sensor rate overtakes the atrial rate and atrial pacing begins, providing AV pacing thereafter.

Although the pacemaker cannot track above the MATR, in most pacemakers the sensor may produce sensor-driven pacing rates above the MATR.

Mode switching. When an atrial tachycardia is detected, the pacemaker automatically switches to a nontracking mode. Some brands switch to VVIR and others to DDIR. The tachycardia is verified for about 10 sec before switching, to avoid erroneously responding to premature atrial contractions (PACs) or interferences.

After the atrial arrhythmia terminates, nontracking may continue for several cycles before the pacemaker switches back to VDD, DDD or DDDR. During this transition time, if the mode is VVIR, there is no AV synchrony, and ventriculoatrial conduction may aggravate the atria. If the mode is DDIR, atrial synchrony is much more likely and ventriculoatrial conduction is unlikely.

Noncompetitive atrial pacing. In unusual situations atrial depolarizations resulting from ventriculoatrial conductions may occur late in the PVARP. At moderate sensor-driven rates the relative refractory period of these depolarizations can extend into the time for the next atrial pace, which increases the risk of inducing atrial arrhythmias. Noncompetitive features can detect these situations and alter the subsequent pacing cycles to lessen the chance of precipitating arrhythmias.

• • •

The foregoing features create very complex ECGs at fast rates. The features are programable and specific to particular brands. During pacemaker evaluations ECGs should always be recorded by the pacemaker's programer because the programer records the pacemaker's timing markers on a separate trace along with the ECG, greatly simplifying analysis.

SPECIAL FEATURES
Pacemaker management of vasovagal and carotid sinus syndromes

These syndromes have two components: cardio-inhibitory induced bradycardia and low stroke volumes resulting from low venous pressures. Pacing can correct the bradycardia, and transiently pacing at a considerably elevated rate can increase cardiac output at small stroke volumes. AV pacing is always used since the atrial contraction aids ventricular filling. Several methods are used.

AV pacing with rate hysteresis. With this feature turned on, the pacing rate is faster than the sensing rate. For example, the pacing rate may be 80 bpm and the sensing rate 50 bpm. At the onset of a cardio-inhibitory event the sinus rate may drop below 50 bpm, initiating pacing at 80 bpm. Later when the natural rate exceeds 80 bpm, sensing resumes. Reviewers of ECGs can identify this feature by noting that the cycle preceding the first atrial pace is longer than the next paced cycle.

Rate-drop response pacing. This feature is designed specifically for treating cardio-inhibitory bradycardias with low filling pressures. The pacemaker monitors a rate range just below the typical lower natural rates of the patient. When the atrial rate drops quickly through this range, a cardio-inhibitory event is assumed and AV pacing is initiated at a fast rate. Pacing continues at the fast rate for several minutes and then decreases gradually until a reasonable natural rate is encountered. Reviewers of ECGs will note sudden drops in native atrial rate, usually to the PLRL, followed by fast atrial paced or AV paced rates.

Sleep rates

Newer pacemakers contain built-in clocks that can be programed to permit lower rates during sleeping hours. A typical case might be where the rate declines gradually during a half hour in the late evening and increases gradually during a half hour in the early morning.

MAXIMIZING ATRIOVENTRICULAR SYNCHRONY WITH VENTRICULAR PACEMAKERS

Many patients who would benefit from AV synchrony received their pacemakers before AV pacing gained acceptance. These pacemakers were almost all ventricular, and many are still functioning. Some of these pacemakers have a feature that allows sensing at a rate less than the pacing rate. This feature allows *rate hysteresis.*

Rate hysteresis stems from the observation that the hemodynamic effects of AV synchrony are superior to the hemodynamic effects of ventricular pacing, especially at low heart rates. It is further observed that some patients do not require pacing all the time and that they frequently have sinus rates between 50 and 70 beats/min with conduction much of the time. For this select group of patients it may be desirable to permit sensing to rates as low as 50 beats/min, since this inhibits pacing and allows the patient's heart to be in synchrony more of the time. Thus a slow rate, the *hysteresis rate,* is applied to sensing. Whenever the rate drops below this rate, pacing begins at the faster rate. Pacing continues at the faster rate until a natural depolarization is sensed above this faster rate; then the lower sensing rate is applied again (Fig. 32-23).

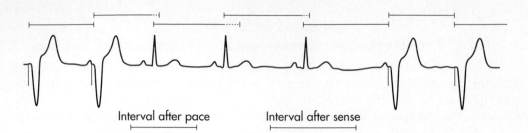

Interval after pace   Interval after sense

Fig. 32-23. Hysteresis. Pacing is occurring at the pacing rate *(shorter interval)*. Sensing of the third complex initiates sensing at the slower hysteresis rate *(longer interval)*. When the native rate becomes less than the hysteresis rate, pacing resumes at the pacing rate *(shorter interval)*.

Retrograde conductions may somewhat reduce the effect of hysteresis by resetting the atria, making it a less frequent occurrence that a natural cycle is fast enough to overcome the pacing rate and reinitiate sensing at the lower rate. Some pacemakers with the feature that allows hysteresis introduce a lengthened cycle periodically during pacing to allow intrinsic cycles, if there are any, to appear. This concept is called *search hysteresis*.

OBTAINING ASSISTANCE

Pacemakers of various brands and models may differ significantly from the preceding general descriptions. Most manufacturers have a 24-hour hotline staffed by experts who are familiar with their brand of pacemakers. These individuals can be quite helpful.

Index

A

A waves, 128, 195, 263, 266, 270, 284
A to C wave interval (jugular venous pulse), 263, 266, 270
A-A intercycle timing, 494, 495
Λ-Λ interval, 501
A-A timing, single chamber (pacing), 495
AAIR (atrial demand pacing with rate modulation), 501
Aberrant ventricular conduction, 178
  defined, 192
  heart rate during, 139
  phase 3, **192-193**
  phase 4, 192
  versus ectopy, **192-215**
Ablation, radiofrequency, 93, 106, 137, 144, 182, 183, 186, 309, 325, **335-336**
ACE inhibitors, 389
Accelerated idiojunctional rhythm, 123, 272
Accelerated idioventricular rhythm (AIVR), 114, **232-237**
  and AV dissociation, 288-289
  clinical implications of, 234-236
  defined, 232
  ECG recognition of, 232-234
  mechanism of, 236-237
  multiform, 234
  during reperfusion, 233-234
  unrelated to reperfusion, 234
  treatment of, 237
Accelerated junctional rhythm, 123
Accentuated antagonism (sinus node), 64
Accessory pathway
  and atrial fibrillation, 10
  atrial insertion site of, 335
  and axis during SVT, 201
  concealed, 304, 305, 306, **317-318**
  defined, 303
  exercise-induced block of, 317
  latent, 304, 305, 306, **314**
  location of, 137, 335
  posteroseptal, 313
  refractory period of, 317
Accessory pathways, two, 334
Action potential, **14-15**
Activation, normal heart, 12
  instant-to-instant, 37
  step-by-step (ECG), 17-20
  summary of, 29
Activation time, normal ventricular, 366
Adenosine, 144
  adverse effects of, 146-147

Adenosine—cont'd
  for paroxysmal supraventricular tachycardia, 146-147, 322
Adenosine-sensitive ventricular tachycardia, 182
Advanced pacing concepts, applications of, **499-505**
Afterdepolarizations
  delayed, 59, 240
  early, 58, 221
AH (atrial-His) interval, 261
AICD (automatic implantable cardioverter-defibrillator), 483
AIVR (accelerated idioventricular rhythm), **232-237**
Alcohol, 65
Altered automaticity, **57-58**
Alternans
  QRS, 139-140
  T wave, 217
Alveolar-arterial oxygen gradient, 436
Aminophylline, 94
Amiodarone, 95, 102
Amyloidosis, 26, 399
AN (atrionodal) region, 124, 262
Aneurysm, ventricular, 397
Angina
  Prinzmetal's, 396-397
  unstable, **342-361**, see also Unstable angina
Anginal pain, 150, **342-343**
  patients' description of, 343
  what it is not, 343-344
Angioplasty, percutaneous transluminal coronary (PTCA), 346, 360
Angiotensin-converting enzyme (ACE) inhibitors, 389
Anisotropic reentry, 56
Anterior fascicular block, see Anterior hemiblock
Antibodies, digoxin, 258
Antidromic circus movement tachycardia (CMT), 137, **133-134**, 205t, 325
Antidromic defined, 133
Antitachycardia stimulation (pacing), 483-486
Antithrombotic therapy, 76, 106, 236, 424-425
Annulus fibrosus, 304
Anxiety, 150
Aortic dissection, 427
Aortic valve disease, 365
Arrhythmogenic mechanisms, **53-60**
  clinical application of, 59-60
  summary of, 60
ART (atrial refractory period), 507
Artifact, ST-T, 397
Aspirin, 358, 389
Athletes, trained, 34, 61, 66, 70, 79, 266, 371
  deconditioning of, 266
Atherosclerotic plaque, 388, 409
ATPase (adenosine triphosphatase) pump, **13**

Page numbers in boldface indicate main discussion; *t* indicates tables.

Atria, activation of, 18
Atrial abnormality
    left, 20, 21, 22, 441, **447-449**
    right, **449-450**
Atrial bradycardia, 501, 503
Atrial enlargement, 20
Atrial event, 494
Atrial flutter, **111-131,** *see also* Flutter, atrial
Atrial-His (AH) interval, 261
Atrial hypertrophy, 20, **451**
Atrial kick, 101, 237
Atrial natriuretic factor, 151
Atrial parasystole, 297-298
Atrial sensing, 507
Atrial septal defect, 24, 365
Atrial standstill, permanent, 73
Atrial tachycardia, *see* Tachycardia, atrial
Atrial tracking rate, maximal (MATR), 499, 511
Atrionodal (AN) region, 124, 262
Atriofascicular bypass tract defined, 304
Atrioventricular, *see* AV
Atropine, 65, 66, 67, 237
Automaticity, **13,** 90
    abnormal, **58,** 156, 176
    altered, 57-58
    clinical suspicion of, 59
    enhanced normal, **57,** 156
AV block, **260-275**
    and AV dissociation, 289-291
    complete, **271-274,** 364, 410, 415
        clinical implications of, 272
        ECG recognition of, 272
        evaluation of site, 260, 272-274
        pathology in, 272
        physical signs of, 272
    in digitalis toxicity, 245-246
    first degree, **261-263**
        clinical implications of, 263
        defined, 260
        ECG recognition, 261
        mechanism of, 261-262
        pediatrics in, 263
        physical signs of, 263
        treatment of, 263
    high grade second degree, 271
    in inferior myocardial infarction, 414-415
    level of noninvasively evaluated, 260
    second degree, **263-271,** 415
        high grade, 271
        two-to-one, 269-271
        type I (AV Wenckebach), 264-267
        type II, 267-268
    summary, 274-275
    third degree, **271-274,** *see also* AV block, complete
    treatment of, 274
    two-to-one, 269-271
    type I (Wenckebach), 264-267
    type II, 267-271
AV conduction
    and carotid sinus massage, 148
    measured, 19
AV delay (pacing), 503
AV dissociation, **284-291**
    and accelerated idioventricular rhythm, 288-289
    and AV block, 289-291
    causes of, 284
    defined, 123-124, 284
    ECG signs of, 196
    in broad QRS tachycardia, **195-199**

AV dissociation—cont'd
    in nonparoxysmal junctional tachycardia, 128, 287-288
    physical signs of, 195-196, 284
    and sinus bradycardia, 285-286
    treatment of, 285
AV interval (pacing), 495, 497, 502
    rate adaptive sense-initiated (RA-SAV), 511
AV junctional anatomy, 124-125
AV node, 15-17
    blood supply to, 390
AV nodal pathways, 15-17
    location of fast and slow, **15-17,** 133-134
AV nodal reentry tachycardia, **133-137,** *see also* Tachycardia, AV nodal reentry
AV node, 15-17
    compact, 15
AV pacing
    rate-drop response, 513
    with rate hysteresis, 513
    sensor-driven rate-modulated, 511
AV pacemakers, 497
AV priority timing (pacing), 503
AV pacing, 495, 498
AV reciprocating tachycardia, 132, **137-144**
    see also circus movement tachycardia
AV ring, 304
AV synchrony, 498
AV valvular problems, 20
AVNRT, **133-137,** *see also* Tachycardia, atrioventricular nodal reentry
Axis
    delta wave, 335
    indeterminate, 40
    lead, **4,** 38-45
    no-man's-land, 40
    summary of in wide complex tachycardia, 201
    in SVT, 201
    in ventricular tachycardia, 200-201
Axis determination, **36-49**
    easy two-step method, 41-45
    exercises for, 43-45
    at a glance, 40
    using hexaxial figure, 47
    importance of, 36-37
    quadrant method for, 45-47
    methods of determining, 37
    summary of, 47

B

Back-to-back PVCs, 164
Baroreceptors, 247
Bazett's formula, 34-35
Beta blockers, 93, 95, 96, **103,** 105, 205*t,* 389, 426
Bezold-Jarisch reflex, 415
Bifascicular block, 363, 381
Bigeminal PACs, 86
Bigeminal PVCs, 163-164
Bigeminal nonconducted PACs, 87-88
Bigeminal rhythms, 243, 267
Bigeminy, rule of, 169
Block
    AV, *see* AV block
    bifascicular, 363
    bundle branch, *see* Bundle branch block
    entrance, 296
    exit, 297
    peri-infarction, **417-418**
    sinoatrial, **68-71**
    trifascicular, 363, **385-386**

Blood gases, arterial, 436
Blood pressure, changing systolic, 195, 196, 284
Blood temperature and pacing, 499
Bradycardia, 34
  atrial, 501, 503
  sinus, **65-67**, 243, 285
Bradycardias, pacemaker therapies for, 480,
  491-514
Broad QRS tachycardia, *see also* Tachycardia,
  broad QRS
  V_1-negative broad QRS tachycardia
    ECG signs of SVT in, 209-211
    ECG signs of ventricular tachycardia in,
      211-212
  V_1-positive broad QRS tachycardia
    ECG signs of SVT in, 206
    ECG signs of ventricular tachycardia in,
      206-207
    Pitfalls in ECG criteria, 207
Brugada, criteria for ventricular tachycardia,
  212
Bundle branch, **302-304**
  left
    blood supply to, 364
    T wave changes in, 393
  right, 362-363
    blood supply to, 364
Bundle branch block, 29, 83, 192, **362-386**
  in acute myocardial infarction **364-365**
  alternating right and left, 377
  chronic, 365
  comparison of right and left in V_1, 365-366
  complete right, 371-372
  incomplete right, 371
  left, 365-366, **372-377**
    cardiac disease in, 376-377
    mechanism 372-373
    with myocardial infarction, 373
    newly acquired, 365
    QRS complex in, 373
    in pediatrics, 365
    physical findings in, 365
  right, 264, **367-371**, 402, 433
    complete versus incomplete, **371**
    with hemiblock, 381-382
    incomplete in athletes and young adults, 371
    intrinsicoid deflection in, 371
    mechanism of, 367-368
    pseudo pattern, 136
    QRS complex in, 368
    with and without myocardial infarction, **368,**
      402
  T wave changes in, 366-367
  with and without myocardial infarction, 368,
    373
Bundle branch reentrant ventricular tachycardia,
  183-187, 205t
  ECG recognition of, 183-184
  emergency treatment of, **186**
  long term treatment of, 186
  mechanism of, 184
  pathophysiology of, 186
  physiologic, 192
  prognosis of, 186
  radiofrequency ablation for, **187**
Bundle of Kent, 303, 304
Bypass graft, coronary artery, 346
Bypass tract
  defined, 304
  intranodal, 340

C

C wave (jugular venous pulse), 263
Caffeine, 65, 85
Calcium channel blockers, **103-104**
  warning for, 104
Calcium channels, 15
Cancer, hypercoagulation state of occult, 432
Cannon A waves, irregular, 195, 263, 284
Capture beats, 201
Cardiac arrhythmia suppression trial (CAST),
  171, 425-426
Cardiac cycle, electrical, 12
Cardiac dilation, right, 432
Cardiac failure, 26
Cardiac injury, and ST segment, 27
Cardiac rotation, 24, 432
Cardiogenic shock, 65
Cardiomegaly, 376
Cardiomyopathy, 58, 176-177, 186, 317, 365
Cardiopulmonary resuscitation, 189
Cardioversion, DC, 102, 104, 105, 144 147, 177,
  186, 189, 205t, 224, 323, 416
Carotid artery bifurcation, 150
Carotid sinus location, 148
Carotid sinus massage, **148-150,** 178
  in atrial flutter, 114, 117-118
  in atrial tachycardia, 90
  caution with, 150
  in nonparoxysmal junctional tachycardia, 128
  procedure for, 150
  in sinus bradycardia, 66
  in sinus tachycardia, 64
  in supraventricular tachycardia, 150, 322
Carotid sinus syndrome, 513
CAST (Cardiac Arrhythmia Suppression Trials),
  171, 425-426
Catecholamine sensitive atrial fibrillation, 99
Catecholamines, 65
Cerebrovascular accident, 393
Cesarean section, 432
Chaotic atrial tachycardia, **93-95,** *see also*
  Tachycardia, multifocal atrial
Chest pain, *see* Anginal pain
Cholecystitis, 427
Chronic obstructive pulmonary disease (COPD),
  94, 445
Cigarette smoking, 189
Circumflex occlusion, 411-413
Circus movement tachycardia (CMT), 137-144,
  318-328, *see also* Tachycardia, circus
  movement
Clockwise rotation of the heart, 24
CMT, **137-144,** *see also* Tachycardia, circus
  movement
Cocaine, 235
Color vision and digitalis, 257
Compensatory pause
  full, 81-82, **158-161**
  less than full, 81-82
  pseudo-full, 84
Complete AV block, 260, **271-274,** 364, 410, 414,
  see also AV block, complete
Compression boots, pneumatic, 437
Compression stockings, graduated, 437
Concealed accessory pathway, 304, 305, 306,
  317-318
  ECG diagnosis of, 318
  incidence of, 317
Concordant pattern, 201-202

Conduction
    aberrant ventricular, 139, 178, **192-215**
    abnormal intraventricular, 362, 399
    concealed, 100
    His-Purkinje, slow, 186
    proven reliable and atrial bradycardia, 501
    retrograde, 123, 158, 159, 199-200, **505-508**
    retrograde concealed, 193-194
    unproven, 501
    unreliable and atrial fibrillation, 505
    unreliable and good atrial rhythm, 501-503
    unreliable and intermittent atrial bradycardia,
        504
    unreliable and constant atrial bradycardia, 504
Conduction disturbances
    intraventricular, 362, 399
    and ST segment deviation, 27
Conduction system, 15
    blood supply to, 364
    idiopathic degenerative diseases of, 365
    trifascicular, 362-364
Conduction time, intraventricular, 24
Congenital heart disease, 20, 91
Congenital long QT syndrome (LQTS), 216,
        217-218
    beta blockers in, 224
    and emergency treatment, 224-225
    of torsades de pointes, 224
Contraceptives, oral, 432
Cool down (automaticity), 90
COPD (chronic obstructive pulmonary disease),
        94, 445
Cor pulmonale, 20
Cornell voltage, 443
Corridor operation, 106
Coronary arteries, **389-391,** 411, 413
Coronary artery
    dominant left and right, 389-391, 411
    left, 391
    right, 390, 411, 413
        AV nodal branch of, 390
        occlusion of, 411, 413
        proximal occlusion of, 411
Coronary artery disease, 26, 176, 189, 365
    chronic, and polymorphic ventricular
        tachycardia, 225-228
    and left bundle branch block, 376
    left main and three vessel, **358,** 360, 397
Coronary artery occlusion
    circumflex, 411
    distal right, 411
    proximal left anterior descending (LAD),
        344-358, 364, 368
    proximal right, 411
    right vs circumflex, 413
Coronary artery spasm, 396
Coronary sinus, 323, 325
Counterclockwise rotation of the heart, 24
Counterpulsation, aortic, 187
Coupling
    exact, fixed, precise, 163, 236, 296, 297
    no fixed, 296
Current of injury, **395-396**

D

DAD mode, 503, 512
DDDR mode, 504, 505, 512
DDIR mode, 505, 512
DDS mode, 503, 505
DVIR mode, 504, 505

Delta wave, 309-310
Depolarization, 13
    abnormal and T wave inversion, 393
    rapid, 14
    slow, 13
    spontaneous, 13
Diastole, electrical, 3, 15
Diastolic current of injury, 395-396
Digitalis, 78, 96, 205t, 240
    dosage of, 242
    and gastrointestinal symptoms, 257
    and ST segment deviation, 27
    and T wave shape, 29
Digitalis dysrhythmias, 158, **239-259**
    alerting features of, 242-243
    mechanisms of, 240-242
    systematic approach to, 242
Digitalis effect, 27, 247, 253
Digitalis toxicity, 235, **239-259**
    atrial fibrillation in, 106
    atrial tachycardia in, 90, 246-249
    atrioventricular block in, 245
    bifascicular ventricular tachycardia in, 254-255
    diagnostic monitoring leads for, **452**
    double tachycardias in, 255-257
    emergency approach to, 258
    fascicular ventricular tachycardia in, 253-255
    and history-taking, 257
    non-cardiac signs of, 257
    nonparoxysmal junctional tachycardia in,
        249-253
    sinoatrial block in, 243-245
    sinus bradycardia in, 243
    summary of, 258
    treatment of, 257-258
Digoxin, **102-103,** 105
    acute myocardial uptake of, 240
    warning, 103
Digoxin antibodies, 258
Dilation, right cardiac, 432
Diltiazem, **103-104**
Disopyramide, 34
Dive reflex, 148
Dobutrex, 187
Dopamine, 187
Drugs, class 1A or 1C, 156
Dual chamber timing (A-A; V-A), 497
Dysrhythmia, term defined, 53

E

ECG
    defined, 3
    normal, 17
ECG grid paper, 31
Echocardiogram, 178, 434-436
Echocardiography, 175
Einthoven, Willem, 4
Einthoven's triangle, 4-6
    electrode placement for, 5-6
Ejection fraction, 175
Elderly, 408
Electrical therapy, tiered, 487-489
Electrocardiogram
    defined, 3
    exercise testing, 174
    normal, 17
    signal averaged, 75, 178, 188, **467-478**
    the 12 lead, **3-11**
    24 hour ambulatory, 174
Electrocardiograph defined, 3

Electrode placement, all leads, 5-10
Electronic modulation, 298
Embolism, acute pulmonary, 24, 65, 426, **431-437**
    differential diagnosis in, 436
    ECG in, 432-434
    echocardiogram in, 434-436
    pathophysiology of, 432
    physical findings in, 432
    precordial T waves in, 393
    prevention of, 437
    risk factors in, 431-432
    Q waves in, 399
    signs and symptoms of, 432
    ST-T changes in, 397
    summary of, 437
    treatment of, 436-437
Emergency treatment
    of broad QRS tachycardia, 177
    of bundle branch reentrant ventricular
        tachycardia, 183-187, 205t
    of torsades de pointes, 223-225
    of idiopathic ventricular tachycardia, 178-183,
        205t
    of myocardial infarction, 420-421
    of paroxysmal supraventricular tachycardia,
        144-150
    of symptomatic bradycardia, 480
Emphysema, 26
End-diastolic PVCs, 164-165
Ensemble averaging, 468-469
Entrainment, 111, 114, 296, 297
Entrance block, 296
Escape
    junctional **129-130,** 266-267
    ventricular, 237-238
Estes criteria, 443
Exit block, 297
Excitable gap, 111, 114
Exercise and pacing, **511-512**
Exercise induced ventricular tachycardia, 186,
    187
Exertion, 65
Eye ball pressure, 148

F

F wave, 97, 111, 115-117
Fab fragments, 258
Fallback (pacing), 510
Fascicular PVCs, 166
Fascicular ventricular tachycardia, 173, 205t,
    253-255
    diagnostic monitoring leads for, 452, 455
Fasciculoventricular pathways defined, 304
Fast Fourier transform, 471
Fibrillation
    atrial, **96-109**
        accessory pathway in, 106, 189, 205t
        acute, 102-104
        in acute MI, 99
        antithrombotic therapy for, 105-106
        catecholamine sensitive, 99
        causes of, 100
        chronic, 105-106
        clinical features of, 99
        controlled, 99-100
        concealed conduction in, 100
        defined, 96
        digitalis toxicity in, 106, 250-253
        ECG recognition of, 96-97
        idiopathic, 96

Fibrillation—cont'd
    atrial—cont'd
        incidence of, 119
        junctional tachycardia in, **250-253**
        lone, 96, 97
        mechanism of, 98-99
        paroxysmal, 96, 98, 99
        in pediatrics, 101
        polyuria in, 151
        postoperative, 99, 106
        physical assessment of, 101-102
        pulse deficit in, 101-102
        radiofrequency ablation for, 106
        regular rhythm in, 102
        risk associated with, 98, 100-101
        subacute, 105
        summary of, 107
        surgery for, 106
        symptoms of, 101
        treatment goals and categories, 102-106
        with two accessory pathways, 334
        types of, 98-99
        uncontrolled, 99-100
        vagal-induced, 99
        ventricular response to, 99-100
        in WPW syndrome, 314, **328-334**
    ventricular, **188-189,** 223
        ECG recognition, 188
        mechanisms, 189
        primary, 174
        prognosis, 189
        symptoms, 189
        treatment, 189
        warning signs of, 176
Flecainide, 102
Flutter
    atrial, **111-131**
        accessory pathway in, 205t
        AV conduction during, 117-119
        with AV dissociation, 113, 114
        common form, 111
        clinical setting in, 119
        differential diagnosis of, 114
        digitalis toxicity in, 253
        ECG recognition of, 111-114
        with group beating, 113, 114
        junctional tachycardia in, 253
        impure, 106-107
        long term treatment of, 120-121
        mechanism of 114-115
        in pediatrics, 120
        short term treatment of, 120
        summary of, 121
        terminology in, 111
        type I, 114, 115
        type II, 114-117
        types of, 111, 112
        uncommon form, 111, 114-117
        Wenckebach conduction during, 119
    ventricular, **188-189**
        ECG recognition, 188
        mechanisms, 189
        prognosis, 189
        symptoms, 189
        treatment, 189
Flutter-fibrillation, atrial (impure flutter), 121,
    106-107
Framingham study, 365, 376
Frequency domain analysis, 470-475
    frequency domain, 471-473

Frequency domain analysis—cont'd
  interpretation of, 475
  methodology, 473-475
Frog sign, 151, 319
Frontal plane leads, 3
Fusion beats (complexes), 201, **292-295**
  atrial, 295, **111-131**
  defined, 292
  ECG recognition of, 292-293
  mechanisms of, 292
  paced, 492-493
  in parasystole, 296
  ventricular, **188-189,** 293-295
  in WPW syndrome, 310, 314, 334

G

Gap, excitable, 111, 114
Gastrointestinal symptoms, and digitalis, 257
Glucose tolerance, impaired, 189
Graft, bypass, 346
Group beating, 113, 114, 242, 243, 249, 251, 258,
    264, 274

H

Hamartoma, 177
Heart, normal electrical activation of, **12-30**
  step-by-step, **17-19**
Heart disease
  congenital, 20, 91
  structural, 150, 186
Heart enlargement, 376
Heart failure, congestive, 29, 65, 150, 408
  and left bundle branch block, 376
Heart rate
  calculation of, 31
  and pacing during exercise, 511-512
  and PR interval, 33-34
Heart rate variability, 67-68
Heart rotation, 24
Heart sounds
  first, 128, 195, 266, 270, 284
  second, 365, 432
    reversed splitting of, 365
  third, 432
  fourth, 432
Hemiblock
  anterior, **377-379,** 402
    versus anterior MI, 383
    ECG recognition of, 378
    clinical implications of, 379
    differential diagnosis in, 382-383
    versus inferior MI, 382-383
    mechanism of, 378
  posterior, **380-381**
    ECG recognition of, 380-381
    clinical implications of, 381
    mechanism of, 380
  with right bundle branch block, 381
  term, 363
Heparin, 349, 358, 437
Hexaxial figure, 37, 47
Hirudin, 360
Hirulog, 360
His-ventricular (HV) interval, 267
History taking, 147
HV (His-ventricular) interval, 267
Hypercoagulation state, 432
Hyperkalemia, 29, **279-283**
  ECG recognition of, 279-282
  mild, 279, 282

Hyperkalemia—cont'd
  moderate, 279-282
  severe, 282
  treatment of, 282
Hyperlipidemia, 189
Hypertension, 20, 29, 189, 365
  acute pulmonary, 432
  and left bundle branch block, 376
Hypertrophic cardiomyopathy, 317
Hypertrophy, **439-451**
  atrial, 20, **451**
  biventricular, 446-447
  left ventricular, **440-443**
    Cornell voltage in, 443
    ECG recognition of, 440-443
    Estes criteria for, 443
    left atrial involvement in, 441
  ventricular, 24, 27, 29, 189, 400, **439-451**
    diagnostic tools for, 439-440
    left, 440-443
    pathogenesis of, 439
    right, 444-445
Hypocalcemia, 29, 58
Hypokalemia, 29, 34, 58, 221, **276-279**
  advanced stage ECG, 276
  causes of 278
  clinical implications of, 278
  ECG recognition of, 276-277
  prevention of, 279
  signs and symptoms of, 279
  treatment of, 279
Hypomagnesemia, 29, 34
Hypotension, hypovolemic post-tachycardia, 151
Hypoxia, 189
Hysteresis, rate, 513

I

Idiojunctional rhythm, accelerated, 123, 272
Idiopathic atrial fibrillation, 96
Idiopathic long QT syndrome (LQTS), 28, 216,
    217, **222-223**
Idiopathic ventricular tachycardia, 173, **178-183,**
    186-187, 205*t*
  clinical implications of, 181
  ECG recognition of 179-180
  emergency treatment of, **182**
  history of, 179
  long term treatment of, 182-183
  prognosis of, 186
  radiofrequency ablation for, **186-187**
  symptoms of, 182
  types of, 179-180
Idioventricular rhythm, 272
  accelerated, 114, **232-237,** 288-289
Infarction
  myocardial, **387-429,** *see also* Myocardial
    infarction
  pulmonary, 432
Injury, current of, **395-396**
Intercycle timing, 494-495
Intranodal bypass tract, 340
Intraventricular conduction, abnormal, 362, 399
Intraventricular conduction time, 24
Intraventricular septum
  activation of, 19
  blood supply to, 390, 391
Intrinsicoid deflection, normal ventricular, 366
Irregularly irregular (irregular irregularity), term
    defined, 98

Ischemia
    myocardial, 28, 29, 58, 65, 189
    nontransmural, 358
    subendocardial, 358, 392
    subepicardial, 392
Isoproterenol, 94

J

J point, **27**, 147
James fiber, 304
Jugular venous distension, 416
Jugular venous pulse, 128, 151, 195, 263, 319
Junctional beats and rhythms, **123-131**
Junctional escape, **129-130**, 266-267
    ECG recognition of, 129
    with retrograde block, 137
    treatment of, 130
Junctional rhythm, 125
    accelerated defined, 123
Junctional tachycardia
    in atrial fibrillation, 250-253
    causes of, 128
    defined, 123
    nonparoxysmal, **126-130**, 249-253
        and AV dissociation, 287-288
        causes of, 128
        in digitalis toxicity, **249-253**
        ECG recognition of, 126-128
        in pediatrics, 128
        physical signs of, 128
        treatment of, 128

K

Kent bundle, 303, 304
Kussmaul's venous sign, 416

L

L-type calcium channels, 15
Lead, defined, 3
Lead I, 5
Lead II, 5
Lead III, 6
Lead axis, **4**, 38-45
Lead V$_{4R}$, 410, **411**, 414, 415-416, 417
Leads
    II and III and location of occlusion, 413
    diagnostic monitoring, **452-463**
        for broad QRS tachycardia, 458-459
        for digitalis intoxication, 452
        for high risk MI, 462-463
        for paroxysmal supraventricular tachycardia, 452-453
        for unstable angina, 458
    electrode placement of, 5-10
    frontal compared to horizontal plane, 3
    horizontal plane, 3
    inferior, 409
    limb, 4
    low voltage limb, 433
    precordial, 6
Leads defined
    bipolar, 3
    MCL, 8-10
    orthogonal, 188
    precordial, 6
    right chest, 8
    unipolar, 3
    unipolar limb, 6
Leads II and III, in inferior MI, 413
Left anterior hemiblock, *see* Hemiblock, anterior

Left posterior hemiblock, *see* Hemiblock, posterior
Lidocaine, 186, 205*t*, 426
    versus procainamide, 178
Limb leads, 4
Long QT syndrome (LQTS), 28, 216, 217, **222-223**
    congenital, 216, **217-218**, 224
    latent, 225
Lown-Ganong-Levine syndrome, 304, **340**
LQTS (long QT syndrome), 28, 216, 217, **222-223**
Lymphocyte activation, transient intermittent, 344

M

Magnesium sulphate or chloride, 94, 187, 205*t*, 224
    advantages of, 224-225
    contraindications for, 224
Magnet mode (pacing), 497
Magnet rate, 497
Mahaim fibers, 304, 336
Marriott, HJL, 9, 53, 232
    sayings of, 69, 158
MATR (maximal atrial tracking rate), 499, 511
Maze procedure, 106
MCL leads, 8-10
Measurement of heart rate and intervals, **31-35**
Mechanisms of arrhythmias, **53-60**
Middle-aged men, and PVCs, 170
Mitral stenosis, 65
Mode switching (pacing), 512
Modulated parasystole, 297, 297-298
Modulation, electronic, 298
Monitoring leads
    for axis shifts and RBBB, 383-385
    for broad QRS tachycardia, 458-459
    for digitalis intoxication, 452
    diagnostic, **452-463**
    for high risk MI, 462-463
    for paroxysmal supraventricular tachycardia, 452-453
    for unstable angina, 353, 355, **458**
    for Wellens syndrome, 355
MSR (maximal sensor rate), 499
Multichannel monitoring, 10
Murmur, pulmonary ejection, 432
Muscular dystrophy, 399
Muscular weakness, 279
Myocardial blood supply, **389-391**
Myocardial disease, 365
    infiltrative and Q waves, 399
Myocardial infarction, acute, 65, 66, 310, **387-429**
    aggressive therapy for high risk, 421
    anterior, acute, 379, 383, **400-407**
        conduction abnormalities in, 407
        ECG identification of high risk in, 402-406
        ECG recognition of, 402
        and hemiblock, 379
        pathologic features of, 406
        reflecting leads in, 400-401
    anterolateral, 401-402
    anteroseptal, 402
    antiarrhythmic drug therapy in, 425-426
    apical, 400
    atrial, **420**
    with bifascicular block, 381-382
    bundle branch block in, 364-365 368, 373
    complications of, 177
    differential diagnosis of, 426-427
    ECG monitoring leads for high risk, 462-463

Myocardial infarction—cont'd
  ECG signs of, **391-399**
  eliminating delayed treatment for, 423-424
  emergency approach to, 420-421
  evolving, 388-389, **391-399**
  inferior, acute, 382-383, **407-414**, 417-418
    conduction abnormalities in, 414-415
    culprit coronary artery in, 411
    ECG recognition of, 409
    ECG and high risk patients in, 410
    locating the occluded artery in, 411-414
    peri-infarction block in, **417-418**
  inferolateral, 418
  left axis shift in, 364
  left bundle branch block in, 373
  locating, 400
  non-Q-wave, 388, 389, **407-409**
    ECG recognition of, 408
    clinical significance of, 408-409
    reflecting leads in, 408
  phases of arrhythmias in, 176
  and polymorphic ventricular tachycardia, 228
  posterior wall, 418
  prior, 176, 195
  prognosis of, 389
  PVCs following, **170-171**
  Q-wave, 389, 391, 398-399, 400-407
  reperfusion arrhythmias in, 67, 176, 235-236,
      422
  right ventricular, **415-417**
    clinical implications of, 416-417
    ECG diagnosis, 415-416
    pathophysiology of, 416
  right bundle branch block in, 368
  ST segment in, **395-396**
  subendocardial, 358, 388
  summary of, 427
  T wave sensitivity in, 28
  transmural, 389
  transportation of, 422-423
  treatment of, 422-426
Myocarditis, 128
Myxedema, 26

N

N (nodal) region, 124, 262
Neck veins in paroxysmal supraventricular
      tachycardia, 151
Neonate, paroxysmal supraventricular
      tachycardia in, 152
Neurohumoral drive and pacing, 499
NH (nodal-His) region, 124, 262
Nicotine, 65
Nitroglycerin, 349
Nodal (N) region, 124
Nodal-His (NH) region, 124
Nodofascicular pathways (fibers), 304, **336-339**
Nodoventricular pathways (fibers), 304, **336-339**
Noncompensatory pause, 81-82
Nonparoxysmal defined, 123
Nose drops, 65

O

Obesity, 189
Open heart surgery, 128
Orthodromic defined, 132
Orthodromic circus movement tachycardia
      (CMT), 137, **318-325**
  with rapidly conducting accessory pathway,
      318-323

Orthodromic circus movement tachycardia
      (CMT)—cont'd
  with slowly conducting accessory pathway,
      323-325
Orthopedic surgery, 432, 437
Overdrive suppression, defined, 83-84, 150, 158,
      160-161, 481
Oversensing, 494
Oxygen gradient, alveolar-arterial, 436

P

P wave, normal, **18,** 20-22
  axis of, 21
  defined, 17
  duration of,20
  height of, 20
  polarity of, 20-21
  shape of, 22
  summary of, 22
P waves in broad QRS tachycardia, 196-199
P' (prime) wave
  defined, 81
  in lead I, 318
  retrograde, 128, 130, 323
P pulmonale, 22
PAC, **81-88,** *see also* Premature atrial complex
Paced fusion, 492-493
Pacemaker
  adaptive-rate, 499
  atrial tracking, 499
  AV, 497
  normal, 15
  rate-modulating, 499
  rate-responsive, 499
  wandering, 78-79
Pacemaker acceleration, 499
Pacemaker blip, 492
Pacemaker block, 2:1, **510**
Pacemaker deceleration, 499
Pacemaker defect, 492
Pacemaker mediated tachycardias (PMT), 506,
      507
Pacemaker modes, 498
  AAIR, 501
  DAD, 503, 512
  DDDR, 504, 505, 512
  DDIR, 505, 512
  DDS, 503, 505
  DVIR, 504, 505
  magnet, 497
  switching of, 512
  VD, 502, 503
  VDDR, 503
  VVIR, 505, 512
Pacemaker sensors, 499
Pacemaker stimuli, 492
Pacemaker therapy, 73, 76, 187, 224, 258, 268,
      323, **479-491**
  automatic implantable cardioverter-defibrillator
      (AICD), 483
  antitachycardia, 483-486
  and arrhythmias, 480*t*
  and blood temperature, 499
  for bradycardia, 480, **491-514**
  goals of, 479-480
  high-energy shock, 482-483
  obtaining assistance for, 514
  for reciprocating tachycardias, 490
  for reentry tachycardias, 482-490
  for tachycardias of cellular origin, 481-482
  tiered therapy of, 487-489

Pacemaker therapy individualized, **501-505**
Pacemaker timing, **494-497**
  intercycle, 494-495
  magnet mode, 497
  mechanisms of, 495-497
Pacemakers
  adaptive-rate, 499
  advanced, 491
  atrial, 491
  atrial tracking, 499
  atrioventricular, 491
  and carotid sinus syndromes, 513
  dual-chamber, 491
  rate-modulating, 499
  rate-responsive, 499
  responsive heart rate and, **498-499**
  sensor-controlled, 499
  sensor-driven, 499
  sensor-rate, 499
  single-chamber, 491
  special features of, 513
  and vasovagal syndromes, 513
Pacing
  advanced, **498**
  atrial, 237
  and blood temperature, 499
  categorizing patients for, 501t
  competitive, 493
  and exercise, **511-512**
  and neurohumoral drive, 499
  noncompetitive atrial, 512
  and respiration 499
  sensor-driven rate-modulated atrioventricular, 511
Pacing concepts, 492
  application of advanced, **499-505**
Palpitations, 150, 307
Pancreatitis, 427
Parasystole, **296-300**
  atrial, 297-298
  clinical implications of, 300
  ECG in, 296
  interectopic intervals in, 297
  modulated, **297-298**
  ventricular, 296
Paralysis, 279
Paroxysmal defined, 133
PAT, *see* Tachycardia, paroxysmal atrial
Pediatrics
  atrial fibrillation in, 101
  atrial flutter in, 120
  atrial tachycardia in, 90
  AV block in, 261
  bundle branch block in, 365
  first degree AV block in, 263
  junctional tachycardia in, 128
  left axis deviation in, 365
  multifocal atrial tachycardia in, 94
  normal sinus rhythm in, 63
  physical signs of, 120
  paroxysmal supraventricular tachycardia in, 152
  PVCs in, 170
  sinus arrhythmia in, 67
  sinus bradycardia in, 65
  sinus tachycardia in, 63
  ventricular tachycardia in, 177
Percutaneous transluminal coronary angioplasty (PTCA), 346, 360
Pericardial disease, 29

Pericardial effusion, 26
Pericarditis, 397, 426
Peri-infarction block, **417-418**
  clinical significance of, 417-418
  ECG recognition of, 418
  history of, 417
Phase 0 to 4, action potential, 14-15
Phenytoin, 258
Physical findings (assessment)
  in atrial fibrillation, 101-102
  in atrial flutter, 120
  in atrial tachycardia, 93
  in AV dissociation 195-196
  in complete AV block, 272
  in bundle branch block, 365
  in hypokalemia, 279
  in nonparoxysmal AV junctional tachycardia, 128
  in pulmonary embolism, acute, 432
  in PVCs, 170
  in two to one AV block, 271
  in type I AV block, 266
  in type II AV block, 268
PJC (premature junctional complex), **125-126**
Plaque, atherosclerotic, 388, 409
Plateau, action potential, 13, **15**
PLRL (programmable lower rate limit), 499, 501, 503, 513
PMT (pacemaker mediated tachycardia, 506, 507, 508
Polymorphic ventricular tachycardia, 174, 205t, **225-229**
Polyuria, 101, 150, 151
Posterior fascicular block, *see* Hemiblock, posterior
Postpartum period, 432
Potassium, 94, 223
  antiarrhythmic functions of, 276
Potassium currents (action potential), 15
Potassium derangements, **276-283**
  summary of, 283
PR interval
  according to age, 308t
  influence of heart rate on, 33-34
  measurement of, 19, 33
  prolonged, 34, 260, **261-263**
  shortened, 34
  in WPW syndrome, 304
PR segment, 18, 33
Precordial thump, 178
Preexcitation
  absence of, 314
  degrees of, 310
  maximal, 313-314
  and ST segment deviation, 27
Preexcitation syndromes, **303-341**
  classification of, 303-304
Precordial thump, 178
Premature atrial complex (PAC), **81-88**
  AV conduction following, 83
  bigeminal 86-88
  causes of, 85
  clinical implications of, 85
  critially timed, 134, 137
  ECG recognition of, 82-83
  mechanism of, 84
  nonconducted, 86
  treatment of, 85
  types of, 86-88

Premature junctional complex (PJC), 125-126
    ECG recognition of, 126
    treatment of, 126
Premature ventricular complex (PVC), **155-172**
    amplitude of, 158
    "back-to-back", 164
    bigeminal, 163-164
    clinical implications of, 170-171
    ECG recognition of, 155-156
    end-diastolic, 164-165
    fascicular, 166
    and full compensatory pause, 158-160
    without heart disease, 170
    interpolated, 165
    mechanism of, 156
    in middle aged men, 170
    multifocal, 161
    in nonsymptomatic, 170
    pairs of, 163-164
    in pediatrics, 170
    physical signs of, 170
    QRS shape in, 157
    QRS width in, 157
    quadrigeminal, 163-164
    R on T, 166-168, 237
    with retrograde conduction, 503, 506
    rule of bigeminy for, 169
    summary of, 171
    T wave of, 158
    treatment of, 171
    trigeminal, 163-164
    types of, 161-169
    "ugly", 161
    unifocal, 161
Prinzmetal's angina, **396-397**
Proarrhythmic defined, 174
Procainamide, 34, 144, 147, 177, 186, 213-214,
        317, 322
    versus lidocaine, 178
Programmable lower rate limit (PLRL), 499, 513
Programmable upper rate limit (PURL), 499, 501,
        511
Propranolol, 78
Pseudofusion, 493
Pseudo r′ wave defined, 135
Pseudo RBBB pattern, 136
Pseudo S wave defined, 135
PSVT, **132-154**, *see also* Tachycardia, paroxysmal
        supraventricular
PTCA (percutaneous transluminal coronary
        angioplasty), 346, 360
Pulmonary disease
    bronchospastic, 95
    chronic obstructive (COPD), 94, 445
Pulmonary ejection murmur, 432
Pulmonary embolism, acute, **431-437**, *see also*
        Embolism, acute pulmonary
Pulse deficit, defined, 101-102
Pure (traditional, classic) parasystole, 296-297
PURL (programmable upper rate limit), 499, 511
PVARP (postventricular atrial refractory period),
        507, 508, 510, 511
PVC, **155-172**, *see also* Premature ventricular
        complex

Q

Q wave, 19, **398-400**
    in acute pulmonary embolism, 399
    in infiltrative myocardial disease, 399
    in intraventricular conduction problems, 399

Q wave—cont'd
    non-MI, 399-400
    normal, 398, 399
    pathologic, 398-399
    in reperfusion, 422
    in ventricular hypertrophy, 400
QRS, normal, 22-27
    amplitude, 26
    best leads for measuring, 25
    duration of, 24
    in limb leads, 22-23
    measurement of, 24-25
    polarity of, 26
    Q wave of, 19, 27
    in precordial leads, 23
    shape of, 26-27
QRS amplitude, PVC, **158**
QRS axis in SVT, 201
    with accessory pathways, 201
    and class IC drugs, 201
QRS axis in ventricular tachycardia, 200-201
    clinical correlations, 200-201
    in idiopathic ventricular tachycardia, 201
    in preexisting bundle branch block, 201
    in previous myocardial infarction, 200
QRS complex
    defined, 17, 19
    evaluation of, **24-27**
    low voltage of, 26
QRS shape in PVCs, **157**
QRS width
    in PVCs, **157**
    in ventricular tachycardia, **200**
QT interval, normal, 34-35
    corrected, (QTc), **34-35**, 217, **225**
    measurement of, 34
Quadrant method (axis), 45-47
Quadrigeminal PVCs 163-164
Quiescence (phase 4), 14
Quinidine therapy, 29, 34, 425-426

R

R-on-T phenomenon, **166-168**, 176
R′ defined, 27
R wave progression, normal, 23
RA-SAV (rate adaptive sense-initiated AV
        intervals, 511
Rabbit ear sign, 207
Radiofrequency ablation, 93, 106, 137, 144, 182,
        183, 186, 309, 325, **335-336**
    for ventricular tachycardia, **186-187**
Rate adaptive sense-initiated AV intervals
        (RA-SAV), 511
Rate-control drugs, 102
Rate limit, upper and lower programmable, 499
Rate-modulating pacemakers, 499
Rate prescriptions, 499
Rate-response curve, 499
Rate-responsive pacemakers, 499
Rate smoothing, 510
Reciprocal changes, 415
Reciprocating defined, 132
Reentrant atrial tachycardia, **91-93**
Reentry, **54-56**, 156, 176, 221
    anatomic, 55-56
    anisotropic, 56
    clinical suspicion of, 59
    functional, 56
    intraatrial, 91
    Lewis model of, 56

Reentry—cont'd
  Mines model of, 55
  SA nodal, 76-78
Reflection, 56-57
Refractory period, 13, 507
  postventricular atrial refractory periods, 507,
    508, 510, 511
Regular irregularity (regularly irregular), defined,
    98
Reperfusion
  ECG evaluation of, 391, **421-422**
  in Wellens syndrome, 348
Reperfusion arrhythmias, 67, 176, 422
Repolarization, **13,** 15, 17, 19
  initial, 14
  normal and abnormal ventricular, 392
  rapid, 14
  slow, 15
Respiration and pacing, 499
Responsive heart rate (pacing), **498-499,** 501
Resuscitation, cardiopulmonary, 67, 180
Retrograde concealed conduction, **193-194**
Retrograde conduction, **505-508**
  defined, 123
  effects of, 505-506
  management of, 506-507
  PVC and, 158, 159
  termination programs for, 507-508
  ventricular tachycardia and, 199-200
Retrograde P' wave, 128, 130, 323
Rosenbaum, M, 363
Rotation of the heart, 24

S

SA (sinoatrial) block, **68-71**
  type I, 68-71
  type II, 71
SA (sinoatrial) nodal reentry, 76-78
  clinical implications of, 77
  differential diagnosis of, 77
  ECG recognition of, 76-77
  mechanism of, 77
  treatment of, 78
SA (sinoatrial) Wenckebach, 68-71
  clinical implications of, 70-71
  ECG recognition of, 70
  mechanism of, 70
  treatment of, 71
SAECG, *see* signal averaged ECG
Sawtooth pattern, 111
Second degree AV block, **263-271,** 415, *see also*
    AV block, second degree
Second heart sound, reversed splitting of, 365
Sensing concepts, **494**
Sensing mechanisms, 494
Sensor-controlled rate determination (pacing),
    498-499
Sensor-driven rate, 49
Sensor-driven rate-modulated atrioventricular
    pacing, 511
Sensor-prescribed rate, 499
Sensor rate, maximal (MSR), 499
Sensor threshold, 499
Sensor varied postventricular atrial refractory
    period, 511
Sensors, pacemaker, 499
Septal activation, normal, 23
Septum
  activation of, 19
  intraventricular, blood supply to, 390, 391

Shock, cardiogenic, 65, 150
Short-long-short sequence, 216, 218
Short PR syndrome, 340
Sick sinus syndrome, 73-76
Signal averaged ECG (SAECG), 175, 178, 188,
    467-478
  frequency domain analysis of, 470-475
  problems analyzing small ECG signals, 467-468
  summary of, 476
  time domain analysis of, 469-470
Signal averaging, 468
Single chamber timing, A-A, 495
Single chamber timing, V-V, 495
Sinoatrial block
  in digitalis toxicity, 243-245
  in pediatrics, 68
  types of, 68
Sinus arrest, **71-73**
  ECG recognition of, 71-73
  treatment of, 73
Sinus arrhythmia, **67-68**
  clinical implications of, 68
  ECG recognition of, 67
  mechanism of, 68
  in pediatrics, 67
  symptoms of, 68
  treatment of, 68
Sinus bradycardia, **65-67**
  and AV dissociation, 285-286
  ECG recognition of, 65
  clinical implications of, 66-67
  in digitalis toxicity, 243
  mechanism of, 66
  in pediatrics, 65
  treatment of, 67
  vagal block in, 66
Sinus nodal arrhythmias, 61-79
  summary of, 79
Sinus nodal dysfunction, **73-76**
  mechanisms of, 75
  pathologic features of, 75-76
  in pediatrics, 73-74
  treatment of, 76
Sinus node
  abnormality, primary, 65
  accentuated antagonism of, 64
Sinus pause, **71-73**
Sinus preference timing, 503
Sinus rhythm, normal, **61-63**
  in pediatrics, 63
  record of after conversion from paroxysmal
    supraventricular tachycardia, 147
Sinus tachycardia, **63-65**
  carotid sinus massage and, 64
  and circus movement tachycardia, 319
  clinical implications of, 65
  ECG recognition of, 63-64
  mechanism of, 65
  pediatrics in, 63
  treatment of, 65
Sleep rates, 513
Slow ventricular tachycardia, 234
Smoking, 85
Sodium channels, fast, 14
Sodium load, 187
Sodium-potassium adenosine triphosphatase
    (ATP) pump, **13,** 240
Sotolol, 102
Spatial averaging, 468
Spectral temporal mapping, 475-476

SSS (sick sinus syndrome), 73-76
ST segment
    in acute injury, **395-396**
    defined, 17, 27
    level of, 27
    normal, 19, 27-28
    in reperfusion, 421, 422
    shape of, 28
ST segment depression, 358, 407
ST segment deviation
    cause of, 27
    causes of other than MI, 397
    in Wellens syndrome, 348
ST segment elevation, 395-397
Stimulation
    concepts of, **492-493**
    mechanisms of, 492
Stimulation concepts, **492-493**
Stimulus artifact, 492
ST-T changes not caused by MI, 396-397
Supraventricular defined, 84
Surgery
    corridor (for atrial fibrillation), 106
    gynecologic cancer, 432, 437
    open heart, 128
    orthopedic, 432, 437
Sustained ventricular tachycardia defined, 174
SVT, *see* Tachycardia, supraventricular
Sympathomimetic agents, 65
Syncope, 66, 68, 150, 151-152, 174
Syndrome(s)
    carotid sinus, 513
    congenital long QT (LQTS), 216, **217-218**
    idiopathic long QT (LQTS), 28, 216, 217,
        222-223
    Lown-Ganong-Levine, 304, **340**
    preexcitation, **303-341**
    short PR, 304, **340**
    sick sinus (SSS), 73-76
    vasovagal, 513
    Wellens, **344-358**, 453t, 457, 458
    Wolff-Parkinson-White, 106, 118, 178, **304-341**,
        426
Systole, electrical defined, 3
Systolic current of injury, 395-396
Systolic stretch, 389

T

T-type calcium channels, 15
T wave
    in bundle branch block, 366-367
    in evolving myocardial infarction, 391-392
    in ischemia, **392**
    hyperacute, 393-394
    normal, 17, 19, 28-29, **392**
    in reperfusion, 421, 422
    in ventricular ectopy, 29
T wave aberration, 217
T wave alternans, 29, 217
T wave humps, 217-218
T wave inversion
    causes of (other than MI), 393
    in Wellens syndrome, 348
T wave peaking, 393-394
Tachycardia
    antidromic circus movement (CMT), 137,
        133-134, 205t, 325
    anti-, 483-486
    atrial, **88-95**, 503
        automatic, 90

Tachycardia—cont'd
    atrial—cont'd
        chaotic, **93-95**
        clinical implications of, 92-93
        differential diagnosis of, 114
        in digitalis toxicity, **246-249**, 452, 453t, 454
        incessant, 91
        managing pacing during, 511
        in pediatrics, 90
        paroxysmal (PAT), **90-93**
        physical findings during, 93
        reentrant, 91-92
        treatment of, 93
    atrial with block, **246-249**
    AV nodal reentry, **133-137**
        anatomical substrate of, 133-134
        clinical implications of, 137
        defined, 133
        ECG recognition of, 135-136
        emergency treatment of, 137, **144**
        mechanism of, 134-135
        and patient education, 137
        radiofrequency ablation for, 137
        uncommon form of, 137
    AV reciprocating, 132, **137-144**
    broad QRS, 177, 453t, 458-461
        axis during, 200-201
        and baseline 12 lead ECG, 212
        classification of, 205t
        differentiating among, **194-195**
        ECG diagnosis of, **200-214**
        ECG monitoring leads for, 453t, 458-459
        fast, broad, irregular, 178
        and history taking, 195
        management of, 177
        P waves in, 196-199
        QRS width during, 200
        summary of, 214-215
        V1-negative, 205t, **209-211**
        V1-positive, 205t, **206-207**
        when in doubt, 213-214
    chaotic atrial, **93-95**, *see also* Multifocal atrial
    circus movement (CMT), 137-144, 318-328
        antidromic, 137, **133-134**, 205t, 325
        clinical implications of, 143
        defined, 133
        ECG recognition, 139-140
        emergency treatment of, 143, **144, 319-323**
        incessant, 137, **143-144**
        initiated by a PAC, 319
        initiated by a PVC, 140, 319
        initiated by sinus tachycardia, 319
        mechanism of, 137-139
        negative ECG signs, 141
        with two accessory pathways, 325-328
        radiofrequency ablation for, 144
        with rapidly conducting accessory pathway,
            318-323
        with slowly conducting accessory pathway,
            143-144
        symptoms during, 307t
    double, **255-257**
    electrical termination of, 482-486
    high-energy shocks for, 482-483
    incessant circus movement, 137, **143-144**
    junctional, 123, 128, 250-253
        nonparoxysmal, **126-130**, 249-253
    multifocal (chaotic) atrial, **93-95**
        causes of 94
        clinical implications of, 94

Tachycardia—cont'd
  multifocal (chaotic) atrial—cont'd
    ECG recognition, 93-94
    mechanism of, 94
    in pediatrics, 94
    treatment of, 94
  orthodromic circus movement (CMT), 137, **318-325**
  pacemaker mediated tachycardia (PMT), 506, 507
  paroxysmal atrial (PAT), **90-93**
    ECG recognition in, 92
    clinical implications of, 92-93
    physical findings in, 93
    treatment of, 93
  paroxysmal supraventricular (PSVT), 90, **132-154**
    adenosine for, 146-147
    diagnostic monitoring leads for, **452-452**, 453t, 456
    differential diagnosis in, 152t
    emergency response to, **144-150**
    in the fetus and neonate, 152
    mechanisms of, 132
    neck veins during, 151
    and nodoventricular fibers, 339
    in pediatrics, 152
    physical signs of, 151-152
    polyuria and, 151
    pulse, blood pressure, and heart sounds during, 151
    rationale of, 144-147
    symptoms of, 150
    syncope during, 151-152
    summary of, 152-153
    terminology in, 132-133
    vagal maneuver for, 145-146
  sinus, **63-65,** 319
  and ST segment deviation, 27
  supraventricular (SVT)
    concordant pattern in, 201-202
    paroxysmal, **132-154**
    with aberrancy, 178
  and T wave inversion, 29
  V1-negative broad QRS, 209-212
  V1-positive broad QRS, 206-207
  ventricular (VT)
    adenosine-sensitive, 182
    bifascicular, **254-255**
    bidirectional, **254-255**
    Brugada's criteria for, 212
    bundle branch reentrant, **183-187,** 205t
    concordant pattern in, 201
    diagnosis of, 174-175
    digitalis induced, 177
    emergency treatment of, 177
    exercise induced, 186, 187
    fascicular, 173, 205t, **253-255**
    hemodynamic decompensation in, 177
    idiopathic, 173, 177, **178-183,** 186-187, 205t
    incidence of, 176
    late after MI, 187
    management of, 177
    mechanisms of, 175-176
    monomorphic, **173-191**
    nonsustained, 174, 176
    in pediatrics, 177
    polymorphic, 174, 205t, **216-231, 225-229**
    primary, 174

Tachycardia—cont'd
  ventricular—cont'd
    prognosis of, 176-177
    QRS morphology in, **202-212**
    radiofrequency ablation for, **186-187**
    "slow", 234
    sustained, 174, 176, 187
    terminology of, 173-174
    treatment of drug related, 187
Tachycardias, double, **255-257**
TARP (total atrial refractory period, 508, 509, **511-512**
Tawara, 363
Terminology, 53, 111, 132-133, 173-174
Tetralogy of Fallot, 177, 365
Thallium exercise testing, 175
Theophylline, 76
Third degree AV block, **271-274,** *see also* AV block, complete
Thromboembolism
  in atrial fibrillation, 100
Thrombolytic therapy, 76, 106, 236, 364, 399, 410, 414-415, 416, **420-425**
Threshold potential, 14
Thrombin generation and formation, 344
Thyroid, 65
Tilt test, upright, 174
Time domain analysis (SAECG), 469-470
  interpretation of, 469-470
Timing mechanisms, 495-497
  single chamber A-A timing, 495
  single chamber V-V timing, 495
Todaro, tendon of, 17
Torsades de pointes, 34, 178, 187, 205t, **216-225**
  causes of acquired, 222
  causes of congenital, 222-223
  ECG diagnosis of, 217
  emergency treatment of, **223-225**
  initiation of, 218
  mechanism of, 221-222
  outcomes of, 223
  prevention of, 223
  and QT prolongation, 217
  quinidine-related, 221
  short-long-short sequence in, 216, 217, **218**
  summary of, 229
  symptoms of, 223
  T waves in, 217-218
  torsade or torsades? 217
  warning signs of, 217-218
Total atrial refractory period (TARP), 508, 509, **511-512**
Transitional zone, 24, 433
Tricuspid regurgitation, 432
Trifascicular block, 363, **385-386**
Trifascicular conduction system, 363
Trigeminal PVCs, 163-164
Triggered activity, **58-59,** 60, 156, 163, 176, 221, 240-242
Triphasic pattern, 206
Two-to-one AV block, **269-271**
  clinical implications of, 271
  ECG recognition of, 269-270
  mechanism of, 271
  physical signs of, 271
Two-step method of axis determination, 41-45
  exercises for, 43-45
Type I AV block (Wenckebach), **264-267**
  and bigeminy, 267
  clinical implications of, 264-266

Type I AV block (Wenckebach)—cont'd
  ECG recognition of, 264
  "footsteps of", 69
  with junctional escape, 266
  mechanism of, 264
  physical signs of, 266
Type I atrial flutter
  F wave morphology in, 115
  mechanism of, 114
Type I sinoatrial block, 68-71
Type II atrial flutter
  F wave morphology in, 115-117
  mechanism of, 114-115
Type II AV block, **267-271**
  clinical implications of, 268
  ECG recognition, 264
  mechanism, 264-265
  physical signs of, 268
Type II sinoatrial block, 71

U

U wave, 17, 29, 34
  prominent, 218, 276-277
Ultrasonography, of leg veins, 436
Undersensing, 494
Upper rate limit, ventricular, 510
Unstable angina, **342-361**, 458
  ECG monitoring leads for, 353, **355**, 453*t*, **458**
  identifying characteristics of, 343
  incidence of, 342
  emergency angiography for, 358
  medical treatment for, 358-360
  pathogenesis, 344
  T wave in, 393
  type of pain in, 342-344
  Wellens syndrome in, 344-358

V

V wave (jugular venous pulse), 263, 266
V$_{4R}$ lead, 410, **411**, 414, 416
V-A intercycle timing, 494, 495
Vagal block
  response of the sinus node to, 66
Vagal maneuvers
  for antidromic CMT, 205*t*
  for atrial flutter, 114, 117-118
  for atrial tachycardia, 90
  for paroxysmal supraventricular tachycardia, 144, 322
  for broad QRS tachycardia, 178
  types of, 322
Vagal stimulation
  see also Carotid sinus massage and vagal maneuvers
  mechanism and methods of, **147-150**
Vagal tone, high, 415
Vagally induced atrial fibrillation, 99
Valsalva's maneuver, 178
Vasovagal syndrome, 513
VD mode, 502, 503
VDDR mode, 503
Vectors, defined 37-38
Ventilation-perfusion (V-Q) disturbance, 432, 436
Ventricular activation time, 366
Ventricular arrhythmias, malignant, 174
Ventricular escape, 237-238

Ventricular event, 494
Ventricular failure, right, 432
Ventricular flutter, **188-189**
Ventricular septal defect, 365
Ventricular standstill, 223
Ventricular synchrony, **513-514**
Ventricular tachycardia, *see* Tachycardia, ventricular
Ventricular upper rate limit, 510
Ventriculoatrial conduction, **505-508**, *see also* Retrograde conduction
Ventriculophasic phenomenon, 88, 111, 247
Verapamil, 78, 93, 95, 96, 103, 105, 147, 178, 205*t*, 213-214, 322
VT, *see* Ventricular tachycardia
Vulnerable period, defined, 28
VV timing, single chamber, 495
VVIR mode, 503, 512

W

Waldo's types of atrial fibrillation, 98
Walking out a rhythm, **81-82**, 158, 297
Wandering pacemaker, 78-79
Warfarin, 437
Warm up (automaticity), 90
Wellens syndrome, **344-358**
  diagnostic monitoring leads for, 355, 453*t*, 457, **458**
  ECG during pain, 349-353
  ECG during pain-free period, 346-349
  ECG recognition of, 349-355
  history of, 346
  time frame for ECG, 353
  treatment of, 358
Wenckebach
  during atrial flutter, 114, 119
  AV, 264-267
  SA (sinoatrial), 68-71
    clinical implications of, 70-71
    ECG recognition of, 70
    mechanism of, 70
    treatment of, 71
Wenckebach-like effect, 551
Wolff-Parkinson-White (WPW) pattern, 304
Wolff-Parkinson-White (WPW) syndrome, 106, 118, 178, **304-341**, 426
  accessory pathways in, 304-305
  anatomic development of, 304
  arrhythmias of, **318-335**
  atrial fibrillation in, 314, **328-334**
  concealed accessory pathways in, 305, **317-318**
  degrees of preexcitation in, 310
  delta wave in, 309-310
  ECG recognition of, 306-310
  genetics of, 306
  and high risk patients, 317
  historical background of, 304
  incidence of, 305-306
  latent accessory pathways in, 305, **314**
  overt, 138, 305, 314
  summary of, 340
  T wave changes in, 317, 393

X

X-ray, chest, 178, 436

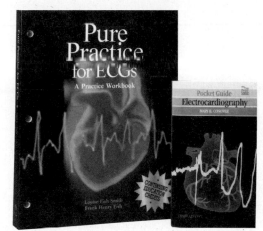
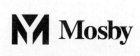